Advances in Musculoskeletal Imaging and Their Applications

Advances in Musculoskeletal Imaging and Their Applications

Editors

Adam Piórkowski
Rafał Obuchowicz
Andrzej Urbanik
Michał Strzelecki

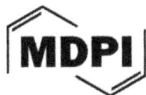 Basel • Beijing • Wuhan • Barcelona • Belgrade • Novi Sad • Cluj • Manchester

Editors

Adam Piórkowski
AGH University of Science
and Technology
Cracow, Poland

Rafał Obuchowicz
Jagiellonian University
Medical College
Cracow, Poland

Andrzej Urbanik
Jagiellonian University
Medical College
Cracow, Poland

Michał Strzelecki
Lodz University of
Technology
Łódź, Poland

Editorial Office
MDPI
St. Alban-Anlage 66
4052 Basel, Switzerland

This is a reprint of articles from the Topic published online in the open access journals *Diagnostics* (ISSN 2075-4418), *Journal of Clinical Medicine* (ISSN 2077-0383), *Tomography* (ISSN 2379-139X), and *Applied Sciences* (ISSN 2076-3417) (available at: https://www.mdpi.com/topics/Musculoskelet_Imaging_Appl).

For citation purposes, cite each article independently as indicated on the article page online and as indicated below:

Lastname, A.A.; Lastname, B.B. Article Title. *Journal Name* **Year**, *Volume Number*, Page Range.

ISBN 978-3-0365-9492-7 (Hbk)
ISBN 978-3-0365-9493-4 (PDF)
doi.org/10.3390/books978-3-0365-9493-4

Cover image courtesy of Adam Piórkowski

© 2023 by the authors. Articles in this book are Open Access and distributed under the Creative Commons Attribution (CC BY) license. The book as a whole is distributed by MDPI under the terms and conditions of the Creative Commons Attribution-NonCommercial-NoDerivs (CC BY-NC-ND) license.

Contents

About the Editors ix

Preface xi

Adam Piórkowski, Rafał Obuchowicz, Andrzej Urbanik and Michał Strzelecki
Advances in Musculoskeletal Imaging and Their Applications
Reprinted from: *J. Clin. Med.* **2023**, *12*, 6585, doi:10.3390/jcm12206585 1

Wei-Cheng Hung, Chin-Jung Hsu, Abhishek Kumar, Chun-Hao Tsai, Hao-Wei Chang and Tsung-Li Lin
Perioperative Radiographic Predictors of Non-Union in Infra-Isthmal Femoral Shaft Fractures after Antegrade Intramedullary Nailing: A Case–Control Study
Reprinted from: *J. Clin. Med.* **2022**, *11*, 3664, doi:10.3390/jcm11133664 11

Nana Maeda, Manabu Maeda and Yasuhito Tanaka
Direct Visualization of Cervical Interlaminar Epidural Injections Using Sonography
Reprinted from: *Tomography* **2022**, *8*, 157, doi:10.3390/tomography8040157 21

Marcin Kozakiewicz
Measures of Corticalization
Reprinted from: *J. Clin. Med.* **2022**, *11*, 5463, doi:10.3390/jcm11185463 33

Agata Giełczyk, Anna Marciniak, Martyna Tarczewska, Sylwester Michal Kloska, Alicja Harmoza, Zbigniew Serafin and Marcin Woźniak
A Novel Lightweight Approach to COVID-19 Diagnostics Based on Chest X-ray Images
Reprinted from: *J. Clin. Med.* **2022**, *11*, 5501, doi:10.3390/jcm11195501 49

Fabio Cofano, Daniele Armocida, Livia Ruffini, Maura Scarlattei, Giorgio Baldari, Giuseppe Di Perna, et al.
The Efficacy of Trabecular Titanium Cages to Induce Reparative Bone Activity after Lumbar Arthrodesis Studied through the 18f-Naf PET/CT Scan: Observational Clinical In-Vivo Study
Reprinted from: *Diagnostics* **2022**, *12*, 2296, doi:10.3390/diagnostics12102296 59

Yen-Yao Li, Shih-Hao Chen, Kuo-Chin Huang, Chien-Yin Lee, Chin-Chang Cheng, Ching-Yu Lee, et al.
High Accuracy and Safety of Intraoperative CT-Guided Navigation for Transpedicular Screw Placement in Revision Spinal Surgery
Reprinted from: *J. Clin. Med.* **2022**, *11*, 5853, doi:10.3390/jcm11195853 71

Tomasz Wach, Małgorzata Skorupska and Grzegorz Trybek
Are Torque-Induced Bone Texture Alterations Related to Early Marginal Jawbone Loss?
Reprinted from: *J. Clin. Med.* **2022**, *11*, 6158, doi:10.3390/jcm11206158 81

Yu-Shin Huang, Yu-Huei Huang, Chiung-Hung Lin, Chang-Fu Kuo and Yun-Ju Huang
Ultrasound Can Be Usefully Integrated with the Clinical Assessment of Nail and Enthesis Involvement in Psoriasis and Psoriatic Arthritis
Reprinted from: *J. Clin. Med.* **2022**, *11*, 6296, doi:10.3390/jcm11216296 97

Daniel Dubinski, Sae-Yeon Won, Bedjan Behmanesh, Daniel Cantré, Isabell Mattes, Svorad Trnovec, et al.
Significance of Temporal Muscle Thickness in Chronic Subdural Hematoma
Reprinted from: *J. Clin. Med.* **2022**, *11*, 6456, doi:10.3390/jcm11216456 109

Ho Young Gil, Wonseok Seo, Gyu Bin Choi, Eunji Ha, Taekwang Kim, Jungyul Ryu, et al.
A New Role for Epidurography: A Simple Method for Assessing the Adequacy of Decompression during Percutaneous Plasma Disc Decompression
Reprinted from: *J. Clin. Med.* 2022, 11, 7144, doi:10.3390/jcm11237144 119

Marcin Kozakiewicz and Tomasz Wach
Exploring the Importance of Corticalization Occurring in Alveolar Bone Surrounding a Dental Implant
Reprinted from: *J. Clin. Med.* 2022, 11, 7189, doi:10.3390/jcm11237189 129

Loreto Ferrández-Laliena, Lucía Vicente-Pina, Rocío Sánchez-Rodríguez, Eva Orantes-González, José Heredia-Jimenez, María Orosia Lucha-López, et al.
Diagnostics Using the Change-of-Direction and Acceleration Test (CODAT) of the Biomechanical Patterns Associated with Knee Injury in Female Futsal Players: A Cross-Sectional Analytical Study
Reprinted from: *Diagnostics* 2023, 13, 928, doi:10.3390/diagnostics13050928 149

Ceyhun Türkmen, Serdar Yılmaz Esen, Zafer Erden and Tülin Düger
Comfort and Support Values Provided by Different Pillow Materials for Individuals with Forward Head Posture
Reprinted from: *Appl. Sci.* 2023, 13, 3865, doi:10.3390/app13063865 161

Mami Iima, Ryo Sakamoto, Takahide Kakigi, Akira Yamamoto, Bungo Otsuki, Yuji Nakamoto, et al.
The Efficacy of CT Temporal Subtraction Images for Fibrodysplasia Ossificans Progressiva
Reprinted from: *Tomography* 2023, 9, 62, doi:10.3390/tomography9020062 179

Rafal Obuchowicz, Karolina Nurzynska, Monika Pierzchala, Adam Piorkowski and Michal Strzelecki
Texture Analysis for the Bone Age Assessment from MRI Images of Adolescent Wrists in Boys
Reprinted from: *J. Clin. Med.* 2023, 12, 2762, doi:10.3390/jcm12082762 187

Ryan Hernandez, Usha Sinha, Vadim Malis, Brandon Cunnane, Edward Smitaman and Shantanu Sinha
Strain and Strain Rate Tensor Mapping of Medial Gastrocnemius at Submaximal Isometric Contraction and Three Ankle Angles
Reprinted from: *Tomography* 2023, 9, 68, doi:10.3390/tomography9020068 205

Claudia Römer, Enrico Zessin, Julia Czupajllo, Thomas Fischer, Bernd Wolfarth and Markus Herbert Lerchbaumer
Effect of Anthropometric Parameters on Achilles Tendon Stiffness of Professional Athletes Measured by Shear Wave Elastography
Reprinted from: *J. Clin. Med.* 2023, 12, 2963, doi:10.3390/jcm12082963 223

Patrick Stein, Felix Wuennemann, Thomas Schneider, Felix Zeifang, Iris Burkholder, Marc-André Weber, et al.
3-Tesla T2 Mapping Magnetic Resonance Imaging for Evaluation of SLAP Lesions in Patients with Shoulder Pain: An Arthroscopy-Controlled Study
Reprinted from: *J. Clin. Med.* 2023, 12, 3109, doi:10.3390/jcm12093109 235

Paweł Kamiński, Rafał Obuchowicz, Aleksandra Stepień, Julia Lasek, Elżbieta Pociask and Adam Piórkowski
Correlation of Bone Textural Parameters with Age in the Context of Orthopedic X-ray Studies
Reprinted from: *Appl. Sci.* 2023, 13, 6618, doi:10.3390/app13116618 249

Karsten Sebastian Luetkens, Jan-Peter Grunz, Andreas Steven Kunz, Henner Huflage, Manuel Weißenberger, Viktor Hartung, et al.
Ultra-High-Resolution Photon-Counting Detector CT Arthrography of the Ankle: A Feasibility Study
Reprinted from: *Diagnostics* **2023**, *13*, 2201, doi:10.3390/diagnostics13132201 263

Tarek Hegazi
Hydroxyapatite Deposition Disease: A Comprehensive Review of Pathogenesis, Radiological Findings, and Treatment Strategies
Reprinted from: *Diagnostics* **2023**, *13*, 2678, doi:10.3390/diagnostics13162678 273

Tomasz Wach, Piotr Hadrowicz, Grzegorz Trybek, Adam Michcik and Marcin Kozakiewicz
Is Corticalization in Radiographs Related to a Higher Risk of Bone Loss around Dental Implants in Smoking Patients? A 5-Year Observation of Radiograph Bone-Texture Changes
Reprinted from: *J. Clin. Med.* **2023**, *12*, 5351, doi:10.3390/jcm12165351 291

Patrick Stein, Felix Wuennemann, Thomas Schneider, Felix Zeifang, Iris Burkholder, Marc-André Weber, et al.
Detection and Quantitative Assessment of Arthroscopically Proven Long Biceps Tendon Pathologies Using T2 Mapping
Reprinted from: *Tomography* **2023**, *9*, 126, doi:10.3390/tomography9050126 307

Marie Schierenbeck, Martin Grözinger, Benjamin Reichardt, Olav Jansen, Hans-Ulrich Kauczor, Graeme M. Campbell and Sam Sedaghat
Detecting Bone Marrow Edema of the Extremities on Spectral Computed Tomography Using a Three-Material Decomposition
Reprinted from: *Diagnostics* **2023**, *13*, 2745, doi:10.3390/diagnostics13172745 323

Hyun-Jin Yoo, Jae-Kyu Choi, Youn-Moo Heo, Sung-Jun Moon and Byung-Hak Oh
Changes in Parameters after High Tibial Osteotomy: Comparison of EOS System and Computed Tomographic Analysis
Reprinted from: *J. Clin. Med.* **2023**, *12*, 5638, doi:10.3390/jcm12175638 333

About the Editors

Adam Piórkowski

Adam Piórkowski obtained a PhD in computer science in 2005. In 2015, he obtained a post-doctoral degree in biomedical engineering, and in 2019, he became a professor at AGH in Krakow. He has been involved in medical image processing since 2003. He is particularly interested in segmentation, normalization and textural analysis of this type of data. He has been involved in medical image processing since 2003. He is particularly interested in segmentation, normalization and textural analysis of this type of data. He conducts scientific projects generally related to medical informatics. He is also an active programmer.

Rafał Obuchowicz

Rafał Obuchowicz currently works in the Department of Radiology of the University Hospital, Krakow, and heads the Imaging Diagnostics department at Lux Med, Krakow. His professional interests are focused on the problems of focal change detection and shape detection in various radiological techniques using classical methods and deep learning machine algorithms. The result of the work undertaken in this direction is the NCBiR project: "XR-AI A diagnostic browser for radiology with computer-aided use of artificial intelligence," of which he is the originator and head of the medical team. He also has a professional interest in analyzing image quality using MR and X-ray techniques, resulting in the completed habilitation procedure entitled: "Analysis and parametrization of information in selected techniques of radiological diagnostics." His hobbies include environmental psychology, history, ecology, and urbanization, and he is the husband of Barbra and father of Isabella and Wiktor.

Andrzej Urbanik

Andrzej Urbanik is a Senior Professor in the Department of Radiology at Jagiellonian University Medical College. He was awarded the title of Radiology Specialist in 1991 and was appointed the Head of the Chair of Radiology (Jagiellonian University Medical College) in 1998. Until 2022, he was the Head of the Radiology Department of the University Hospital, Krakow. During this period, he also served as the Head of the Department of Diagnostic Imaging at the University Hospital in Krakow. Moreover, he founded the Electroradiology field at the Medical Faculty of the University of Rzeszów. He has produced 344 publications during his scientific activities, including peer-reviewed Polish and international journal articles, book chapters, and video/CD films. He has published 716 abstracts of presentations at Polish (459) and international (257) congresses, has supervised the completion of 24 doctoral theses, and is the tutor of four professors. Furthermore, he supervises five habilitation programs and is the head of specialization internships for 18 doctors.

Michał Strzelecki

Prof. Michał Strzelecki has been employed at the Institute of Electronics, Lodz University of Technology (TUL) since 1988, and since 2007 has been a Full Professor. In the years 2004–2019, he was Deputy Director of the Institute for Teaching and Research. He also served as Vice Dean for Research at the Faculty of Electrical, Electronic, Computer and Control Engineering, TUL until 2020. His scientific interests include the processing and analysis of biomedical signals and images, data analysis methods, and artificial intelligence. In particular, he is interested in issues related to image texture analysis and the applications and hardware implementations of artificial neural networks. He also works on the development of software aimed at support of medical imaging diagnostics. Within these interests, Prof. Strzelecki conducts extensive cooperation with domestic and foreign medical universities on the construction and development of systems supporting the diagnostic process. He has participated in numerous international research programs, including COST B21, BM1103, TD1007 (a member of the Management Committee), DGF, 7FP and projects funded by the National Science Centre (Poland) and the National Centre for Research and Development (Poland). He is the author and co-author of more than 200 scientific publications. In 2006–2008, he was employed at the Jeonbuk National University, Jeonju, Republic of Korea as a Visiting Professor.

Preface

We are pleased to provide readers with a fascinating book describing the latest achievements in the field of musculoskeletal imaging. This book is a collection of carefully selected scientific works on modern methods of processing and analyzing images of the human musculoskeletal system aimed at extracting quantitative information supporting its diagnosis. Our goal was to demonstrate that diagnostic information can be formalized and standardized from acquired images and then further explored using features that are not necessarily intuitive, easy to describe, or even visible to the naked eye. Individual contributions present original and latest methods for assessing a wide range of modalities—from X-ray and Fluoroscopy, through Conventional or Spectral Computed Tomography, Magnetic Resonance Imaging, Ultrasound and Elastography, and ending with PET/CT.

The book is of interest to an advanced and broad interdisciplinary readership, including medical doctors, researchers, and engineers representing both medical, and engineering viewpoints. We believe that this book will be inspiring not only for doctors involved in the diagnosis and treatment of the musculoskeletal system, but also for other experts.

Adam Piórkowski, Rafał Obuchowicz, Andrzej Urbanik , and Michał Strzelecki
Editors

Editorial

Advances in Musculoskeletal Imaging and Their Applications

Adam Piórkowski [1,*], Rafał Obuchowicz [2], Andrzej Urbanik [2] and Michał Strzelecki [3]

1. Department of Biocybernetics and Biomedical Engineering, AGH University of Science and Technology, 30-059 Krakow, Poland
2. Department of Diagnostic Imaging, Jagiellonian University Medical College, 31-008 Krakow, Poland; rafalobuchowicz@su.krakow.pl (R.O.); aurbanik@mp.pl (A.U.)
3. Institute of Electronics, Lodz University of Technology, 93-590 Lodz, Poland; michal.strzelecki@p.lodz.pl
* Correspondence: adam.piorkowski@agh.edu.pl

1. Introduction

Modern medical imaging systems provide ever-more information about the patient's health condition. Precision, resolution, and sensitivity are increasing, and new possibilities of differentiating the condition of tissue appear. Such advances are also taking place in musculoskeletal imaging. Ever-more accurate imaging in various modalities allows us to discover new relationships between the image and the diagnosis. It is, therefore, important to use all this information to best serve the patient, hence research related to the analysis of medical images is so important, because it allows us to indicate what is invisible to the naked eye or quantify what has so far been measured by humans or subject to discretionary assessment.

This collection includes 25 works related to the analysis of images created during diagnostics of the musculoskeletal system using various modalities, starting with X-ray and fluoroscopy, before moving onto conventional or spectral computed tomography, magnetic resonance imaging, ultrasound, and elastography and PET/CT and ending with systems for analyzing patient mechanics. Research was carried out related to the detection of various conditions, parameterization of clinical and population phenomena, and detection of image–clinical condition relationships. Despite the current popularity of machine learning techniques [1], the collection is made up of classic engineering methods related to image processing. Several works use textural analysis, which has not been appreciated so far and is particularly useful in relation to the imaging of the structure, especially the bones.

2. Texture Analysis in Musculoskeletal Imaging

Recently, radiomics has played an increasing role in analysis of biomedical images, being a tool for the quantitative description of digital image content. Radiomic features can be divided into histogram-based, texture-based, and shape-based features [2]. Of most interest are texture-based parameters that describe the structure and properties of visualized tissues and organs. Such parameters, if properly selected and repeatable, are very useful for reliable characterization of internal human organs independently of the image modality used. It has been demonstrated that texture analysis can be usefully implemented for classifying median nerves in carpal tunnel syndrome in echo images [3], diagnosis of cysts and granulomas in intra-oral radiographs [4] or quality assessment of MR images [5]. There is also free software available for texture feature evaluation, such as MaZda [6] and its successor qMaZda [7], widely used by many researchers to facilitate texture analysis in many medical image processing tasks. Such an approach is also present in some of the papers included in this Special Issue.

In [8,9], the research question discussed whether corticalization in radiographs is related to a higher risk of bone tissue loss adjacent to dental implants in smoking patients. Dental implant research has frequently delved into the factors that contribute to implant failure due to marginal bone loss. Smoking, known for its detrimental effects on health and bone structure, plays a role in impacting oral health and jawbone condition. The study is aimed at exploring how tobacco smoking influences the peri-implant jawbone's corticalization. Texture features were analyzed for radiographs, and corticalization around the implant was investigated. MaZda software was employed for this task. The study that covers a 5-year observation of radiograph bone texture established a link between smoking and alterations in the tissue structure near dental implants. The corticalization phenomenon, which can be immediately detected post-implantation, is a crucial marker. It may serve as an early indicator of the implant's likelihood of success. Understanding the correlation between smoking and resulting changes in bone structure around dental implants allows physicians to make more informed decisions about the viability of implants for smokers versus non-smokers. Physicians can provide tailored advice and counseling to patients who smoke, highlighting dental implants' potential risks and outcomes. This can potentially lead to better patient compliance and health outcomes.

Research described in [10] aimed to elucidate the reasons behind marginal bone loss (MBL) post-dental implant insertion without functional loading, focusing on understanding bone alterations surrounding the implant neck. A noticeable association between MBL and higher torques was evident after 3 months, albeit exclusively in the mandible. Over time, the radiographic texture features—sum average, entropy, difference entropy, long-run emphasis, short-run emphasis, and discrete wavelet decomposition transform attributes—underwent alterations. The study found that MBL correlates with the torque level applied during the dental implant insertion and the procedure's anatomical placement. Understanding the relationship between torque during implant insertion and MBL provides physicians with valuable information to optimize their technique and minimize MBL in patients. Using insights from the study, physicians can ensure that patients have the best potential outcomes from dental implant procedures, especially in terms of minimizing bone loss.

The author of [11] investigates the behavior of bone index (BI) values in regions of bone loss characterized by radiographically translucent non-trabecular areas to propose alternative indices specifically designed for detecting corticalization in living bone via the use of textural analyses. The study provides clinicians with valuable insights into the changes that occur in peri-implant bone over time after dental implant insertion. By understanding how bone index (BI) values change and the phenomenon of corticalization, clinicians can make more informed assessments of bone health surrounding dental implants. The study introduces objective measures, such as mean optical density, entropy, and differential entropy, which can help clinicians to quantitatively assess changes in peri-implant bone. These measures provide clinicians with reliable data to accurately track bone changes and monitor the progression of bone remodeling.

The objective of the research presented in [12] was to discern a link between textural characteristics discerned in X-ray skeletal images and the ages of the subjects. Through rigorous visual scrutiny of the images, the study sought correlations between textural attributes and chronological age. The investigation pinpointed five specific anatomical landmarks for analysis on both sides of the body, which were the iliac wing, femoral neck, greater trochanter, ischium, and femoral shaft. Each landmark's textural attributes were systematically measured. Of all landmarks, the left femoral neck showcased the most pronounced relationships. Specifically, the textural patterns derived from the histogram of oriented gradients and the gray-level co-occurrence matrix were most correlated with age, presenting a correlation coefficient (ρ) of -0.52 and a significant p-value of 4.95×10^{-14}. The primary revelation from this investigation is that age-related structural variations in the femoral neck region are more profound compared to other femoral components. By understanding the correlations between textural features in X-ray images and age, physicians can make more informed diagnoses linked to bone health- and age-related changes. The methodology proposed can be pivotal in enabling the early identification of osteoporosis. Early detection enables timely interventions, which can improve outcomes and reduce the risk of fractures.

Another paper [13] considers the bone age evaluation of adolescent wrists in boys from MRI Images. Such a bone age is typically X-ray assessed. It makes possible the assessment of the child's development and is an important parameter of the child's proper growth. However, diagnosing a specific disease is not enough. Diagnoses and prognoses often depend on the degree to which the selected case varies from the bone age norms. The bone age examination could then become a standard screening test. Replacing the technique for the bone age evaluation would also protect the patient against harmful dose of ionizing radiation, which results in a less invasive test. The experiments performed have shown that MRI texture representing wrist region ensures robust results in the determining of bone age while the patient is not exposed to ionizing radiation. Since MRI does not involve ionizing radiation, doctors can recommend it without concerns about exposing their patients, especially younger ones, to potential radiation risks. This finding means that repeat examinations, if necessary, are safer. The potential to normalize bone age evaluations as standard screenings would offer physicians a consistent method to track and evaluate developmental progress.

3. Applications of Image Analysis in Musculoskeletal Imaging

For patients with medial open-wedge high tibial osteotomy (MOWHTO), unintended distal tibial rotation is observed [14]. While computed tomography (CT) is conventionally used for lower limb alignment assessments, the novel low-dose EOS system now offers automated three-dimensional limb modeling and alignment measurement. This research juxtaposed alignment modifications, post-MOWHTO, detected through the EOS system and CT. This finding highlights the EOS system's potential as a viable alternative to CT in evaluating specific pre- and post-surgical parameters. The propensity of the distal tibia to undergo internal rotation post-MOWHTO was verified, albeit without identifying the significant factors contributing to this deformation.

One potential benefit for physicians is that the EOS system, being a low-dose imaging modality, exposes patients to significantly less radiation compared to standard CT scans. This allows physicians to more frequently order imaging if required without subjecting patients to high radiation doses. Three-dimensional limb modeling gives physicians a comprehensive view of the limb, which could be essential for surgical planning and assessment. Automation feature in EOS can potentially save physicians time, as manual measurement can be time-consuming and prone to human error. As the study suggested that there was negligible variation between CT and EOS in terms of capturing pre- and post-operative changes, physicians can feel confident using the EOS system as a reliable diagnostic tool. Lower radiation exposure and potentially shorter imaging time can enhance the patient's comfort and experience, which indirectly benefits the physician by facilitating easier patient management and improved patient compliance. Depending on the physical setup and equipment requirements, the EOS system might offer benefits in terms of space utilization or ease of operation compared to traditional CT systems. Incorporating advanced imaging technologies like the EOS system can enhance the systems' diagnostic capabilities, patient care, and operational efficiency for physicians.

Bone marrow edema (BME), indicative of acute fractures, is difficult to discern using traditional computed tomography (CT) scans [15]. The efficacy of the three-material decomposition (TMD) method for identifying traumatic BME in extremities using spectral computed tomography (SCT) has been studied. The bone compartments analyzed included the distal radius, proximal and distal tibia, proximal femur and fibula, and the long bone diaphysis. Two radiologists, uninformed of the BME status, reviewed these cases in a randomized sequence to determine BME presence. Consistency between the two raters was high, with an inter-rater reliability of 0.84 ($p < 0.001$). Individual bone compartments demonstrated sensitivities ranging from 86.7 to 93.8% and specificities ranging from 84.2 to 94.1%. Positive predictive values varied from 82.4 to 94.7%, while negative predictive values were between 87.5 and 93.3%. The proposed TMD method offers robust diagnostic accuracy in detecting BME in extremities, suggesting its potential as a routine diagnostic tool in emergency scenarios.

The TMD method on SCT provides high sensitivity and specificity, enabling physicians to make confident and accurate diagnoses of BME and acute fractures. With a reliable method to detect BME, physicians can quickly determine the best course of treatment for patients, potentially leading to faster recovery times. Given the highlighted potential of this approach in emergency situations, it could be invaluable for physicians in these settings, where time-sensitive decisions are crucial.

T2 mapping has been studied for its capability to detect and quantify anomalies in the long biceps tendon (LBT) [16]. The research aimed to understand how effectively T2 mapping can identify arthroscopically confirmed LBT pathologies and measure T2 values in both healthy and damaged tendons. On the generated T2 maps, precise regions of interest were identified, targeting the sulcal segment of the LBT, to measure average T2 values. Healthy tendons showcased an average T2 value of 23.3 ± 4.6 ms, while tendinopathy-afflicted tendons displayed an increased value of 47.9 ± 7.8 ms. This differentiation yielded a sensitivity and specificity rate of 100% for all diagnostic thresholds between 29.6 and 33.8 ms. T2 mapping is effective in discerning and quantifying healthy and pathological LBTs. This technique can offer insights into the ultra-structural health of tendons, facilitating the timely detection of anomalies.

Physicians can benefit from the study because the clear distinction between healthy and pathological tendons, as demonstrated by the T2 values, allows early and accurate diagnosis of tendon anomalies. With specific T2 values associated with healthy and pathological tendons, physicians can quantitatively track the progress of treatments, whether conservative or surgical.

Hydroxyapatite deposition disease (HADD) is a complex condition marked by the deposition of hydroxyapatite crystals in soft tissues, resulting in inflammation and pain [17]. This review delves into the intricate etiology of HADD, its progression stages, radiological manifestations, differential diagnosis, and treatment options. The role of imaging specialists in its management is also underscored. The evolution of HADD is charted across three distinct phases: pre-calcification, during calcification, and post-calcification. HADD, though intricate, can be effectively diagnosed and managed with a comprehensive understanding of its origins, progression, and imaging characteristics. As imaging plays a central role in both diagnosis and treatment, the expertise of imaging specialists remains invaluable. This review aspires to offer clinicians a holistic perspective on HADD, ensuring optimal patient outcomes.

The review provides a holistic understanding of HADD, ranging from its etiology to treatment, allowing physicians to deepen their knowledge of the disease. By understanding the radiological findings and the potential of HADD to mimic other diseases, physicians can make more accurate diagnoses, reducing the chance of misdiagnosis.

The objective of study [18] was to evaluate the image fidelity of ultra-high-resolution arthrography of the ankle using a photon-counting detector CT. In this experiment, arthrograms were bilaterally captured from four cadaveric samples using both full-dose (10 mGy) and reduced-dose (3 mGy) scanning protocols. Three distinct convolution kernels, characterized by varying spatial frequencies, were employed for the purpose of image reconstruction (ρ50; Br98: 39.0, Br84: 22.6, Br76: 16.5 lp/cm). Optimal osseous tissue representation was observed using the Br98 ultra-sharp kernel ($S \leq 0.043$). However, cartilage visualization was enhanced with diminishing modulation transfer functions across dose protocols ($p \leq 0.014$). Remarkably, the reduced-dose Br76 exhibited a CNR comparable to the full-dose Br84 ($p > 0.999$) and surpassed Br98 ($p < 0.001$) across all tissues. Utilizing a photon-counting detector CT for ankle arthrography with ultra-high-resolution collimation offers remarkable image clarity and detailed tissue analysis, augmenting the inspection of intricate anatomical structures. While osseous structures were best depicted using an ultra-sharp convolution kernel, soft tissues notably benefited from a convolution kernel with a reduced spatial frequency.

The ultra-high-resolution capability ensures that the clinician obtains unparalleled clarity in images, essential for discerning minute anatomical variations or potential pathology. The flexibility to choose between different convolution kernels based on spatial frequencies means that clinicians can optimize image quality based on the specific tissue or structure that they are investigating. The capability of the reduced-dose (3 mGy) Br76 to offer comparable CNR to the full-dose Br84 and even surpass Br98 indicates that clinicians can achieve high-quality images while reducing radiation exposure to the specimen or patient.

Study [19] probed the efficacy of T2 mapping in terms of evaluating the glenoid labrum and distinguishing between intact labral substances and superior labral anterior posterior (SLAP) lesions, utilizing arthroscopy as the benchmark standard. The established mean T2 value for unblemished labral substances was denoted as 20.8 ± 2.4 ms, while it was found to be 37.7 ± 10.63 ms for subjects presenting with SLAP lesions. These findings propose that the methodological assessment and quantification of labral (ultra)structural constitution via T2 mapping may capacitate the differentiation between arthroscopically verified SLAP lesions and a pristine glenoid labrum.

The ability of T2 mapping to distinguish between healthy labral substances and SLAP lesions with high sensitivity and specificity provides physicians with a reliable diagnostic tool. This helps in performing accurate assessment, reducing the risk of misdiagnosis. Before the potential confirmation via arthroscopy, T2 mapping offers a non-invasive method to detect SLAP lesions. This can save patients from unnecessary invasive procedures and related complications.

Shear wave elastography (SWE) is an emergent diagnostic modality employed to discern tissue abnormalities [20]. Within the realm of preventive medicine, the capability of SWE to identify early structural alterations preceding functional deficits offers considerable promise. The study aimed to discern the effect of anthropometric determinants on Achilles tendon rigidity using SWE. Additionally, the influence of diverse sports activities on tendon stiffness was probed to devise preventive medical strategies for elite athletes. Notable gender-based disparities in AT stiffness are evident across distinct sporting disciplines. Sprinters demonstrated the pinnacle of AT rigidity, a crucial aspect to be considered during clinical evaluations. Prospective research endeavors should explore the potential advantages of undertaking musculoskeletal SWE evaluations both before and after sports seasons.

Thanks to performed research, physicians have improved their understanding of how differential stiffness in Achilles tendons based on gender and sport specificity can refine diagnostic accuracy, ensuring that anomalies are not just dismissed as sport- or gender-related norms. By being aware of the normal stiffness ranges for different groups, clinicians can more effectively identify individuals who might be at increased risk of injuries or other tendon pathologies. For interventions such as physiotherapy or surgical procedures, a clear understanding of typical stiffness values can guide treatment modalities and expected outcomes, ensuring optimum patient care.

Study [21] provides insights into the kinematics of the medial gastrocnemius during isometric contractions. This knowledge can be instrumental in understanding muscle performance, adaptations, and potential injury mechanisms, especially for activities that demand a lot from the calf muscles.

The analysis of the differential muscle deformation and force at various ankle angles can guide rehabilitation exercises, strength training, and sport-specific training to optimize performance and reduce injury risks. The identification of increased force generation at dorsiflexion ankle angles due to higher fiber cross-section deformation asymmetry and higher shear strains can guide clinicians in prescribing exercises or interventions, ensuring that the foot's position is optimized to achieve specific therapeutic goals.

Study [22] aimed to ascertain the potential benefits of CT temporal subtraction (TS) images in enhancing the detection of developing or enlarging ectopic bone lesions among fibrodysplasia ossificans progressiva (FOP) patients. A retrospective analysis of four FOP patients was conducted. By subtracting registered prior CT scans from more recent scans,

TS images were generated. Utilizing TS augmented the detection sensitivity for evolving or enlarging ectopic bone lesions in FOP patients for all interpreters.

It was demonstrated that TS provides improved sensitivity in detecting emerging or enlarging ectopic bone lesions, especially in conditions like fibrodysplasia ossificans progressiva (FOP). This can facilitate earlier intervention or treatment adjustments. By leveraging the augmented ability to detect changes over time using TS, physicians can make more informed decisions regarding treatment plans, allowing tailored interventions based on the progression of the condition. By comparing changes over time in one set of images, physicians can quickly identify areas of concern without having to manually compare previous and current scans.

Study [23] was designed to ascertain the optimal pillow choice for individuals with forward head posture (FHP) by analyzing pressure distributions across the head, neck, upper body and the support provided to the spine in various sleeping postures. Participants were assessed using five distinct pillow types: viscose, fiber, cotton, goose feather, and wool. The material composition of a pillow significantly impacted the comfort and support experienced by users, especially in the context of specific spinal alignments, like FHP. Furthermore, an individual's preferred sleeping orientation influences the efficacy of a pillow material in terms of spinal support and overall comfort.

Physicians can provide evidence-based recommendations on pillow choice to patients presenting with forward head posture (FHP) based on their preferred sleeping position. This can enhance the therapeutic interventions designed for patients with neck or spine issues. Understanding the relationship between pillow material, sleeping position, and spinal alignment enables physicians to tailor advice and treatments for individual patients, optimizing outcomes.

Study [24] sought to discern kinematic variances at the point of initial contact between female futsal athletes with and without antecedent knee injuries through a functional motor pattern assessment. The ancillary objective was to juxtapose kinematic variations between the dominant limb (typically used for kicking) and the non-dominant limb across the entire cohort using the aforementioned test. Athletes devoid of knee injury antecedents demonstrated kinematic profiles more attuned to physiologically optimal stances to circumvent the valgus collapse mechanism, especially in parameters like hip adduction, internal rotation, and pelvic rotation in the dominant limb. Notably, the dominant limb caused increased knee valgus across participants, indicating heightened injury susceptibility for this limb.

The study resulted in the authors understanding the kinematic differences between injured and non-injured female futsal players that physicians must consider. They can identify at-risk players by observing their motor patterns during specific movements. This allows early intervention strategies, possibly preventing further injuries. For players recovering from knee injuries, the findings can guide physiotherapy and rehabilitation interventions, emphasizing the importance of achieving more physiological positions during movement to avoid the valgus collapse mechanism.

Percutaneous plasma disc decompression (PPDD) serves as a minimally invasive intervention strategy for discogenic lumbar pain and symptoms related to disc herniation [25]. Yet, the procedure currently lacks established variables to predict its outcomes. The correlation between the enhancements in epidurographic imagery and procedure success rate was meticulously assessed. Both the Numerical Rating Scale (NRS) and the Oswestry Disability Index (ODI) were employed to gauge pain intensity and functional impairment, respectively, being used preoperatively and one-month post-intervention. Remarkably, groups with improved epidurographic findings displayed significantly superior pain alleviation and procedural success rates compared to those without such enhancements.

Understanding the potential role of epidurography as an outcome predictor can aid clinicians in making better-informed treatment decisions. If a patient demonstrates epidurographic improvement, they may be more likely to benefit from PPDD. Using epidurography as a predictive tool, physicians can better identify which patients are more likely to benefit from the procedure, leading to higher treatment success rates. By recognizing the potential end-point of the PPDD procedure through epidurography, doctors can avoid over- or under-treating, leading to optimized results and reduced patient discomfort or risk of developing a worsened condition.

The diminished thickness of the temporal muscle (TMT) has been identified as an adverse prognostic factor in patients with brain tumors [26]. Separately, chronic subdural hematoma (CSDH) is a neurosurgical condition notorious for its high recurrence and elusive outcome prediction models. The thickness of the temporal muscle could serve as a tangible prognostic marker, potentially aiding in identifying CSDH patients at heightened risk.

The Identification of temporal muscle thickness (TMT) as a potential prognostic indicator can help physicians to quickly stratify patients based on the risk of poor outcomes. Understanding which patients are more vulnerable allows more informed clinical decision-making. Understanding the association between reduced TMT and outcomes such as hematoma volume and post-operative performance can guide surgeons in their approach, post-operative care, and setting realistic expectations for patients and their families.

The primary goal of this research was to scrutinize and juxtapose ultrasonographic findings in the nails and entheses of patients diagnosed with psoriasis and psoriatic arthritis [27]. Disparities were found in the Nail Psoriasis Severity Index scores and the scores derived from the Glasgow Ultrasound Enthesitis Scoring System when comparing patients with psoriasis to those with psoriatic arthritis. Ultrasonographic assessments revealed more pronounced nail abnormalities in individuals with psoriasis, whereas enthesopathic changes in the lower extremities were more prominent in subjects with psoriatic arthritis.

The use of ultrasonography for the examination of nails and entheses can assist in the early detection of abnormalities in patients with psoriasis and psoriatic arthritis. This is vital for making a timely and accurate diagnosis. Understanding the variations in ultrasonographic findings between psoriasis and psoriatic arthritis allows physicians to design more tailored treatment plans based on the specific condition and its severity.

Intraoperative CT-navigation (iCT-navigation) has shown efficacy in enhancing the precision and safety of transpedicular screw insertion during primary spinal operations [28]. Nonetheless, the challenges associated with altered bone structures and fibrotic tissues make revision spinal surgeries complex. The study aimed to assess the fidelity and safety of iCT-navigation during screw insertion at untouched sites compared to previously operated sites in revision thoracolumbar spinal procedures.

The study illustrates that iCT-navigation can enhance the precision of screw placements, even in revision sites, which are traditionally more challenging due to the disrupted anatomy. The utilization of iCT-navigation appears to reduce the risk of complications, as evidenced by the lack of neurological injuries in the patients studied. The iCT-navigation allows the instantaneous identification of unaccepted screws, permitting their immediate adjustment during the same operation, potentially reducing the need for further revision surgeries.

Titanium trabecular cages (TTCs) have been developed as promising implants with the intent to ensure both immediate and long-lasting spinal stability via rapid osseointegration [29]. However, robust radiological and clinical evidence affirming their effectiveness was lacking. The study aimed to assess the reactive bone behavior at plates adjacent to custom-designed TTCs in lumbar interbody operations using positron emission tomography (PET)/computed tomography (CT) with 18F sodium fluoride (18F-NaF). The 18F-NaF PET/CT has been validated as an effective modality to probe the metabolic repair reaction post-TTC implantation, radiographically illustrating the cage's capacity to incite reparative osteoblastic activity on the vertebral endplate surface.

The study provides clinicians with valuable insights into the reactive bone behavior adjacent to titanium trabecular cages (TTCs) used in lumbar interbody fusion surgeries. This knowledge may aid in better understanding the osseointegration process and inform surgical planning, potentially leading to improved patient outcomes. The use of 18F sodium fluoride (18F-NaF) PET/CT as a tool to assess metabolic–reparative reactions offers clinicians a scientifically rigorous approach to evaluate the success of implantation. This evidence-based assessment can guide clinical decisions related to patient management and treatment adjustments.

Study [30] introduces an innovative and lightweight machine learning-based approach aimed at facilitating the diagnosis of COVID-19 through the analysis of X-ray images. The proposed method offers a rapid and effective means of diagnosing COVID-19 based on medical imaging. The proposed approach has potential as a valuable tool to assist radiologists in enhancing the diagnostic workflow for COVID-19. The method showcased effectiveness and speed in providing accurate diagnoses.

The introduced schema serves as an additional support tool for radiologists in COVID-19 diagnosis. It assists radiologists by offering a structured method for evaluating X-ray images and potentially reducing the workload associated with manual image interpretation. The lightweight nature of the approach allows the quick processing and analysis of X-ray images. This speed can significantly expedite the diagnostic process, enabling doctors to promptly make informed decisions about patient care.

An innovative technique for conducting cervical interlaminar epidural steroid injections (CILESIs) guided via ultrasound (US), which eliminates the reliance on the loss-of-resistance approach for identifying the epidural space, was presented in [31].

The employment of this novel ultrasound-guided technique for cervical interlaminar epidural steroid injections (CILESIs) offers physicians increased accuracy and precision during the procedure. The direct visualization of anatomical structures aids in precise needle placement, minimizing the risk of complications and optimizing treatment outcomes. The use of ultrasound imaging allows physicians to monitor the administration of injectable substances in real time, ensuring that the medication is delivered accurately and without causing inadvertent damage to surrounding tissues. This heightened level of safety can lead to a decrease in adverse events and complications associated with cervical epidural injections.

Antegrade intra-medullary (IM) nailing remains the typical treatment for femoral shaft fractures, yet non-union rates remain high for infra-isthmal femoral shaft fractures based on this approach [32]. Thus, a retrospective case–control study aimed at identifying perioperative radiographic factors linked to non-union in these cases after antegrade IM nailing was performed.

The results of this retrospective case–control study provide physicians with valuable insights into the radiographic risk factors associated with non-union after antegrade intra-medullary (IM) nailing for infra-isthmal femoral shaft fractures. Armed with this knowledge, physicians can make more informed treatment decisions by considering these risk factors and tailoring their approach to reduce the likelihood of non-union. By understanding the radiographic elements that contribute to non-union, physicians can adopt strategies to mitigate these risks during the treatment process. This proactive approach can lead to improved patient outcomes, reduced complications, and enhanced recovery rates, thereby bolstering the physician's reputation and patient satisfaction.

4. Conclusions

We hope that all readers will appreciate this Special Issue and that the collection of the articles will be useful in a clinical or scientific way, as well as inspire further investigations into the domain of musculoskeletal imaging. We would also like to encourage doctors to use various quantitative image processing and analysis methods and expand cooperation with computer scientists and biomedical engineers in this area. New information obtained thanks to such analyses will improve the efficiency and repeatability of the diagnostic process.

Author Contributions: Conceptualization, R.O., A.P. and M.S.; methodology, R.O., A.P. and M.S.; software, A.P.; validation, R.O., A.P. and M.S.; formal analysis, A.U.; investigation, R.O., A.P. and M.S.; resources, A.U.; data curation, A.U.; writing—original draft preparation, R.O., A.P. and M.S.; writing—review and editing, R.O., A.P. and M.S.; visualization, A.P.; supervision, R.O.; project administration, A.P. and R.O.; funding acquisition, R.O. All authors have read and agreed to the published version of the manuscript.

Conflicts of Interest: The authors declare no conflict of interest.

References

1. Strzelecki, M.; Badura, P. Machine Learning for Biomedical Application. *Appl. Sci.* **2022**, *12*, 2022. [CrossRef]
2. Mayerhoefer, M.E.; Materka, A.; Langs, G.; Häggström, I.; Szczypiński, P.; Gibbs, P.; Cook, G. Introduction to Radiomics. *J. Nucl. Med.* **2020**, *61*, 488–495. [CrossRef] [PubMed]
3. Obuchowicz, R.; Kruszyńska, J.; Strzelecki, M. Classifying median nerves in carpal tunnel syndrome: Ultrasound image analysis. *Biocybern. Biomed. Eng.* **2021**, *41*, 335–351. [CrossRef]
4. Pociask, E.; Nurzynska, K.; Obuchowicz, R.; Bałon, P.; Uryga, D.; Strzelecki, M.; Izworski, A.; Piórkowski, A. Differential Diagnosis of Cysts and Granulomas Supported by Texture Analysis of Intraoral Radiographs. *Sensors* **2021**, *21*, 7481. [CrossRef]
5. Strzelecki, M.; Piórkowski, A.; Obuchowicz, R. Effect of Matrix Size Reduction on Textural Information in Clinical Magnetic Resonance Imaging. *J. Clin. Med.* **2022**, *11*, 2526. [CrossRef] [PubMed]
6. Szczypiński, P.M.; Strzelecki, M.; Materka, A.; Klepaczko, A. MaZda—The software package for textural analysis of biomedical images. *Adv. Intell. Soft Comput.* **2009**, *65*, 73–84.
7. Szczypinski, P.M.; Klepaczko, A.; Kociolek, M. QMaZda—Software tools for image analysis and pattern recognition. In Proceedings of the Signal Processing—Algorithms, Architectures, Arrangements, and Applications Conference Proceedings, Poznan, Poland, 20–22 September 2017; pp. 217–221.
8. Wach, T.; Hadrowicz, P.; Trybek, G.; Michcik, A.; Kozakiewicz, M. Is Corticalization in Radiographs Related to a Higher Risk of Bone Loss around Dental Implants in Smoking Patients? A 5-Year Observation of Radiograph Bone-Texture Changes. *J. Clin. Med.* **2023**, *12*, 5351. [CrossRef]
9. Kozakiewicz, M.; Wach, T. Exploring the Importance of Corticalization Occurring in Alveolar Bone Surrounding a Dental Implant. *J. Clin. Med.* **2022**, *11*, 7189. [CrossRef]
10. Wach, T.; Skorupska, M.; Trybek, G. Are Torque-Induced Bone Texture Alterations Related to Early Marginal Jawbone Loss? *J. Clin. Med.* **2022**, *11*, 6158. [CrossRef]
11. Kozakiewicz, M. Measures of Corticalization. *J. Clin. Med.* **2022**, *11*, 5463. [CrossRef]
12. Kamiński, P.; Obuchowicz, R.; Stępień, A.; Lasek, J.; Pociask, E.; Piórkowski, A. Correlation of Bone Textural Parameters with Age in the Context of Orthopedic X-ray Studies. *Appl. Sci.* **2023**, *13*, 6618. [CrossRef]
13. Obuchowicz, R.; Nurzynska, K.; Pierzchala, M.; Piorkowski, A.; Strzelecki, M. Texture Analysis for the Bone Age Assessment from MRI Images of Adolescent Wrists in Boys. *J. Clin. Med.* **2023**, *12*, 2762. [CrossRef]
14. Yoo, H.; Choi, J.; Heo, Y.; Moon, S.; Oh, B. Changes in Parameters after High Tibial Osteotomy: Comparison of EOS System and Computed Tomographic Analysis. *J. Clin. Med.* **2023**, *12*, 5638. [CrossRef] [PubMed]
15. Schierenbeck, M.; Grözinger, M.; Reichardt, B.; Jansen, O.; Kauczor, H.; Campbell, G.; Sedaghat, S. Detecting Bone Marrow Edema of the Extremities on Spectral Computed Tomography Using a Three-Material Decomposition. *Diagnostics* **2023**, *13*, 2745. [CrossRef] [PubMed]
16. Stein, P.; Wuennemann, F.; Schneider, T.; Zeifang, F.; Burkholder, I.; Weber, M.; Kauczor, H.; Rehnitz, C. Detection and Quantitative Assessment of Arthroscopically Proven Long Biceps Tendon Pathologies Using T2 Mapping. *Tomography* **2023**, *9*, 1577–1591. [CrossRef]
17. Hegazi, T. Hydroxyapatite Deposition Disease: A Comprehensive Review of Pathogenesis, Radiological Findings, and Treatment Strategies. *Diagnostics* **2023**, *13*, 2678. [CrossRef]
18. Luetkens, K.; Grunz, J.; Kunz, A.; Huflage, H.; Weißenberger, M.; Hartung, V.; Patzer, T.; Gruschwitz, P.; Ergün, S.; Bley, T.; et al. Ultra-High-Resolution Photon-Counting Detector CT Arthrography of the Ankle: A Feasibility Study. *Diagnostics* **2023**, *13*, 2201. [CrossRef]
19. Stein, P.; Wuennemann, F.; Schneider, T.; Zeifang, F.; Burkholder, I.; Weber, M.; Kauczor, H.; Rehnitz, C. 3-Tesla T2 Mapping Magnetic Resonance Imaging for Evaluation of SLAP Lesions in Patients with Shoulder Pain: An Arthroscopy-Controlled Study. *J. Clin. Med.* **2023**, *12*, 3109. [CrossRef]
20. Römer, C.; Zessin, E.; Czupajllo, J.; Fischer, T.; Wolfarth, B.; Lerchbaumer, M. Effect of Anthropometric Parameters on Achilles Tendon Stiffness of Professional Athletes Measured by Shear Wave Elastography. *J. Clin. Med.* **2023**, *12*, 2963. [CrossRef]
21. Hernandez, R.; Sinha, U.; Malis, V.; Cunnane, B.; Smitaman, E.; Sinha, S. Strain and Strain Rate Tensor Mapping of Medial Gastrocnemius at Submaximal Isometric Contraction and Three Ankle Angles. *Tomography* **2023**, *9*, 840–856. [CrossRef]
22. Iima, M.; Sakamoto, R.; Kakigi, T.; Yamamoto, A.; Otsuki, B.; Nakamoto, Y.; Toguchida, J.; Matsuda, S. The Efficacy of CT Temporal Subtraction Images for Fibrodysplasia Ossificans Progressiva. *Tomography* **2023**, *9*, 768–775. [CrossRef]
23. Türkmen, C.; Esen, S.; Erden, Z.; Düger, T. Comfort and Support Values Provided by Different Pillow Materials for Individuals with Forward Head Posture. *Appl. Sci.* **2023**, *13*, 3865. [CrossRef]

24. Ferrández-Laliena, L.; Vicente-Pina, L.; Sánchez-Rodríguez, R.; Orantes-González, E.; Heredia-Jimenez, J.; Lucha-López, M.; Hidalgo-García, C.; Tricás-Moreno, J. Diagnostics Using the Change-of-Direction and Acceleration Test (CODAT) of the Biomechanical Patterns Associated with Knee Injury in Female Futsal Players: A Cross-Sectional Analytical Study. *Diagnostics* **2023**, *13*, 928. [CrossRef] [PubMed]
25. Gil, H.; Seo, W.; Choi, G.; Ha, E.; Kim, T.; Ryu, J.; Kim, J.; Choi, J. A New Role for Epidurography: A Simple Method for Assessing the Adequacy of Decompression during Percutaneous Plasma Disc Decompression. *J. Clin. Med.* **2022**, *11*, 7144. [CrossRef] [PubMed]
26. Dubinski, D.; Won, S.; Behmanesh, B.; Cantré, D.; Mattes, I.; Trnovec, S.; Baumgarten, P.; Schuss, P.; Freiman, T.; Gessler, F. Significance of Temporal Muscle Thickness in Chronic Subdural Hematoma. *J. Clin. Med.* **2022**, *11*, 6456. [CrossRef] [PubMed]
27. Huang, Y.; Huang, Y.; Lin, C.; Kuo, C.; Huang, Y. Ultrasound Can Be Usefully Integrated with the Clinical Assessment of Nail and Enthesis Involvement in Psoriasis and Psoriatic Arthritis. *J. Clin. Med.* **2022**, *11*, 6296. [CrossRef]
28. Li, Y.; Chen, S.; Huang, K.; Lee, C.; Cheng, C.; Lee, C.; Wu, M.; Huang, T. High Accuracy and Safety of Intraoperative CT-Guided Navigation for Transpedicular Screw Placement in Revision Spinal Surgery. *J. Clin. Med.* **2022**, *11*, 5853. [CrossRef]
29. Cofano, F.; Armocida, D.; Ruffini, L.; Scarlattei, M.; Baldari, G.; Di Perna, G.; Pilloni, G.; Zenga, F.; Ballante, E.; Garbossa, D.; et al. The Efficacy of Trabecular Titanium Cages to Induce Reparative Bone Activity after Lumbar Arthrodesis Studied through the 18f-Naf PET/CT Scan: Observational Clinical In-Vivo Study. *Diagnostics* **2022**, *12*, 2296. [CrossRef]
30. Giełczyk, A.; Marciniak, A.; Tarczewska, M.; Kloska, S.; Harmoza, A.; Serafin, Z.; Woźniak, M. A Novel Lightweight Approach to COVID-19 Diagnostics Based on Chest X-ray Images. *J. Clin. Med.* **2022**, *11*, 5501. [CrossRef]
31. Maeda, N.; Maeda, M.; Tanaka, Y. Direct Visualization of Cervical Interlaminar Epidural Injections Using Sonography. *Tomography* **2022**, *8*, 1869–1880. [CrossRef]
32. Hung, W.; Hsu, C.; Kumar, C.; Tsai, C.; Chang, H.; Lin, T. Perioperative Radiographic Predictors of Non-Union in Infra-Isthmal Femoral Shaft Fractures after Antegrade Intramedullary Nailing: A Case-Control Study. *J. Clin. Med.* **2022**, *11*, 3664. [CrossRef] [PubMed]

Disclaimer/Publisher's Note: The statements, opinions and data contained in all publications are solely those of the individual author(s) and contributor(s) and not of MDPI and/or the editor(s). MDPI and/or the editor(s) disclaim responsibility for any injury to people or property resulting from any ideas, methods, instructions or products referred to in the content.

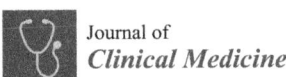

Article

Perioperative Radiographic Predictors of Non-Union in Infra-Isthmal Femoral Shaft Fractures after Antegrade Intramedullary Nailing: A Case–Control Study

Wei-Cheng Hung [1,†], Chin-Jung Hsu [1,2,†], Abhishek Kumar [1,3], Chun-Hao Tsai [1,4], Hao-Wei Chang [1] and Tsung-Li Lin [1,4,5,*]

1. Department of Orthopedics, China Medical University Hospital, Taichung 404327, Taiwan; d24645@mail.cmuh.org.tw (W.-C.H.); d5983@mail.cmuh.org.tw (C.-J.H.); kumar@aior.co.in (A.K.); d7940@mail.cmuh.org.tw (C.-H.T.); d22067@mail.cmuh.org.tw (H.-W.C.)
2. School of Chinese Medicine, China Medical University, Taichung 404333, Taiwan
3. Anup Institute of Orthopedics and Rehabilitation, Patna 800020, India
4. Department of Sports Medicine, College of Health Care, China Medical University, Taichung 406040, Taiwan
5. Graduate Institute of Biomedical Sciences, China Medical University, Taichung 404333, Taiwan
* Correspondence: d18144@mail.cmuh.org.tw; Tel.: +886-4-2205-2121
† These authors contributed equally to this work.

Abstract: Antegrade intramedullary (IM) nailing is the gold standard treatment for femoral shaft fractures; however, the non-union rate of infra-isthmal femoral shaft fractures is still high after antegrade IM nailing. This retrospective case–control study aimed to determine the association between perioperative radiographic factors and the non-union of infra-isthmal femoral shaft fractures after antegrade IM nailing. Univariate and multivariate analyses were used to evaluate the radiographic risk factors of non-union. Ninety-three patients were included, with thirty-one non-unions and sixty-two matched controls between 2007 and 2017. All were regularly followed up for 2 years. Receiver operating characteristic analysis revealed that a ratio of the unfixed distal segment > 32.5% was strongly predictive of postoperative non-union. The risk factors for non-union were AO/OTA type B and C (odds ratio [OR]: 2.20), a smaller ratio of the distal fragment (OR: 4.05), a greater ratio of the unfixed distal segment (OR: 7.16), a higher ratio of IM canal diameter to nail size at the level of fracture (OR: 6.23), and fewer distal locking screws (OR: 2.31). The radiographic risk factors for non-union after antegrade IM nailing for infra-isthmal femoral shaft fractures were unstable fractures, shorter distal fragments, longer unfixed distal fragments, wider IM canal, and fewer distal locking screws. Surgeons must strive to avoid non-union with longer and larger nails and apply more distal locking screws, especially for unstable, wider IM canal, and shorter distal fragment fractures.

Keywords: infra-isthmal femoral shaft fracture; non-union; antegrade intramedullary nailing

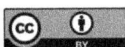

1. Introduction

Femoral shaft fractures are common in orthopedic high-energy injuries. Their worldwide annual incidence ranges from 10 to 21 cases per 100,000 individuals [1,2]. For decades, antegrade intramedullary (IM) nailing has been the gold standard treatment for acute adult femoral shaft fractures. As the indications for nailing have expanded to include more complex situations, the rates of non-union of acute femoral shaft fractures after antegrade IM nailing have also increased to 4.1–12.5% [3–7]. Various studies have reported the risk factors of non-union; these include open fractures, unreamed antegrade IM nailing, bone loss, soft tissue interposition, open reduction, the distraction of the fracture site, insufficient fixation, smoking, nonsteroidal anti-inflammatory drug (NSAID) usage, and delayed weight-bearing [3–5].

Park et al. categorized femoral shaft fractures into supra-isthmal, isthmal, and infra-isthmal fractures [8]. The infra-isthmal region has a thin cortex and poor bone stock. The distal fragment of an infra-isthmal fracture is difficult to stabilize, and instability may develop after the nailing procedure. In the infra-isthmus femoral region, the mechanical stiffness of the bone–implant complex diminishes during metaphysis-diaphysis transition [9]. Kim et al. demonstrated the statistically significant differences in non-union between isthmal and non-isthmal fracture sites [10]. Yang et al. reported that a greater ratio of fracture site to isthmus diameter as a preoperative predictive factor was associated with a higher postoperative complication rate, such as non-union [11]. Watanabe et al. reported that distal fragments shorter than 43% of the femoral length are a risk factor for aseptic non-union in femoral nailing [12].

To the best of our knowledge, no studies have identified the factors for non-union in infra-isthmal femoral shaft fractures after antegrade IM nailing. We hypothesized the unstable fracture pattern, shorter length of the distal fragment, wider IM canal at the level of fracture, and insufficient distal fixation would predict non-union in such fractures. Therefore, the purpose of this retrospective case–control study was to evaluate the perioperative radiographic risk factors for non-union in infra-isthmal femoral shaft fractures.

2. Materials and Method

This single-center, retrospective case–control study was conducted at the department of orthopedic surgery in a tertiary healthcare hospital. We identified patients with infra-isthmal femoral shaft fractures (ICD-9-CM codes 821.20) who were treated with antegrade IM nailing via closed reduction surgery between June 2007 and June 2017. A total of 93 patients met the following criteria for study inclusion: (1) age > 20 years, (2) infra-isthmal fractures, (3) isolated unilateral fractures, (4) acute and close fractures, (5) fixation within 3 weeks, and (6) follow-up > 2 years after the surgery. We excluded cases in which bony union may have been influenced by the following factors: (1) multiple fractures, (2) combined femoral neck fractures, (3) segmental fractures, (4) periprosthetic fractures, (5) pathological fractures, (6) open fractures, (7) brain injury, (8) open reduction, and (9) postoperative infections.

Age- and body mass index-matched skeletally mature adults who underwent interlocking nailing for an infra-isthmal femoral shaft fracture during the same study period as the test patients were selected from the orthopedic registry and included in the union and non-union groups. The case–control ratio was set to 1:2. The infra-isthmal region was defined as the region between the upper border of the transepicondylar width of the knee joint and the isthmus [13]. Fellow-trained orthopedic surgeons performed all surgeries via the standard approach of a closed reduction with IM nailing.

Bony union can be defined by bridging callus formation in at least three of the four cortices (as seen on radiographs), absence of motion or pain during physiological stress to the fracture, or presence of full weight-bearing ability [14]. Radiological non-union was classified as hypertrophic or atrophic [15] and was defined by a lack of cortical continuity on more than two cortices, lack of bridging callus formation, persistent fracture lines, or absence of signs of progression to healing for 3 months.

During the study period, eight parameters were measured in the anteroposterior (AP) and lateral views of preoperative and immediate postoperative radiographs to evaluate the radiographic risk factors for non-union. Preoperative radiographs were evaluated to classify the fracture types in accordance with the AO Foundation/Orthopaedic Trauma Association (AO/OTA) classification system [16]. Goniometric measurements were performed using immediate postoperative radiographs to determine the coronal plane angulation on AP radiographs and the sagittal plane angulation on lateral radiographs (the long axes of the proximal and distal fragment's diaphyses intersect). The ratio of the distal fragment was measured using immediate postoperative radiographs in accordance with the protocol by Watanabe et al. (Figure 1). The ratio of the unfixed distal segment, as well as the ratio of IM canal diameter to nail size at the level of fracture (C/N ratio) (Figure 2), and the number of distal locking screws and poller screws were also measured.

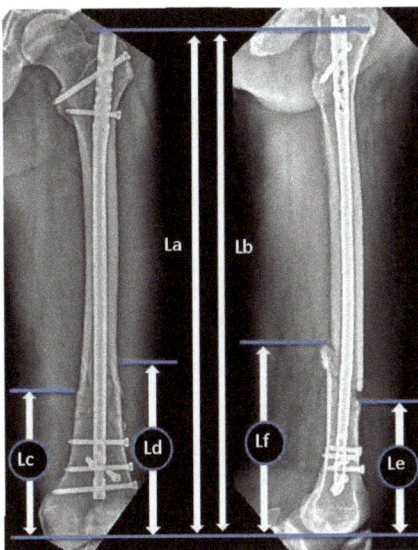

Figure 1. Ratio of the distal fragment: D/L, L: (La + Lb)/2, D: (Lc + Ld + Le + Lf)/4. D: Main distal fragment length, L: femur length, La: distance from the tip of the greater trochanter to the intercondylar notch in the AP view, Lb: distance from the tip of the greater trochanter to the intersection of the Blumensaat line and the trochlear groove line in the lateral view, Lc: distance from the intercondylar notch to the distal fracture line at the lateral site in the AP view, Ld: distance from the intercondylar notch to the distal fracture line at the medial site in the AP view, Le: distance from the intercondylar notch to the distal fracture line at the anterior site in the lateral view, Lf: distance from the intercondylar notch to the distal fracture line at the posterior site in the lateral view.

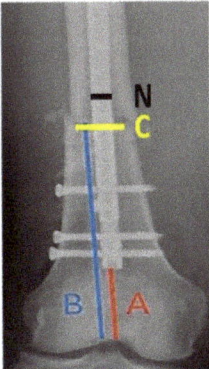

Figure 2. Ratio of the unfixed distal segment: A/B. A: Distance from the tip of the nail to the intercondylar notch in the AP view, B: main distal fragment length from the proximal fracture line to the intercondylar notch in the AP view. Ratio of the IM canal diameter to nail size at the level of fracture: C/N. C: IM canal diameter at the level of fracture in the AP view, N: nail size in the AP view.

Statistical Analysis

Statistical analyses were performed using IBM SPSS Statistics (version 23.0; SPSS Inc., Armonk, NY, USA). Descriptive statistics are presented as means and 95% confidence intervals (CIs) for continuous variables and as counts and percentages for categorical variables. The chi-squared test was performed for the nominal scale, while one-way analysis of variance was performed for the ratio scale. The areas under the curves were obtained using receiver operating characteristic (ROC) to predict the ratio of the unfixed distal segment and C/N ratio for postoperative non-union. Univariate and multivariate logistic regression analysis was performed for all variables to determine their relationship with the development of non-union after antegrade IM nailing. Statistical significance was defined as $p < 0.05$.

3. Results

Ninety-three patients (70 men, 23 women) were included in this study. The mechanism of injury was high-energy trauma in all 93 patients. The following four types of antegrade nails were used in the treatment: (1) Zimmer Natural Nail (Zimmer-Biomet, Warsaw, IN, USA), (2) Targon femoral nail (Aesculap, Tuttlingen, Germany), (3) Expert Asian Femoral Nail (A2FN; Synthes, Solothurn, Switzerland), and (4) King Bo femur interlocking nail (Syntec Scientific Co, Changhwa, Taiwan). Figure 3 show the "Strengthening the Reporting of Observational Studies in Epidemiology" flowchart, which details the study design.

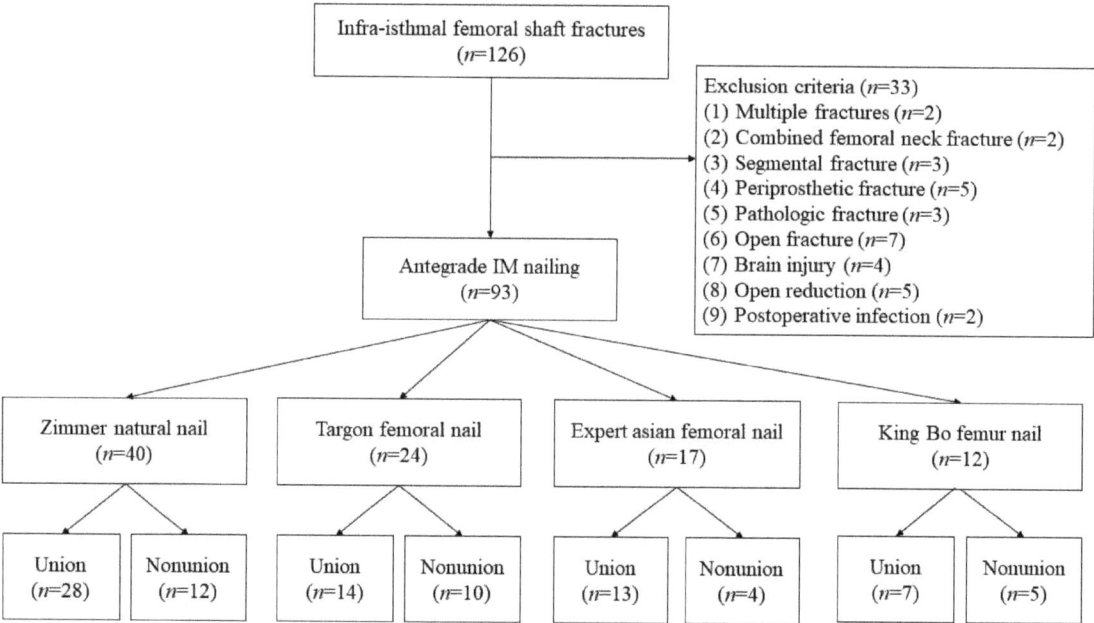

Figure 3. "Strengthening the Reporting of Observational Studies in Epidemiology" flowchart detailing the design of this study.

Based on the radiological classification, there were 25 hypertrophic non-union and 6 atrophic non-union cases. Bony unions took an average of 23.1 weeks to complete in the united cohort. The demographic and radiographic characteristics of the study participants are presented in Table 1.

Table 1. Study variables and their association with non-union and union of fractures.

	Non-Union (n = 31)	Union (n = 62)	p-Value
Age, years (95% CI)	28.6 (20–34)	28.2 (20–35)	0.687
Male, n (%)	23 (74.2)	47 (75.8)	0.672
Right laterality, n (%)	18 (58.1)	40 (64.5)	0.514
BMI, kg/m² (95% CI)	23.6 (18.4–33.8)	24.1 (18.8–34.2)	0.761
AO/OTA classification			0.004
Type A, n (%)	11 (35.5)	42 (67.7)	
Type B and C, n (%)	20 (64.5)	20 (32.3)	
Postoperative coronal deformity, degree (95% CI)	7.0 (2–10)	6.7 (3–9)	0.341
Postoperative sagittal deformity, degree (95% CI)	3.6 (2–9)	2.8 (2–10)	0.412
Ratio of the distal fragment, % (95% CI)	34.6 (28–40)	44.5 (37–47)	0.021
Ratio of the unfixed distal fragment, % (95% CI)	32.3 (24.1–41.8)	23.8 (16.4–28.7)	0.013
C/N ratio, (95% CI)	2.2 (1.9–2.4)	1.9 (1.8–2.1)	0.028
Distal locking screws, n (95% CI)	2.1 (2–4)	3.4 (2–4)	0.033
Poller screws, n (95% CI)	0.69 (0–2)	0.93 (0–4)	0.086

CI: confidence interval; n, number; BMI, body mass index; AO/OTA, AO Foundation/Orthopaedic Trauma Association; C/N, IM canal diameter to nail size at the level of fracture.

A ratio of the unfixed distal segment > 32.5% was substantially predictive of postoperative non-union, according to ROC curve analysis (Figure 4). Furthermore, the ROC curve indicated that the C/N ratio > 2.1 had sensitivity and specificity of 69% and 70%, respectively, in predicting non-union.

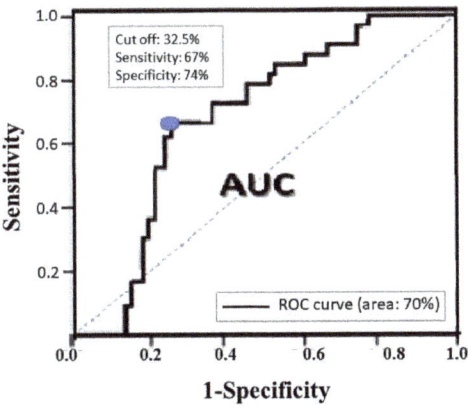

Figure 4. ROC curve for non-union. ROC analysis revealed that the summation of sensitivity and specificity was the greatest at the point indicated by the blue circle; it corresponds to a ratio of the unfixed distal segment that is 32.5% of the main distal fragment length.

Table 2 present univariate risk factors for the non-union of infra-isthmal femoral shaft fractures after antegrade nailing. On multivariate logistic regression analysis, AO/OTA classification types B and C, ratio of the distal fragment < 43%, ratio of the unfixed distal fragment > 32.5%, C/N ratio > 2.1, and distal locking screws < 3 were identified as independent risk factors for non-union after antegrade nailing (Table 3).

Table 2. Risk factors for non-union after antegrade nailing (univariate analysis).

Risk Factor	Odds Ratio (95% CI)	p-Value
AO/OTA classification type B and C	2.87 (0.67–5.84)	0.028
Ratio of the distal fragment < 43%	5.41 (2.09–10.65)	0.002
Ratio of the unfixed distal fragment > 32.5%	9.23 (3.44–24.06)	<0.001
C/N ratio > 2.1	8.71 (2.07–21.27)	0.001
Distal locking screws < 3	3.16 (1.94–9.17)	0.004

AO/OTA, AO Foundation/Orthopaedic Trauma Association; CI, confidence interval; C/N, IM canal diameter to nail size at the level of fracture.

Table 3. Independent risk factors for non-union after antegrade nailing (multivariate analysis).

Risk Factor	Adjusted Odds Ratio (95% CI)	p-Value
AO/OTA classification type B and C	2.20 (0.47–4.13)	0.037
Ratio of the distal fragment < 43%	4.05 (1.43–7.12)	0.018
Ratio of the unfixed distal fragment > 32.5%	7.16 (2.37–17.96)	0.031
C/N ratio > 2.1	6.23 (1.94–17.38)	0.017
Distal locking screws < 3	2.31 (1.08–6.18)	0.013

AO/OTA, AO Foundation/Orthopaedic Trauma Association; CI, confidence interval; C/N, IM canal diameter to nail size at the level of fracture.

4. Discussion

This is the first retrospective case–control study to evaluate the perioperative radiographic predictors of non-union in infra-isthmal femoral shaft fractures after antegrade IM nailing; these included unstable fractures (AO/OTA classifications B and C), shorter distal fragments, longer unfixed distal fragments, wider IM canal, and fewer distal locking screws. Moreover, the most noteworthy finding of this study was that a ratio of the unfixed distal segment > 32.5% was substantially predictive of postoperative non-union.

For long bone fractures, retrospective studies revealed comminution and increasing displacement as the potential risk factors of non-union [17], while prospective studies confirmed the unstable fracture type as a significant risk factor for non-union [18]. In this study, we found that the AO/OTA classifications demonstrated a significant difference between the union and non-union groups. This may explain why the non-union rates depended on the unstable and comminuted fracture patterns.

The rotational instability of infra-isthmal fractures is due to the movements of the gastrocnemius and hamstring tendons that occur during motion. Furthermore, it is also attributed to the fact that the medullary cavity of the infra-isthmal fragment has a diameter that is substantially larger than that of the nail employed [10,19]. Thus, the infra-isthmal area of the femur is thought to be responsible for reducing the mechanical stiffness of the bone-implant constructs [9]. Yang et al. reported that the ratio of fracture site to isthmus canal diameter ≥ 2 was a reliable preoperative parameter to predict non-union [11]. In the current study, C/N ration > 2.1, as a postoperative parameter which revealed a significant difference between the union and non-union groups, was similar to Yang's finding. This finding could explain why the wider IM diameter at the fracture site is related to a higher non-union rate after antegrade IM nailing.

Watanabe et al. noted that if the length of the distal fragment is less than 43% of the total femoral length, further surgical fixation can be considered [12]. Ha et al. reported that the instability of distal fragments leads to higher failure rates in non-union cases [20]. According to our results, the ratio of the distal fragment differed significantly between the non-union and union groups; this could partially explain why a smaller distal fragment ratio was the predictor of non-union in the current study.

The fixation strength is thought to be enhanced when the nail's tip is as close to the Blumensaat line as possible [10]. The current study's findings revealed a significant difference between the union and non-union groups when the ratio of the unfixed distal segment was over 32.5%. Furthermore, the ratio of the distal fragment and the ratio of the unfixed distal fragment predicted the development of non-union after antegrade nailing. These two predictors support the importance of nail length in the risk of non-union.

Multiple surgical tools can augment bone-implant stability in distal femoral fragments, such as poller screws and more distal locking screws. Bryan et al. discussed the effect of poller screws with retrograde nails on distal fragment stability [21,22]. Kim et al. reported that exchange nailing in infra-isthmal femoral shaft non-union with a more secure distal fixation, such as with poller screws and additional interlocking screws, may be an effective and reliable treatment option [10]. In the current study, the distal screw density was significantly different between the union and non-union groups, whereas the poller screws did not show any obvious intergroup differences. This suggests that increasing the distal screw density may be an effective way to reduce the likelihood of non-union.

There are several treatments for non-union of infra-isthmal femoral shaft fractures following an internal fixation; however, their outcomes remain debatable. Pihlajamäki et al. stated that exchange nailing without bone grafting was the best method for treating non-union after an index femoral nailing surgery [4]. Brinker et al. reported their experience of exchanging preexisting nails with nails that were at least 1 mm larger than the previous nails or up to 4 mm in size (if the previous nail was undersized) for treating non-union [23]. Park et al. reported that augmentation plating with autogenous bone grafting might be a better option than exchange nailing [8]. Various studies have reported that replacing the original nail with a retrograde nail can improve distal fragment stability [21,22]. Indeed, the advantages of retrograde IM nailing are a longer working length, adequate fixation of the distal fragment through the use of more interlocking screws, and easier reduction of the short distal fragment. Furthermore, Auston et al. reported that a retrograde IM nail combined with long segment blocking screws significantly increased stability by eliminating the "Bell-Clapper effect" in patients with distal femur fracture who had low bone quality, such as the elderly [24]. However, the disadvantages of this surgical method include cartilage damage to the femoral condyle and postoperative knee pain. Several studies have compared the functional outcomes and knee pain incidence between antegrade and retrograde nailing; however, these are currently inconclusive with debatable findings [6,25,26].

This study had several limitations. First, this was a retrospective case–control study with a limited number of patients and different surgeons, which could have led to some bias. Second, we only mentioned radiographic risk factors; other risk factors, such as smoking, effects of reaming, the timing of weight-bearing, and NSAID usage, were not considered. Third, four types of antegrade IM nail systems were utilized for fixation, giving rise to potential implant bias. Therefore, larger clinical studies are required to tackle these limitations.

5. Conclusions

The perioperative radiographic predictors of non-union in infra-isthmal femoral shaft fractures after antegrade IM nailing were unstable fractures, shorter distal fragments, longer unfixed distal fragments, higher C/N ratio, and fewer distal locking screws. A ratio of the unfixed distal segment > 32.5% is a reliable parameter for predicting instability and non-union after surgery. We recommended the use of longer and larger nails with more distal locking screws when treating infra-isthmal femoral shaft fractures, especially those with an unstable pattern, wider IM canal, and shorter distal fragments.

Author Contributions: Conceptualization, T.-L.L. and C.-J.H.; methodology, C.-J.H. and A.K.; software, W.-C.H.; validation, W.-C.H.; formal analysis, W.-C.H. and H.-W.C.; investigation, W.-C.H. and H.-W.C.; resources, C.-J.H.; data curation, W.-C.H.; writing—original draft preparation, W.-C.H. and T.-L.L.; writing—review and editing, T.-L.L., H.-W.C., T.-L.L. and C.-H.T.; visualization, W.-C.H.; supervision, T.-L.L. and C.-J.H.; project administration, C.-J.H. All authors have read and agreed to the published version of the manuscript.

Funding: This research received no external funding.

Institutional Review Board Statement: The study was conducted according to the guidelines of the Declaration of Helsinki and approved by the local institutional review board of China Medical University & Hospital Research Ethics Committee (CMUH111-REC2-097).

Informed Consent Statement: Informed consent was obtained from all subjects involved in the study.

Data Availability Statement: All the available data have been presented in this study. Details regarding data supporting the reported results can be requested at the following e-mail address: jeffrey59835983@gmail.com.

Conflicts of Interest: The authors declare no conflict of interest.

References

1. Weiss, R.J.; Montgomery, S.M.; Al Dabbagh, Z.; Jansson, K.A. National Data of 6409 Swedish Inpatients with Femoral Shaft Fractures: Stable Incidence Between 1998 and 2004. *Injury* **2009**, *40*, 304–308. [CrossRef] [PubMed]
2. Agarwal-Harding, K.J.; Meara, J.G.; Greenberg, S.L.; Hagander, L.E.; Zurakowski, D.; Dyer, G.S. Estimating the Global Incidence of Femoral Fracture from Road Traffic Collisions: A Literature Review. *J. Bone Jt. Surg. Am.* **2015**, *97*, e31. [CrossRef] [PubMed]
3. Taitsman, L.A.; Lynch, J.R.; Agel, J.; Barei, D.P.; Nork, S.E. Risk Factors for Femoral Nonunion after Femoral Shaft Fracture. *J. Trauma* **2009**, *67*, 1389–1392. [CrossRef] [PubMed]
4. Pihlajamäki, H.K.; Salminen, S.T.; Böstman, O.M. The Treatment of Nonunions Following Intramedullary Nailing of Femoral Shaft Fractures. *J. Orthop. Trauma* **2002**, *16*, 394–402. [CrossRef] [PubMed]
5. Canadian Orthopaedic Trauma Society. Nonunion Following Intramedullary Nailing of the Femur with and without Reaming. Results of a Multicenter Randomized Clinical Trial. *J. Bone Jt. Surg. Am.* **2003**, *85*, 2093–2096. [CrossRef]
6. Ricci, W.M.; Bellabarba, C.; Evanoff, B.; Herscovici, D.; DiPasquale, T.; Sanders, R. Retrograde Versus Antegrade Nailing of Femoral Shaft Fractures. *J. Orthop. Trauma* **2001**, *15*, 161–169. [CrossRef]
7. Selvakumar, K.; Saw, K.Y.; Fathima, M. Comparison Study Between Reamed and Unreamed Nailing of Closed Femoral Fractures. *Med. J. Malaysia* **2001**, *56*, 24–28.
8. Park, J.; Kim, S.G.; Yoon, H.K.; Yang, K.H. The Treatment of Nonisthmal Femoral Shaft Nonunions with IM Nail Exchange Versus Augmentation Plating. *J. Orthop. Trauma* **2010**, *24*, 89–94. [CrossRef]
9. Song, S.H. Radiologic Outcomes of Intramedullary Nailing in Infraisthmal Femur-Shaft Fracture with or without Poller Screws. *Biomed. Res. Int.* **2019**, *2019*, 9412379. [CrossRef]
10. Kim, J.W.; Yoon, Y.C.; Oh, C.W.; Han, S.B.; Sim, J.A.; Oh, J.K. Exchange Nailing with Enhanced Distal Fixation is Effective for the Treatment of Infraisthmal Femoral Nonunions. *Arch. Orthop. Trauma Surg.* **2018**, *138*, 27–34. [CrossRef]
11. Yang, T.C.; Tzeng, Y.H.; Wang, C.S.; Lin, C.C.; Chang, M.C.; Chiang, C.C. "Ratio of fracture site diameter to isthmus femoral canal diameter" as a predictor of complication following treatment of infra-isthmal femoral shaft fracture with antegrade intramedullary nailing. *Injury* **2021**, *52*, 961–966. [CrossRef] [PubMed]
12. Watanabe, Y.; Takenaka, N.; Kobayashi, M.; Matsushita, T. Infra-isthmal Fracture is a Risk Factor for Nonunion After Femoral Nailing: A Case-Control Study. *J. Orthop. Sci.* **2013**, *18*, 76–80. [CrossRef] [PubMed]
13. Yang, K.H.; Kim, J.R.; Park, J. Nonisthmal Femoral Shaft Nonunion as a Risk Factor for Exchange Nailing Failure. *J. Trauma Acute Care Surg.* **2012**, *72*, E60–E64. [CrossRef] [PubMed]
14. Frölke, J.P.; Patka, P. Definition and Classification of Fracture Non-unions. *Injury* **2007**, *38*, S19–S22. [CrossRef]
15. Weber, B.G.; Brunner, C. The Treatment of Nonunions without Electrical Stimulation. *Clin. Orthop. Relat. Res.* **1981**, *161*, 24–32. [CrossRef]
16. Fracture and Dislocation Compendium. Orthopaedic Trauma Association Committee for Coding and Classification. *J. Orthop. Trauma* **1996**, *10* (Suppl. 1: V-ix), 1–154.
17. Nicholson, J.A.; Makaram, N.; Simpson, A.; Keating, J.F. Fracture Nonunion in Long Bones: A Literature Review of Risk Factors and Surgical Management. *Injury* **2021**, *52*, S3–S11. [CrossRef]
18. Zura, R.; Mehta, S.; Della Rocca, G.J.; Steen, R.G. Biological Risk Factors for Nonunion of Bone Fracture. *JBJS Rev.* **2016**, *4*, e5. [CrossRef]
19. Reis, N.D.; Hirschberg, E. The Infra-isthmic Fracture of the Shaft of the Femur. *Injury* **1977**, *9*, 8–16. [CrossRef]
20. Ha, S.S.; Oh, C.W.; Jung, J.W.; Kim, J.W.; Park, K.H.; Kim, S.M. Exchange Nailing for Aseptic Nonunion of the Femoral Shaft after Intramedullary Nailing. *J. Trauma Inj.* **2020**, *33*, 104–111. [CrossRef]
21. Zhang, X.; Zhong, B.; Sui, S.; Yu, X.; Jiang, Y. Treatment of Distal Femoral Nonunion and Delayed Union by Using a Retrograde Intramedullary Interlocking Nail. *Chin. J. Traumatol.* **2001**, *4*, 180–184. [PubMed]
22. Van Dyke, B.; Colley, R.; Ottomeyer, C.; Palmer, R.; Pugh, K. Effect of Blocking Screws on Union of Infraisthmal Femur Fractures Stabilized With a Retrograde Intramedullary Nail. *J. Orthop. Trauma* **2018**, *32*, 251–255. [CrossRef] [PubMed]
23. Brinker, M.R.; O'Connor, D.P. Exchange Nailing of Ununited Fractures. *J. Bone Jt. Surg Am.* **2007**, *89*, 177–188. [CrossRef]

24. Auston, D.; Donohue, D.; Stoops, K.; Cox, J.; Diaz, M.; Santoni, B.; Mir, H. Long Segment Blocking Screws Increase the Stability of Retrograde Nail Fixation in Geriatric Supracondylar Femur Fractures: Eliminating the "Bell-Clapper Effect". *J. Orthop. Trauma* **2018**, *32*, 559–564. [CrossRef] [PubMed]
25. Yu, C.K.; Singh, V.A.; Mariapan, S.; Chong, S.T. Antegrade Versus Retrograde Locked Intramedullary Nailing for Femoral Fractures: Which Is Better? *Eur. J. Trauma Emerg. Surg.* **2007**, *33*, 135–140. [CrossRef] [PubMed]
26. Tornetta, P.; Tiburzi, D. Antegrade or Retrograde Reamed Femoral Nailing. A Prospective, Randomised Trial. *J. Bone Jt. Surg. Br.* **2000**, *82*, 652–654. [CrossRef]

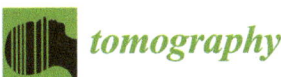

Case Report

Direct Visualization of Cervical Interlaminar Epidural Injections Using Sonography

Nana Maeda [1], Manabu Maeda [1,*] and Yasuhito Tanaka [2]

1. Maeda Orthopaedic Clinic, 864-1 Kidera-cho, Nara 630-8306, Japan; nana-k@mvd.biglobe.ne.jp
2. Department of Orthopedics, Nara Medical University, 840 Shijo-cho Kashihara, Nara 634-8521, Japan; yatanaka@naramed-u.ac.jp
* Correspondence: mmaeda@ktj.biglobe.ne.jp

Abstract: In this case series, we describe a novel ultrasound (US)-guided cervical interlaminar epidural steroid injections (CILESIs) procedure that does not depend on the loss-of-resistance method for epidural space identification. A needle is introduced into three US-identified structures (triple bar sign), the interspinal ligament, ligamentum flavum, and dura mater. The injectants are monitored using superb microvascular imaging during injection. Here, we demonstrate the use of US-guided CILESIs in nine cases and propose the use of sonography, rather than conventional methods, for easier and safer cervical epidural injections. Sonography for direct visualization of cervical epidural injection may allow for outpatient injections.

Keywords: ultrasound; epidural injection; cervical; steroid; superb microvascular imaging

1. Introduction

A major concern for cervical epidural injection (CEDI) in patients with neck pain and cervical radiculopathy is the safety and effectiveness of the procedure. Reports of serious complications such as spinal cord injury have led to concerns regarding this procedure's safety [1–3]. Fluoroscopy or computed tomography (CT) guidance aims to reduce the risks of epidural injection, such as dural puncture or spinal cord injury. However, although both guidance approaches improve safety, they cannot completely aid in advancing the tip of the needle into the epidural space, as these approaches cannot visualize the entire intrusion route [2–5].

It is also important to examine the placement of the needle tip and the spread of the injectant to ensure its effectiveness [6]. The loss-of-resistance (LOR) method is performed for blinded or fluoroscopic epidural injections. However, it is limited by false-positive LOR before the needle enters the epidural space [7,8]. CT guidance uses high radiation exposure to carefully check the needle tip position, which also poses a problem [9]. However, CT cannot image the epidural space without a contrast medium, which can cause adverse effects [10]. Furthermore, CT emits ionizing radiation, which can cause cancer [11].

Sonography offers an alternative method for performing cervical interlaminar epidural steroid injections (CILESIs). It could help reduce the risk of injury, avoid the pitfall of false-positive LOR, and avoid radiation exposure or the use of contrast media by allowing direct visualization of the location of the needle tip during the procedure with cross-sectional imaging [6].

However, the technique for ultrasound (US)-guided CILESIs has not been reported, and no case series has described the safety of this technique in cervical lesions. Herein, we report cases of US-guided CILESIs without fluoroscopy.

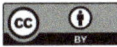

2. Materials and Methods

2.1. Patients

This study was performed at the Maeda Orthopedic Clinic and was approved by its institutional review board (Commission of Ethics approval number 00000003).

Patients provided written informed consent for the cervical epidural block and the publication of this report. Overall, nine patients presented to the Maeda Orthopedic Clinic between August 2021 and January 2022. All patients underwent US-guided CEDI for the treatment of neck pain or interscapular radicular pain due to cervical disc herniation, cervical discopathy, cervical canal stenosis, or thoracic disc herniation.

2.2. US-Guided CEDI

This novel US-guided CILESIs was performed as follows. First, the axial image of the interspinal ligament, ligamentum flavum, and dura mater as a triple bar sign was identified using a posterolateral with transverse scan approach by a PVI-475BX convex probe (Aplio i800 systems; Canon Medical System, Tochigi, Japan) (Figure 1). To optimize this image, the patient was placed in the prone position, and a pillow was placed under their chest. The patient was then asked to place their forehead on the bed and flex their neck to the maximum extent possible (Figure 2). For needle placement, the tip of the needle was advanced into the ligamentum flavum, tangential to the dura mater, under US guidance using an in-plane technique (Figure 1, Video S1). At first, while inserting and removing the needle, the needle was translocated from the caudal (or cranial) side to the correct plane where the triple bar sign is seen clearly (Figure 3A; view from the side of the body). The needle direction should be corrected if needed. Red arrows indicate an inappropriate needle direction, with an extension line (indicated by dashed arrows) facing the spinal cord or the interspinal ligament. The needle trajectory should be corrected from those indicated by the red arrows to that indicated by the blue arrow (Figure 3B; view from the caudal side of the body). As no critical arteries or nerves are passed using this approach, the needle orbit correction can be repeated just before the needle tip reaches the ligamentum flavum. As a result, accurate needle placement is possible.

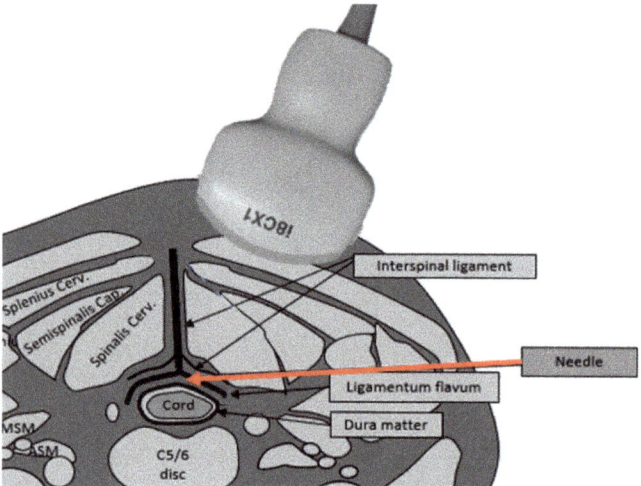

Figure 1. The illustration shows the needle insertion route on the cross-sectional image of the neck. The main structures are the cord, dura mater, interspinous ligament, and ligamentum flavum. The epidural space exists between the dura mater and the ligamentum flavum. The needle (red arrow) is introduced tangentially in between the ligamentum flavum and dura matter.

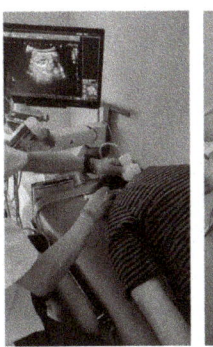 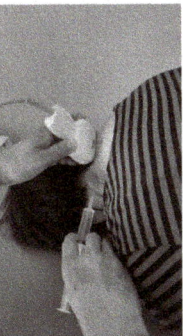

Figure 2. The patient is placed in the prone position, and the pillow is placed under the patient's chest. Then, the patient is asked to place their forehead on the bed and flex their neck to the maximum extent possible.

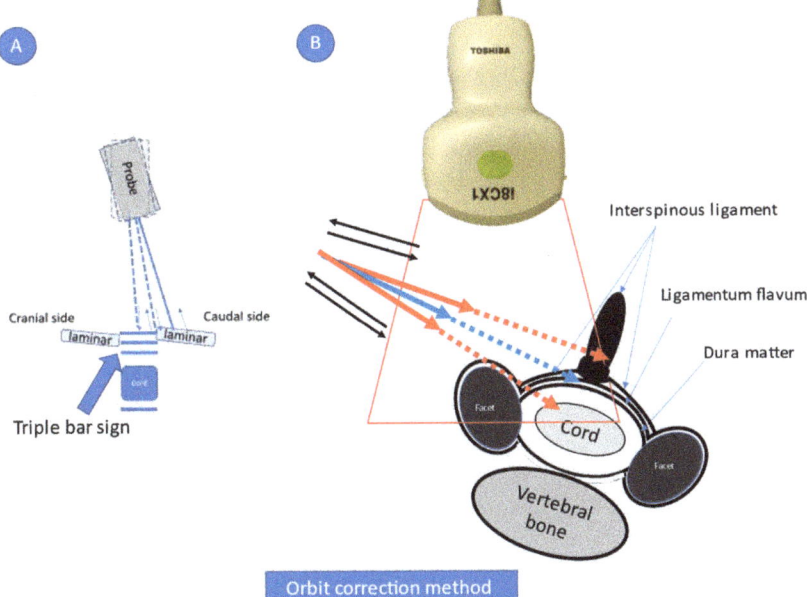

Figure 3. Orbit correction method.

Video S1. The needle tip is advanced tangentially between the ligamentum flavum and dura matter under ultrasonography (US) guidance. This can be confirmed by the resistance of the needle tip when reaching the complex of the ligamentum flavum felt by the practitioner's hand when checking the US monitor.

While being inserted and removed, the needle is translocated from the caudal (or cranial) side to the correct plane where a triple bar sign is seen clearly (Figure 3A). Next, the needle direction is corrected. Red arrows indicate inappropriate needle directions, with extension lines (indicated by dashed arrows) facing the spinal cord or interspinal ligament. The needle orbit should be corrected from the red to the blue trajectory (Figure 3B, view from the caudal side of the body).

Using a posterolateral approach, the needle is visible from the insertion point to the epidural space between the ligamentum flavum and dura matter. At first, while being inserted and removed (indicated by blue arrows in the figure), the needle is translocated from the caudal (or cranial) side to the correct plane where a triple bar sign (which is composed of the interspinal ligament, ligamentum flavum, and dura matter) is seen clearly (Figure 3A; view from the side of the body). Next, the needle direction is corrected. Red arrows indicate inappropriate needle directions, with extension lines (indicated by dashed arrows) facing the spinal cord or interspinal ligament. The needle orbit should be corrected from the red to the blue trajectory (Figure 3B; view from the caudal side of the body). Because there are no critical arteries and nerves through this approach, the needle orbit correction can be repeated just before the needle tip reaches the ligamentum flavum. As a result, accurate injection is possible.

Confirmation that the needle tip had reached the ligamentum flavum was achieved based on resistance according to the pressure felt by the operator whilst observing the US monitor. We then applied gentle pressure to the syringe plunger as the needle was slowly advanced into the space between the ligamentum flavum and dura mater reaching approximately two-thirds of the triple bar sign, where easy flow of the injectant was facilitated (Figure 4, Video S2). If the needle tip was located more superficially than the ligamentum flavum, any attempt to inject the injectant would be evident in the surrounding muscle tissue or the pseudo-epidural space, such as the space of Okada (Figure 5, Video S3).

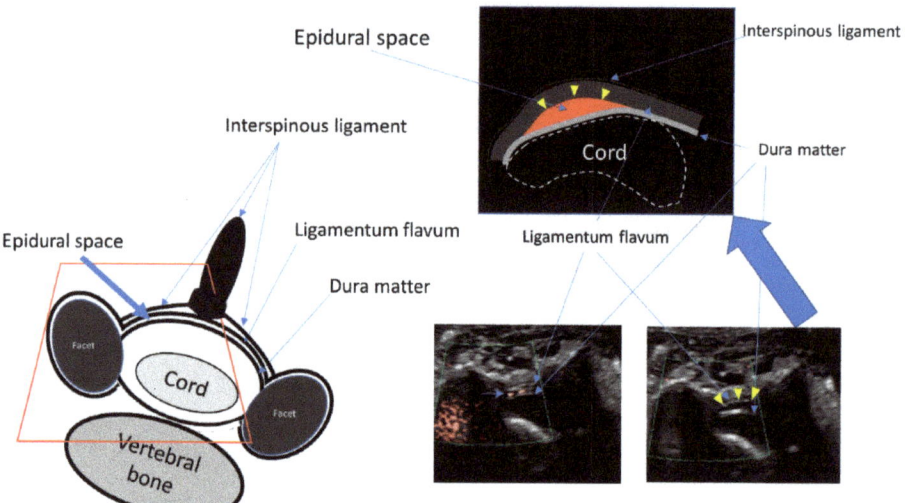

Figure 4. The illustration shows the cross section of the spinal canal. The main structures are the cord, the dura mater, the interspinous ligament, and the ligamentum flavum. The epidural space exists between the dura mater and the ligamentum flavum. The space of Okada exists between the interspinous ligament and the ligamentum flavum. Ultrasound data show the superb microvascular imaging signal during injection (left picture) and the enlargement of the epidural space after injection (upper illustration and right picture).

Video S2. The needle is gradually advanced while applying pressure to the plunger. If the needle tip is located more superficially than the epidural space, microvascular imaging (SMI) shows that there is no flow of injectant into it. However, once the dense fibrous ligamentum flavum is pierced, the injectant flows. This is immediately confirmed using SMI. Subsequently, the epidural space is gradually enlarged by epidural injection.

Once the dense fibrous ligamentum flavum was pierced, the injectant was able to flow into the epidural space; this was immediately confirmed using superb microvascular imaging (SMI) (Figure 4, Video S2). Lastly, the practitioner verified the epidural space enlargement using the epidural injection. We used 4 mg of dexamethasone in 6 mL of 0.25% lidocaine for CEDI.

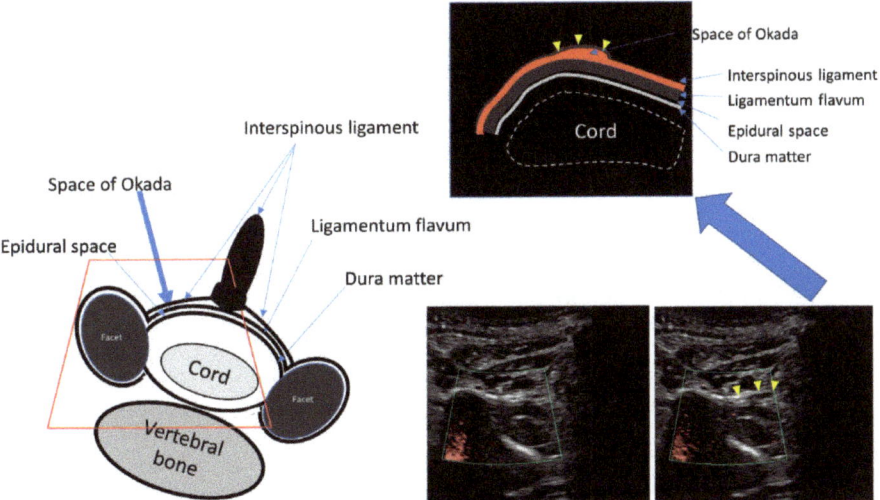

Figure 5. The pseudo-epidural space is enlarged by a small dose of injection. The space between the interspinous ligament and ligamentum flavum, such as the space of Okada, is observed sonographically. If the needle tip is located more superficially than the ligamentum flavum, the injectant will appear in the space of Okada or in the spinalis cervicalis muscle once administered.

2.3. CT Epidurography

To confirm the accuracy of US-guided CEDI, we chose one patient (case 4) and two other patients (a 78-year-old male patient with cervical canal stenosis (Supplementary Materials S1) and a 58-year-old female patient with cervical disc herniation (Supplementary Materials S2) who were not included in this case series because they could not be followed up for >2 months). We performed US-guided CEDI at the C4/5 level. We used a contrast medium instead of dexamethasone (3.5 mL iohexol-240 [Omnipaque-240; GE Healthcare Pharma, Tokyo, Japan]) in 3.5 mL of 0.25% lidocaine. Immediately after injection of the contrast medium, anterior–posterior and lateral epidurograms of the cervical spine were captured. Subsequently, the patients were placed in the prone position within the gantry of the CT scanner (Aquilion Start Canon medical system, Tochigi, Japan) and CT was performed from C1 to L1 5 min after injection. The two orthopedic surgeons and the author have 32, 38, and 24 years of experience, respectively. Technical success was determined by reviewing CT epidurograms for the presence of epidural contrast. The spread of contrast within the epidural space was also assessed on CT epidurograms.

2.4. Pain Intensity

Pain intensity was evaluated using the visual analog scale (VAS). All patients were instructed on how to use the VAS prior to the cervical epidural block (0, no pain; 10, worst pain conceivable). Before the procedure, an interventional orthopedic doctor questioned the patients regarding their baseline VAS scores for pain. The patients were discharged on the day of the procedure and asked to revisit 1 week and 2 months later for evaluation of side effects and pain scores, respectively. If the pain persisted, we treated patients with an additional block and rechecked their pain scores.

2.5. Functional Ability

Functional ability was evaluated using the neck disability index (NDI). The NDI is a 10-item self-administered disease-specific questionnaire that evaluates the impact of neck pain on a patient's daily life and the corresponding disability. The questionnaire scores range from 0 to 50; the higher the score, the greater the disability. The validity and reliability of this scale have been previously established [12].

Symptom improvement was assessed before and 2 months after the injection using the VAS and the Japanese version of the NDI. Any potential complications, including headache, increased neck pain, or stiffness, were monitored. Moreover, functional ability was rechecked in patients treated with an additional block.

Patients were asked about their opioid consumption, any additional cervical spine injections, and progression to surgery during the follow up period, and the answers were documented in their profile.

3. Results

During the study period, nine participants with radicular pain underwent US-guided CEDI. The radicular pain in one, two, three, and three patients was caused by thoracic disc herniation, cervical disc herniation, cervical discopathy, and cervical canal stenosis, respectively. These patients were followed up from 60 to 348 days after the procedure. Their baseline data are presented in Table 1. The baseline and demographic characteristics of the patients were recorded, and the mean age of patients was 51.2 years (range, 23–74 years). Six participants were men and three were women. The mean body mass index was 24.2 km/m^2 (range, 19.3–31.2 km/m^2). At the 2-month follow-up, there were significant reductions in NDI from 44.4 to 15.6 points in Table 2. The mean VAS score of neck pain was 8.3 at before the procedure and 1.8 at the 2-month follow-up in Table 2. Among those who reported having recurrent pain (four patients), no patient used opioids for analgesia, four patients reported receiving additional injections, and no patient underwent surgery. During the follow-up period, one patient was able to discontinue opioids.

Table 1. Clinical and demographic characteristics.

Case	Age (years)	Sex	Body Mass Index (kg/m^2)	Diagnosis
1	24	M	24	Th1/2 Disc herniation
2	45	M	31.2	C2/3, 5/6, 6/7 Disc herniation
3	51	M	20.9	Cervical discopathy
4	73	F	19.3	Cervical canal stenosis
5	73	M	24.7	Cervical canal stenosis
6	63	F	28.8	C5/6 Disc herniation
7	74	F	21.4	Cervical canal stenosis
8	35	M	26.2	Cervical discopathy
9	23	M	21	Cervical discopathy

Table 2. Pain intensity and functional ability before and after ultrasound-guided epidural injection.

Case	Injection Site	Pre Visual Analog Scale Scores	Post Visual Analog Scale Scores	Neck Disability Index	Additional Injection (Times)	Additional Opioid Consumption (Times)
1	C6/7	10	2.5	40%→4%	0	0
2	C5/6	10	5	70%→26%	0	0
3	C5/6	4	2	16%→20%	0	0
4	C4/5	10	2	94%→34%	20	0
5	C5/6	5.9	0	8%→2%	0	0
6	C4/5	9	0	48%→10%	0	0
7	C3/4	10	5	54%→28%	4	0
8	C6/7	9	0	28%→4%	4	0
9	C5/6	6.5	0	42%→12%	2	0

Vascular or subdural injections were not confirmed in any of the patients during the procedure. Furthermore, we did not encounter any significant complications, including stroke or persistent neurological deficits, during the procedure or 2-month follow-up. Nausea and general fatigue were observed after epidurography using a contrast media (case 4); however, the symptoms resolved within a day.

CT epidurograms revealed that the procedure was technically successful in all three patients from whom they were obtained, including case 4. The spread of contrast was confirmed from the C2 vertebra level to the Th5 vertebra level according to the axial CT epidurogram.

SMI was performed with a small injection. An appropriate epidural space was detected using SMI after the needle was advanced. The epidural space was then enlarged by means of an additional injection directed to the area where the SMI signal was detected (Figure 4, Video S3).

Video S3. The retrodural space of Okada is gradually enlarged by epidural injection. This lesion is not a true space in the epidural space. The loss-of-resistance method cannot differentiate between the space of Okada and the epidural space.

3.1. Representative Cases

3.1.1. Case 4

A 73-year-old woman presented with severe posterior cervical pain and right shoulder pain. The pain did not resolve with the use of medications (an opioid, an anti-inflammatory analgesic, and a muscle relaxant). Magnetic resonance imaging revealed cervical canal stenosis. Her pain persisted for 3 weeks; therefore, US-guided C3/4 interlaminar CEDI of 1 mL dexamethasone (4 mg) and 6 mL 0.25% lidocaine was administered. In the examination room, SMI was used to confirm that the parenteral solution had spread throughout the epidural space. Subsequently, the VAS score decreased from 10 to 5. An additional four blocks were performed for 2 months, and the VAS decreased from 5 to 2.

After 2 months, she experienced exacerbations and remission of symptoms. She received US-guided epidural blocks 20 times in total. We confirmed the 20th US-guided injection using CT epidurography (Figure 6).

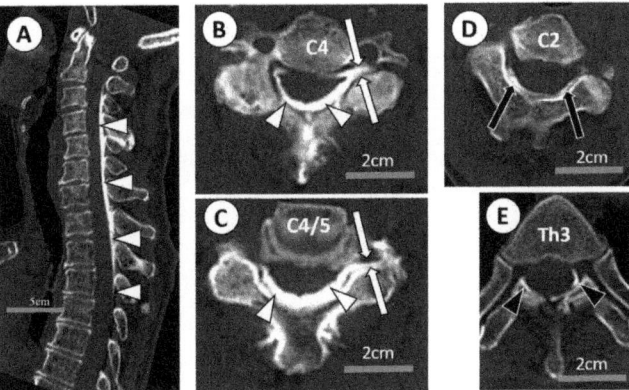

Figure 6. CT epidurogram after C4/5 US-guided epidural injection administered to a 73-year-old female with severe posterior cervical pain and right shoulder pain (case 4) associated with cervical canal stenosis. (**A**) Sagittal view of CT epidurogram. Dorsal spread (white arrow heads) between C2 and Th3 are confirmed. (**B,C**) Axial view of CT epidurogram (a slice of C4 vertebra and C4/5 disc; injection site). Dorsal spread (white arrow heads) and C5 root filling (white arrows) were confirmed. (**D,E**) Axial view of CT epidurogram at C2 and Th3 vertebra). Cephalad spread (black arrows) was confirmed up to C2 vertebra level and caudal spread (black arrow heads) was confirmed down to Th3 vertebra level.

3.1.2. Case 5

A 73-year-old man presented with severe pain in his right shoulder and arm. Radiographs revealed that the patient had severe cervical spondylosis. Considering that severe night pain and insomnia had persisted for 2 weeks, US-guided C5/6 interlaminar CEDI of 1 mL dexamethasone (4 mg) and 6 mL 0.25% lidocaine was administered. Subsequently, the VAS score decreased from 10 to 1. No additional blocks were administered. No recurrence of pain was observed at the 8-month follow-up.

3.1.3. Case 9

A 23-year-old man presented with severe pain in his right neck and interscapular region. The pain persisted despite diagnostic facet joint blocks (right Th5/6, right C3/4, and right C4/5 facet blocks). Magnetic resonance imaging revealed no vertebral bone injury; however, damage to the C3/4 and C4/5 discs was observed. The pain persisted for 3 months; therefore, US-guided C5/6 interlaminar CEDI of 1 mL dexamethasone (4 mg) and 6 mL 0.25% lidocaine was administered. In the examination room, SMI was used to confirm that the parenteral solution had spread throughout the epidural space. Subsequently, the VAS score decreased from 10 to 1. Two additional blocks were administered over 7 weeks, leading to the resolution of his pain. No recurrence of pain was observed at the 3-month follow-up.

4. Discussion

Reports of serious complications such as spinal cord injury have led to concerns regarding the safety of CEDI [1–3]. Epidural injections can be performed with or without a guide (blinded injection). Fluoroscopy or CT guidance aims to reduce the risks of epidural injection, such as dural puncture or spinal cord injury [13–16].

In the interlaminar approach, a guide is used to advance the needle tip just before the epidural space [13].

CT guidance in interlaminar ESI improves the evaluation of the proper positioning of the needle owing to its high resolution and cross-sectional imaging [13]. However, the introduction of the needle into the epidural space cannot be visualized according to the movement of the needle during the procedure. US, as an alternative method for performing CILESI, could help reduce the risk of injury by allowing direct visualization of the location of the needle tip during the procedure with cross-sectional imaging. However, a technique for US-guided CILESI has not been reported, and no case series have described its safety because US has some limitations in neuraxial (epidural or intrathecal) procedures as it has a limited resolution at deep levels and near bony surfaces that affect image quality, and it is not possible to visualize the real-time propagation of the injectable in the epidural or intrathecal space [17].

CEDI is based on the LOR method [2,7]. The epidural space is closed by negative pressure unless there is an abscess or bleeding. It is approximately 1–2 mm in diameter at levels above C6-C7 and is less dependent on individual variation, including the presence of spinal stenosis [14,15]. Thus, the safety zone for interlaminar CEDI is very narrow [16]. In reviews of malpractice claims between 2005 and 2008, 64 cases involved cervical interventions, 20 of which resulted in direct spinal cord injury associated with interlaminar CEDI [5,9].

The needle tip position must be visualized throughout the procedure to ensure accurate injection into the epidural space. Clinical practice guidelines recommend fluoroscopic guidance in all CEDIs [18]. However, fluoroscopic guidance methods are limited because they use bones as landmarks. Therefore, it is difficult to guide the needle tip into the gap of the ligamentum flavum and dura mater safely, as it is approximately 1 mm thick and permeable to X-rays, without direct visualization.

For the accurate insertion of the needle, the US monitor, the affected area, and the practitioner should be in a straight line. However, this is not always possible during outpatient examinations because the size of the examination room is limited. Furthermore, since the needle is inserted deeply, needle orbit correction is often needed. As there are no critical arteries or nerves beyond the ligamentum flavum through this approach, the needle orbit correction can be repeated just before the needle tip reaches the ligamentum flavum. As a result, accurate injection is possible with our US guided method.

The LOR technique relies on penetration of the ligamentum flavum. However, up to 74% of the ligamenta flava are discontinuous in the midline of the cervical region [19]. Dural puncture cannot be prevented based on bony landmarks or the LOR technique because the needle is inserted near the midline under conventional method. Furthermore, the safety of the CEDI procedure is highly dependent on the operator's experience. In contrast, US can easily identify the ligamentum flavum, dura mater, and the needle tip independent of the operator's experience.

If the needle is advanced deeply, dural puncture or spinal injury can be avoided because the needle is tangentially advanced with respect to the dura. Even in cases of inappropriate injection, the practitioner could use the US image to confirm and terminate the inappropriate injection from the beginning, if necessary. Therefore, serious complications, such as total spine anesthesia or spinal injury, could be avoided. The direction of the needle has two advantages. The first is improved needle visibility by bringing the needle closer to the probe in parallel. The second is the avoidance of dural puncture and spinal cord injury.

Unlike US guidance, fluoroscopy and CT guidance (Figure 7) cannot accurately visualize the needle tip position. Fluoroscopy-guided CEDI can only confirm whether the LOR method is performed correctly based on contrast, identifying the epidural space after the trial of LOR. Additionally, CT-guided CEDI cannot show needle movement in real-time as the procedure progresses. The placement of the needle tip is only confirmed after needle insertion. SMI methods have been used to identify slow blood flow in the body. Unlike CT and fluoroscopy, SMI helps visualize not only microvessels with slow blood flow but also the movement of liquid (injectant) flow without contrast injection [20], and it can be a useful tool to confirm if the needle tip is in proper anatomical position e.g., the epidural space. Under SMI, the spread of the injectant can be visualized using US while simultaneously confirming the proper placement of the tip of the needle between the ligamentum flavum and dura matter (Figure 3) [6]. The major difference is that it offers real-time, radiation-free guidance for interventions.

The LOR method can also be used to precisely detect the epidural space using SMI signals. However, the LOR method is associated with false-positive LOR before the needle enters the epidural space. False-positive LOR occurs in 29.4% of patients who undergo CEDI under conventional fluoroscopic guidance [7]. The retrodural space of Okada is a potential space dorsal to the ligamentum flavum that allows communication between the bilateral facet joints and interspinous bursa [8,21,22]. In the current study, the space of Okada on the ligamentum flavum was visible using US (Figure 5, Video S3).

US guidance allows better positional relationships between the needle tip and anatomical structures (e.g., lamina, space of Okada, and epidural space) in cross-sectional imaging such as CT guidance. A previous investigation examining conventional fluoroscopy-guided lumbar interlaminar ESI demonstrated that many non-target injections in the retrodural space of Okada are likely to go unnoticed at the time of the procedure [21]. This may be because conventional fluoroscopy contrast material in the retrodural space of Okada can mimic true dorsal epidural spread as these two spaces run parallel to each other and may therefore overlap in standard lateral and anteroposterior projections [21,22]. Our US data also revealed that the space is too close to be identified by fluoroscopy. This suggested that inappropriate injection by LOR could be avoided using US.

Riveros-Perez et al. introduced color Doppler imaging to confirm the correct position of the epidural needle in the lumbar spine [23]. However, this method has not been applied to CEDI [17]. For cervical epidural injection, Zhang et al. reported transforaminal epidural steroid injections using sonography [24]. However, they did not employ color Doppler imaging to confirm the correct position of the needle and neither did they visualize the spinal cord, its nutrient vessels, or the radicular artery during the procedure. Serious complications such as spinal cord injury, either directly or indirectly via injury of its nutrient vessels, have been reported in transforaminal epidural steroid injections [1–3]. We visualized the spinal cord and surrounding vessels during the interlaminar epidural injection using the SMI method. To the best of our knowledge, our study is the first to achieve direct visualization of not only the entry route of the needle but also of the spinal cord and surrounding vessels during the CILESIs procedure.

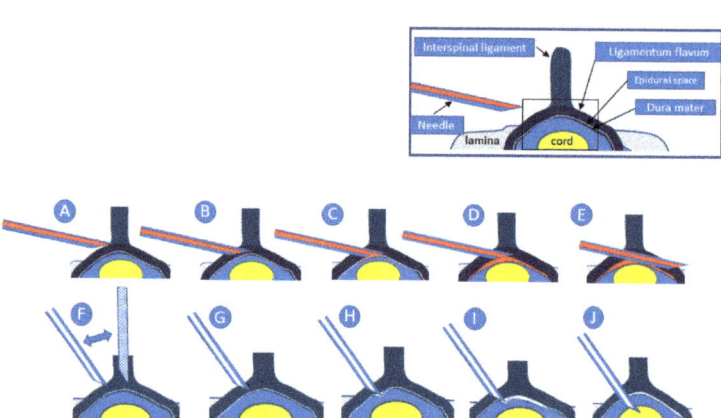

Figure 7. Upper figures show our cervical epidural injection (CEDI) method in which the needle is inserted tangentially into the dura (**A–E**). Lower figures show the conventional CEDI method wherein the needle is inserted nearly perpendicular to the dura (**F–J**). In both methods, loss of resistance may be confirmed before and after the insertion into the flavum (**A,C,F,H**). The closer the needle is inserted vertically, the higher the risk of dural puncture because the safety margin between the flavum and the dura becomes narrower (**G,H**). The risk of dural puncture can be avoided if the needle is inserted tangentially into the dura (**C,D**). In the conventional method (**J**), when the needle is advanced deeply, dural puncture cannot be avoided. Meanwhile, in our method, dural puncture can be avoided because the needle penetrates tangentially to the dura (**E**). The flow of the injectant into the epidural space is visualized in real-time under ultrasound-guided epidural injection (**C**).

5. Conclusions

In conclusion, we propose the possible use of US for easier and safer CILESIs compared with conventional methods. US for the direct visualization of CILESIs may allow for safer outpatient injections.

Supplementary Materials: The following are available online at https://www.mdpi.com/article/10.3390/tomography8040157/s1, Figure S1: a 78-year-old male patient with cervical canal stenosis, Figure S2: a 58-year-old female patient with cervical disc herniation, Video S1: Approach of US guided cervical epidural injection, Video S2: Enlargement of the space of OKADA, Video S3: Spread of the epidural space during epidural injection.

Author Contributions: Conceptualization, M.M. and N.M.; methodology, N.M.; investigation, M.M.; resources, M.M.; data curation, M.M.; writing—original draft preparation, N.M.; writing—review and editing, Y.T.; visualization, M.M.; supervision, Y.T. All authors have read and agreed to the published version of the manuscript.

Funding: This research received no external funding.

Institutional Review Board Statement: This study was performed at the Maeda Orthopedic Clinic and was approved by its institutional review board (Commission of Ethics), 00000003.

Informed Consent Statement: The patients provided written informed consent for a cervical epidural block and the publication of this report.

Data Availability Statement: The data that supports the findings of this study are available in the supplementary material of this article.

Acknowledgments: The authors appreciate Ichiro Higashiyama for correcting data of CT-epidurography.

Conflicts of Interest: The authors declare no conflict of interest.

References

1. Stout, A. Epidural Steroid Injections for Cervical Radiculopathy. *Phys. Med. Rehabil. Clin. N. Am.* **2011**, *22*, 149–159. [CrossRef] [PubMed]
2. Abbasi, A.; Malhotra, G.; Malanga, G.; Elovic, E.P.; Kahn, S. Complications of interlaminar cervical epidural steroid injections: A review of the literature. *Spine* **2007**, *32*, 2144–2151. [CrossRef] [PubMed]
3. Huston, C.W. Cervical epidural steroid injections in the management of cervical radiculitis: Interlaminar versus transforaminal. A review. *Curr. Rev. Musculoskelet. Med.* **2009**, *2*, 30–42. [CrossRef] [PubMed]
4. Provenzano, D.A.; Fanciullo, G. Cervical transforaminal epidural steroid injections: Should we be performing them? *Reg. Anesth. Pain Med.* **2007**, *32*, 168, author reply 169–170. [CrossRef]
5. Kim, J.; Kim, K.; Lee, M.; Kim, S. Correlation Between Intravascular Injection Rate, Pain Intensity, and Degree of Cervical Neural Foraminal Stenosis During a Cervical Transforaminal Epidural Block. *J. Pain Res.* **2021**, *14*, 3017–3023. [CrossRef]
6. Maeda, M.; Maeda, N.; Masuda, K.; Nagano, T.; Tanaka, Y. Ultrasound-Guided Cervical Intervertebral Disc Injection without Fluoroscopy. *J. Ultrasound Med.* **2022**, in press. [CrossRef]
7. Kim, Y.U.; Kim, D.; Park, J.Y.; Choi, J.-H.; Kim, J.H.; Bae, H.-Y.; Joo, E.-Y.; Suh, J.H. Method to Reduce the False-Positive Rate of Loss of Resistance in the Cervical Epidural Region. *Pain Res. Manag.* **2016**, *2016*, 9894054. [CrossRef]
8. Okada, K. Studies on the cervical facet joints using arthrography of the cervical facet joint. *Nihon Seikeigeka Gakkai Zasshi* **1981**, *55*, 563–580. (In Japanese)
9. Lustig, J.P.; Aubry, S.; Vidal, C.; Pazart, L.; Moreau-Gaudry, A.; Bricault, I. Body interventional procedures: Which is the best method for CT guidance? *Eur. Radiol.* **2020**, *30*, 1593–1600. [CrossRef]
10. Ha, S.O.; Kim, D.Y.; Sohn, Y.D. Clinical characteristics of adverse reactions to nonionic low osmolality contrast media in patients transferred from the CT room to the emergency room. *SpringerPlus* **2016**, *5*, 929. [CrossRef]
11. Wylie, J.D.; Jenkins, P.A.; Beckmann, J.T.; Peters, C.L.; Aoki, S.K.; Maak, T.G. Computed Tomography Scans in Patients with Young Adult Hip Pain Carry a Lifetime Risk of Malignancy. *Arthrosc. J. Arthrosc. Relat. Surg.* **2018**, *34*, 155–163.e3. [CrossRef] [PubMed]
12. Takeshita, K.; Oshima, Y.; Ono, T.; Kato, S.; Hosono, N.; Kawaguchi, Y.; Hasegawa, K.; Isomura, T.; Oshina, M.; Oda, T.; et al. Validity, reliability and responsiveness of the Japanese version of the Neck Disability Index. *J. Orthop. Sci.* **2013**, *18*, 14–21. [CrossRef]
13. Kranz, P.; Raduazo, P.; Gray, L.; Kilani, R.; Hoang, J. CT Fluoroscopy-Guided Cervical Interlaminar Steroid Injections: Safety, Technique, and Radiation Dose Parameters. *Am. J. Neuroradiol.* **2012**, *33*, 1221–1224. [CrossRef] [PubMed]
14. Amrhein, T.J.; Parivash, S.N.; Gray, L.; Kranz, P.G. Incidence of Inadvertent Dural Puncture During CT Fluoroscopy–Guided Interlaminar Epidural Corticosteroid Injections in the Cervical Spine: An Analysis of 974 Cases. *Am. J. Roentgenol.* **2017**, *209*, 656–661. [CrossRef] [PubMed]
15. Hogan, Q.H. Epidural anatomy examined by cryomicrotome section. Influence of age, vertebral level, and disease. *Reg. Anesth. J. Neural Blockade Obstet. Surg. Pain Control.* **1996**, *21*, 395–406.
16. House, L.M.; Barrette, K.; Mattie, R.; McCormick, Z.L. Cervical epidural steroid injection: Techniques and evidence. *Phys. Med. Rehabil. Clin.* **2018**, *29*, 1–17. [CrossRef]
17. Moreno, B.; Barbosa, J. Ultrasound-Guided Procedures in the Cervical Spine. *Cureus* **2021**, *13*, e20361. [CrossRef]
18. Hurley, R.W.; Adams, M.C.; Barad, M.; Bhaskar, A.; Bhatia, A.; Chadwick, A.; Deer, T.R.; Hah, J.; Hooten, W.M.; Kissoon, N.R.; et al. Consensus practice guidelines on interventions for cervical spine (facet) joint pain from a multispecialty international working group. *Pain Med.* **2022**, *47*, 3–59. [CrossRef]
19. Lirk, P.; Kolbitsch, C.; Putz, G.; Colvin, J.; Colvin, H.P.; Lorenz, I.; Keller, C.; Kirchmair, L.; Rieder, J.; Moriggl, B. Cervical and High Thoracic Ligamentum Flavum Frequently Fails to Fuse in the Midline. *Anesthesiology* **2003**, *99*, 1387–1390. [CrossRef]
20. Maeda, M.; Maeda, N.; Nagano, T. Diagnosis of sternal fracture using static and stressed ultrasonography. *J. Jpn. Soc. Orthop. Ultrason.* **2018**, *30*, 210–219.
21. Kranz, P.; Joshi, A.; Roy, L.; Choudhury, K.; Amrhein, T. Inadvertent Intrafacet Injection during Lumbar Interlaminar Epidural Steroid Injection: A Comparison of CT Fluoroscopic and Conventional Fluoroscopic Guidance. *Am. J. Neuroradiol.* **2016**, *38*, 398–402. [CrossRef] [PubMed]
22. Kim, M.J.; Choi, Y.S.; Suh, H.J.; Kim, Y.J.; Noh, B.J. Unintentional lumbar facet joint injection guided by fluoroscopy during interlaminar epidural steroid injection: A retrospective analysis. *Korean J. Pain* **2018**, *31*, 87–92. [CrossRef] [PubMed]

23. Riveros-Perez, E.; Albo, C.; Jimenez, E.; Cheriyan, T.; Rocuts, A. Color your epidural: Color flow Doppler to confirm labor epidural needle position. *Minerva Anestesiol.* **2019**, *85*, 376–383. [CrossRef] [PubMed]
24. Zhang, X.; Shi, H.; Zhou, J.; Xu, Y.; Pu, S.; Lv, Y.; Wu, J.; Cheng, Y.; Du, D. The effectiveness of ultrasound-guided cervical transforaminal epidural steroid injections in cervical radiculopathy: A prospective pilot study. *J. Pain Res.* **2018**, *12*, 171–177. [CrossRef]

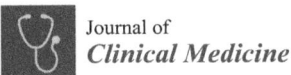

Article
Measures of Corticalization

Marcin Kozakiewicz

Department of Maxillofacial Surgery, Medical University of Lodz, 113 Żeromskiego Str., 90-549 Lodz, Poland; marcin.kozakiewicz@umed.lodz.pl; Tel.: +48-42-6393422

Abstract: After the insertion of dental implants into living bone, the condition of the peri-implant bone changes with time. Implant-loading phenomena can induce bone remodeling in the form of the corticalization of the trabecular bone. The aim of this study was to see how bone index (BI) values behave in areas of bone loss (radiographically translucent non-trabecular areas) and to propose other indices specifically dedicated to detecting corticalization in living bone. Eight measures of corticalization in clinical standardized intraoral radiographs were studied: mean optical density, entropy, differential entropy, long-run emphasis moment, BI, corticalization index ver. 1 and ver. 2 (CI v.1, CI v.2) and corticalization factor (CF). The analysis was conducted on 40 cortical bone image samples, 40 cancellous bone samples and 40 soft tissue samples. It was found that each measure distinguishes corticalization significantly ($p < 0.001$), but only CI v.1 and CI v.2 do so selectively. CF or the inverse of BI can serve as a measure of peri-implant bone corticalization. However, better measures are CIs as they are dedicated to detecting this phenomenon and allowing clear clinical deduction.

Keywords: dental implants; long-term results; long-term success; functional loading; peri-implant bone; intra-oral radiographs; radiomics; texture analysis; corticalization; bone remodeling

1. Introduction

The functional loading of dental implants induces permanent changes in the alveolar crest [1,2]. The functional loading of intraosseous dental implants causes significant changes in the structure of the alveolar marginal bone, observed radiographically [3]. There was corticalization and associated marginal bone loss relentlessly progressing over the five and ten years of observation presented previously [3]. It is expressed in the loss of trabeculation (lower entropy of bone radiostructure) in favor of the unification of the arrangement of bone components and their massification (increase of long elements in radiograph). Both of these structural changes are summarized in the bone index (BI). The conducted analysis strongly suggests that the phenomenon of corticalization is a nonbeneficial alteration of the bone around the implants (at least in the scope disclosed in this study). It means that marginal bone loss will increase as corticalization progresses.

The trabecular structure disappears and is successively replaced by cortical bone-like tissue. These observations were made on the digital analysis of peri-implant bone structure in intraoral radiographs. For this, the bone index [4,5] was used, or, strictly speaking, the inverse of this index since BI is used to detect trabecular bone. Due to the fact of dichotomous deduction possibilities (cancellous bone vs. cortical bone), 1/BI was proposed for detecting corticalization.

However, BI is oriented toward detecting cancellous bone. In trabecular structure radiographs, BI reaches the highest values. In contrast, it reaches low values in other bone structures. The author suspects that low BIs occur not only in images of cortical and corticalized bone but also in areas of bone atrophy (uniformly radiologically translucent). This suspicion is related to the structure of the BI [4,6] since there is a measure in its structure that highlights the existence of long strings of pixels of similar brightness (in other words, of similar radiographic translucency). This measure is not related to high brightness (optical density) only but shows both high and low optical density regions. BI cannot be the only measure for evaluating bone at dental implant site. Unfortunately, BI does not indicate whether a clinically suspicious site is corticalization or bone loss. This is a significant disadvantage. To avoid it, each examined site or radiograph should be subjected to visual inspection, which precludes the automation of the analysis and completely excludes the use of radiomics.

The aim of this study was to see how BI behaves in areas of bone atrophy (radiologically translucent non-trabecular areas) and to propose other indices specifically dedicated to detecting corticalization in living bone.

2. Materials and Methods

The source of the scientific material included in this study was digital intraoral radiographs [7] taken with the Digora Optima system (Soredex, Helsinki, Finland): 7 mA, 70 kV an 0.1 s (Focus apparatus—Instrumentarium Dental, Tuusula, Finland). Positioner Rinn (Densply, Charlotte, NC, USA) was used for the 90° angle of X beam to the surface of phosphor plate. Storage phosphor plates were read immediately after exposure.

Square areas of 3844 pixels (62 × 62), i.e., regions of interest (ROIs) in 8-bit, greyscale images were included in the study, numbering 40 for the compact (cortical) bone images, 40 for the cancellous (trabecular) bone images and 40 soft tissue images (Figure 1). A total of 120 ROIs were analyzed.

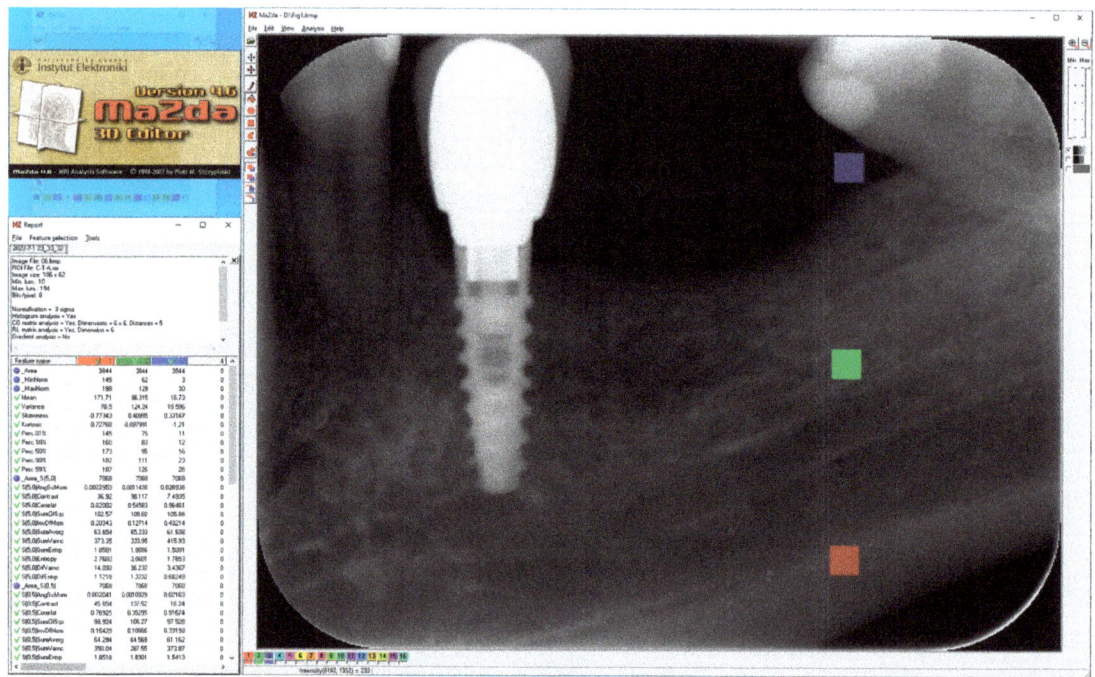

Figure 1. Regions of interest were located in cortical bone (ROI 1), trabecular bone (ROI 2) and soft tissue (ROI 3) in main window of MaZda. Next, a series of textural features was extracted (MZ Reports—on the left) and exported in comma-separated vector format (CSV).

This provided information on three unique regions: cortical bone, trabecular bone and soft tissue. The textures of the X-ray images were analyzed in MaZda 4.6 freeware invented by the University of Technology in Lodz [8] to test measures of corticalization in control environments of trabecular bone (representing original bone before implant-dependent alterations) and soft tissue (representing product of marginal bone loss). MaZda provides both first-order (mean optical density) and second-order (entropy, differential entropy (DifEntr), long-run emphasis moment (LngREmph)) data. Due to the fact that the second-order data are given for four directions in the image, and in the present study, the author did not wish to search for directional features, the arithmetic mean of these four primary data was included for further analysis. The regions of interest (ROIs) were normalized ($\mu \pm 3\sigma$) to share the same average (μ) and standard deviation (σ) of optical density within the ROI. To eliminate noise, [9] worked on data reduced to 6 bits. For analysis in a co-occurrence matrix, a spacing of 5 pixels was chosen. In the formulas that follow, $p(i)$ is a normalized histogram vector (i.e., histogram whose entries are divided by the total number of pixels in ROI), $i = 1,2,..., N_g$ denotes the number of optical density levels. Mean optical density (only a first-order feature) is calculated as follows:

$$\mu = \sum_{i=1}^{N_g} i p(i) \tag{1}$$

Second-order features are found by:

$$Entropy = -\sum_{i=1}^{N_g} \sum_{j=1}^{N_g} p(i,j) \log(p(i,j)) \tag{2}$$

$$DifEntr = -\sum_{i=1}^{N_g} p_{x-y}(i) \log(p_{x-y}(i)) \tag{3}$$

where Σ is sum, Ng is the number of levels of optical density in the radiograph, i and j are optical density of pixels 5-pixel distant one from another, p is probability and log is common logarithm [10]. The differential entropy calculated in this way is a measure of the overall scatter of bone structure elements in a radiograph. Its high values are typical for cancellous bone [4,11,12]. Next, the last primary texture feature was calculated (Figure 2):

$$LngREmph = \frac{\sum_{i=1}^{Ng} \sum_{k=1}^{Nr} k^2 p(i,k)}{\sum_{i=1}^{Ng} \sum_{k=1}^{Nr} p(i,k)} \tag{4}$$

where Σ is sum; Nr is the number of series of pixels with density level i and length k; Ng is the number of levels for image optical density; Nr is the number of pixel in the series; and p is probability [13,14]. This texture feature describes thick, uniformly dense, radio-opaque bone structures in intraoral radiograph images [4,12].

The equations for DifEntr and LngREmph were subsequently used for the index construction [4–6,12]. The bone index (BI), which represents the ratio of the diversity of the structure observed in the radiograph to the measure of the presence of uniform longitudinal structures, was calculated:

$$Bone\ Index = \frac{DifEntr}{LngREmph} \tag{5}$$

Two more formulas were developed with the intention that they would describe the intuitive increases in their values together with the progression of corticalization and that they would suppress the results for cancellous and soft-tissue sites by representing such sites with low values:

$$Corticalization\ Index\ ver.1 = \frac{LngREmph \cdot Mean}{DifEntr} \tag{6}$$

$$Corticalization\ Index\ ver.2 = \frac{LngREmph \cdot Mean}{Entropy} \tag{7}$$

The Kruskal–Wallis test was used for the comparison of medians between cortical, and trabecular or soft tissue radiograph (Statgraphics–StatPoint Technologies, Inc., The Plains, VA, USA). Factor analysis was used to find the statistically supported next measure for the corticalization process product. Input vectors: mean optical density, texture entropy, DifEntrp, and LngREmph. The procedure was performed for factors of eigenvalue ≥ 1. A probabilistic neural network (PNN) to classify cases into different ROI was applied. Rate of correctly classified ROIs by the network was evaluated.

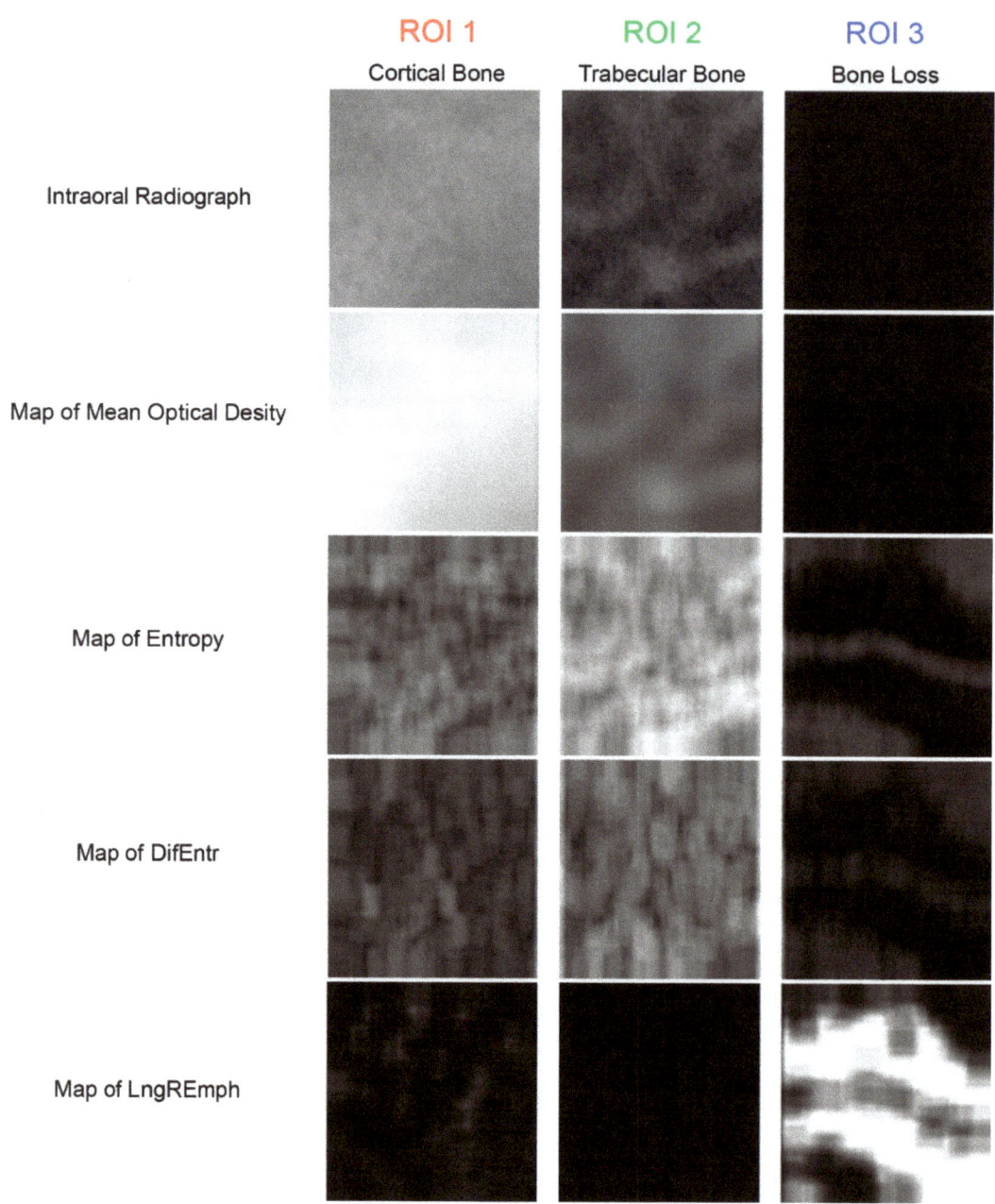

Figure 2. The source material and the primary texture features extracted from it. The meanings of the ROIs are the same as in Figure 1. Maps of the local intensity of the studied features are below the original radiographs. The map is created from square boxes of nine pixels. In the maps of features, lighter areas indicate higher local intensity of the feature, while darker areas indicate lower intensity of the feature.

3. Results

Calculations for selected measures of corticalization in radiographs of three types of tissue representing the corticalization phenomenon, bone loss and the reference region of cancellous bone are shown in Table 1. The results of the primary bone imaging features are shown in Figure 3. These consisted of one first-order feature (mean optical density) and two second-order features (DifEntr and LngREmph).

Table 1. Numerical results of the investigation of selected measures of corticalization.

Measure of Corticalization	ROI 1 Cortical Bone	ROI 2 Trabecular Bone	ROI 3 Bone Loss	Note
Mean Optical Density	132 ± 27	91 ± 15	34 ± 15	$p < 0.001$ [1]
Entropy	2.68 ± 0.15	2.74 ± 0.19	1.79 ± 0.27	$p < 0.001$ [2]
Differential Entropy	1.10 ± 0.09	1.28 ± 0.10	0.81 ± 0.15	$p < 0.001$ [1]
LngREmph	1.66 ± 0.21	1.55 ± 0.18	3.01 0.97	$p < 0.001$ [3]
Bone Index	0.67 ± 0.13	0.84 ± 0.15	0.31 ± 0.14	$p < 0.001$ [1]
Corticalization Index ver.1	200 ± 42	112 ± 28	115 ± 26	$p < 0.001$ [4]
Corticalization Index ver.2	81 ± 15	53 ± 13	52 ± 12	$p < 0.001$ [4]
Corticalization Factor	114 ± 23	80 ± 12	29 ± 14	$p < 0.001$ [1]

[1] Statistically significant difference found between all the ROIs compared with each other; [2] ROI 3 is significantly lower than ROI 1 as well ROI 2; [3] ROI 3 is significantly higher than ROI 1 as well as ROI 2; [4] ROI 1 is significantly higher than ROI 2 as well as ROI 3. ROI—region of interest; LngREmph—long-run emphasis moment.

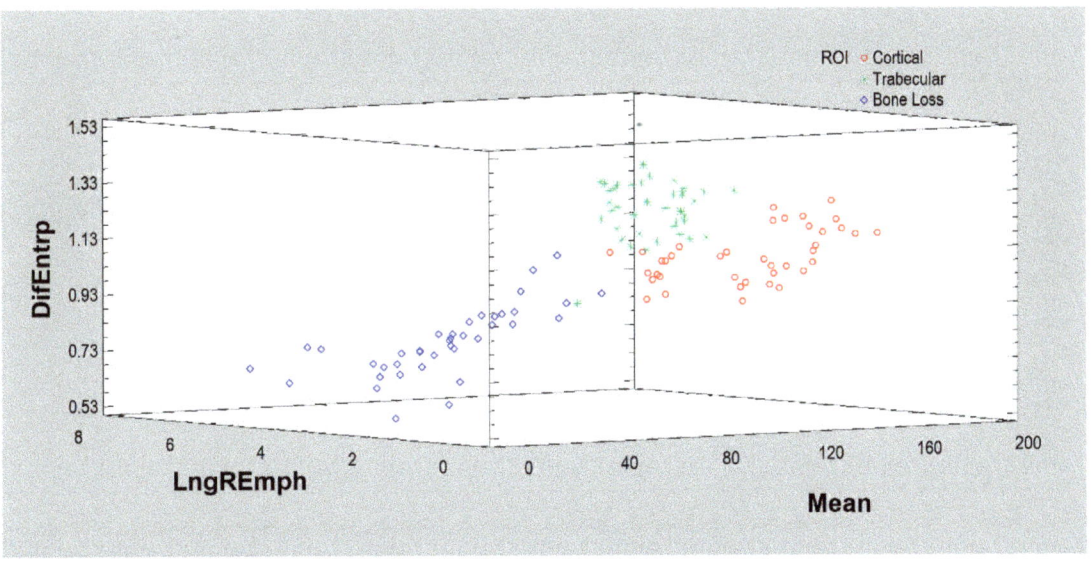

Figure 3. Based on the above three features (DifEntrp, Mean optical density, LngREmph), the algorithm manages to initially separate the results for the three tissues (ROIs), but corticalization (Cortical) is not well discriminated here. It is worth noting that the simple measure of mean optical density itself shows the differences between the regions of interest studied.

The constructed indices were then examined in three ROIs: bone index (Figure 4), corticalization index ver. 1 (Figure 5) and corticalization index ver. 2 (Figure 6).

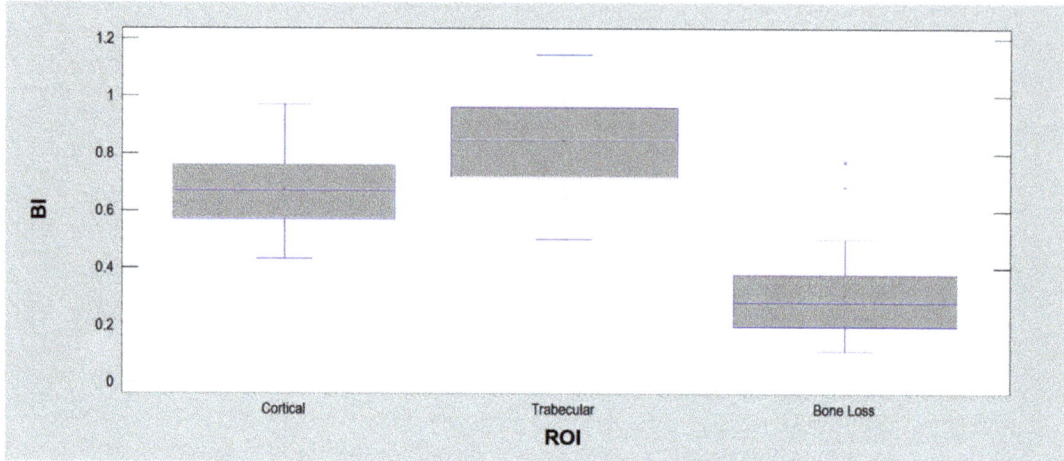

Figure 4. The bone index (BI) was calculated for the detection of normal bone (i.e., trabecular bone) within dental alveolus during guide bone regeneration. That is why BI reaches the highest values in ROI 2 representing trabecular bone. There are significant statistical differences between each ROI.

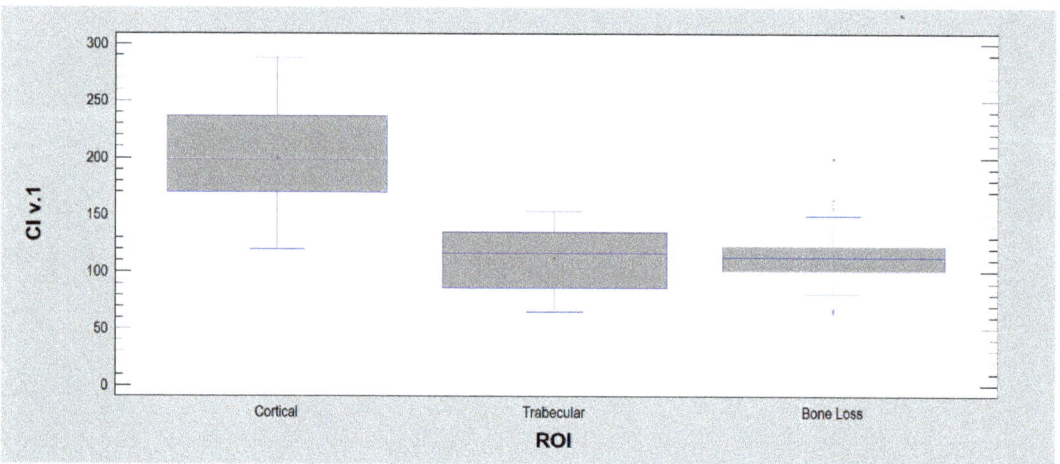

Figure 5. Corticalization index ver. 1 (CI v. 1) is based on two components included in BI and mean optical density. The components are arranged inversely to the BI to emphasize the corticalization sites rather than trabeculation, and the mean optical density enhances this effect because it is located in the numerator and is highest in the cortical bone.

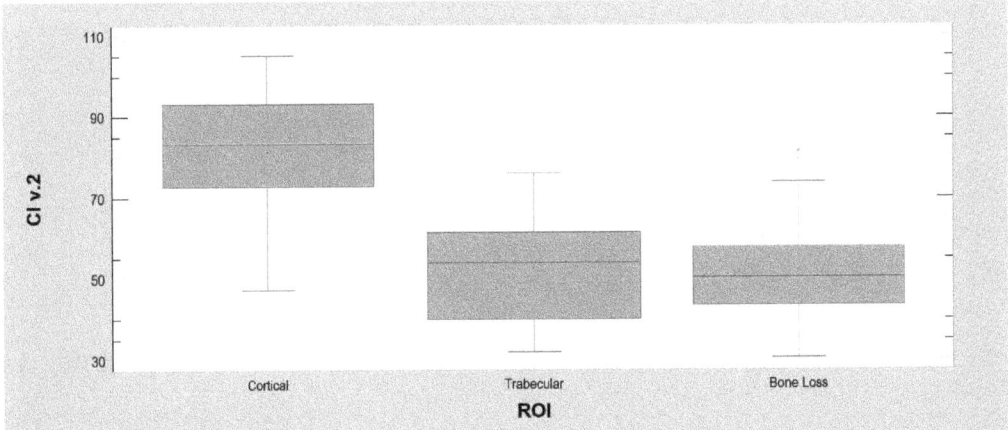

Figure 6. Corticalization index ver. 2 (CI v. 2). This corticalization measure differs from version 1 by replacing differential entropy (ver. 1) in the denominator with entropy (here, ver. 2). This was dictated by the good statistical separation of ROI 1 from the other two ROIs by entropy. However, due to the greater spread of entropy in ROIs than differential entropy, the separation between ROIs is weaker here (but still highly statistically significant: $p < 0.001$).

The purpose of the factor analysis was to obtain a small number of factors that would account for most of the variability in the four textural features (mean optical density, texture entropy, DifEntrp, and LngREmph). In this case, the factor was extracted with a high eigenvalue, 3.30 (much greater than or equal to 1.0). It accounted for 82.4% of the variability in the original texture data. Since principal components was selected, the initial communality estimates were set to assume that all of the variability in the data was due to common factors. Moreover, the Kaiser–Meyer–Olkin measure of sampling adequacy (KMO) was above 0.6 for that set of input features. This factorability test indicates whether or not it is likely to be worthwhile attempting to extract factors from a set of variables. The KMO statistic provides an indication of how much common variance is present. For factorization to be worthwhile, KMO should normally be at least 0.6. Since KMO = 0.768, factorization was likely to provide interesting information about any underlying factors. The equation that estimated the common factor (the corticalization factor, CF) was performed to represent the factor loadings:

$$CF = 0.8446 \cdot Mean + 0.9555 \cdot Entropy + 0.9066 \cdot DifEntr - 0.9211 \cdot LngREmph \qquad (8)$$

where the values of the variables in the equation are standardized by subtracting their means and dividing by their standard deviations. It also shows the estimated communalities, which can be interpreted as estimating the proportion of the variability in each variable attributable to the extracted factors.

Factor analysis indicated that by placing the main emphasis on the simple measurement of mean optical density and measuring the amount of chaoticity in the texture, it is possible to more than adequately detect corticalization sites in the bone image (high CF = 114 ± 23) with simultaneous indication of normal trabecular structure (intermediate values 80 ± 12) and sites that are no longer bone, such as those affected by marginal bone loss (lower values 29 ± 14). The presence of pixel long series of similar optical density is minimized in this corticalization evaluation technique. However, removing LngREmph from the analysis lowers the KMO to 0.618. Thus, one should suspect that short pixel series (i.e., the inverse of LngREmph) is more important in assessing corticalization. A second conclusion from this relationship is the essentiality of evaluating pixel series for indicating corticalization sites.

Thus, the last of the corticalization measures examined here was obtained from factor analysis: CF (Figure 7). It was strongly stratified and allowed for good discrimination of cortical bone from cancellous bone, cancellous bone from soft tissue, and soft tissue from cortical bone ($p < 0.001$).

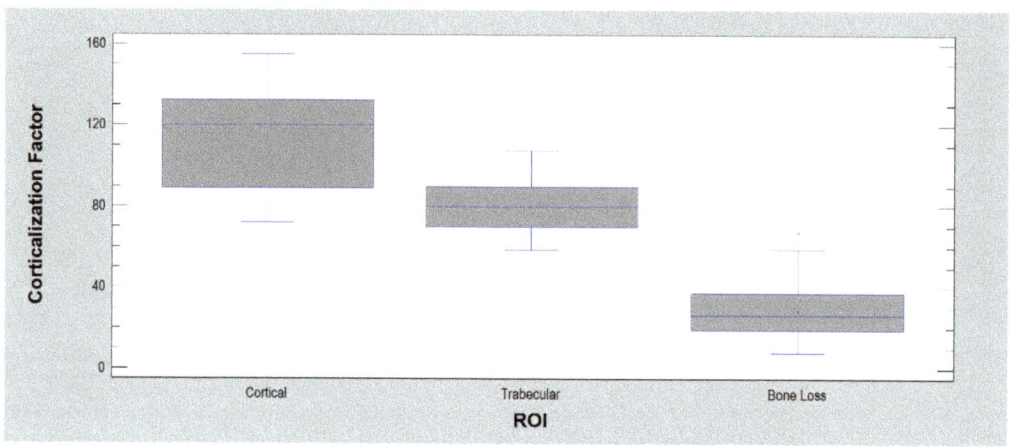

Figure 7. Corticalization Factor (CF). It has statistical features similar to BI, but it is most strongly expressed in cortical sites, weaker in trabecular bone and weakest in soft tissues.

The relationships of the corticalization index with the bone index and corticalization factor are shown in Figure 8 below.

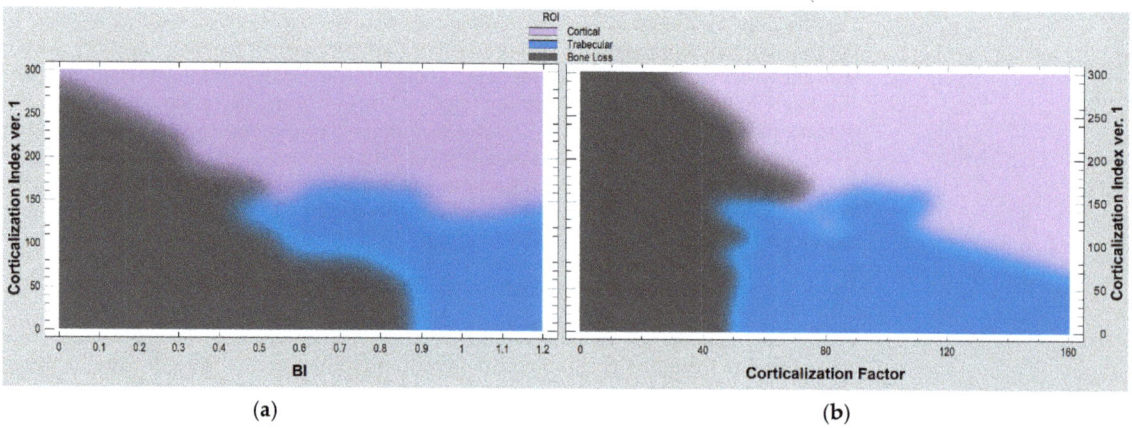

Figure 8. The relationships of selected corticalization measures in the evaluation of intraoral radiographs. (**a**) Corticalization index ver.1 with bone index (BI). A probabilistic neural network (PNN) used to classify cases into different three structures in radiograph (cortical, trabecular, bone loss), based on two input variables (corticalization index ver.1 and bone index). Of the 120 ROIs, 93% were correctly classified by the network. (**b**) Corticalization index ver.1 with corticalization factor. Among the 120 ROIs used, 94% were correctly classified in this pair of corticalization evaluators.

4. Discussion

It is worth noting that a simple measure derived from radiograph histogram analysis (i.e., mean optical density) has been used in dentomaxillofacial radiology for decades [9,15–24].

It carries a great deal of clinically useful information but does not allow the automation feature of radiomics [25–28] because it requires an analog context for understanding the significance of local density changes. A second argument is the vast amount of other information coming from the radiograph beyond the histogram data. In dentistry, more than 10,000 texture features computing from the determined ROIs are now possible [29]. A final issue is the non-specificity of the mean optical density for assessing bone corticalization since residual granules of biomaterial previously implanted into bone, for example, can be detected by this feature [30,31].

In peri-implant bone, optical density increases on plain intraoral radiography in patients treated with immediate-loading implants [1,32]. Similar observations were made for late-loaded implants in the same time horizon (12 months of functional loading) that were noted in the peri-implant bone texture structure [33]. The sum of squares, a feature from the co-occurrence matrix, was studied, and it was found that there is a significant decrease in the value of this texture feature around the integrated dental implant at 12 months after prosthetic loading. This indicates a homogenization of the bone texture and a decrease in its intrinsic contrast [33]. These are the initial reports describing the phenomenon of corticalization of the alveolar crest caused by dental implants.

How to measure the product quantity derived from corticalization process in peri-implant bone in a clinical situation is a critical question. In recent years, the occurrence of corticalization in peri-implant bone was mentioned in scientific literature [32,34–36], and attempts are being made to describe this phenomenon [3] and get to know its clinical significance.

The importance of the standardization of images and ROI should be emphasized first. The approach to this issue depends on the tools used later. When digital radiographic subtraction is used [7,9,16–18,21,22], geometric alignment is necessary first because two radiographs of the same implant but taken at different times are superimposed. Rotational, translational, scale and affine distortions need to be corrected. Next, alignment and contrast brightness are needed. This is best achieved by aligning the histograms of the reference locations [20,23]. In the research presented in this study, this second range of alignment is essential. An alignment algorithm is introduced in the MaZda program consists of standardizing the ROI. The ROIs were adjusted ($\mu \pm 3\sigma$) to share the same average (μ) and standard deviation (σ) of optical density within the ROI.

Bone index (BI) is a good measure for determining the qualitative changes occurring in the cancellous bone of the jaw. A decrease in its value indicates the disappearance of the structure characteristic of trabecular bone. This is most likely related to corticalization since low BI precedes the appearance of marginal trabecular bone in dental implantology by years. There was a strong association of low BI (0.41 ± 0.19) present in the fifth year of implant use with marginal bone loss at that time ($p < 0.0001$) [3]. Bone index also well describes the results of guided bone regeneration inside the alveolus [4]. It highlights the appearance of bone trabeculae at the site of biomaterial implantation. Inferences based on the BI also seem to work well in other disciplines, i.e., in the analysis of bone consolidation quality [37], where a low BI is present at post-fracture sites because the islands of bone densities are more homogeneous (compact) than cancellous bone. This results in a less-chaotic structure, i.e., entropy is reduced (and this entropy is the numerator of the fraction forming the BI). For the same reasons, the bone image here has broad and uniform radio-opaque fields, where long lines of pixels of the same optical density can be found. This causes a high LngREmph, and this is the denominator of the fraction that forms BI. Thus, it affects the reduction of the final BI to 0.70–0.79. Unfortunately, LngREmph (as well BI) cannot describe the pixel series as high optical density (bone apposition) or low optical density (bone loss) points in an image (BI is also low in homogenous radiologically translucent regions).

Moreover, in a study of corticalization, one would need a tool indicating the sites of corticalization rather than the inverse, a tool indicating trabeculation, since bone loss is much more strongly represented in this index (i.e., 1/BI) than corticalization itself. Corticalization index ver. 1 is based on up to the inverse of the described bone index enhanced by the mean optical density result in the ROI. Corticalization index ver. 2 in its design is similar to the inverse of the texture index described previously [5].

The presence of statistically significant differences between the ROIs of the corticalization measures studied indicates that they are all useful to some degree. However, the three tissues tested differed from each other in mean optical density, differential entropy, bone index, corticalization factor). This does not provide a simple measure indicating the site of corticalization searched for in this study. Nevertheless, it should be stated here that both mean optical density and corticalization factor are highest at the site of corticalization. Entropy, on the other hand, is uniformly elevated in both bone tissues (i.e., corticalized and trabecular) relative to soft tissue, which is almost lacking a chaotically scattered texture pattern (Table 1). The next one-element group is the long-run emphasis moment (LngREmph), whose value is highest in soft tissue and lowest in both bone types studied ($p < 0.001$). Yet other measures studied here (both corticalization indices) unambiguously indicate that a given site is corticalized and significantly different from both trabecular bone and well bone loss (i.e., soft tissue). Thus, these two measures do not have the interpretive contamination of random bone loss detection introduced inside. High values here indicate only a corticalization phenomenon, in contrast to the low values, which indicate everything else, i.e., trabecular bone and bone loss. Therefore, these two measures also cannot be used for evaluating the results of guided bone regeneration (the bone index is great for this purpose), nor can they be used to study sites of bone loss. It will be possible in the future to select the best measure for studying a particular phenomenon in peri-implant bone. However, for the considerations in this study, the indices of corticalization (CI ver.1 and CI ver. 2) are the most interesting measures selected.

It seems appropriate to present a dedicated index for detecting corticalization as a phenomenon important for the long-term success of implant treatment. The purpose of this paper is to present such an index for clinical application. The interpretation inconvenience of 1/BI can be resolved by associating the index with high brightness (i.e., high optical density) as typically found in radiographic images of compact (cortical) bone. This gave the idea to include in the index the first-order feature of mean brightness/optical density, i.e., the mean from the histogram of the examined region of interest.

Both versions of CI allow for distinguishing corticalization from atrophy and, of course, also from trabecular bone. The question is whether it is better to rely on BI in the assessment of corticalization, which after all is designed to search for trabecular bone in X-ray images and which also distinguishes bone atrophy well (BI for cancellous bone is the highest, for cortical bone, it is statistically significantly lower and for the site of bone loss, it is significantly lower to corticalized bone). Or is it better to rely on a CI that indicates only corticalization and describes trabecular bone and bone loss together at an equal level i.e., CI ver.1 approx. 114, CI ver.2 approx. 52 for non-corticalization sites.

When considering these aspects of the analysis, it should be emphasized that marginal bone loss has already been very well described in the literature, and the methods to diagnose it are known and evident [38–43]. It is also known to be an unequivocally unfavorable phenomenon for implant success [44–46]. Corticalization itself is suspected as a potentially unfavorable prognostic factor [3]. Thus, it seems best at this stage of the understanding of this phenomenon to focus on the dichotomous separation of the peri-implant bone image structure: corticalized versus other (i.e., cancellous or affected by loss).

As is well known, cortical structural changes can have very serious adverse effects, as in patients treated with antiresorptive therapy (MRONJ) [47], less severe as it seems after a decade of monitoring bone transformation around dental implants [3] or perhaps have a positive effect as in the case of immediate loading of dental implants [32].

The phenomenon described here is so pronounced in the jaws because the bone appositional index here is one of the highest in the body [48]. It is certainly higher than in the iliac bone, femur or vertebrae. In the mandible, the bone apposition rate is 0.086–0.088 μm per hour. This process guarantees the osseointegration of the dental implants in the first phase but is probably responsible in later years for the corticalization of the surrounding area modulated by the permanent loading of the bone by biting and chewing forces. The remodeling and the superimposition of new osteons to the older [49]. This late effect at sufficiently high levels can lead to increased bone fragility and brittleness through the mechanism of osteon hypermineralization, which is related to the process of bone apposition [50]. However, in the jawbone, the phenomenon occurs on a microscale. Whether it is a negative process for the long-term maintenance of functioning dental implants is uncertain. Perhaps for this reason, it is worth thinking about other methods of building measures to describe bone corticalization.

A new approach is the use of factor analysis to evaluate peri-implant bone. The hopes placed in it are based on good predictive experiences from other surgical teams [51,52]. The advantage is the statistically reliable combination of information flowing from several texture features into a single number (corticalization factor) describing the variation occurring in, for example, four features: mean optical density, the frequency of long series of pixels of similar optical density (LngREmph) and two measures of texture pattern scattering (entropy and differential entropy). This aforementioned reliability relies on high eigenvalues and KMO statistics.

Information describing the triplet variation (cortical vs. trabecular vs. bone loss) can reduce the number of features while retaining their internal information by the factor analysis and equation for the corticalization factor (8). It turns out that based on the factor calculated in this way (CF), statistically significant differences ($p < 0.05$) can be indicated between corticalization site roentgenograph (value approx. 120) and cancellous bone (value about 80) versus bone loss (value less than 40). Both analyses (Figure 8) indicate the possibility of the direct transition of cancellous bone to atrophy and of cortical bone to atrophy. Based on the presented methods for the detection of corticalization, there is no indication of a transition state between cancellous bone and bone loss. It is certainly not a corticalized bone. Bone loss can arise directly from one or the other bone tissue.

On the other hand, when considering the interpretive convenience in a study of only corticalization, it is more comfortable to use a tool that gives dichotomously differentiated results, i.e., yes or no for corticalization, and such measures are presented above: the corticalization indices.

It is important and interesting to validate the corticalization measures presented here on a wide range of patients in variable clinical situations (e.g., different implants [53,54], different surgical protocols [55], bone compression screws [56,57], different prosthetic work [58], vitamin D3 levels [47] and molecular signaling modulation [59]). This will allow for choosing the best applications for particular measures. Or perhaps it will prove advisable to use several measures simultaneously, e.g., for monitoring remodeling of the cancellous and cortical substance. It is also important to test the usefulness in other parts of skeletal surgery such as hand [60], foot [61], thoracic [62], orthognathic [63], spine [64], joint replacements [35,65] and rehabilitation [66,67].

One should not forget other measures of corticalization being developed in dentistry itself like fractal dimension and multifractal spectra [53,68–70]. It seems that this valuable and interesting source may in the future bring very useful measures of peri-implant bone remodeling.

This study provides important clinical considerations for dentistry (especially dental implantology). First, it systematizes the possibilities of assessing bone remodeling. It will be possible in the future to select the most suitable index in relation to the observed bone remodeling processes. Second, it is important to relate an objective measure of bone condition with the prediction of dental implant maintenance in normal function. The proposed measures of corticalization are applicable for monitoring bone health around the dental abutments associated with bridges and crowns and the results of guided bone regeneration and tissue bone regeneration in implantology and perioodontology. The clinical relevance of this study can also be seen in monitoring antiresorptive therapy in the treatment of osteoporosis and controlling the metastasis of malignant tumors to bone. Orthopedists, neurosurgeons and hand surgeons who also use metal stabilizers, screws, cages and joint replacements may also benefit. Many fields of medicine need evaluators that assess the condition of bone and its transformation as a function of time. In these example fields of medicine, for example, the use of the corticalization index is being looked at.

5. Conclusions

The corticalization factor, or inverse of bone index, can serve as a measure of peri-implant bone corticalization. However, better measures are the corticalization indices as these are dedicated to detecting corticalization and allowing for clear clinical deduction.

Funding: This research was funded by the Medical University of Lodz (grant numbers 503/5-061-02/503-51-001-18, 503/5-061-02/503-51-001-17 and 503/5-061-02/503-51-002-18).

Institutional Review Board Statement: The study was conducted according to the guidelines of the Declaration of Helsinki and approved by the Institutional Ethics Committee of the Medical University of Lodz, PL (protocol no. RNN 485/11/KB and date of approval: 14.6.2011).

Informed Consent Statement: Informed consent was obtained from all subjects involved in the study.

Data Availability Statement: The data on which this study is based will be made available upon request at https://www.researchgate.net/profile/Marcin-Kozakiewicz access on 30 June 2022.

Acknowledgments: The author would like to thank Andrzej Materka and Michał Strzelecki (Lodz University of Technology, Poland) very much for his valuable comments and consultation of image analysis techniques.

Conflicts of Interest: The author declares no conflict of interest.

References

1. Carneiro, L.S.; da Cunha, H.A.; Leles, C.R.; Mendonça, E.F. Digital subtraction radiography evaluation of longitudinal bone density changes around immediate loading implants: A pilot study. *Dentomaxillofac. Radiol.* **2012**, *41*, 241–247. [CrossRef] [PubMed]
2. Hartman, G.A.; Cochran, D.L. Initial implant position determines the magnitude of crestal bone remodeling. *J. Periodontol.* **2004**, *75*, 572–577. [CrossRef] [PubMed]
3. Kozakiewicz, M.; Skorupska, M.; Wach, T. What Does Bone Corticalization around Dental Implants Mean in Light of Ten Years of Follow-Up? *J. Clin. Med.* **2022**, *11*, 3545. [CrossRef] [PubMed]
4. Kozakiewicz, M.; Szymor, P.; Wach, T. Influence of General Mineral Condition on Collagen-Guided Alveolar Crest Augmentation. *Materials* **2020**, *13*, 3649. [CrossRef]
5. Kozakiewicz, M.; Wach, T. New oral surgery materials for bone reconstruction—A comparison of five bone substitute materials for dentoalveolar augmentation. *Materials* **2020**, *13*, 2935. [CrossRef]
6. Kozakiewicz, M.; Gabryelczak, I. The Osteosynthesis of the Mandibular Head, Does the Way the Screws Are Positioned Matter? *J. Clin. Med.* **2022**, *11*, 2031. [CrossRef]
7. Kozakiewicz, M.; Wilamski, M. Technika standaryzacji wewnątrzustnych zdjęć rentgenowskich [Standardization technique for intraoral radiographs]. *Czas. Stomat.* **1999**, *52*, 673–677.
8. Szczypiński, P.M.; Strzelecki, M.; Materka, A.; Klepaczko, A. MaZda-A software package for image texture analysis. *Comput. Methods Programs Biomed.* **2009**, *94*, 66–76. [CrossRef]
9. Kozakiewicz, M.; Bogusiak, K.; Hanclik, M.; Denkowski, M.; Arkuszewski, P. Noise in subtraction images made from pairs of intraoral radiographs: A comparison between four methods of geometric alignment. *Dentomaxillofac. Radiol* **2008**, *37*, 40–46. [CrossRef]
10. Kołaciński, M.; Kozakiewicz, M.; Materka, A. Textural entropy as a potential feature for quantitative assessment of jaw bone healing process. *Arch. Med. Sci.* **2015**, *11*, 78–84. [CrossRef]
11. Wach, T.; Kozakiewicz, M. Are recent available blended collagen-calcium phosphate better than collagen alone or crystalline calcium phosphate? Radiotextural analysis of a 1-year clinical trial. *Clin. Oral Investig.* **2021**, *25*, 3711–3718. [CrossRef] [PubMed]
12. Wach, T.; Kozakiewicz, M. Fast-Versus Slow-Resorbable Calcium Phosphate Bone Substitute Materials—Texture Analysis after 12 Months of Observation. *Materials* **2020**, *13*, 3854. [CrossRef] [PubMed]
13. Haralick, R. Statistical and Structural Approaches to Texture. *Proc. IEEE* **1979**, *67*, 786–804. [CrossRef]
14. Materka, A.; Strzelecki, M. *Texture Analysis Methods—A Review, COST B11 Report (Presented and Distributed at MC Meeting and Workshop in Brussels, June 1998)*; Technical University of Lodz: Lodz, Poland, 1998.
15. Appleton, R.S.; Nummikoski, P.V.; Pigno, M.A.; Cronin, R.J.; Chung, K.-H. A radiographic assessment of progressive loading on bone around single osseointegrated implants in the posterior maxilla. *Clin. Oral Implants Res.* **2005**, *16*, 161–167. [CrossRef]
16. Brägger, U. Digital imaging in periodontal radiography. A review. *J. Clin. Periodontol.* **1988**, *15*, 551–557. [CrossRef] [PubMed]

17. Brägger, U.; Bürgin, W.; Marconi, M.; Häsler, R.U.; Lang, N.P. Influence of contrast enhancement and pseudocolor transformation on the diagnosis with digital subtraction images (DSI). *J. Periodontal. Res.* **1994**, *29*, 95–102. [CrossRef]
18. Brägger, U.; Pasquali, L. Color conversion of alveolar bone density changes in digital subtraction images. *J. Clin. Periodontol.* **1989**, *16*, 209–214. [CrossRef]
19. Dudek, D.; Kozakiewicz, M. Szerokość beleczek kostnych w szczęce i żuchwie człowieka na podstawie cyfrowych radiologicznych zdjęć wewnątrzustnych [Bone trabecula width in the human maxilla and mandible based on digital intraoral radiographs]. *Mag. Stomat.* **2012**, *236*, 77–80.
20. Duinkerke, A.S.; van de Poel, A.C.; Doesburg, W.H.; Lemmens, W.A. Densitometric analysis of experimentally produced periapical radiolucencies. *Oral Surg. Oral Med. Oral Pathol.* **1977**, *43*, 782–797. [CrossRef]
21. Gröndahl, H.G.; Gröndahl, K.; Webber, R.L. A digital subtraction technique for dental radiography. *Oral Surg. Oral Med. Oral Pathol.* **1983**, *55*, 96–102. [CrossRef]
22. de Molon, R.S.; Batitucci, R.G.; Spin-Neto, R.; Paquier, G.M.; Sakakura, C.E.; Tosoni, G.M.; Scaf, G. Comparison of changes in dental and bone radiographic densities in the presence of different soft-tissue simulators using pixel intensity and digital subtraction analyses. *Dentomaxillofac. Radiol.* **2013**, *42*, 20130235. [CrossRef] [PubMed]
23. da Silva, R.; Duailibi Neto, E.F.; Todescan, F.F.; Ruiz, G.M.; Pannuti, C.M.; Chilvarquer, I. Evaluation of cervical peri-implant optical density in longitudinal control of immediate implants in the anterior maxilla region. *Dentomaxillofac. Radiol.* **2020**, *49*, 20190396. [CrossRef] [PubMed]
24. Webber, R.L.; Ruttimann, U.E.; Heaven, T.J. Calibration errors in digital subtraction radiography. *J. Periodontal. Res.* **1990**, *25*, 268–275. [CrossRef]
25. Bogowicz, M.; Vuong, D.; Huellner, M.W.; Pavic, M.; Andratschke, N.; Gabrys, H.S.; Guckenberger, M.; Tanadini-Lang, S. CT radiomics and PET radiomics: Ready for clinical implementation? *Q. J. Nucl. Med. Mol. Imaging* **2019**, *63*, 355–370. [CrossRef] [PubMed]
26. Mayerhoefer, M.E.; Materka, A.; Langs, G.; Häggström, I.; Szczypiński, P.; Gibbs, P.; Cook, G. Introduction to Radiomics. *J. Nucl. Med.* **2020**, *61*, 488–495. [CrossRef] [PubMed]
27. Noortman, W.A.; Vriens, D.; Grootjans, W.; Tao, Q.; de Geus-Oei, L.F.; Van Velden, F.H. Nuclear medicine radiomics in precision medicine: Why we can't do without artificial intelligence. *Q. J. Nucl. Med. Mol. Imaging* **2020**, *64*, 278–290. [CrossRef]
28. Reuzé, S.; Schernberg, A.; Orlhac, F.; Sun, R.; Chargari, C.; Dercle, L.; Deutsch, E.; Buvat, I.; Robert, C. Radiomics in Nuclear Medicine Applied to Radiation Therapy: Methods, Pitfalls, and Challenges. *Int. J. Radiat. Oncol. Biol. Phys.* **2018**, *102*, 1117–1142. [CrossRef]
29. Pociask, E.; Nurzynska, K.; Obuchowicz, R.; Bałon, P.; Uryga, D.; Strzelecki, M.; Izworski, A.; Piórkowski, A. Differential Diagnosis of Cysts and Granulomas Supported by Texture Analysis of Intraoral Radiographs. *Sensors* **2021**, *21*, 7481. [CrossRef]
30. Kozakiewicz, M.; Marciniak-Hoffman, A.; Denkowski, M. Long term comparison of application of two betatricalcium phosphates in oral surgery. *Dent. Med. Probl.* **2009**, *46*, 284–388.
31. Kozakiewicz, M.; Marciniak-Hoffman, A.; Olszycki, M. Comparative Analysis of Three Bone Substitute Materials Based on Co-Occurrence Matrix. *Dent. Med. Probl.* **2010**, *47*, 23–29.
32. Linkevicius, T.; Linkevicius, R.; Gineviciute, E.; Alkimavicius, J.; Mazeikiene, A.; Linkeviciene, L. The influence of new immediate tissue level abutment on crestal bone stability of subcrestally placed implants: A 1-year randomized controlled clinical trial. *Clin. Implant Dent. Relat. Res.* **2021**, *23*, 259–269. [CrossRef] [PubMed]
33. Dudek, D. Ocena Przebudowy Kości Obciążonej Wszczepami Zębowymi z Zastosowaniem Cyfrowej Analizy Tekstur Obrazu Radiologicznego [Evaluation of Dental Implants Loaded Bone Remodeling Using Digital Texture Analysis in Radiographic Images]. Doctorate Thesis, Medical University of Lodz, Lodz, Poland, 2012.
34. Baer, R.A.; Nölken, R.; Colic, S.; Heydecke, G.; Mirzakhanian, C.; Behneke, A.; Behneke, N.; Gottesman, E.; Ottria, L.; Pozzi, A.; et al. Immediately provisionalized tapered conical connection implants for single-tooth restorations in the maxillary esthetic zone: A 5-year prospective single-cohort multicenter analysis. *Clin. Oral Investig.* **2022**, *26*, 3593–3604. [CrossRef]
35. Dowgierd, K.; Pokrowiecki, R.; Borowiec, M.; Kozakiewicz, M.; Smyczek, D.; Krakowczyk, Ł. A Protocol for the Use of a Combined Microvascular Free Flap with Custom-Made 3D-Printed Total Temporomandibular Joint (TMJ) Prosthesis for Mandible Reconstruction in Children. *Appl. Sci.* **2021**, *11*, 2176. [CrossRef]
36. Kinaia, B.M.; Shah, M.; Neely, A.L.; Goodis, H.E. Crestal bone level changes around immediately placed implants: A systematic review and meta-analyses with at least 12 months' follow-up after functional loading. *J. Periodontol.* **2014**, *85*, 1537–1548. [CrossRef] [PubMed]
37. Kozakiewicz, M.; Gabryelczak, I. Bone Union Quality after Fracture Fixation of Mandibular Head with Compression Magnesium Screws. *Materials* **2022**, *15*, 2230. [CrossRef] [PubMed]
38. Dowgierd, K.; Pokrowiecki, R.; Borowiec, M.; Sokolowska, Z.; Dowgierd, M.; Wos, J.; Kozakiewicz, M.; Krakowczyk, Ł. Protocol and Evaluation of 3D-Planned Microsurgical and Dental Implant Reconstruction of Maxillary Cleft Critical Size Defects in Adolescents and Young Adults. *J. Clin. Med.* **2021**, *10*, 2267. [CrossRef]
39. Kütan, E.; Bolukbasi, N.; Yildirim-Ondur, E.; Ozdemir, T. Clinical and Radiographic Evaluation of Marginal Bone Changes around Platform-Switching Implants Placed in Crestal or Subcrestal Positions: A Randomized Controlled Clinical Trial. *Clin. Implant Dent. Rel. Res.* **2014**, *17*, e364–e375. [CrossRef]

40. Moraschini, V.; Poubel, L.A.D.C.; Ferreira, V.F.; Barboza, E.D.S.P. Evaluation of survival and success rates of dental implants reported in longitudinal studies with a follow-up period of at least 10 years: A systematic review. *Int. J. Oral Maxillofac. Surg.* **2015**, *44*, 377–388. [CrossRef]
41. Pellicer-Chover, H.; Díaz-Sanchez, M.; Soto-Peñaloza, D.; Peñarrocha-Diago, M.A.; Canullo, L.; Peñarrocha-Oltra, D. Impact of crestal and subcrestal implant placement upon changes in marginal peri-implant bone level. A systematic review. *Med. Oral Patol. Oral Cir. Bucal* **2019**, *24*, e673–e683. [CrossRef]
42. Pokrowiecki, R.; Szałaj, U.; Fudala, D.; Zaręba, T.; Wojnarowicz, J.; Łojkowski, W.; Tyski, S.; Dowgierd, K.; Mielczarek, A. Dental Implant Healing Screws as Temporary Oral Drug Delivery Systems for Decrease of Infections in the Area of the Head and Neck. *Int. J. Nanomed.* **2022**, *17*, 1679–1693. [CrossRef] [PubMed]
43. von Wilmowsky, C.; Moest, T.; Nkenke, E.; Stelzle, F.; Schlegel, K.A. Implants in bone: Part II. Research on implant osseointegration: Material testing, mechanical testing, imaging and histoanalytical methods. *Oral Maxillofac. Surg.* **2014**, *18*, 355–372. [CrossRef]
44. Kowalski, J.; Łapińska, B.; Nissan, J.; Łukomska-Szymanska, M. Factors Influencing Marginal Bone Loss around Dental Implants: A Narrative Review. *Coatings* **2021**, *11*, 865. [CrossRef]
45. Sargolzaie, N.; Zarch, H.H.; Arab, H.; Koohestani, T.; Ramandi, M.F. Marginal bone loss around crestal or subcrestal dental implants: Prospective clinical study. *J. Korean Assoc. Oral Maxillofac. Surg.* **2022**, *48*, 159–166. [CrossRef] [PubMed]
46. Chrcanovic, B.R.; Albrektsson, T.; Wennerberg, A. Reasons for failures of oral implants. *J. Oral Rehabil.* **2014**, *41*, 443–476. [CrossRef]
47. Wiesner, A.; Szuta, M.; Galanty, A.; Paśko, P. Optimal Dosing Regimen of Osteoporosis Drugs in Relation to Food Intake as the Key for the Enhancement of the Treatment Effectiveness-A Concise Literature Review. *Foods* **2021**, *29*, 720. [CrossRef] [PubMed]
48. Tam, C.S.; Harrison, J.E.; Reed, R.; Cruickshank, B. Bone apposition rate as an index of bone metabolism. *Metabolism* **1978**, *27*, 143–150. [CrossRef]
49. Pazzaglia, U.E.; Congiu, T.; Marchese, M.; Spagnuolo, F.; Quacci, D. Morphometry and Patterns of Lamellar Bone in Human Haversian Systems. *Anat. Rec. Adv. Integr. Anat. Evol. Biol.* **2012**, *295*, 1421–1429. [CrossRef]
50. Nyssen-Behets, C.; Arnould, V.; Dhem, A. Hypermineralized lamellae below the bone surface: A quantitative microradiographic study. *Bone* **1994**, *15*, 685–689. [CrossRef]
51. Jabłoński, S.; Brocki, M.; Kordiak, J.; Misiak, P.; Terlecki, A.; Kozakiewicz, M. Acute mediastinitis: Evaluation of clinical risk factors for death in surgically treated patients. *ANZ J. Surg.* **2013**, *83*, 657–663. [CrossRef]
52. Jabłoński, S.; Brocki, M.; Krzysztof, K.; Wawrzycki, M.; Santorek-Strumiłło, E.; Łobos, M.; Kozakiewicz, M. Evaluation of prognostic value of selected biochemical markers in surgically treated patients with acute mediastinitis. *Med. Sci. Monit.* **2012**, *18*, CR308–CR315. [CrossRef]
53. Hadzik, J.; Kubasiewicz-Ross, P.; Simka, W.; Gębarowski, T.; Barg, E.; Cieśla-Niechwiadowicz, A.; Trzcionka Szajna, A.; Szajna, E.; Gedrange, T.; Kozakiewicz, M.; et al. Fractal Dimension and Texture Analysis in the Assessment of Experimental Laser-Induced Periodic Surface Structures (LIPSS) Dental Implant Surface-In Vitro Study Preliminary Report. *Materials* **2022**, *15*, 2713. [CrossRef] [PubMed]
54. Jaźwiecka-Koscielniak, E.; Kozakiewicz, M. A new modification of the individually designed polymer implant visible in X-ray for orbital reconstruction. *J. Cranio-Maxillofac. Surg.* **2014**, *42*, 1520–1529. [CrossRef] [PubMed]
55. Wach, T.; Kozakiewicz, M. Comparison of Two Clinical Procedures in Patient Affected with Bone Deficit in Posterior Mandible. *Dent. Med. Probl.* **2016**, *53*, 22–28. [CrossRef]
56. Kozakiewicz, M. Change in Pull-Out Force during Resorption of Magnesium Compression Screws for Osteosynthesis of Mandibular Condylar Fractures. *Materials* **2021**, *14*, 237. [CrossRef]
57. Kozakiewicz, M. Small-diameter compression screws completely embedded in bone for rigid internal fixation of the condylar head of the mandible. *Br. J. Oral Maxillofac. Surg.* **2018**, *56*, 74–76. [CrossRef]
58. Alhammadi, S.H.; Burnside, G.; Milosevic, A. Clinical outcomes of single implant supported crowns versus 3-unit implant-supported fixed dental prostheses in Dubai Health Authority: A retrospective study. *BMC Oral Health* **2021**, *21*, 171. [CrossRef]
59. Cheng, X.; Zhou, X.; Liu, C.; Xu, X. Oral Osteomicrobiology: The Role of Oral Microbiota in Alveolar Bone Homeostasis. *Front. Cell Infect. Microbiol.* **2021**, *11*, 751503. [CrossRef]
60. Lee, J.H.; Kim, G.H.; Park, M.J. Clinical outcomes of open-wedge corrective osteotomy using autogenous or allogenic bone grafts for malunited distal radius: A novel parameter for measuring the rate of bone union. *Acta Orthop. Traumatol. Turc.* **2022**, *56*, 199–204. [CrossRef]
61. Fox, J.; Enriquez, B.; Bompadre, V.; Carlin, K.; Dales, M. Observation Versus Cast Treatment of Toddler's Fractures. *J. Pediatr. Orthop.* **2022**, *42*, e480–e485. [CrossRef]
62. Reindl, S.; Jawny, P.; Girdauskas, E.; Raab, S. Is it Necessary to Stabilize Every Fracture in Patients with Serial Rib Fractures in Blunt Force Trauma? *Front Surg.* **2022**, *9*, 845494. [CrossRef]
63. Dowgierd, K.; Borowiec, M.; Kozakiewicz, M. Bone changes on lateral cephalograms and CBCT during treatment of maxillary narrowing using palatal osteodistraction with bone-anchored appliances. *J. Craniomaxillofac. Surg.* **2018**, *46*, 2069–2081. [CrossRef] [PubMed]
64. Cai, Y.; Khanpara, S.; Timaran, D.; Spence, S.; McCarty, J.; Aein, A.; Nunez, L.; Arevalo, O.; Riascos, R. Traumatic spondylolisthesis of axis: Clinical and imaging experience at a level one trauma center. *Emerg. Radiol.* **2022**, *29*, 715–722. [CrossRef] [PubMed]

65. Egol, K.A.; Walden, T.; Gabor, J.; Leucht, P.; Konda, S.R. Hip-preserving surgery for nonunion about the hip. *Arch. Orthop. Trauma Surg.* **2022**, *142*, 1451–1457. [CrossRef]
66. Dowgierd, K.; Lipowicz, A.; Kulesa-Mrowiecka, M.; Wolański, W.; Linek, P.; Myśliwiec, A. Efficacy of immediate physiotherapy after surgical release of zygomatico-coronoid ankylosis in a young child: A case report. *Physiother Theory Pract.* **2021**, *15*, 1–7. [CrossRef]
67. Stowers, J.M.; Black, A.T.; Kavanagh, A.M.; Mata, K.; Bohm, A.; Katchis, S.D.; Weiner, L.S.; Spielfogel, W.; Rahnama, A. Predicting Nonunions in Ankle Fractures Using Quantitative Tibial Hounsfield Samples From Preoperative Computed Tomography: A Multicenter Matched Case Control Study. *J. Foot Ankle Surg.* **2022**, *61*, 562–566. [CrossRef] [PubMed]
68. Borowska, M.; Bębas, E.; Szarmach, J.; Oczeretko, E. Multifractal characterization of healing process after bone loss. *Biomed. Signal Process. Control* **2019**, *52*, 179–186. [CrossRef]
69. Borowska, M.; Szarmach, J.; Oczeretko, E. Fractal texture analysis of the healing process after bone loss. *Comput. Med. Imaging Graph.* **2015**, *46*, 191–196. [CrossRef]
70. Kozakiewicz, M.; Chaberek, S.; Bogusiak, K. Using fractal dimension to evaluate alveolar bone defects treated with various bone substitute materials. *Open Med.* **2014**, *8*, 776–789. [CrossRef]

Journal of Clinical Medicine

Article

A Novel Lightweight Approach to COVID-19 Diagnostics Based on Chest X-ray Images

Agata Giełczyk [1,*], Anna Marciniak [1,2], Martyna Tarczewska [1], Sylwester Michal Kloska [2], Alicja Harmoza [2], Zbigniew Serafin [2] and Marcin Woźniak [2]

1. Faculty of Telecommunications, Computer Science and Electrical Engineering, Bydgoszcz University of Science and Technology, 85-796 Bydgoszcz, Poland
2. Faculty of Medicine Ludwik Rydygier Collegium Medicum in Bydgoszcz, Nicolaus Copernicus University in Torun, 85-067 Bydgoszcz, Poland
* Correspondence: agata.gielczyk@pbs.edu.pl

Abstract: Background: This paper presents a novel lightweight approach based on machine learning methods supporting COVID-19 diagnostics based on X-ray images. The presented schema offers effective and quick diagnosis of COVID-19. Methods: Real data (X-ray images) from hospital patients were used in this study. All labels, namely those that were COVID-19 positive and negative, were confirmed by a PCR test. Feature extraction was performed using a convolutional neural network, and the subsequent classification of samples used Random Forest, XGBoost, LightGBM and CatBoost. Results: The LightGBM model was the most effective in classifying patients on the basis of features extracted from X-ray images, with an accuracy of 1.00, a precision of 1.00, a recall of 1.00 and an F1-score of 1.00. Conclusion: The proposed schema can potentially be used as a support for radiologists to improve the diagnostic process. The presented approach is efficient and fast. Moreover, it is not excessively complex computationally.

Keywords: features extraction; X-ray images; COVID-19; machine learning; image processing

1. Introduction

COVID-19 is a disease caused by the SARS-CoV-2 virus. It has a wide range of symptoms, most of which affect the respiratory tract. It can lead to serious inflammation of the lungs and, consequently, pneumonia [1]. The COVID-19 pandemic has exposed healthcare problems around the world. The large number of patients to diagnose and the limited number of tests and staff available turned out to be a significant problem. As a result, the number of diagnostic tests performed was very often too low. The diagnostic method that turned out to be the gold standard for the confirmation of SARS-CoV-2 infection was the polymerase chain reaction (PCR) test. However, this method is not error free and sometimes gives false results [2]. Another difficulty comes from the fact that some people, despite being infected with the SARS-CoV-2 virus, do not develop symptoms of the disease [3] and are not referred for PCR testing. This can cause problems with the correct diagnosis of the disease. Despite its latency, the disease can cause serious changes in the lungs. In these cases, the diagnosis is possible on the basis of an X-ray of the lungs. For this reason, machine learning methods have been used to detect COVID-19 infections on X-ray images. Methods based on machine learning (ML) turned out to be effective and useful during the analysis and assessment of the impact of diseases (e.g., COVID-19 or pneumonia) on X-ray images of the lungs [4–6]. The major contributions of this paper are as follows:

- We propose a novel approach to chest X-ray image analysis in order to diagnose COVID-19 using an original CNN-based features extraction method.

- We obtained a new dataset containing samples from confirmed COVID-19 cases as well as from uninfected patients. The infection status of both groups was confirmed by a PCR test. We performed an augmentation in order to increase the dataset's size.
- We implemented the proposed features extraction for different classifiers, obtaining promising results.

Further parts of this paper are constructed in the following manner: (a) a brief review of the state-of-the-art is presented in Section 2; (b) in Section 3, we describe the dataset, augmentation process and the proposed approach to the classification; (c) in Section 4, we present the obtained results; (d) in Section 5 (the Discussion) we compare our results with other state-of-the-art approaches, we pull out some conclusions, and we present perspectives for future work on this topic.

2. Related Work

To combat the challenges posed by the pandemic to the healthcare service, Khan et al. [7] proposed a deep-learning-based method of accurate and quick diagnosis of COVID-19 using X-ray images. They proposed a method consisting of two novel deep learning frameworks: Deep Hybrid Learning (DHL) and Deep Boosted Hybrid Learning (DBHL). The use of both of these frameworks led to an improvement in their COVID-19 diagnostic methods. The result was a model capable of identifying COVID-19 in X-ray images with over 98% accuracy on a previously unseen dataset. This method has been shown to be effective in reducing both false positives and false negatives and has proven to be a useful supportive tool for radiologists.

Tahir et al. [8] proposed a model based on a convolutional neural network (CNN) capable of lung segmentation and localization of specific changes caused by COVID-19. The dataset used consisted of nearly 34,000 X-ray images, including lung images of people with COVID-19 and pneumonia and of healthy people. An important element of the study was the appropriate marking of photos by specialists. This method recognized COVID-19 and its effects on the lung image with sensitivity and specificity values over 99%.

In [9], Brunese et al. used transfer learning to create a model capable of detecting COVID-19 changes in X-ray images of the lungs. This model is applicable (1) to the classification of healthy people and patients with changes in lung X-ray images; (2) to distinguish between COVID-19 and other lung diseases; and (3) to distinguish lung lesions caused by the SARS-CoV-2 infection. This model was based on the VGG-16 (16-layered convolutional neural network) and underwent transfer learning. This study included 6523 X-ray images from healthy individuals, patients with various lung diseases and patients with COVID-19. The model trained on this dataset achieved a sensitivity equal to 0.96 and a specificity of 0.98 (accuracy of 0.96) for distinguishing between healthy individuals and patients with lung diseases, and a sensitivity of 0.87 and a specificity equal to 0.94 (accuracy of 0.98) for distinguishing lung diseases from COVID-19. The image analysis process itself is extremely fast and takes only about 2.5 s. The data presented by the authors indicate that the developed model achieves good and reliable results.

Chakraborty et al. [10] presented a COVID-19 detection method based on a Deep Learning Method (DLM) using X-ray images. The authors used different architectures of deep neural networks in order to achieve optimal results. They combined several pretrained models such as ResNet18, AlexNet, DenseNet, VGG16, etc. This approach showed to be effective and cost significantly less than standard laboratory diagnostic methods. The dataset consisted of 10,040 chest X-ray images, which included a normal/healthy population, COVID-19 patients and patients with pneumonia. The presented model was highly accurate (96.43%) and sensitive (93.68%). This work showed the high usefulness of ML models for determining changes in X-ray images, which can facilitate the work of radiologists who, as a result of this quick method, can refer patients directly to treatment.

Civit-Masot et al. [11] noted that traditional tests to identify SARS-CoV-2 infection are invasive and time consuming. Imaging, on the other hand, is a useful method for assessing disease symptoms. Due to the limited number of trained medical doctors who can reliably assess X-ray images, it is necessary to invent ways to facilitate this type of assessment. The authors used the VGG-16-based Deep Learning model to identify pneumonia and COVID-19. The presented results indicate high accuracy (close to 100%) and specificity of the model, which qualify it as an effective screening test.

It is also worth mentioning that ML-based methods can support not only radiology specialists. In [12], we can see the transfer learning approach to discovering the impact of the stringency index on the number of deaths caused by the SARS-Cov-2 virus. As presented in [13], ML can be also implemented in order to predict the COVID-19 diagnosis based on symptoms. Statistical analyses revealed that the most frequent and significant predictive symptoms are fevers (41.1%), coughs (30.3%), lung infections (13.1%) and runny noses (8.43%). A total of 54.4% of people examined did not develop any symptoms that could be used for diagnosis. Moreover, ML can also be a useful tool in vaccine discovering, as presented in [14].

Recently, numerous ML-based approaches for rapid diagnostics have been published. In addition, they have gathered increasingly more attention from some government and international agencies. For example, the European Commission published a White Paper entitled 'On Artificial Intelligence—A European approach to excellence and trust [15]. Seven key requirements were identified and are described in the document:

- Human agencies and oversight;
- Technical robustness and safety;
- Privacy and data governance;
- Transparency;
- Diversity, non-discrimination and fairness;
- Societal and environmental well-being;
- Accountability.

The following statement in the EC publication is worth noting: AI can and should itself critically examine resource usage and energy consumption and should be trained to make choices that are positive for the environment. It follows from the above citation that it is extremely important to focus on providing solutions that are not only cost and time effective but also that spare energy used for computations. This kind of approach to AI has become introduced as the 'GreenAI' [16] and has gathered increasingly more attention recently [17]. Research working on the GreenAI have also proposed some novel metrics [18]. As a result of this metric, researchers can compare not only the accuracy and precision of the proposed method, but also its sustainability and eco-friendliness.

3. Materials and Methods

The general overview of the proposed method is presented in Figure 1. The image presents an example of the data obtained from the hospital and some consequential steps: the augmentation process and pre-processing of the sample. In Figure 1, the features extraction and classification steps are presented. Finally, the proposed method gives the answer of *"true"* for the COVID-19-positive sample and *"false"* for the healthy sample. Each step of the process is described in detail in this section. All experiments were carried out with the use of Python 3.7 and the TensorFlow platform. Among others, we used the following libraries: scikit-learn, Xgboost, Lightgbm and Catboost.

3.1. Dataset

In this research, anonymized real data were used. The data were obtained from Antoni Jurasz University Hospital No. 1 in Bydgoszcz, Department of Radiology and Imaging Diagnostics. A total of 60 chest X-ray images were obtained; 30 were from healthy individuals, and 30 had COVID-19 confirmed by a PCR test. The images were provided in the DICOM format. The images were in a raw form, without masks. Some samples from the dataset are presented in Figure 2.

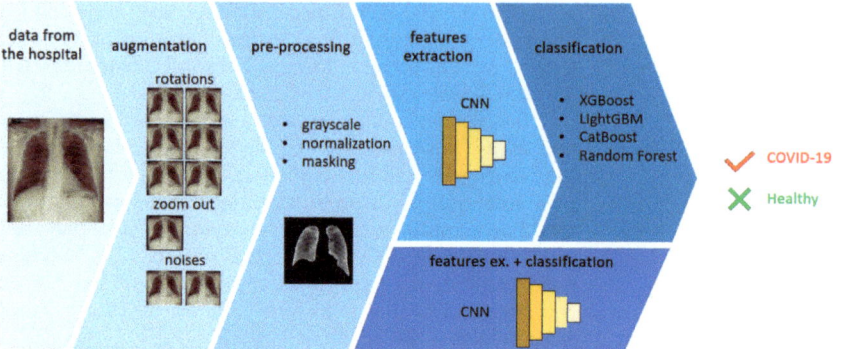

Figure 1. The following steps of processing in the proposed method: data acquisition, data augmentation, sample pre-processing, features extraction and binary classification of COVID-19 as positive or negative (healthy).

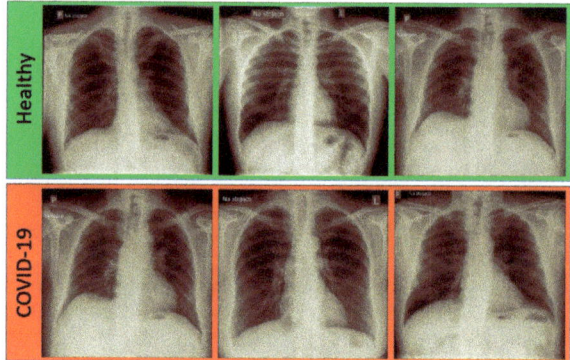

Figure 2. The exemplary images from the dataset divided into two classes: Healthy and COVID-19 confirmed by a PCR test.

3.2. Data Augmentation

In order to perform training, the dataset was divided into 3 disjointed subsets: the training set (80%), validation set (10%) and testing set (10%). Unfortunately, the quantity of samples was not enough to use any ML technique. Thus, we decided to use augmentation for increasing the size of the training dataset. As a result of the augmentation, 10 samples from one single image were obtained. The initial proper balance in the dataset was unchanged, and as a result, the dataset was still well balanced. The following methods for augmentation were implemented:

- rotations—1°, 2° and 3° both clockwise and anti-clockwise;
- noises—a random Gaussian noise and a salt and pepper noise were added;
- zooming out—the image was resized to obtain 95% of its original size.

3.3. Data Pre-Processing

First of all, the samples were moved to grayscale images and were normalized. The goal of normalization was to improve the quality of the images, e.g., by enhancing the contrast, as described in [19]. The data obtained from the hospital were not masked. Thus, the essential step of processing was to provide proper masks to help in selecting the region of interest. The goal of this step was to prevent the ML-based model from learning information that is useless from the point of view of COVID-19 diagnostics, such as images of a collar bone or a stomach. Hand crafting masks would be time consuming, and it would require the involvement of a specialist. On the other hand, proposing a novel method of segmentation can be treated as a separate scientific problem, as presented in [20,21]. Therefore, it was decided to use the pretrained model, which is widely available and very powerful in masking X-ray images [22].

3.4. ML-Based Methods

ML-based methods were used in two steps of processing, namely features extraction and classification. As a baseline, a convolutional neural network (CNN) was used for both steps. Then, almost the same CNN architecture was used solely for extracting features, since it was reported as very promising and efficient [23,24].

The features extraction step can be an essential one for the whole image processing system. It can reduce the complexity of the problem, and consequently, it can make the proposed approach more efficient, require less computing time and, therefore, more eco-friendly. The general schema of the CNN is presented in Figure 3. The input in this architecture was grayscale images with sizes of 512 × 512 pixels. Then, three pairs of convolutional layers and max pooling layers were used. Each of them was responsible for performing operations between the filters and the input of each corresponding layer. The convolutional layers consisted of 64, 128 and 256 filters, respectively. On each layer, an ReLU activation function was used to implement and perform nonlinear transformations. Then, the flattened layer and the dense layer were used. The proposed neural networks against the dense layer neuron quantity were examined. The values, with a range of [5,200], were tested. Involving the validation subset, it was observed that the most promising was using 57 features. This features extraction type was qualified for further research and development. Then, numerous classifiers were examined: XGBoost [25], Random Forest [26], LightGBM [27] and CatBoost [28]. It was decided to use these classifiers due to some reasons. First of all, they are tree-based algorithms, and they perform very well in binary classification problems. Secondly, they have been already used in similar applications, as presented in [29–31], providing promising results.

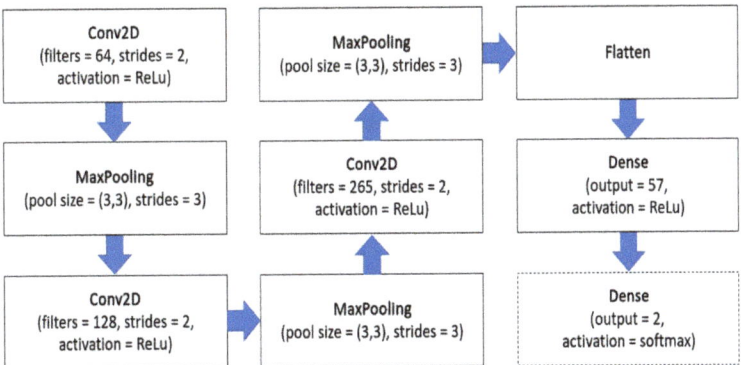

Figure 3. The architecture of the CNN used in the research. In dashed lines, the added Dense network was in solely a CNN-based approach.

The approach based on solely CNN both for features extraction and for classification had one change in the architecture. In this case, the next dense layer with the softmax activation function (presented in Figure 3 in dashed line) was added. It enabled the binary classification of COVID-19 positive or negative. This approach was trained, validated and tested using the above-mentioned training, validation and testing datasets, respectively. The training parameters were: 50 epochs, a learning rate equal to 0.00001 and a loss function set to SparseCategoricalCrossentropy.

4. Results

Since the hospital data represent two classes (COVID-19 positive and healthy), the problem of the disease diagnostics can be treated as a binary classification. In this research, the confusion matrices were used in order to evaluate and compare the ML-based methods. Four measures were defined, as follows:

- TP—true positives—COVID-19-infected patients classified as sick;
- FP—false positives—healthy patient images classified as COVID-19 infected;
- FN—false negatives—COVID-19-infected patients classified as healthy;
- TN—true negatives—healthy patients classified as healthy.

Each model in the research was evaluated using accuracy (Equation (1)), precision (Equation (2)), recall (Equation (3)) and F1-score (Equation (4)), which use the abovementioned measures of TP, FP, FN and TN.

$$\text{Acc} = \frac{TP + TN}{TP + TN + FP + FN},\tag{1}$$

$$\text{Precision} = \frac{TP}{TP + FP},\tag{2}$$

$$\text{Recall} = \frac{TP}{TP + FN},\tag{3}$$

$$\text{F1-score} = \frac{2 \cdot \text{Precision} \cdot \text{Recall}}{\text{Precision} + \text{Recall}},\tag{4}$$

All experiments were performed using a Tesla with GPU support. As a result of its enormous computing power, low price, relatively low demand for electricity and the CUDA environment support, Tesla systems have become an attractive alternative to traditional high-power computing systems, such as CPU clusters and supercomputers. This kind of device can be extremely helpful in image processing and also in medicine diagnostics.

The obtained results from all the experiments are provided in Table 1. All the evaluated metrics are given: accuracy, precision, recall and F1-score. The approach using the CNN both for features extraction and for classification provided the less promising results. Two examined classifiers provided the highest results: XGBoost and LightGBM, with accuracy = 1.0, precision = 1.0, recall = 1.0 and F1-score = 1.0. For selecting the optimal classifier for the presented solution, the computational time for both classifiers, namely the training time and prediction time for a single image, was compared. It was decided to use this parameter for optimization because the goal was to provide a light, sustainable and eco-friendly solution. For XGBoost, the average training time was equal to 242 ms, and the prediction time for a single image was above 11ms. For LightGBM, those times were 132 ms and less than 2 ms, respectively. That is why LightGBM is marked in bold in Table 1.

Table 1. Obtained results: accuracy, precision, recall and F1-score for all experiments.

F. Extractor	Classifier	Accuracy	Precision	Recall	F1-Score
CNN	CNN	0.86	0.75	1.00	0.86
CNN	XGBoost	1.00	1.00	1.00	1.00
CNN	Random Forest	0.91	0.86	1.00	0.92
CNN	LightGBM	1.00	1.00	1.00	1.00
CNN	CatBoost	0.91	0.86	1.00	0.92

One could ask 'what makes LightGBM faster than XGBoost?'. The following are the features of LightGBM that affect its effectiveness and the mathematics (Equation (5)) behind LightGBM that allow one to understand the answer to this question [32,33].

$$V_j(d) = \frac{1}{n}\tag{5}$$

where $A_l = \{x_i \in A : x_{ij} \leq d\}$, $A_r = \{x_i \in A : x_{ij} > d\}$, $B_l = \{x_i \in B : x_{ij} \leq d\}$, $B_r = \{x_i \in B : x_{ij} > d\}$, d is the point in the data where the split is calculated to find the optimal gain in variance and the coefficient $\frac{1-a}{b}$ is used to normalize the sum of the gradients over B back to the size of A^C.

LightGBM produces trees and finds the leaves with the greatest variance to perform division with the use of leaf-sage techniques. LightGBM achieves the optimal number of leaves in the trees and uses the minimum amount of data in the tree.

5. Discussion

ML methods can be valuable tool for COVID-19 diagnosis. ML-based methods cannot replace an experienced medical doctor in the final diagnosis, but they help significantly in the process, relieving the burden on health care and improving the diagnostic process. Screening with X-ray images is less expensive and faster than PCR testing [34]. This is one of the reasons why it is worth developing ML-based techniques to assist specialists in diagnostics.

In [35], the authors paid particular attention to the explainability AI (xAI), as it is essential in clinical applications. Explainable approaches increase the confidence and trust of the medical community in AI-based methods. They noted that X-ray imaging was not a method of choice when diagnosing COVID-19. However, the changes visible in the X-ray images of the lungs allow for the detection of pathological changes at an early stage of their development. For this reason, the authors indicated the usefulness of models supporting radiologists in their work and improving the decision-making process. The dataset of X-ray images used by the authors contained nearly 900 X-ray images of both COVID-19 patients and healthy patients, which was a significantly bigger dataset than that presented in this paper. Therefore, it could learn a wider range of differences between the images. In this work, the authors used pre-trained networks (ResNet-18 and DenseNet-121) to perform image classification with the best AUC score of 0.81. The sensitivity and specificity results obtained by authors were significantly lower than ours, however, which may be caused by dataset size differences. The model proposed in this research is fast, efficient and does not require high computing power; thus, it can be used in ordinary computers in hospital laboratories. The presented model obtained satisfactory results of evaluation metrics, which confirm its accuracy. These results are comparable and potentially better than those reported in the state-of-the-art review (Section 2). Some detailed results provided in the literature are presented in Table 2. However, our concern remains on the small number of original images that formed the basis of the database used. We believe that the method of data augmentation used may introduce bias; however, with such a small amount of data, this step was necessary. We believe that this is an aspect that could be improved in the course of further cooperation with hospitals that would provide more learning data.

Table 2. Results compared to other state-of-the-art methods, namely accuracy, precision, recall, F1-score and AUC. The results not provided by the authors are marked with '-'.

Authors	Method	Acc.	Prec.	Rec.	F1	AUC
Rajagopal [27]	CNN + SVM	0.95	0.95	0.95	0.96	-
Júnior et al. [30]	VGG19 + XGBoost	0.99	0.99	0.99	0.99	-
Nasari et al. [29]	DenseNet169 + XGBoost	0.98	0.98	0.92	0.97	-
Ezzoddin et al. [36]	DenseNet169 + LightGBM	0.99	0.99	1.00	0.99	-
Laeli et al. [28]	CNN + RF	0.99	-	-	-	0.99
Proposed	CNN + LightGBM	1.00	1.00	1.00	1.00	1.00

Table 2 presents numerous approaches providing comparable results. It is essential to mention that some of them are based on very complex architectures, use an extremely big number of training parameters, need excessive computational power and require long training. However, we decided to use fewer than 60 features and a light, fast classifier in our approach. Thus, the approach proposed in this paper is lightweight, efficient and fast. In the literature, we can observe very complex and resource-consuming approaches (such as COVID-Net, as proposed in [37], or ResNet, as implemented in [38]). It is worth emphasizing that the proposed solution is lighter but still equally or more efficient. Unfortunately, it is very difficult to compare the eco-friendliness of different computing-based diagnostic approaches, as it is not customary to provide such information in scientific publications. Hopefully, in the near future, the sustainability of the proposed methods will become more significant for researchers and editors.

We are also aware that there are some future improvements required for the presented model. It is necessary to validate the model on a larger, different dataset. X-ray images made with the use of various equipment exhibit different features, which may be an obstacle to the universality of the presented model. It is worth checking how the model performs on a new set of data from the same hospital and, alternatively, on a set from a different source. Likely, the additional pre-processing can help to make all samples uniform. Another potential extension of this work is providing the xAI. Its main aim is not only giving the classification but also providing an explanation of why such a decision was made by a ML-based method. Implementing the xAI can allow radiologist doctors to evaluate the model and verify whether it makes the decisions based on real COVID-19 lesions.

Author Contributions: Conceptualization, A.G., M.T. and A.M.; methodology, A.G.; software, M.T.; validation, A.M., Z.S. and S.M.K.; formal analysis, M.W.; investigation, A.M. and S.M.K.; resources, Z.S. and A.H.; data curation, M.W. and A.H.; writing—original draft preparation, S.M.K.; writing—review and editing, A.G.; visualization, M.T.; supervision, M.W.; project administration, A.G.; funding acquisition, A.G and A.M. All authors have read and agreed to the published version of the manuscript.

Funding: This research was funded by Bydgoszcz University of Science and Technology grant number DNM 32/2022. Part of this research was supported by the National Centre for Research and Development of Poland (Narodowe Centrum Badań i rozwoju, NCBR) with project number POWR.03.02.00-00-I019/16-00.

Institutional Review Board Statement: The project was approved by the Ethics Committee of the Nicolaus Copernicus University in Toruń Collegium Medicum in Bydgoszcz (decision no. KB 454/2022.)

Informed Consent Statement: Not applicable.

Data Availability Statement: The data used in the research in a raw, anonymized form are available at https://github.com/UTP-WTIiE/Xray_data.git (accessed on 2 August 2022).

Conflicts of Interest: The authors declare no conflict of interest.

References

1. Zheng, J. SARS-CoV-2: An Emerging Coronavirus that Causes a Global Threat. *Int. J. Biol. Sci.* **2020**, *16*, 1678–1685. [CrossRef] [PubMed]
2. Tahamtan, A.; Ardebili, A. Real-time RT-PCR in COVID-19 detection: Issues affecting the results. *Expert Rev. Mol. Diagn.* **2020**, *20*, 453–454. [CrossRef] [PubMed]
3. Pang, L.; Liu, S.; Zhang, X.; Tian, T.; Zhao, Z. Transmission Dynamics and Control Strategies of COVID-19 in Wuhan, China. *J. Biol. Syst.* **2020**, *28*, 543–560. [CrossRef]
4. Momeny, M.; Neshat, A.A.; Hussain, M.A.; Kia, S.; Marhamati, M.; Jahanbakhshi, A.; Hamarneh, G. Learning-to-augment strategy using noisy and denoised data: Improving generalizability of deep CNN for the detection of COVID-19 in X-ray images. *Comput. Biol. Med.* **2021**, *136*, 104704. [CrossRef]
5. Kassania, S.H.; Kassanib, P.H.; Wesolowskic, M.J.; Schneidera, K.A.; Detersa, R. Automatic Detection of Coronavirus Disease (COVID-19) in X-ray and CT Images: A Machine Learning Based Approach. *Biocybern. Biomed. Eng.* **2021**, *41*, 867–879. [CrossRef]
6. Jain, G.; Mittal, D.; Thakur, D.; Mittal, M.K. A deep learning approach to detect Covid-19 coronavirus with X-ray images. *Biocybern. Biomed. Eng.* **2020**, *40*, 1391–1405. [CrossRef]
7. Khan, S.H.; Sohail, A.; Khan, A.; Hassan, M.; Lee, Y.S.; Alam, J.; Basit, A.; Zubair, S. COVID-19 detection in chest X-ray images using deep boosted hybrid learning. *Comput. Biol. Med.* **2021**, *137*, 104816. [CrossRef]
8. Tahir, A.M.; Chowdhury, M.E.; Khandakar, A.; Rahman, T.; Qiblawey, Y.; Khurshid, U.; Kiranyaz, S.; Ibtehaz, N.; Rahman, M.S.; Al-Maadeed, S.; et al. COVID-19 infection localization and severity grading from chest X-ray images. *Comput. Biol. Med.* **2021**, *139*, 105002. [CrossRef]
9. Brunese, L.; Mercaldo, F.; Reginelli, A.; Santone, A. Explainable Deep Learning for Pulmonary Disease and Coronavirus COVID-19 Detection from X-rays. *Comput. Methods Programs Biomed.* **2020**, *196*, 105608. [CrossRef]

10. Chakraborty, S.; Murali, B.; Mitra, A.K. An Efficient Deep Learning Model to Detect COVID-19 Using Chest X-ray Images. *Int. J. Environ. Res. Public Health* **2022**, *19*, 2013. [CrossRef]
11. Civit-Masot, J.; Luna-Perejón, F.; Domínguez Morales, M.; Civit, A. Deep Learning System for COVID-19 Diagnosis Aid Using X-ray Pulmonary Images. *Appl. Sci.* **2020**, *10*, 4640. [CrossRef]
12. Ayesha, S.; Yu, Z.; Nutini, A. COVID-19 Variants and Transfer Learning for the Emerging Stringency Indices. *Neural Process. Lett.* **2022**, 1–10. [CrossRef]
13. Ahamad, M.M.; Aktar, S.; Rashed-Al-Mahfuz, M.; Uddin, S.; Liò, P.; Xu, H.; Summers, M.A.; Quinn, J.M.W.; Moni, M.A. A machine learning model to identify early stage symptoms of SARS-Cov-2 infected patients. *Expert Syst. Appl.* **2020**, *160*, 113661. [CrossRef] [PubMed]
14. Kannan, S.; Subbaram, K.; Ali, S.; Kannan, H. The role of artificial intelligence and machine learning techniques: Race for covid-19 vaccine. *Arch. Clin. Infect. Dis.* **2020**, *15*, e103232. [CrossRef]
15. EC. On Artificial Intelligence—A European Approach to Excellence and Trusty. Available online: https://ec.europa.eu/info/sites/default/files/commission-white-paper-artificial-intelligence-feb2020_en.pdf/ (accessed on 2 July 2022).
16. Schwartz, R.; Dodge, J.; Smith, N.A.; Etzioni, O. Green ai. *Commun. ACM* **2020**, *63*, 54–63. [CrossRef]
17. Yigitcanlar, T. Greening the artificial intelligence for a sustainable planet: An editorial commentary. *Sustainability* **2021**, *13*, 13508. [CrossRef]
18. Lenherr, N.; Pawlitzek, R.; Michel, B. New universal sustainability metrics to assess edge intelligence. *Sustain. Comput. Inform. Syst.* **2021**, *31*, 100580. [CrossRef]
19. Giełczyk, A.; Marciniak, A.; Tarczewska, M.; Lutowski, Z. Pre-processing methods in chest X-ray image classification. *PLoS ONE* **2022**, *17*, e0265949. [CrossRef]
20. Hasan, M.J.; Alom, M.S.; Ali, M.S. Deep learning based detection and segmentation of COVID-19 & pneumonia on chest X-ray image. In Proceedings of the 2021 International Conference on Information and Communication Technology for Sustainable Development (ICICT4SD), Dhaka, Bangladesh, 27–28 February 2021; IEEE: Piscataway, NJ, USA, 2021; pp. 210–214.
21. Munusamy, H.; Muthukumar, K.J.; Gnanaprakasam, S.; Shanmugakani, T.R.; Sekar, A. FractalCovNet architecture for COVID-19 chest X-ray image classification and CT-scan image segmentation. *Biocybern. Biomed. Eng.* **2021**, *41*, 1025–1038. [CrossRef]
22. Alimbekov, R.; Vassilenko, I.; Turlassov, A. Lung Segmentation Library. Available online: https://github.com/alimbekovKZ/lungs_segmentation/ (accessed on 15 May 2022).
23. Rajagopal, R. Comparative analysis of COVID-19 X-ray images classification using convolutional neural network, transfer learning, and machine learning classifiers using deep features. *Pattern Recognit. Image Anal.* **2021**, *31*, 313–322. [CrossRef]
24. Laeli, A.R.; Rustam, Z.; Pandelaki, J. Tuberculosis Detection based on Chest X-rays using Ensemble Method with CNN Feature Extraction. In Proceedings of the 2021 International Conference on Decision Aid Sciences and Application (DASA), Sakheer, Bahrain, 7–8 December 2021; IEEE: Piscataway, NJ, USA, 2021; pp. 682–686.
25. Chen, T.; Guestrin, C. Xgboost: A scalable tree boosting system. In Proceedings of the 22nd ACM SIGKDD International Conference on Knowledge Discovery and Data Mining, San Francisco, CA, USA, 13–17 August 2016; Association for Computing Machinery: New York, NY, USA, 2016; pp. 785–794.
26. Breiman, L. Bagging predictors. *Mach. Learn.* **1996**, *24*, 123–140. [CrossRef]
27. Ke, G.; Meng, Q.; Finley, T.; Wang, T.; Chen, W.; Ma, W.; Ye, Q.; Liu, T. Lightgbm: A highly efficient gradient boosting decision tree. In Proceedings of the Advances in Neural Information Processing Systems, Long Beach, CA, USA, 4–9 December 2017; Volume 30.
28. Prokhorenkova, L.; Gusev, G.; Vorobev, A.; Dorogush, A.V.; Gulin, A. CatBoost: Unbiased boosting with categorical features. In Proceedings of the Advances in Neural Information Processing Systems, Montreal, QC, Canada, 3–8 December 2018; Volume 31.
29. Nasiri, H.; Hasani, S. Automated detection of COVID-19 cases from chest X-ray images using deep neural network and XGBoost. *Radiography* **2022**, *28*, 732–738. [CrossRef] [PubMed]
30. Júnior, D.A.D.; da Cruz, L.B.; Diniz, J.O.B.; da Silva, G.L.F.; Junior, G.B.; Silva, A.C.; de Paiva, A.C.; Nunes, R.A.; Gattass, M. Automatic method for classifying COVID-19 patients based on chest X-ray images, using deep features and PSO-optimized XGBoost. *Expert Syst. Appl.* **2021**, *183*, 115452. [CrossRef] [PubMed]
31. Jawahar, M.; Prassanna, J.; Ravi, V.; Anbarasi, L.J.; Jasmine, S.G.; Manikandan, R.; Sekaran, R.; Kannan, S. Computer-aided diagnosis of COVID-19 from chest X-ray images using histogram-oriented gradient features and Random Forest classifier. *Multimed. Tools Appl.* **2022**, 1–18. [CrossRef] [PubMed]
32. Machado, M.R.; Karray, S.; Sousa, I.T.D. LightGBM: An effective decision tree gradient boosting method to predict customer loyalty in the finance industry. In Proceedings of the 14th International Conference Science and Education, Toronto, ON, Canada, 19–21 September 2019.
33. Misshuari, I.W.; Herdiana, R.; Farikhin, A.; Saputra, J. Factors that Affect Customer Credit Payments During COVID-19 Pandemic: An Application of Light Gradient Boosting Machine (LightGBM) and Classification and Regression Tree (CART). In Proceedings of the 11th Annual International Conference on Industrial Engineering and Operations Management, Singapore, 7–11 March 2021.
34. Nikolaou, V.; Massaro, S.; Fakhimi, M.; Stergioulas, L.; Garn, W. COVID-19 diagnosis from chest x-rays: Developing a simple, fast, and accurate neural network. *Health Inf. Sci. Syst.* **2021**, *9*, 1–11. [CrossRef]
35. Barbano, C.A.; Tartaglione, E.; Berzovini, C.; Calandri, M.; Grangetto, M. A two-step explainable approach for COVID-19 computer-aided diagnosis from chest x-ray images. *arXiv* **2021**, arXiv:2101.10223.

36. Ezzoddin, M.; Nasiri, H.; Dorrigiv, M. Diagnosis of COVID-19 Cases from Chest X-ray Images Using Deep Neural Network and LightGBM. In Proceedings of the 2022 International Conference on Machine Vision and Image Processing (MVIP), Ahvaz, Iran, 23–24 February 2022; IEEE: Piscataway, NJ, USA, 2022; pp. 1–7.
37. Wang, L.; Lin, Z.Q.; Wong, A. Covid-net: A tailored deep convolutional neural network design for detection of covid-19 cases from chest x-ray images. *Sci. Rep.* **2020**, *10*, 19549. [CrossRef] [PubMed]
38. Rajpal, S.; Lakhyani, N.; Singh, A.K.; Kohli, R.; Kumar, N. Using handpicked features in conjunction with ResNet-50 for improved detection of COVID-19 from chest X-ray images. *Chaos Solitons Fractals* **2021**, *145*, 110749. [CrossRef]

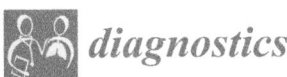

Study Protocol

The Efficacy of Trabecular Titanium Cages to Induce Reparative Bone Activity after Lumbar Arthrodesis Studied through the 18f-Naf PET/CT Scan: Observational Clinical In-Vivo Study

Fabio Cofano [1,2], Daniele Armocida [3,*], Livia Ruffini [4], Maura Scarlattei [4], Giorgio Baldari [4], Giuseppe Di Perna [1], Giulia Pilloni [5], Francesco Zenga [1], Elena Ballante [6,7], Diego Garbossa [1] and Fulvio Tartara [8]

1. Neurosurgery Unit, Department of Neuroscience, University of Turin, 10124 Turin, Italy
2. Spine Surgery Unit, Humanitas Gradenigo, 10153 Turin, Italy
3. Neurosurgery Unit, Department of Human Neuroscience, Sapienza Università of Rome, 00185 Rome, Italy
4. Nuclear Medicine Unit, University Hospital of Parma, 43100 Parma, Italy
5. Neurosurgery Unit ASST Fatebenefratelli Sacco, 20121 Milan, Italy
6. BioData Science Center, IRCCS Mondino Foundation, 27100 Pavia, Italy
7. Department of Mathematics, University of Pavia, 27100 Pavia, Italy
8. Neurosurgery Unit, ICCS Città Studi, 20131 Milan, Italy
* Correspondence: danielearmocida@yahoo.it; Tel.: +39-39-3287-4496

Abstract: *Background:* Titanium trabecular cages (TTCs) are emerging implants designed to achieve immediate and long-term spinal fixation with early osseointegration. However, a clear radiological and clinical demonstration of their efficacy has not yet been obtained. The purpose of this study was to evaluate the reactive bone activity of adjacent plates after insertion of custom-made titanium trabecular cages for the lumbar interbody with positron emission tomography (PET)/computed tomography (CT) 18F sodium fluoride (18F-NaF). *Methods:* This was an observational clinical study that included patients who underwent surgery for degenerative disease with lumbar interbody fusion performed with custom-made TTCs. Data related to the metabolic-reparative reaction following the surgery and its relationship with clinical follow-up from PET/CT performed at different weeks were evaluated. PET/CTs provided reliable data, such as areas showing abnormally high increases in uptake using a volumetric region of interest (VOI) comprising the upper (UP) and lower (DOWN) limits of the cage. *Results:* A total of 15 patients was selected for PET examination. Timing of PET/CTs ranged from one week to a maximum of 100 weeks after surgery. The analysis showed a negative correlation between the variables SUVmaxDOWN/time (r = −0.48, p = 0.04), ratio-DOWN/time (r = −0.53, p = 0.02), and ratio-MEAN/time (r = −0.5, p = 0.03). Shapiro–Wilk normality tests showed significant results for the variables ratio-DOWN (p = 0.002), ratio-UP (0.013), and ratio-MEAN (0.002). *Conclusions:* 18F-NaF PET/CT has proven to be a reliable tool for investigating the metabolic-reparative reaction following implantation of TTCs, demonstrating radiologically how this type of cage can induce reparative osteoblastic activity at the level of the vertebral endplate surface. This study further confirms how electron-beam melting (EBM)-molded titanium trabecular cages represent a promising material for reducing hardware complication rates and promoting fusion.

Keywords: lumbar arthrodesis; titanium trabecular cages

1. Introduction

Vertebral fusion is the most common and effective intervention for the treatment of lumbar disc degeneration [1], and the introduction of minimally-invasive techniques has gained popularity, lowering surgery-related traumatic insult [2,3]. However, the occurrence of failed-back-surgery syndrome after arthrodesis still remains a problem in 5% to 15% of lumbar-spine-fusion cases [4]. To reduce the rate of failure, scientists have, in recent decades, moved to investigating new concepts concerning techniques and instrumentation. Further, the evaluation of the sagittal balance and pelvic parameters has assumed increasing value becoming an element of analysis and discussion. High pelvic incidence-lumbar-lordosis mismatch has been shown to be associated with adjacent segment degeneration, increased risk of revision surgery, and residual or worsened postoperative symptoms [5–7]. For these reasons, the restoration and long-term preservation of segment lordosis (SL) is now considered one of the major goals of vertebral-fusion procedures. The use of interbody fusion with intersomatic cages is the most widely used and effective method to increase and correct SL [8]. Restoration of intervertebral-disc lordosis and height with iperlordotic-cage insertion produces a significant axial load [9] on the vertebral endplate, enhancing sagittal correction [8].

The most frequent complication of interbody fusion is the cage subsidence within vertebral endplates with consequent reduction of disc height and loss of segmental lordotic correction [9,10]. This also results in a reduced mechanical stability leading to pseudoarthrosis and poorer clinical outcomes. Time of subsidence has been reported as varying from some weeks to several months and many factors can contribute to its occurrence, including bone quality, cage morphology, and materials [11–13]. Therefore, the need to generate stable lordotic corrections has also brought attention to the use of materials able to guarantee primary stability and rapid biological-integration capacity. In this regard trabecular metal cages present remarkable aspects of interest [14].

Trabecular titanium is emerging as a valuable candidate to achieve immediate and long-term spinal correction and stability through effective early osteo-integration.

Recent in vitro studies [15,16] demonstrated that trabecular titanium is a biocompatible surface able to induce mesenchymal stem cell adhesion, proliferation, and differentiation towards the osteogenic lineage, even without the addition of osteogenic factors [17]. Trabecular titanium had a sufficient roughness to allow cell attachment, migration, and proliferation suggesting interesting biological behaviors of the scaffold. It appears very likely that the highly porous contact area between the cage and the vertebral endplates assures an optimal ground for bone ingrowth [18,19].

However, in vivo clinical studies directly demonstrating the effectiveness of the osteo-integrative activity of these materials and their role in preventing subsidence are still lacking. Fluorine-18-sodium fluoride (F-NaF) PET/CT is a relatively new high-resolution bone imaging technique that measures turnover. 18F-NaF PET has previously been shown to correlate with histomorphometric parameters [20] and the osteo-integration capacity of different materials and their use has been increasingly used to accurately assess the images and provide awareness of the normal distribution and major artifacts in imaging [21]. This study aimed to evaluate reactive adjacent endplate bony activity after trabecular titanium cage (TTC) placement in order to assess, in vivo, the potential for implant osteo-integration through the analysis of data extracted from positron-emission tomography/computed tomography (PET/CT) obtained at varying times after surgery using 18F-sodium fluoride (18F-NaF), a tracer chemically absorbed into hydroxyapatite in the bone matrix by osteoblasts able to reflect bone re-modeling.

2. Materials and Methods

This was an observational study analyzing prospectively collected data of consecutive patients undergoing single- or multi-level lumbar interbody fusion surgery using TTC for degenerative diseases of the lumbar spine who underwent additional imaging examination with 18F-NaF PET/CT for diagnostic evaluation in cases of persistent/recurrent low back pain to investigate the reactive bone activity of the vertebral endplates adjacent to the implanted cage, where standard imaging (MRI or CT) was inconclusive and showed no common signs of cage failure. Patients were recruited over a period from March 2017 to June 2019. The study was then approved by the ethics committee at our institution (Numb. 15092, 8 April 2019).

Due to the cost of the diagnostic procedure, recruitment stopped when the maximum number of patients approved by the committee was reached. Written informed consent was obtained from each patient prior to their enrolment in the study.

2.1. Inclusion and Exclusion Criteria

All consecutive patients scheduled for lumbar-spinal-fixation surgery were eligible for this study.

Patients were included in the study if they underwent a lumbar-spine stabilization procedure in the absence of comorbidities and bone disease. Patients were included if, in the postoperative period, they could undergo and sustain an appropriated follow-up program. Patients evaluated had each had implanted the same type of custom-made TTC: TTCs modeled by CAD/CAM technology by means of electron-beam melting (EBM) technology (MT Ortho s.r.l., Aci Sant'Antonio, CT, Italy) for lumbar interbody fusion performed through a lateral transpsoas (XLIF) and/or anterior retroperitoneal (ALIF) approach. Other inclusion criteria were: a previous surgery for degenerative disease with lumbar or lumbosacral interbody fusion performed with TTCs during the investigation period, spontaneous acceptance and informed consent for execution of 18F-NaF PET/CT, absence of comorbidities that contraindicate the execution of the examination, and full availability to achieve at least one year of follow-up.

Exclusion criteria were: (1) patients aged below 16 years; (2) those who were undergoing scoliosis surgery; (3) patients who had a previous surgical history entailing laminectomy or the application of osteosynthesis material at the target levels; (4) patients with incomplete or incorrect data on clinical, radiological, surgical, or follow-up records; (5) patients with ongoing infectious, traumatic, or oncological spinal diseases; and (6) patients with diagnosed osteoporosis (a T-score less than -2.5 on dual-energy X-ray absorptiometry bone densitometry measurements).

All patients underwent a general medical, neurological, and oncologic evaluation at admission. For all the included patients, we recorded patient-related variables such as sex, age, timing of surgery and PET/CT scan, type of surgery, clinical status before and after surgery with the Oswestry Disability Index (ODI) and NRS score for back pain with at least one year follow-up, and PET/CT data (see below the imaging protocol paragraph). Each patient underwent only one PET examination to limit exposure to radioisotopes.

18F-NaF PET/CT was used in the enrolled patients for clinical assessment in cases of persistent/recurrent back pain to investigate reactive bony activity of the vertebral endplates adjacent to implanted porous titanium cage, when standard imaging (MRI or CT) was inconclusive and did not show common signs of cage subsidence.

2.2. Interbody Implants and Surgery

All patients underwent interbody fusion with TTCs via the lateral transpsoas or anterior retroperitoneal approach. After radical discectomy and careful preparation of the vertebral endplates, intervertebral cages (MT Ortho s.r.l., Aci Sant'Antonio, CT, Italy) (Figure 1), were inserted into the disc space. The upper and lower vertebrae were fixed using transpedicular screws connected to titanium rods for primary stabilization. The choice of posterior instrumentation with percutaneous or open technique was made according to the need for open decompression or in degenerative, multilevel coronal misalignment. No anterior plates were used with anterior approaches. The specific design features, such as anterior height, individual lordosis correction angle, and footprint are provided by the medical prescriber; moreover, each device is designed exclusively for specific patient since the upper and lower cage surfaces match perfectly with the respective endplate morphology. The shape of the cage was designed in order to restore local lordosis and to respect the harmony of individual spino-pelvic parameters and the pelvic incidence, pelvic tilt, and lumbar lordosis [20,21]. Neuromonitoring was always used during lateral approaches [22]. All interventions were performed by a single surgeon (F.T.) with extensive experience in anterior and lateral approaches.

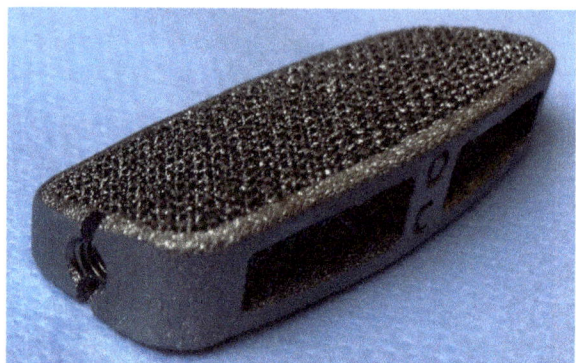

Figure 1. Custom-made trabecular titanium cage for XLIF surgery.

2.3. 18F-NaF PET/CT Imaging Protocol

The preoperative 18F-NaF PET/CT scan was performed in accordance to the European Association of Nuclear Medicine (EANM) guidelines for bone imaging [23] and the Society of Nuclear Medicine (SNM) practice guidelines for 18F-NaF PET/CT bone scan 1.0. [24] Patients were well hydrated before the study and during the uptake time to enhance renal excretion, reducing radiation exposure. Metal objects were removed to prevent attenuation artifacts. PET/CT images were acquired on a 3D integrated PET/CT system Discovery IQ (GE Healthcare, Milwaukee, WI, USA).

Dynamic PET images of the target vertebral region were acquired in list mode for 30 min (frames/time 6×5 s, 3×10 s, 9×60 s, 10×120 s) immediately after i.v. injection of 18F-NaF (1.5–3.7 mbq /kg) diluted in 3–5 mL of saline as a 60 s bolus and flushed with saline. Whole-body PET/CT (WB-PET/CT) was acquired in supine position 60 min after tracer injection. Patients voided immediately prior to the scan to reduce bladder activity and were positioned supine on the tomographic bed with arms elevated over the head. WB-PET/CT protocol included a topogram to define the field of view (FOV) from the base of the skull to the pelvis, followed by a low-dose CT scan (120 kV, 140 mA, pitch 1, collimation 16×1.25) for attenuation correction and anatomical correlation, and a PET emission scan (3 min per bed position, diagonal FOV 70 cm, 512×512 matrix size). Acquired data were reconstructed by Q Clear (GE Healthcare), a Bayesian penalized-likelihood reconstruction algorithm (strength 350). Images were corrected for injected dose, tracer decay, patient body-weight, and attenuation using the low-dose CT scan. Late 18F-NaF PET/CT image of the site of cages was acquired 90 min after tracer injection.

2.4. Metabolic Parameters

Imaging review and analysis of attenuation-corrected PET and CT images were performed using an Advantage Workstation 4.4. (GE Healthcare, Milwaukee, WI, USA).

18F-NaF PET/CT scans were analyzed by three nuclear medicine physicians (M.S., L.R., and G.B.) who were blinded to patients' clinical history and differences between readers were resolved through consensus.

Areas with abnormally high uptake increases—focal, well-circumscribed, and clearly above the background reference area—were identified and contoured using a volumetric region of interest (VOI) encompassing the upper (UP) and lower (DOWN) cage limit (vertebral endplates).

Standardized uptake values (SUVs) were obtained by normalizing the 18F-NaF concentration in the bone region of interest for injected activity and body weight (SUV = kbq/mL × body weight (kg)/injected activity (mbq)) [25].

The maximum SUV value (SUVmax) as the hottest voxel within the VOI was calculated for the UP and DOWN VOIs (SUVmaxUP and SUVmaxDOWN) [26]. Mean values between SUVmaxUP and SUVmaxDOWN were evaluated and classified as M-SUV.

Uptake of both UP and DOWN VOIs, as well as the mean between them, were normalized (ratio-UP, ratio-DOWN, ratio-MEAN) relatively to 18F-NaF uptake (SUVmax) in the right hip bone, measured within a VOI placed on the normal-appearing bone, encompassing both the cortex and the marrow space, in order to obtain a baseline uptake of the patient and allow a reliable comparison among patients.

2.5. Size, Statistics, and a Potential Source of Bias

The study size was given by the selection of the inclusion criteria. As previously stated, we addressed no missing data because incomplete records were an exclusion criterion. The sample was analyzed with SPSS v18 (SPSS Inc., Released 2009, PASW Statistics for Windows, Version 18.0, Chicago, IL, USA) to outline potential correlations between the investigated variables. Comparisons between nominal variables were made with the chi-square test. The threshold of statistical significance was considered as $p < 0.05$.

As a first step only the most caudal level of fusion was analyzed in order to guarantee the independence of observations. The choice to include in this analysis the most caudal level was due to the greatest load borne. The correlation between time and all the considered variables was evaluated by a Pearson correlation analysis (Pearson coefficient and p-value of the related test are reported to evaluate the significance). Scatter plots were drawn to visualize the relationship with a regression line. Then all the dataset was analyzed with a mixed-effects model which can handle non-independent observations, and Shapiro–Wilk tests were performed on the variables to satisfy the normality assumption of the models. This model analyzes the influence of the variable time on the target variable, where the variable subject is considered as the random factor. Final models were fitted using the restricted maximum likelihood (REML) method and the general Satterthwaite approximation for the degrees of freedom.

3. Results

A total number of 38 patients underwent arthrodesis with EBM TTCs between March 2017 and June 2019. After selection with the previously described criteria, 15 selected cases (7 M, 8 F) underwent lumbar PET/CT with 18F-NaF. Descriptive data are summarized in Table 1. A total of 35 interbody fusions (26 XLIF, 9 ALIF) were performed in these patients. The most frequently treated level was L4-L5 (12/35). In the 35 patients, 18F-NaF PET/CTs were performed within 6 months of the surgical procedure. In four patients PET/CT examination was performed more than one year after surgery, despite radiological evidence of fusion, because of recurrent back pain revealing no complications involving the arthrodesis. No toxicity or adverse reactions to the tracer were reported by patients However, PET/CTs did not reveal any complication involving the arthrodesis. In one case, L3-L5 arthrodesis was followed by L5-S1 elongation two years later; the patient was submitted to PET/CT 11 weeks after L4-L5 surgery and 4 weeks after elongation.

All patients achieved fusion with clinical improvement of their back pain at the last follow-up when compared to the pre-op evaluation, and no subsidence or surgical revisions was reported, preserving the homogeneity of the sample and the interpretation of 18F-NaF PET data.

Study of Metabolic Results

Mean value of SUVmax was 20 ± 8.9 for the UP-VOI and 21.8 ± 9.6 for the DOWN-VOI.

The mean value of the ratio-UP was 1.4 ± 1.1 and of the ratio-DOWN was 1.6 ± 1.3. Mean follow-up time was 22.2 months (min/max 13/32). (Table 1). Fusion was achieved and registered in all the cases at one-year follow-up. Considering Pearson correlation, the analysis showed a negative correlation between the variables SUVmaxDOWN/time ($r = -0.48$, $p = 0.04$), ratio-DOWN/time ($r = -0.53$, $p = 0.02$), and ratio-MEAN/time ($r = -0.5$, $p = 0.03$). The p was not significant for the variables SUVmaxUP/time ($p = 0.15$), M-SUV/time ($p = 0.07$), or ratio-UP/time ($p = 0.058$) (Figure 2).

Table 1. Descriptive Data.

Patients	15 (7 M, 8 F)
Age (mean/min/max)	61/41/77
Levels	4 L1-L2 (11.5%) 6 L2-L3 (17.1%) 7 L3-L4 (20%) 12 L4-L5 (34.3%) 6 L5-S1 (17.1%)
Type of fusion	XLIF (26), ALIF (9)
Number of levels of surgery	4 Single level (26.7%) 6 Two levels (40%) 2 Three levels (13.3%) 2 Four levels (13.3%) 1 Five levels (6.7%)
Follow-up (mean/min/max)	22.2/13/32

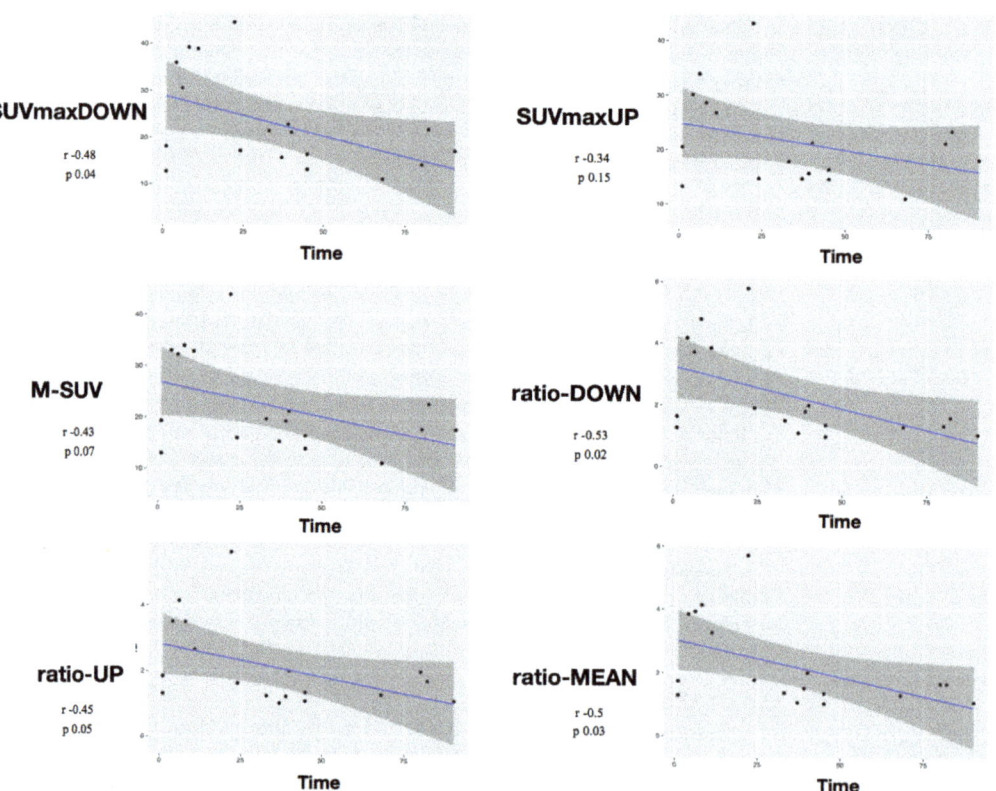

Figure 2. Pearson correlation analysis between all considered variables and time. Scatter plots were drawn to visualize the relationship with a regression line.

Shapiro–Wilk normality tests showed significant results considering the variables ratio-DOWN ($p = 0.002$), ratio-UP ($p = 0.01$), and ratio-MEAN ($p = 0.002$). The p was not significant considering as variables SUVmaxDOWN ($p = 0.05$), SUVmaxUP ($p = 0.93$), or M-SUV ($p = 0.33$) (Figure 3).

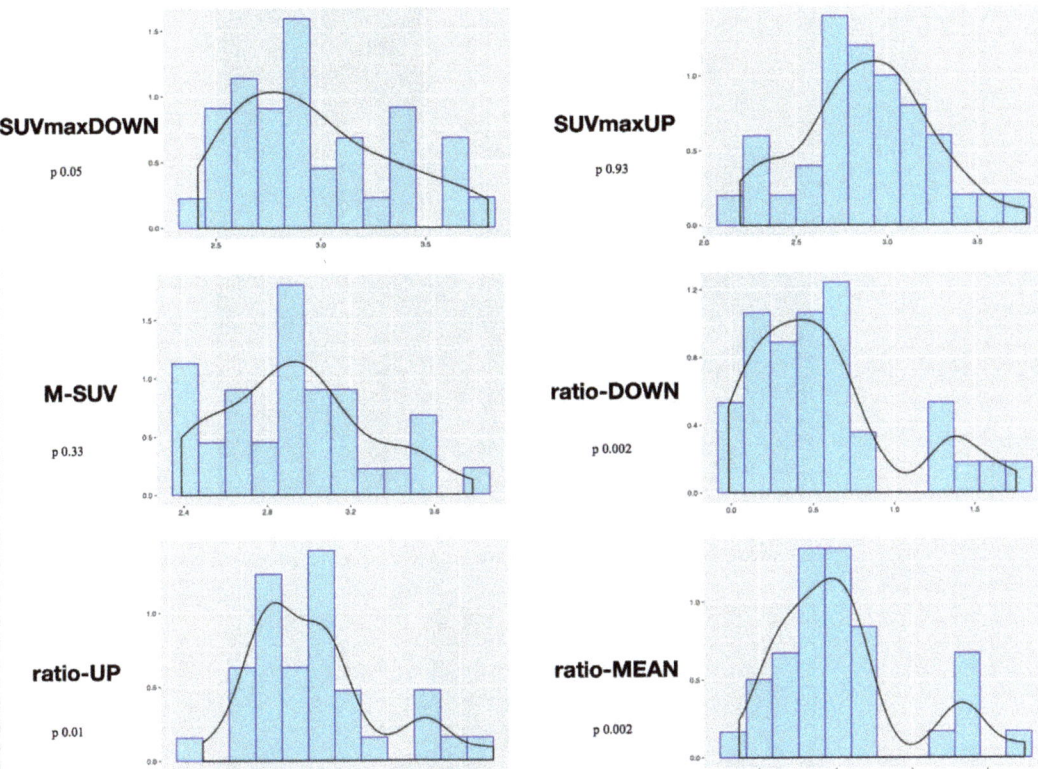

Figure 3. Mixed-effects model analysis with the considered variables and time.

4. Discussion

Trabecular titanium was developed to take advantage of its increased porosity and interconnectivity in order to enable greater bone growth and tissue differentiation [27]. The reason for its wide use is due to its biocompatibility, corrosion resistance, low density, and capacity for osteo-integration [28–31]. Early preclinical studies [15–17] on TTCs showed good adhesion and proliferation of mesenchymal cells on the surface of the scaffold [32,33], suggesting an effective cell-material interaction [15–17] with a favorable contribution to improved fusion.

In this study the use of 18F-NaF PET/CT provided some adjunctive information about the metabolic-reparative reaction following the implantation of an interbody fusion cage during clinical follow-up; PET/CT supports the evidence regarding the ability of the cage to reach effective early osteo-integration.(Figures 4 and 5) and provide some indications regarding the time required for the bone-remodeling process (the patients underwent PET examinations at different times and this has undoubtedly helped to give value to the final results).

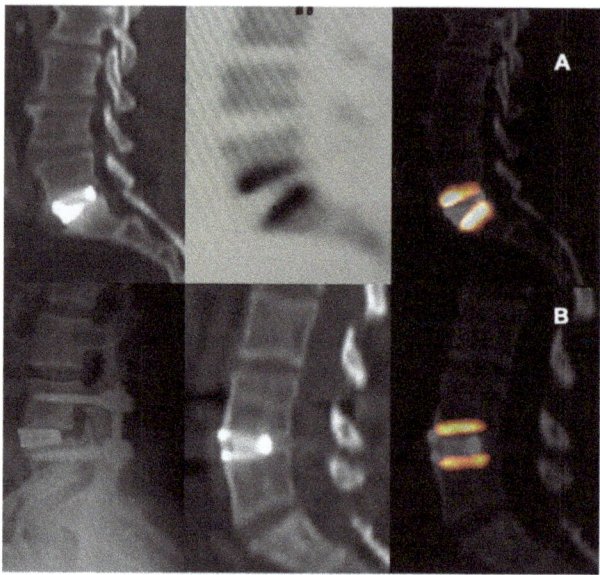

Figure 4. CT and PET images showing metabolic activity on vertebral plates after arthrodesis surgery with trabecular titanium cage. L5-S1 ALIF, 11 weeks (**A**); L4-L5 XLIF, 27 weeks (**B**).

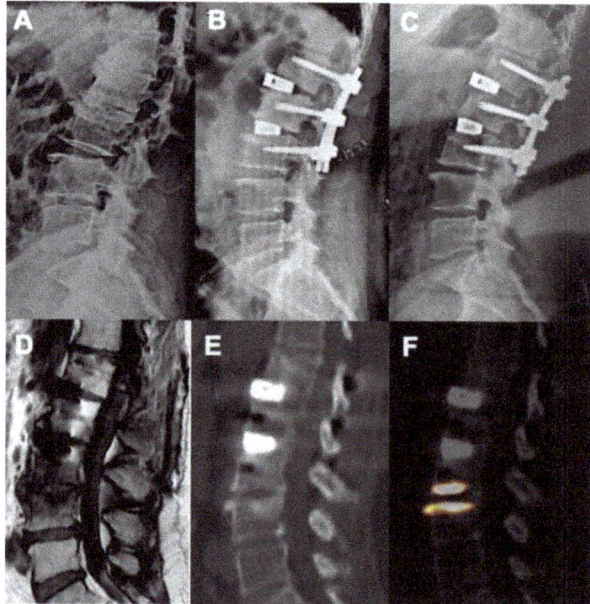

Figure 5. Pre-operative standing X-ray (**A**), immediate postoperative (**B**), and 58 weeks follow-up (**C**) showing good sagittal correction after L1-L2 and L2-L3 XLIF surgery. PET (**F**) and CT (**E**) images showed no activity at the level of the implanted vertebral plates suggesting a proper integration with the bone. Appearance of L3-L4 activity was related to the occurrence of degenerative junctional pathology as also shown by T1-weighted MRI sequences with Modic I signal (**D**).

The investigation was performed to obtain metabolic information related to surgical implant with regard to clinical status. Ratio values of upper and lower endplates, as well as mean ratio showed, in both the Pearson correlation and in Shapiro–Wilk normality tests, that an increase of regional blood flow and bone formation activity is registered after surgery for arthrodesis.

According to our results, tracer uptake was already visible in the first week after implantation. This first finding is probably related to the increase in blood flow after preparation of the vertebral endplate and to the consequent bone-cell activation at the contact surface. Therefore the metabolic activity, probably linked to the osteogenic activity, increases progressively until reaching a peak between approximately the 3rd and 4th month after surgery (Figures 2 and 3). This progressive increase in activity can be correlated, as supported by in vitro studies, to the migration, adhesion, and growth of cells from the vertebral bone tissue and to consequent osteoblastic activity with apposition of the bone matrix within the cage pores [34]. In the later stages, the metabolic hyperactivity on the vertebral endplates decreases progressively and tends to disappears around the 10th–12th month after surgery (Figures 2 and 3). This reduction may be the expression of a lower need for bone remodeling caused by sufficient acquired interbody fusion and stability [35,36]. The reparative phase could tend to run out after the formation of bone bridges between the cages and the vertebral plate. The growth of tissue inside the cage can be the basis for a real osteo-integration avoiding delayed subsidence and ensuring stability of the obtained correction.

Few studies have reported the use of 18F-NaF PET for clinical reasons after spinal fusion. Fischer et al. [37] investigated successful incorporation of cervical and lumbar cages after fusion with the use of PET/CT demonstrating that an unsuccessful fusion with residual stress and micro instability was characterized by increased 18F-NaF uptake [37] This is why some studies started reporting associations between tracer uptake and failed implant incorporations [38]. PET hyperactivity was described by Brans et al. [39] in patients with persisting symptoms after lumbar surgery and was connected to concomitant CT findings of subsidence. An increased uptake has also been registered in other studies of cases with screw-loosening with a specificity of 97.4% in patient-based analysis [40]. A relationship with painful pseudarthrosis was suggested by Peters et al. in a retrospective series of 36 patients, because after surgery 18F-NaF activity was reported to be significantly higher in patients with worse functional scores [41]. Abnormal foci of uptake appear to be related to the patient's source of pain and could be located at various sites involved in arthrodesis (cages, screws, rods, or bone grafts) helping surgeons to choose the best management and strategy if a surgical revision is considered mandatory [42,43].

In this series, implant stability and fusion were finally confirmed by radiological exams (X-rays of CT), helping us to adequately validate our results. As described by previous studies, the presence of pseudarthrosis, subsidence, or implants loosening could result in abnormal uptake, increasing over time and helping to discriminate between asymptomatic and symptomatic cases requiring revision [41–43]. According with our preliminary results [36], the use of custom-made TTCs is confirmed to represent a promising approach in order to achieve good stability promoting active osteo-integration and fusion, while minimizing subsidence rates.

We argue that customization for cages and the use of TTCs allows surgeons to take advantage of implant stability by maximizing the contact surface area, and also to plan appropriate SL restoration when necessary.

The innate osteo-inductive capability of the porous titanium scaffold has been suggested from these data. Cells were able to migrate and colonize the inner portions of the cages indicating that trabecular titanium represents a suitable material with appealing properties in terms of biological behavior. In addition, we can clinically confirm that the use of a fully porous device allows for an homogeneous biomechanical distribution of axial load—thus reducing the risks of subsidence of hollow cages filled with bone substitutes—and for the bone matrix to grow into the cage, rapidly stabilizing the implant, confirming what was shown in pre-clinical studies [34–37].

Zhang et al. [34] verified, at first, the satisfactory biomechanical properties of TTCs compared with standard solid cages in a finite-element analysis and McGilvray et al. also demonstrated a statistically significant range of motion of 3D printed TTCs compared with PEEK or porous PEEK coated with titanium [35].

In conclusion, 18F-NaF PET/CT proved to be a reliable tool to assess incorporation of spinal implants after surgery, providing some adjunctive confirmation about the metabolic-reparative reaction [44] following the implantation of a TTC.

Limitations and Further Studies

This is the first prospective study of the radiological demonstration of TTCs using PET/TC.

The main limitations of the study were the exiguity of the sample and the variability of the number of treated levels that empowered the clinical burden of the radiological analysis. In order to avoid unethical exposure of control patients to radioisotopes, there was no control group of standard titanium/PEEK cages. The inclusion of such a control group would also not have supported the aim of the study. PET studies were performed at different times after surgery but not at previously well-defined times. The different timings definitely contributed to the value of the statistical analysis and results. The correlation between data obtained with PET and the data obtained from in vitro experiments was largely based on abstract rational associations.

Among future perspectives, other than its already-described role in diagnosing symptomatic subsidence and implant failure or loosening, the use of 18F-NaF PET/CT could be of importance in the correct clinical diagnosis of adjacent-segment disease and especially in identifying symptomatic discs in the context of a multilevel degenerated spine, playing the part of the outdated spinal discography (Figure 5).

5. Conclusions

18F-NaF PET/CT proved to be a reliable tool for investigating the metabolic-reparative reaction following the implantation of an interbody fusion cage. Customization of cages and the use of TTCs allows surgeons to take advantage of implant stability by maximizing the contact surface area, and also, when necessary, to plan appropriate SL restoration. 18F-NaF PET/CT demonstrates that TTCs have a good capacity for induction, over time, of reparative osteoblastic activity at the vertebral endplate surface reaching a peak after 3–4 months, with metabolic activity later progressively decreasing until fusion is achieved, probably after 10–12 months.

This aspect was associated with stability and absence of subsidence at radiological follow-up, confirming that EBM-printed TTCs represent a promising material for reducing hardware complication rates and promoting fusion.

Author Contributions: Conceptualization and methodology, F.T.; software and formal analysis, E.B.; investigation, G.B., G.P. and F.Z.; writing—original draft preparation, F.C., G.D.P., L.R. and M.S.; writing—review and editing, D.A.; visualization, D.G.; project administration, coordination of the study group, and supervision: F.C., D.G. and F.T. All authors have read and agreed to the published version of the manuscript.

Funding: This research received no external funding.

Institutional Review Board Statement: The study was conducted in accordance with the Declaration of Helsinki, and approved by the Institutional Review Board (Azienda Ospedaliero-Universitaria di Parma) Number 15092, 8 April 2019.

Informed Consent Statement: Informed consent was obtained from all subjects involved in the study.

Data Availability Statement: Not applicable.

Conflicts of Interest: The authors declare no conflict of interest.

References

1. Andersson, G.B. Epidemiological features of chronic low-back pain. *Lancet* **1999**, *354*, 581–585. [CrossRef]
2. Mobbs, R.J.; Phan, K.; Malham, G.; Seex, K.; Rao, P.J. Lumbar interbody fusion: Techniques, indications and comparison of interbody fusion options including PLIF, TLIF, MI-TLIF, OLIF/ATP, LLIF and ALIF. *J. Spine Surg.* **2015**, *1*, 2–18. [CrossRef] [PubMed]
3. Mehren, C.; Mayer, H.M.; Siepe, C.; Grochulla, F.; Korge, A. The minimally invasive anterolateral approach to L2-5. *Oper. Orthop. Traumatol.* **2010**, *22*, 221–228. [CrossRef] [PubMed]
4. Chun, D.S.; Baker, K.C.; Hsu, W.K. Lumbar pseudarthrosis: A review of current diagnosis and treatment. *Neurosurg. Focus* **2015**, *39*, E10. [CrossRef]
5. Rothenfluh, D.A.; Mueller, D.A.; Rothenfluh, E.; Min, K. Pelvic incidencelumbar lordosis mismatch predisposes to adjacent segment disease after lumbar spinal fusion. *Eur. Spine J.* **2015**, *24*, 1251–1258. [CrossRef]
6. Matsumoto, T.; Okuda, S.; Maeno, T.; Yamashita, T.; Yamasaki, R.; Sugiura, T.; Iwasaki, M. Spinopelvic sagittal imbalance as a risk factor for adjacent-segment disease after single-segment posterior lumbar interbody fusion. *J. Neurosurg. Spine* **2017**, *26*, 435–440. [CrossRef]
7. Makino, T.; Kaito, T.; Fujiwara, H.; Honda, H.; Sakai, Y.; Takenaka, S.; Yoshikawa, H.; Yonenobu, K. Risk factors for poor patientreported quality of life outcomes after posterior lumbar interbody fusion: An analysis of two-year follow-up. *Spine* **2017**, *42*, 1502–1510. [CrossRef]
8. Uribe, J.S.; Smith, D.A.; Dakwar, E.; Baaj, A.A.; Mundis, G.M.; Turner, A.W.L.; Cornwall, G.B.; Akbarnia, B.A. Lordosis restoration after anterior longitudinal ligament release and placement of lateral hyperlordotic interbody cages during the minimally invasive lateral transpsoas approach: A radiographic study in cadavers. *J. Neurosurg. Spine* **2012**, *17*, 476–485. [CrossRef]
9. Beutler, W.J.; Peppelman, W.C., Jr. Anterior lumbar fusion with paired BAK standard and paired BAK Proximity cages: Subsidence incidence, subsidence factors, and clinical outcome. *Spine J.* **2003**, *3*, 289–293. [CrossRef]
10. Choi, J.Y.; Sung, K.H. Subsidence after anterior lumbar interbody fusion using paired stand-alone rectangular cages. *Eur. Spine J.* **2006**, *15*, 16–22. [CrossRef]
11. Le, T.V.; Baaj, A.A.; Dakwar, E.; Burkett, C.J.; Murray, G.; Smith, D.A.; Uribe, J.S. Subsidence of polyetheretherketone intervertebral cages in minimally invasive lateral retroperitoneal transpsoas lumbar interbody fusion. *Spine (Phila Pa 1976)* **2012**, *37*, 1268–1273. [CrossRef] [PubMed]
12. Marchi, L.; Abdala, N.; Oliveira, L.; Amaral, R.; Coutinho, E.; Pimenta, L. Radiographic and clinical evaluation of cage subsidence after stand-alone lateral interbody fusion. *J. Neurosurg. Spine* **2013**, *19*, 110–118. [CrossRef] [PubMed]
13. Armocida, D.; Pesce, A.; Cimatti, M.; Proietti, L.; Santoro, A.; Frati, A. Minimally invasive transforaminal lumbar interbody fusion using expandable cages: Increased risk of late postoperative subsidence without a real improvement of perioperative outcomes: A clinical monocentric study. *World Neurosurg.* **2021**, *156*, e57–e63. [CrossRef] [PubMed]
14. Warburton, A.; Girdler, S.J.; Mikhail, C.M.; Ahn, A.; Cho, S.K. Biomaterials in Spinal Implants: A Review. *Neurospine* **2019**, *4*, 101–110. [CrossRef]
15. Bari, E.; Tartara, F.; Cofano, F.; Di Perna, G.; Garbossa, D.; Perteghella, S.; Sorlini, M.; Mandracchia, D.; Giovannelli, L.; Gaetani, P.; et al. Freeze-dried secretome (lyosecretome) from mesenchymal stem/stromal cells promotes the osteoinductive and osteoconductive properties of titanium cages. *Int. J. Mol. Sci.* **2021**, *22*, 8445. [CrossRef]
16. Ragni, E.; Orfei, C.P.; Bidossi, A.; De Vecchi, E.; Francaviglia, N.; Romano, A.; Maestretti, G.; Tartara, F.; de Girolamo, L. Superior osteo-inductive and osteo-conductive properties of trabecular titanium vs. PEEK scaffolds on human mesenchymal stem cells: A proof of concept for the use of fusion cages. *Int. J. Mol. Sci.* **2021**, *22*, 2379. [CrossRef]
17. Caliogna, L.; Bina, V.; Botta, L.; Benazzo, F.M.; Medetti, M.; Maestretti, G.; Mosconi, M.; Cofano, F.; Tartara, F.; Gastaldi, G. Osteogenic potential of human adipose derived stem cells (hASCs) seeded on titanium trabecular spinal cages. *Sci. Rep.* **2020**, *10*, 18284. [CrossRef]
18. McGilvray, K.C.; Easley, J.; Seim, H.B.; Regan, D.; Berven, S.H.; Hsu, W.K.; Mroz, T.E.; Puttlitz, C.M. Bony ingrowth potential of 3D-printed porous titanium alloy: A direct comparison of interbody cage materials in an in vivo ovine lumbar fusion model. *Spine J.* **2018**, *18*, 1250–1260. [CrossRef]
19. Olivares-Navarrete, R.; Gittens, R.A.; Schneider, J.M.; Hyzy, S.L.; Haithcock, D.A.; Ullrich, P.F.; Schwartz, Z.; Boyan, B.D. Osteoblasts exhibit a more differentiated phenotype and increased bone morphogenetic protein production on titanium alloy substrates than on poly-ether-ether-ketone. *Spine J.* **2012**, *12*, 265–272. [CrossRef]
20. Aaltonen, L.; Koivuviita, N.; Seppänen, M.; Burton, I.S.; Kröger, H.; Löyttyniemi, E.; Metsärinne, K. Bone histomorphometry and 18F-sodium fluoride positron emission tomography imaging: Comparison between only bone turnover-based and unified TMV-based classification of renal osteodystrophy. *Calcif. Tissue Int.* **2021**, *109*, 605–614. [CrossRef]
21. Sarikaya, I.; Elgazzar, A.H.; Sarikaya, A.; Alfeeli, M. Normal bone and soft tissue distribution of fluorine-18-sodium fluoride and artifacts on 18F-NaF PET/CT bone scan: A pictorial review. *Nucl. Med. Commun.* **2017**, *38*, 810–819. [CrossRef] [PubMed]
22. Lamartina, C.; Berjano, P. Classification of sagittal imbalance based on spinal alignment and compensatory mechanisms. *Eur. Spine J.* **2014**, *23*, 1177–1189. [CrossRef]
23. Schwab, F.J.; Diebo, B.G.; Smith, J.S.; Hostin, R.A.; Shaffrey, C.I.; Cunningham, M.E.; Mundis, G.M.; Ames, C.P.; Burton, D.C.; Bess, S.; et al. Fine-tuned surgical planning in adult spinal deformity: Determining the lumbar lordosis necessary by accounting for both thoracic kyphosis and pelvic incidence. *Spine J.* **2014**, *14*, S73. [CrossRef]

24. Cofano, F.; Zenga, F.; Mammi, M.; Altieri, R.; Marengo, N.; Ajello, M.; Pacca, P.; Melcarne, A.; Junemann, C.; Ducati, A.; et al. Intraoperative neurophysiological monitoring during spinal surgery: Technical review in open and minimally invasive approaches. *Neurosurg. Rev.* **2019**, *42*, 297–307. [CrossRef] [PubMed]
25. Beheshti, M.; Mottaghy, F.M.; Paycha, F.; Behrendt, F.F.F.; Van den Wyngaert, T.; Fogelman, I.; Strobel, K.; Celli, M.; Fanti, S.; Giammarile, F.; et al. (18)F-NaF PET/CT: EANM procedure guidelines for bone imaging. *Eur. J. Nucl. Med. Mol. Imaging* **2015**, *42*, 1767–1777. [CrossRef] [PubMed]
26. Segall, G.; Delbeke, D.; Stabin, M.G.; Even-Sapir, E.; Fair, J.; Sajdak, R.; Smith, G.T. SNM practice guideline for sodium 18F-fluoride PET/CT bone scans 1.0. *J. Nucl. Med.* **2010**, *51*, 1813–1820. [CrossRef]
27. Kinahan, P.E.; Fletcher, J.W. Positron emission tomography-computed tomography standardized uptake values in clinical practice and assessing response to therapy. *Semin. Ultrasound CT MR* **2010**, *31*, 496–505. [CrossRef]
28. Boellaard, R. Standards for PET image acquisition and quantitative data analysis. *J. Nucl. Med.* **2009**, *50* (Suppl. 1), 11S–20S. [CrossRef]
29. Rao, P.J.; Pelletier, M.H.; Walsh, W.R.; Mobbs, R.J. Spine interbody implants: Material selection and modification, functionalization and bioactivation of surfaces to improve osseointegration. *Orthop. Surg.* **2014**, *6*, 81–89. [CrossRef]
30. Ramakrishna, S.M.J.; Wintermantel, E.; Leong, K.W. Biomedical applications of polymer-composite materials: A review. *Compos. Sci. Technol.* **2001**, *61*, 1189–1224. [CrossRef]
31. Stadelmann, V.A.; Terrier, A.; Pioletti, D.P. Microstimulation at the bone-implant interface upregulates osteoclast activation pathways. *Bone* **2008**, *42*, 358–364. [CrossRef] [PubMed]
32. Park, H.W.; Lee, J.K.; Moon, S.J.; Seo, S.K.; Lee, J.H.; Kim, S.H. The efficacy of the synthetic interbody cage and Grafton for anterior cervical fusion. *Spine (Phila Pa 1976)* **2009**, *34*, E591–E595. [CrossRef] [PubMed]
33. Kurtz, S.M.; Devine, J.N. PEEK biomaterials in trauma, orthopedic, and spinal implants. *Biomaterials* **2007**, *28*, 4845–4869. [CrossRef] [PubMed]
34. Fujibayashi, S.; Takemoto, M.; Neo, M.; Matsushita, T.; Kokubo, T.; Doi, K.; Ito, T.; Shimizu, A.; Nakamura, T. A novel synthetic material for spinal fusion: A prospective clinical trial of porous bioactive titanium metal for lumbar interbody fusion. *Eur. Spine J.* **2011**, *20*, 1486–1495. [CrossRef] [PubMed]
35. Takemoto, M.; Fujibayashi, S.; Neo, M.; So, K.; Akiyama, N.; Matsushita, T.; Kokubo, T.; Nakamura, T. A porous bioactive titanium implant for spinal interbody fusion: An experimental study using a canine model. *J. Neurosurg. Spine* **2007**, *7*, 435–443. [CrossRef] [PubMed]
36. Zhang, Z.; Li, H.; Fogel, G.R.; Liao, Z.; Li, Y.; Liu, W. Biomechanical analysis of porous additive manufactured cages for lateral lumbar interbody fusion: A finite element analysis. *World Neurosurg.* **2018**, *111*, e581–e591. [CrossRef]
37. Tartara, F.; Bongetta, D.; Pilloni, G.; Colombo, E.V.; Giombelli, E. Custom-made trabecular titanium implants for the treatment of lumbar degenerative discopathy via ALIF/XLIF techniques: Rationale for use and preliminary results. *Eur. Spine J.* **2020**, *29*, 314–320. [CrossRef]
38. Fischer, D.R.; Zweifel, K.; Treyer, V.; Hesselmann, R.; Johayem, A.; Stumpe, K.D.M.; Von Schulthess, G.K.; Hany, T.F.; Strobel, K. Assessment of successful incorporation of cages after cervical or lumbar intercorporal fusion with [(18)F]fluoride positron-emission tomography/computed tomography. *Eur. Spine J.* **2011**, *20*, 640–648. [CrossRef]
39. Ayubcha, C.; Zirakchian Zadeh, M.; Stochkendahl, M.J.; Al-Zaghal, A.; Hartvigsen, J.; Rajapakse, C.S.; Borja, A.J.; Arani, L.S.; Gerke, O.; Werner, T.J.; et al. Quantitative evaluation of normal spinal osseous metabolism with 18F-NaF PET/CT. *Nucl. Med. Commun.* **2018**, *39*, 945–950. [CrossRef] [PubMed]
40. Brans, B.; Weijers, R.; Halders, S.; Wierts, R.; Peters, M.; Punt, I.; Willems, P. Assessment of bone graft incorporation by 18F-fluoride positron-emission tomography/computed tomography in patients with persisting symptoms after posterior lumbar interbody fusion. *EJNMMI Res.* **2012**, *2*, 42. [CrossRef]
41. Seifen, T.; Rodrigues, M.; Rettenbacher, L.; Piotrowski, W.; Holzmannhofer, J.; Mc Coy, M.; Pirich, C. The value of (18)F-fluoride PET/CT in the assessment of screw loosening in patients after intervertebral fusion stabilization. *EJNMMI* **2015**, *42*, 272–277.
42. Peters, M.; Willems, P.; Weijers, R.; Wierts, R.; Jutten, L.; Urbach, V.; Arts, J.; Van Rhijn, L.; Brans, B. Pseudarthrosis after lumbar spinal fusion: The role of 18F-fluoride PET/CT. *EJNMMI* **2015**, *42*, 1891–1898. [CrossRef] [PubMed]
43. Pouldar, D.; Bakshian, S.; Matthews, R.; Rao, V.; Manzano, M.; Dardashti, S. Utility of 18F sodium fluoride PET/CT imaging in the evaluation of postoperative pain following surgical spine fusion. *Musculoskelet Surg.* **2017**, *101*, 159–166. [CrossRef] [PubMed]
44. Quon, A.; Dodd, R.; Iagaru, A.; de Abreu, M.R.; Hennemann, S.; Neto, J.M.A.; Sprinz, C. Initial investigation of 18F-NaF PET/CT for identification of vertebral sites amenable to surgical revision after spinal fusion surgery. *EJNMMI* **2012**, *39*, 1737–1744. [CrossRef]

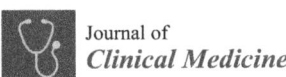

Article

High Accuracy and Safety of Intraoperative CT-Guided Navigation for Transpedicular Screw Placement in Revision Spinal Surgery

Yen-Yao Li [1,2,*], Shih-Hao Chen [3], Kuo-Chin Huang [1,2], Chien-Yin Lee [1,4], Chin-Chang Cheng [5], Ching-Yu Lee [6,7], Meng-Huang Wu [6,7] and Tsung-Jen Huang [6,7]

1. Department of Orthopaedic Surgery, Chang Gung Memorial Hospital at Chiayi, Chiayi County 613016, Taiwan
2. Department of Medicine, College of Medicine, Chang Gung University, Taoyuan City 333323, Taiwan
3. Department of Orthopedics, Buddhist Tzu-chi General Hospital at Dahlin, Chiayi County 622401, Taiwan
4. Department of Nursing, Chang Gung University of Science and Technology, Taoyuan City 333324, Taiwan
5. Department of Orthopedics, St Martin de Porres Hospital, Chiayi City 600044, Taiwan
6. Department of Orthopedics, Taipei Medical University Hospital, Taipei City 110301, Taiwan
7. Department of Orthopedics, School of Medicine, College of Medicine, Taipei Medical University, Taipei City 110301, Taiwan
* Correspondence: yao.ortho@gmail.com; Tel.: +886-5-362-1000

Abstract: Background: Intraoperative CT-guided navigation (iCT-navigation) has been reported to improve the accuracy and safety of transpedicular screw placement in primary spinal surgery. However, due to a disrupted bony anatomy and scarring tissue, revision spinal surgery can be challenging. The purpose of this study was to evaluate the accuracy and safety of iCT-navigation for screw placement at the virgin site versus the revision site in revision thoracolumbar spinal surgery. Method: In total, 254 screws were inserted in 27 revision surgeries, in which 114 (44.9%) screws were inserted at the site with previous laminectomy or posterolateral fusion (the revision site), 64 (25.2%) were inserted at the virgin site, and 76 (29.9%) were inserted to replace the pre-existing screws. CT scans were conducted for each patient after all screws were inserted to intraoperatively confirm the screw accuracy. Results: In total, 248 (97.6%) screws were considered accepted. The rate of accepted screws at the virgin site was 98.4% (63/64) versus 95.6% (109/114) at the revision site (p: 0.422). There were six (2.4%) unaccepted screws, which were immediately revised during the same operation. There was no neurological injury noted in our patients. Conclusion: With the use of iCT-navigation, the rate of accepted screws at the revision site was found to be comparable to that at the virgin site. We concluded that iCT-navigation could achieve high accuracy and safety for transpedicular screw placement in revision spinal surgery and allow for the immediate revision of unaccepted screws.

Keywords: thoracolumbar spine; revision spinal surgery; intraoperative computed tomography; navigation; transpedicular screw

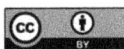

1. Introduction

The transpedicular screw (TPS) system is one of the most widely used fixation devices in spinal surgery. It provides a three-column fixation [1] of the spine. It is essential to ensure the optimal trajectory of TPS insertion to offer the strongest bony purchase and prevent nerve tissue injury. TPS insertion can be challenging in revision spinal surgery [2], because the anatomical features used to identify the entry of a TPS may have been destroyed or obscured by the fusion mass or abundant scar tissue, causing a standard fluoroscopy to be insufficient to identify the proper entry of a TPS due to blurry images for altered or fused anatomy [2–4].

Several advanced image-guided techniques have emerged in the past two decades, including three-dimensional (3D) fluoroscopy [5,6], O-arm [7,8] and intraoperative computed tomography (iCT) [9,10]. One study [11] reported that the accuracy of the TPS was comparable for both primary and revision spine surgery using O-arm-guided navigation. However, some of the TPS placements in revision spinal surgery were performed at the virgin site for the extension of posterior instrumentation, instead of right over the revision site. Thus, the accuracy of TPS placement at the revision site could be different from that of the whole revision spine surgery. In the current study, we aimed to evaluate the accuracy and safety of iCT-navigation for TPS placement right over the revision site versus the virgin site in complex revision thoracolumbar spinal surgery.

2. Materials and Methods

We enrolled 27 consecutive patients who underwent TPS placement assisted with intraoperative CT (Siemens, Munich, Germany) integrated with navigation (Brainlab, Munich, Germany) for revision thoracolumbar spinal surgeries. The study was approved by the Institutional Review Board of the Chang Gung Memorial Hospital.

There were 27 patients (13 women and 14 men) in the present study, with an average age of 67 years (range 47–92 years). A total of 254 TPSs was inserted during the revision spinal surgeries, which were categorized into 3 groups: "revision site" screws (no. = 114) inserted over a previous laminectomy or posterolateral fusion field; "virgin site" screws (64) inserted at a site away from previous laminectomy or posterolateral fusion for the extension of posterior instrumentation; and "exchanged" screws (76), inserted to replace pre-existing screws with screws of a different style or brand through the previous trajectories.

2.1. Surgical Technique

After general anesthesia, the patient was positioned prone on a Wilson radiolucent frame (Mizuho OSI, California, CA, USA) on a Jackson table. A midline incision with paraspinal muscle stripping was performed to expose the previous operation site and extended to the virgin level if necessary. The pre-existing screws were exchanged for screws of a different brand, if necessary, which were inserted manually through previous trajectories without using iCT-navigation. Thereafter, the superior articular processes of the facets through which we planned to insert new TPSs were exposed. The reference array was then securely fixed at a vertebra distal to the expected lowest instrumented vertebra (usually L5 or S1) by tightly clamping its spinal process.

The operative field was scanned with the intraoperative CT, and the image data were transferred to the navigation system. A straight drilling guide was then registered to guide a 2.7 mm in diameter drill bit to create the optimal track for the TPS under iCT-navigation by checking the axial, sagittal and coronal views (Figure 1). A TPS with an optimal length and diameter was chosen and inserted through the pedicle trajectory after being adequately tapped. After completing all TPS placements, CT scans were conducted to confirm whether the TPSs were in the optimal position, which we called confirmatory CT scans (Figure 2).

2.2. Assessment of TPS Placement

Intraoperatively, with the aid of the confirmatory CT scan, we evaluated the TPS accuracy and divided the results into 2 conditions: "accepted" and "unaccepted". An accepted screw was defined as having a medial pedicle breach of ≤ 3 mm or a lateral pedicle or body wall breach of ≤ 3 mm. The position of the TPS was considered biomechanically optimal and safe from neurologic injury. An unaccepted screw was defined as having a medial pedicle breach of >3 mm or a lateral pedicle or body wall breach of >3 mm (Figure 3); the TPS could be biomechanically suboptimal and create a risk of nerve tissue injury, and, therefore, was immediately revised under iCT-navigation. After replacing the unaccepted screw, the second confirmatory CT scan was performed to ensure that the screw was in an accepted position.

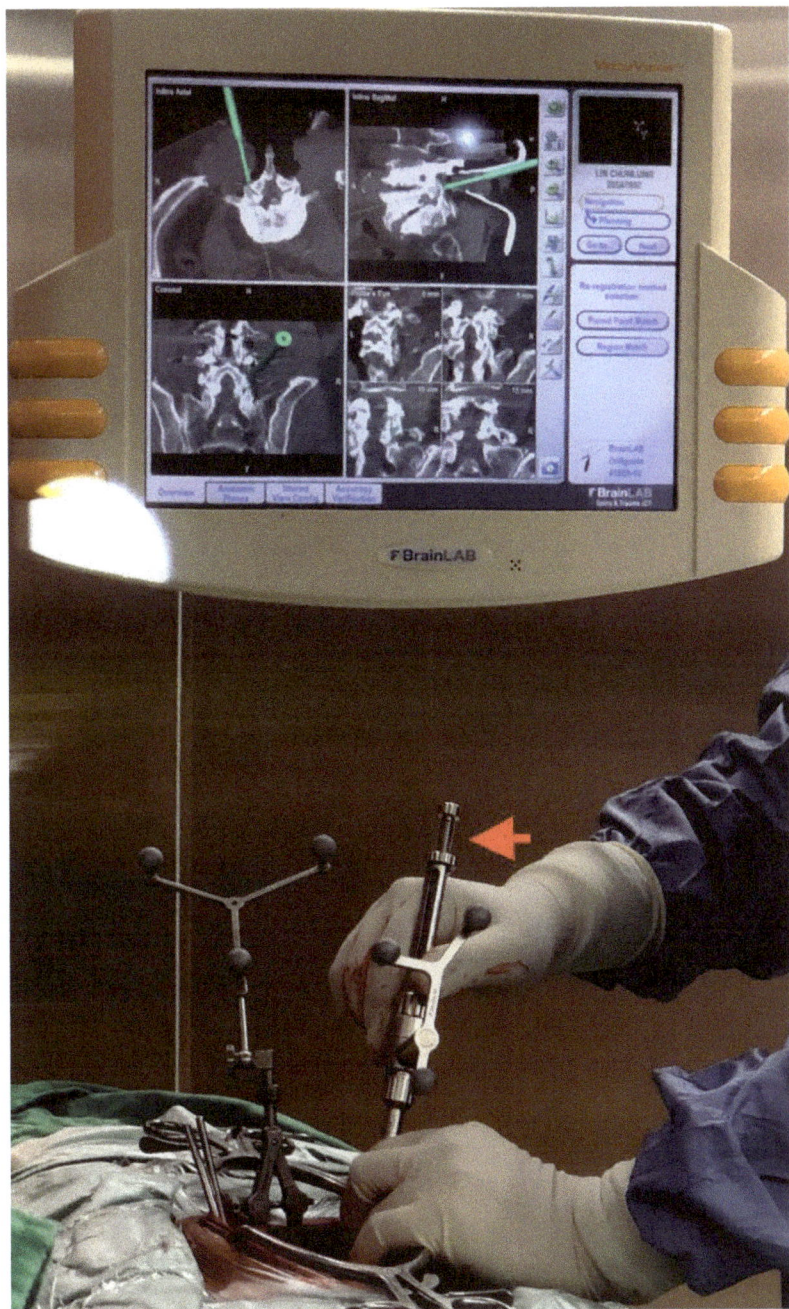

Figure 1. The straight drilling guide (red arrow) was used to guide a 2.7 mm in diameter drill bit to create the optimal TPS track under iCT-navigation by checking the axial, sagittal and coronal views.

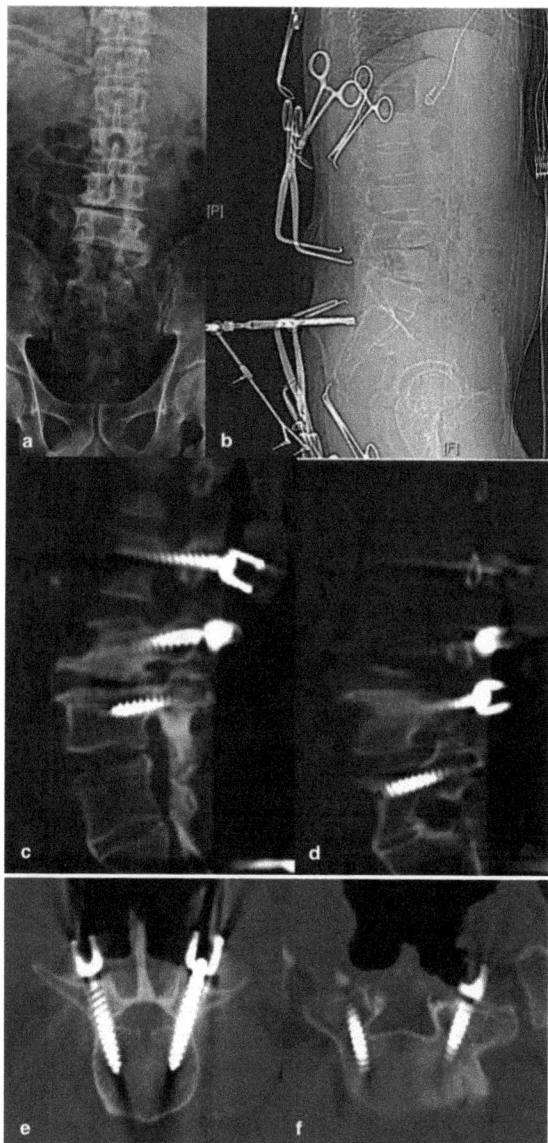

Figure 2. A 55-year-old male patient with post-laminectomy instability and spinal stenosis; X-ray (**a**) showed previous laminectomy of L4, L5 and partial L3. This patient underwent revision spinal surgery with the use of iCT-navigation; X-ray (**b**) showed the reference array fixed at the spinal process of S1 for iCT-navigation. Intraoperatively, after all screws were inserted, the confirmatory CT scan demonstrated sagittal and axial views of screws (**c,e**) at the virgin site and (**d,f**) at the revision site.

2.3. Radiographic and Clinical Analyses

The accuracy of the TPS placement was assessed with the first confirmatory CT. The rates of accepted screws and unaccepted screws were calculated for comparison between the virgin site and the revision site. Perioperative medical records were collected retrospectively, and postoperative neurological complications were evaluated.

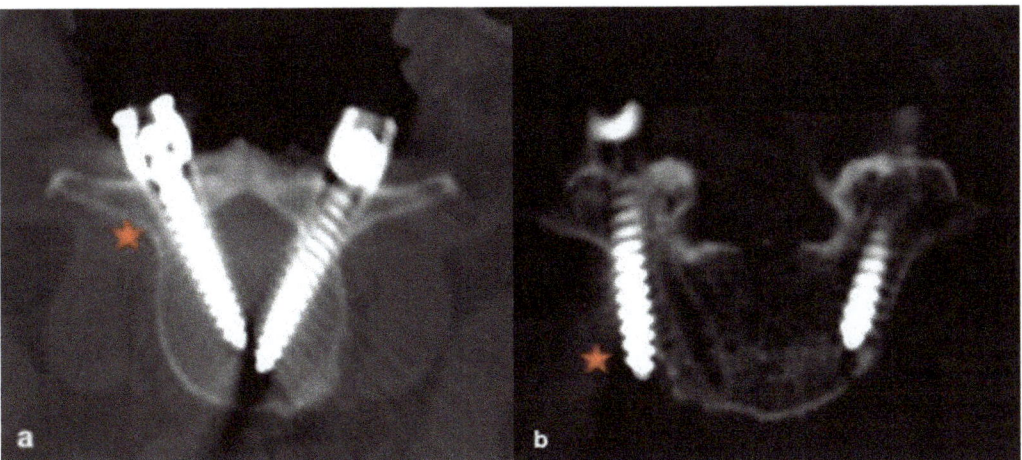

Figure 3. Unaccepted screw (red star) was defined as (**a**) a medial pedicle breach of >3 mm or (**b**) a lateral pedicle or body wall breach of >3 mm.

2.4. Statistical Analysis

Descriptive statistics were reported as percentages to describe the rates of accepted screws and unaccepted screws. Fisher's exact test was used to compare the rates of accepted and unaccepted screws between the virgin site and the revision site. The test was considered significant if $p < 0.05$.

3. Results

In total, 27 patients were categorized using the etiology for revision spine surgery: 12 patients (44.4%) were diagnosed with postlaminectomy instability with or without posterolateral fusion; 9 (33.3%) patients had adjacent segmental disease with spinal stenosis or instability; 4 (14.8%) patients had malpositions of a previous TPS with clinical neurologic symptoms; and the remaining 2 (7.4%) patients had a refractory postoperative infection (Supplementary Table S1).

Of the total 254 TPSs, 248 screw placements were considered accepted (97.6%) by the first confirmatory CT, including all of the "exchanged screws" (N = 76). The rates of accepted screws were comparable both at the virgin site (63, 98.4%) and the revision site (109, 95.6%). There was no significant difference between both groups ($p = 0.422$).

There were six screws (2.4%) considered unaccepted: one (1.6%) at the virgin site with a medial pedicle breach; and five (4.4%) at the revision site, including two with a medial pedicle breach and three with a lateral pedicle or body wall breach. The rates of unaccepted screws trended higher at the revision site than at the virgin site, but were not significantly different. All the unaccepted screws were revised immediately with the assistance of iCT-navigation, and, then, each proved to be accepted with a secondary confirmatory CT. No postoperative neurologic deterioration was observed related to the screw placement.

4. Discussion

With the use of iCT-navigation for revision spinal surgery, the rate of accepted screws was 97.6%, which was comparable to other studies [2,11] for revision surgery. Hsieh et al. [11] adopted an O-arm with navigation to guide TPS placement. They reported "good or fair" rates of screw placement (pedicle breach <3 mm) as 98.7% in the primary surgery group and 98.6% in the revision surgery group, which were not significantly different. Even compared with our previous studies for primary surgery [10,12], which reported the accuracy of TPS placement was 96–98%, the accuracy in the current study for revision surgery was comparable. However, we divided our series of TPS placements into two groups for comparison: the revision site and the virgin site. The rate of accepted screws was 98.4% (63/64) at the virgin site and 95.6% (109/114) at the revision site ($p = 0.422$). There was one (1.6%) unaccepted screw noted at the virgin site, and five (4.4%) at the revision site. The rates of unaccepted screws trended higher at the revision site than at the virgin site, but were not significantly different. We assumed that some of the TPSs in revision spinal surgery could be inserted at the virgin site for the extension of posterior instrumentation instead of right over the revision site. Thus, the accuracy of TPS placement at the revision site could be different from or inferior to that at the virgin site across the whole revision spinal surgery.

In the current study, most of the unaccepted screws were noted at the revision site. We considered dense postoperative fibrotic tissue or scarring to be the principal causes resulting in screw malpositioning at the revision site. Once the navigation device bent around the dense scar during the process of TPS placement, the navigation had the potential to fail. The scar tissue caused excessive pressure on the instrument and usually resulted in the medial deviation of the screw trajectory. Furthermore, if the surgeon exerted excessive bending force on the instrument (the drill or awl) to apply soft tissue pressure, the instrument could skive off the pedicle and result in the lateral skidding of the trajectory. The skiving effect might explain why there were more unaccepted screws presenting with a lateral wall breach (3, 60%) at the revision site. We suggest that the skiving effect could be diminished with the adequate release of soft tissue tension, and by using a high-speed drill with a shard bit for drilling [13].

There have been few studies focused on the feasibility or accuracy of TPS placement in revision spinal surgery. Kim et al. [2] reported that the accuracy of TPS placement in revision surgery was excellent with the free-hand technique. The revision rates of misplaced screws were 1.1% in the virgin site screw group and 2.9% in the revision site group, which were not significantly different. However, the TPSs were evaluated with plain radiography, not CT, which might have underestimated the number of misplaced screws. Free-hand TPS insertions in revision spinal surgery are technically demanding, and it is laborious to identify the entry point of the TPS when anatomic features are distorted. With the use of iCT-navigation in the current study, surgeons were able to confidently insert the TPSs during revision spinal surgery. Hsieh et al. [11] adopted an O-arm (Medtronic, Inc., Minneapolis, MN, USA) with navigation to guide TPS placement. They collected postoperative CT scans to evaluate screw accuracy in revision spinal surgery. Interestingly, for the purpose of decreasing radiation, confirmatory intraoperative CT scans were not routinely performed in their study, unless there was concern for screw malpositioning. There were six poor screws (1.4%, pedicle breach of > 3 mm) found postoperatively in their study; fortunately, none caused neurological deficits and, thus, were not revised. In our study, unaccepted screws were identified intraoperatively with the first confirmatory CT. After the secondary confirmatory CT, all the revised screws were accepted.

Since unaccepted screws may not always result in neurologic deficits, it might not be necessary to revise all of them intraoperatively. Laine et al. [14] reported that no screw caused neurological problems if the pedicle breach was less than 4.0 mm on the postoperative CT scan. Castro et al. [15] found that a TPS with medial pedicle breach of more than 6 mm created a high risk of nerve root damage. In the current study, the criteria to revise a screw was a medial pedicle breach of > 3mm or a lateral pedicle or body wall of >3 mm, which might be appropriate. However, we should keep in mind that even a medial 2 mm breach can be symptomatic, whereas a lateral breach of approximately 5 mm often remains asymptomatic in some extreme case. Although all unaccepted screws were revised intraoperatively and successfully, the use of a secondary confirmatory CT increased the patients' exposure to radiation. Intraoperative neuromonitoring was available in the current study, by which the authors could have avoided revising some of the unaccepted screws and rescued a TPS with a pedicle breach of <3 mm and abnormal neuromonitoring alerts.

In spinal surgery with posterior instrumentation, the free-hand technique combined with intraoperative fluoroscopy is commonly used to confirm the entry point and trajectory of the TPS. The reported incidence of misplaced screws ranged from 10.5% to 21% [14,16–18]. Two-dimensional (2D) fluoroscopy may not provide sufficient image information to safely insert TPSs in spinal deformities [12,17,18] due to a remodeled bony structure or spinal fractures [10,16] because of hypermobile spinal segments and disrupted anatomy, such as facets or pedicle fractures. Furthermore, it would be technically challenging to use fluoroscopy for TPS placement in revision spine surgery due to the altered anatomy, indistinct bony landmarks and excessive scar tissue [2]. CT scans can provide adequate image information to evaluate TPS position, including the axial, coronal and sagittal planes [14], and is, therefore, the better choice for guiding TPS placement in cases of compromised spine anatomy, such as deformity, trauma, and revision spine surgery.

In the last two decades, several advanced imaging techniques have emerged that are able to provide 3D images. Usually, 3D fluoroscopy is limited by a small "field-of-view" scan area and an inferior image quality, with a screw accuracy inferior to iCT [19]. The O-arm is a cone-beam computed tomography, which has higher rates for screws revised intraoperatively [20], but has a similar accuracy for postoperative screw placement as compared with iCT. Therefore, we believe that iCT is the imaging technology of choice to provide the optimal image resolution for TPS placement. However, it cannot provide real-time imaging to immediately determine the screw trajectory and may further expose the patients to a greater radiation dosage.

Certain navigation techniques enable the diminution of CT scans for guiding TPS placement, while providing virtual but real-time images to guide TPS placement. The iCT-navigation technique is an effective method for TPS placement in complex spinal surgery for patients with spinal deformities [12] and unstable thoracolumbar spine fractures, with a high TPS accuracy of up to 98% [9,10]. It also allows for the immediate revision of unaccepted TPSs during surgery, followed by a secondary confirmatory CT scan. This option is highly practical in the case of immediate intraoperative revision, because returning to another surgery for screw revision would increase the risk for the patient. Although the confirmatory CT scan exposes patients to radiation, the medical staff are protected from radiation in a lead-shielded room.

There were several limitations in our study. It might be relatively expensive to set up the iCT-navigation system; however, the installation charge should be considered against the cost of reoperation for patients with misplaced screws. We should have measured the dose of radiation to which patients were exposed, which might have been relatively high, since the entire workflow of iCT-navigation surgery contained at least two CT scans, including the registration scan and confirmatory scan. According to our previous studies [10] for primary surgery, the mean dose of patient radiation exposure was 15.8 mSv, and the mean dose per single level was 2.7 mSv. Fortunately, according to the recommendation by the International Commission on Radiological Protection, the annual maximum permissible dose is 20 mSv per year with no single year exceeding 50 mSv. Hence, the radiation dose to the patient in our study might have been within the limit. Furthermore, although this study was purely an imaging-based investigation and did not focus on functional outcomes, it was found that there were no immediate postoperative neurologic deficits.

5. Conclusions

The use of iCT-navigation for TPS placement in revision thoracolumbar spinal surgery was a useful technique for improving the accuracy and safety of TPS placement and allowed for the immediate intraoperative revision of unaccepted screws. The rate of accepted screws at the revision site was comparable to that at the virgin site in revision spinal surgery, although the rate of unaccepted screws at the revision site trended higher than at the virgin site. No postoperative neurological injury was noted in our patients.

Supplementary Materials: The following supporting information can be downloaded at: https://www.mdpi.com/article/10.3390/jcm11195853/s1, Table S1: Demographic and Perioperative Data.

Author Contributions: Conceptualization, Y.-Y.L.; methodology, Y.-Y.L. and S.-H.C., software, C.-C.C. and C.-Y.L. (Chien-Yin Lee); validation, K.-C.H.; formal analysis, C.-Y.L. (Ching-Yu Lee) and M.-H.W.; supervision, T.-J.H. All authors have read and agreed to the published version of the manuscript.

Funding: This research received no external funding.

Institutional Review Board Statement: This study was approved by the ethics committee of the Chang-Gung Memorial Hospital, Taiwan (approval no. 202100339B0).

Informed Consent Statement: Informed consent from individual patients was waived because of the retrospective study with anonymized data.

Data Availability Statement: The original data generated during the study are included in the article. Further inquiries can be directed to the corresponding author.

Conflicts of Interest: The authors declare no conflict of interest.

References

1. Suk, S.; Lee, S.M.; Chung, E.R.; Kim, J.H.; Kim, S.S. Selective thoracic fusion with segmental pedicle screw fixation in the treatment of thoracic idiopathic scoliosis: More than 5-year follow-up. *Spine* **2005**, *30*, 1602–1609. [CrossRef] [PubMed]
2. Kim, Y.W.; Lenke, L.G.; Kim, Y.J.; Bridwell, K.H.; Kim, Y.B.; Watanabe, K.; Watanabe, K. Free-hand TPS placement during revision spinal surgery analysis of 552 screws. *Spine* **2008**, *33*, 1141–1148. [CrossRef] [PubMed]
3. Kim, Y.J.; Lenke, L.G.; Cheh, G.; Riew, K.D. Evaluation of pedicle screw placement in the deformed spine using intraoperative plain radiographs: A comparison with computerized tomography. *Spine* **2005**, *30*, 2084–2088. [CrossRef] [PubMed]
4. Hicks, J.M.; Singla, A.; Shen, F.H.; Arlet, V. Complications of pedicle screw fixation in scoliosis surgery: A systematic review. *Spine* **2010**, *35*, E465–E470. [CrossRef] [PubMed]
5. Acosta, F.L., Jr.; Thompson, T.L.; Campbell, S.; Weinstein, P.R.; Ames, C.P. Use of intraoperative isocentric C-arm 3D fluoroscopy for sextant percutaneous pedicle screw placement: Case report and review of the literature. *Spine J.* **2005**, *5*, 339–343. [CrossRef] [PubMed]
6. Holly, L.T.; Foley, K.T. Three-dimensional fluoroscopy-guided percutaneous thoracolumbar pedicle screw placement technical note. *J. Neurosurg. Spine* **2003**, *99*, 324–329. [CrossRef] [PubMed]
7. Oertel, M.F.; Hobart, J.; Stein, M.; Schreiber, V.; Scharbrodt, W. Clinical and methodological precision of spinal navigation assisted by 3D intraoperative O-arm radiographic imaging. *J. Neurosurg. Spine* **2011**, *14*, 532–536. [CrossRef] [PubMed]
8. Silbermann, J.; Riese, F.; Allam, Y.; Reichert, T.; Koeppert, H.; Gutberlet, M. Computed tomography assessment of pedicle screw placement in lumbar and sacral spine: Comparison between free-hand and O-arm based navigation techniques. *Eur. Spine J.* **2011**, *20*, 875–881. [CrossRef] [PubMed]
9. Lee, M.H.; Lin, M.H.; Weng, H.H.; Cheng, W.C.; Tsai, Y.H.; Wang, T.C.; Yang, J.T. Feasibility of Intraoperative Computed Tomography Navigation System for Pedicle Screw Insertion of the Thoracolumbar Spine. *J. Spinal. Disord Tech.* **2013**, *26*, E183–E187. [CrossRef] [PubMed]
10. Lee, C.Y.; Wu, M.H.; Li, Y.Y.; Cheng, C.C.; Hsu, C.H.; Huang, T.J.; Hsu, R.W. Intraoperative computed tomography navigation for transpedicular screw fixation to treat unstable thoracic and lumbar spine fractures. *Medicine* **2015**, *94*, e757. [CrossRef] [PubMed]
11. Hsieh, J.C.; Drazin, D.; Firempong, A.O.; Pashman, R.; Johnson, P.; Kim, T.T. Accuracy of intraoperative computed tomography image-guided surgery in placing pedicle and pelvic screws for primary versus revision spine surgery. *Neurosurg. Focus* **2014**, *36*, e2. [CrossRef] [PubMed]
12. Li, Y.Y.; Lee, C.Y.; Wu, M.H.; Huang, T.J.; Cheng, C.C.; Lee, C.Y. Intraoperative computed tomography navigation for transpedicular screw in posterior instrumentation and correction of adolescent idiopathic scoliosis. *Formosan. J. Musculoskelet Disord* **2016**, *7*, 57–62.
13. Tsai, T.H.; Tzou, R.D.; Su, Y.F.; Wu, C.H.; Tsai, C.Y.; Lin, C.L. Pedicle screw placement accuracy of bone-mounted miniature robot system. *Medicine* **2017**, *96*, e5835. [CrossRef]
14. Laine, T.; Makitalo, K.; Schlenzka, D.; Tallroth, K.; Poussa, M.; Alho, A. Accuracy of pedicle screw placement: A prospective CT study in 30 consecutive low back patients. *Eur. Spine J.* **1997**, *6*, 402–405. [CrossRef] [PubMed]
15. Castro, W.H.; Halm, H.; Jerosch, J.; Malms, J.; Steinbeck, J.; Blasius, S. Accuracy of pedicle screw placement in lumbar vertebrae. *Spine* **1996**, *21*, 1320–1324. [CrossRef] [PubMed]
16. Carbone, J.J.; Tortolani, P.J.; Quartararo, L.G. Fluoroscopically assisted pedicle screw fixation for thoracic and thoracolumbar injuries: Technique and short-term complications. *Spine* **2003**, *28*, 91–97. [CrossRef] [PubMed]
17. Lehman, R.A.; Lenke, L.G.; Keeler, K.A.; Kim, Y.J.; Cheh, G. Computed tomography evaluation of pedicle screws placed in the pediatric deformed spine over an 8-year period. *Spine* **2007**, *32*, 2679–2684. [CrossRef] [PubMed]

18. Samdani, A.F.; Ranade, A.; Saldanha, V.; Yondorf, M.Z. Learning curve for placement of thoracic pedicle screws in the deformed spine. *Neurosurgery* **2010**, *66*, 290–295. [CrossRef] [PubMed]
19. Hecht, N.; Yassin, H.; Czabanka, M.; Fohre, B.; Arden, K.; Liebig, T.; Vajkoczy, P. Intraoperative computed tomography versus 3D C-arm imaging for navigated spinal instrumentation. *Spine* **2018**, *43*, 370–377. [CrossRef] [PubMed]
20. Scarone, P.; Vincenzo, G.; Distefano, D.; Grande, F.D.; Cianfoni, A.; Presilla, S.; Reinert, M. Use of the Airo mobile intraoperative. CT system versus the O-arm for transpedicular screw fixation in the thoracic and lumbar spine: A retrospective cohort study of 263 patients. *J. Neurosurg. Spine* **2018**, *29*, 397–406. [CrossRef] [PubMed]

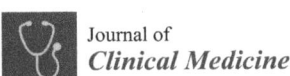

Article

Are Torque-Induced Bone Texture Alterations Related to Early Marginal Jawbone Loss?

Tomasz Wach [1,*], Małgorzata Skorupska [1] and Grzegorz Trybek [2]

[1] Department of Maxillofacial Surgery, Medical University of Lodz, 113 Zeromskiego Str., 90-549 Lodz, Poland
[2] Department of Oral Surgery, Pomeranian Medical University in Szczecin, 70-111 Szczecin, Poland
* Correspondence: tomasz.wach@umed.lodz.pl; Tel.: +48-42-639-3422

Abstract: The reason why marginal bone loss (MBL) occurs after dental implant insertion without loading has not yet been clearly investigated. There are publications that confirm or reject the notion that there are factors that induce marginal bone loss, but no research investigates what exactly occurs in the bone surrounding the implant neck. In this study, 2196 samples of dental implant neck bone radiographs were analyzed. The follow-up period was 3 months without functional loading of the implant. Marginal bone loss was evaluated in relation to the torque used during the final phase of implant insertion. Radiographic texture features were also analyzed and evaluated. The analyses were performed individually for the anterior and posterior part of the alveolar crest in both the mandible and maxilla. After 3 months, an MBL relation with higher torque (higher than 40 Ncm; $p < 0.05$) was observed, but only in the lower jaw. The texture features Sum Average (SumAverg), Entropy, Difference Entropy (DifEntr), Long-Run Emphasis (LngREmph), Short-Run Emphasis (ShrtREmph), and discrete wavelet decomposition transform features were changed over time. This study presents that MBL is related to the torque value during dental implant insertion and the location of the procedure. The increasing values of SumAverg and LngREmph correlated with MBL, which were 64.21 to 64.35 and 1.71 to 2.01, respectively. The decreasing values of Entr, DifEntr, and ShrtREmph also correlated with MBL, which were 2.58 to 2.47, 1.11 to 1.01, and 0.88 to 0.84, respectively. The analyzed texture features may become good indicators of MBL in digital dental surgery.

Keywords: dental implant; torque; marginal bone loss; intraoral radiographs; radiomics; texture analysis; bone remodeling

1. Introduction

Presently, the most common procedure in oral surgery after wisdom tooth extraction are dental implants [1]. With the increasing number of dental implant placements, more and more post-operative complications also occur. One of the major complications is marginal bone loss (MBL) next to the dental implant neck [2]. Marginal bone loss is a condition where the bone surrounding the implant neck atrophies. It is affected by different factors, e.g., smoking, diabetes mellitus, vitamin D and 25-hydroxycholecaliferol level, implant placement technique, region of the jaw, and also torque during the surgical procedure [3–6]. MBL may occur after few years, but also after the first 3 months of healing. The osteotomy techniques used for implant placement may also differ and may affect MBL [7]. MBL that occurs after a few years may be a condition related to more factors, e.g., prosthetic restoration and gingival vertical and horizontal width. MBL may be associated with a high torque value [8,9] if the correct procedure steps have not been followed and the appropriate primary stability of the implant has occurred [10].

The visual assessment of the surrounding implant neck bone on radiographs may not be sufficient or reliable. Another way to evaluate radiographic images is to check how the radiographic textures change over time—the shade level of the pixels can be analyzed.

This analysescan be used, for example, to check how the texture of the bone substitute materials have changed after several months, translating this change into healing process progress [11–14].

The first aim of this study is to check whether torque and the location of the implant have an influence on MBL and to determine whether there is a change of radiographic texture in the bone surrounding the implant neck. The second aim is to check how the radiographic texture near the implant neck changes over time and to determine the prognostic factors of MBL in image texture.

2. Materials and Methods

In this study, 2196 samples of neck area implants were included and analyzed. A total of 504 males and 496 females aged between 15 and 86 years old were included in the study. All patients had undergone the same surgical procedure, namely, bone-level dental implant placement under local anesthesia (4% articaine with 1:100,000 adrenaline, 3 M ESPE AG, Seefeld, Germany). The patients were divided into two groups depending on whether MBL occurred after 3 months or not, and also into a mandible and maxilla group where the anterior and posterior parts were distinguished:

MBL appearance (YES) if MLB is >0
MBL appearance (NO) if MBL is =0

The inclusion criteria were two-dimensional radiographs taken immediately after surgery and 3 months later, the measurement of torque value immediately after dental implant placement, and laboratory tests to check patients' vitamin levels, ions, and hormones: parathormone (PTH), where the norm is 10 to 60 pg/mL; thyrotropin (TSH), where the norm is 0.23–4.0 µU/mL; calcium in serum (Ca^{2+}), where the norm is 9–11 mg/dL; glycated hemoglobin (HbA1c), where the norm is <5%; and vitamin 25(OH)D3 (D3), where the norm is 31–50 ng/mL. Spine densitometry, where the T-score can be examined, was also considered. The T-score shows the ratio between the bone mineral density (BMD) of the examined patient and the average BMD for young patients. A normal value for normal bone is >-1.0, osteopenia is indicated by values between -1.0 and -2.5, and scores < -2.5 indicate osteoporosis. The exclusion criteria included a lack of X-rays, defective X-ray images in the visual assessment, lack of a clear torque value, and lack of laboratory tests. In this study, only patients with proper values from the laboratory tests were included.

Surgery was done under local anesthesia, Septanest + A 1:100.00, by one surgeon according to the recommended protocols. The healing process was carried out under a closed mucoperiosteal flap, unloaded in two-stage implants. The thickness of the soft tissue did not affect the healing process or MBL in the first stage of healing. Table 1 presents the implants used in this study and their technical features. The data were confirmed at www.spotimplant.com/en/dental-implant-identification, accessed on 5 March 2022.

Two-dimensional X-ray images were taken immediately after surgery (00M) and 3 months later (03M). Radiographs were taken using the DIGORA OPTIME radiography system (TYPE DXR-50, SOREDEX, Helsinki, Finland). The radiographs were taken in the standardized way [15] with the following parameters: 7 mA, 70 mV, and 0.1 s (the focus apparatus was from Instrumentarium Dental, Tuusula, Finland). Positioners were used to take images repeatedly, with the X-ray beam at a 90° angle to the surface of the phosphor plate. The texture of the X-ray images was analyzed in the MaZda 4.6 software, developed by the University of Technology in Łódź, Poland [16], to check how the features changed over the 3 months of observation. A limitation of the study is that the laboratory tests were not checked after 3 months.

Table 1. Names and features of implants used.

Implant Name	Titanium Alloy No.	Insertion Level	Connection Type	Connection Shape	Neck Shape	Neck Microthreads	Body Shape	Body Threads	Apex Shape	Apex Hole	Apex Groove
AB Dental Devices I5	Grade 5	Bone level	Internal	Hexagon	Straight	No	Tapered	Square	Flat	No hole	Yes
ADIN Dental Implants Touareg	Grade 5	Bone level	Internal	Hexagon	Straight	Yes	Tapered	Square	Flat	No hole	Yes
Alpha Bio ATI	Grade 5	Bone level	Internal	Hexagon	Straight	Yes	Straight	Square	Flat	No hole	Yes
Alpha Bio OCI	Grade 5	Bone level	Internal	Hexagon	Straight	No	Straight	No Threads	Dome	Round	No
Alpha Bio DFI	Grade 5	Bone level	Internal	Hexagon	Straight	Yes	Tapered	Square	Flat	No hole	Yes
Alpha Bio SFB	Grade 5	Bone level	Internal	Hexagon	Straight	No	Tapered	V-shaped	Flat	No hole	Yes
Alpha Bio SPI	Grade 5	Bone level	Internal	Hexagon	Straight	Yes	Tapered	Square	Flat	No hole	Yes
Argon Medical Prod. K3pro Rapid	Grade 4	Subcrestal	Internal	Conical	Straight	Yes	Tapered	V-shaped	Dome	No hole	Yes
Bego Semados RI	Grade 4	Bone level	Internal	Hexagon	Straight	Yes	Tapered	Reverse buttress	Cone	No hole	Yes
Dentium Super Line	Grade 5	Bone level	Internal	Conical	Straight	No	Tapered	Buttress	Dome	No hole	Yes
Friadent Ankylos C/X	Grade 4	Subcrestal	Internal	Conical	Straight	No	Tapered	V-shaped	Dome	No hole	Yes
Implant Direct InterActive	Grade 5	Bone level	Internal	Conical	Straight	Yes	Tapered	Reverse buttress	Dome	No hole	Yes
Implant Direct Legacy 3	Grade 5	Bone level	Internal	Hexagon	Straight	Yes	Tapered	Reverse buttress	Dome	No hole	Yes
MIS BioCom M4	Grade 5	Bone level	Internal	Hexagon	Straight	No	Straight	V-shaped	Flat	No hole	Yes
MIS C1	Grade 5	Bone level	Internal	Conical	Straight	Yes	Tapered	Reverse buttress	Dome	No hole	Yes
MIS Seven	Grade 5	Bone level	Internal	Hexagon	Straight	Yes	Tapered	Reverse buttress	Dome	No hole	Yes
Osstem Implant Company GS III	Grade 5	Bone level	Internal	Conical	Straight	Yes	Tapered	V-shaped	Dome	No hole	Yes
SGS Dental P7N	Grade 5	Bone level	Internal	Hexagon	Straight	Yes	Tapered	V-shaped	Flat	No hole	Yes
TBR Implanté	Grade 5	Bone level	Internal	Octagon	Straight	No	Straight	No threads	Flat	Round	Yes
Wolf Dental Conical Screw-Type	Grade 4	Bone level	Internal	Hexagon	Straight	No	Tapered	V-shaped	Cone	No Hole	Yes

The analyses were performed in a few steps: first, all of the X-rays were edited (leveled) (Figure 1); next, the MBL near the implant neck area was measured (Figure 2), and then the X-ray image was loaded into MaZda in a bitmap file format. Next, the region of interest (ROI) was marked near the neck on the mesial and/or distal side of the implant (5–6 mm height) (Figure 3a). The ROI was marked on the RTG image immediately after inserting the dental implant and after 3 months of healing (Figure 3b). Any bone loss after 3 months was evaluated through radiographic analysis, as the vertical differences between the implant platforms and the first bone contact with the implant surface. The ROIs were normalized ($\mu \pm 3\sigma$) to share the same average (μ) and standard deviation (σ) of optical density within the ROI. The selected image texture features—sum of squares (SumOfSqrs), sum of average (SumAverg), entropy, different entropy (DifEntr), long-run emphasis moment (LngREmph), and short-run emphasis moment (ShrtREmph)—in the ROIs were calculated for the reference bone and for the bone near the implant neck. The Haar wavelet decomposition (LH, HL, LL, HH) was also performed and statistically analyzed after 3 months of observation. All features were gathered from four angles: 0°, 45°, 90°, and 135° from done pixel and the average value was later calculated.

$$SumAverg = \sum_{i=1}^{2N_g} ip_{x+y}(i)$$

$$SumOfSqrs = \sum_{N_g}^{N_g} \cdot \sum_{j=1}^{N_g} (i - \mu_x)^2 \, p(i,j)$$

$$Entropy = -\sum_{i=1}^{N_g} \sum_{j=1}^{N_g} p(i,j) \log(p(i,j))$$

$$DifEntr = -\sum_{i=1}^{N_g} p_{x-y}(i) \log(p_{x-y}(i))$$

where Σ is sum, N is the number of levels of optical density in the radiograph, i and j are the optical density of pixels five-image-point distant one from another, p is probability, and log is logarithm [11].

$$LngREmph = \left(\sum_{i=1}^{N_g} \sum_{j=1}^{N_r} j^2 p(i,j)\right)/C$$

$$ShrtREmph = \left(\sum_{i=1}^{N_g} \sum_{j=1}^{N_r} j^{-2} p(i,j)\right)/C$$

where Σ is sum, N is the number of series of pixels with density level i and length j. N_g is the number of levels for image density (8 bits, i.e., 256 gray levels), N_r is the number of pixels in series, p is the probability, and C is the coefficient, as below:

$$C = \sum_{j=1}^{N_r} \sum_{i=1}^{N_g} p(i,j)$$

Statistical Analysis

The Kruskal–Wallis test (to compare time-dependent alternations in medians) was applied for statistical analysis. Next, a multiple comparison procedure was used to determine which means were significantly different from the others. The method discriminates among the variables Fisher's least significant difference (LSD) procedure. The difference was considered significant if $p < 0.05$. Stargraphics Centurion XVI (Statgraphics-StatPoint Technologies, Inc., The Plains, VA, USA) was used for the statistical analyses.

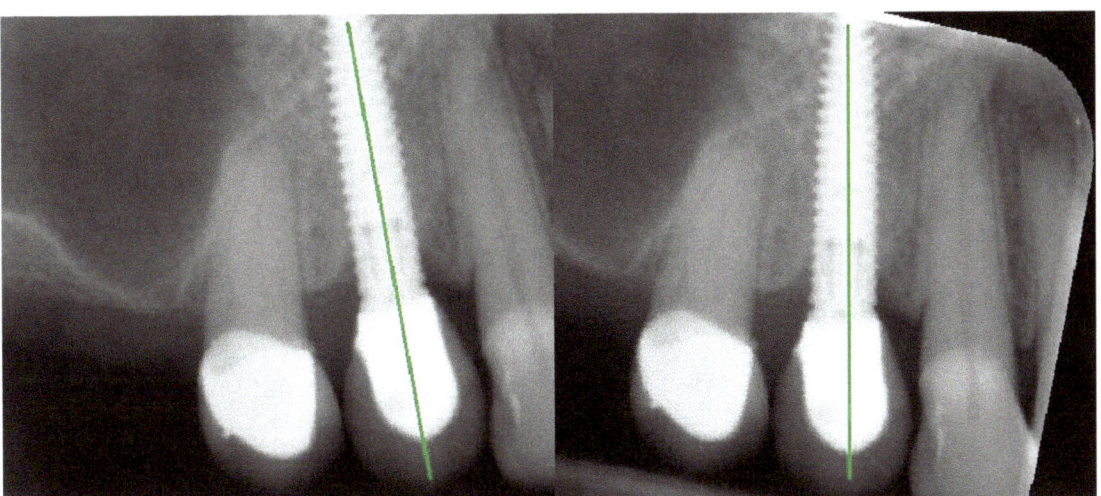

Figure 1. Geometrical alignment of radiograph image. The green line marked on the implants indicates the long axis of the implant.

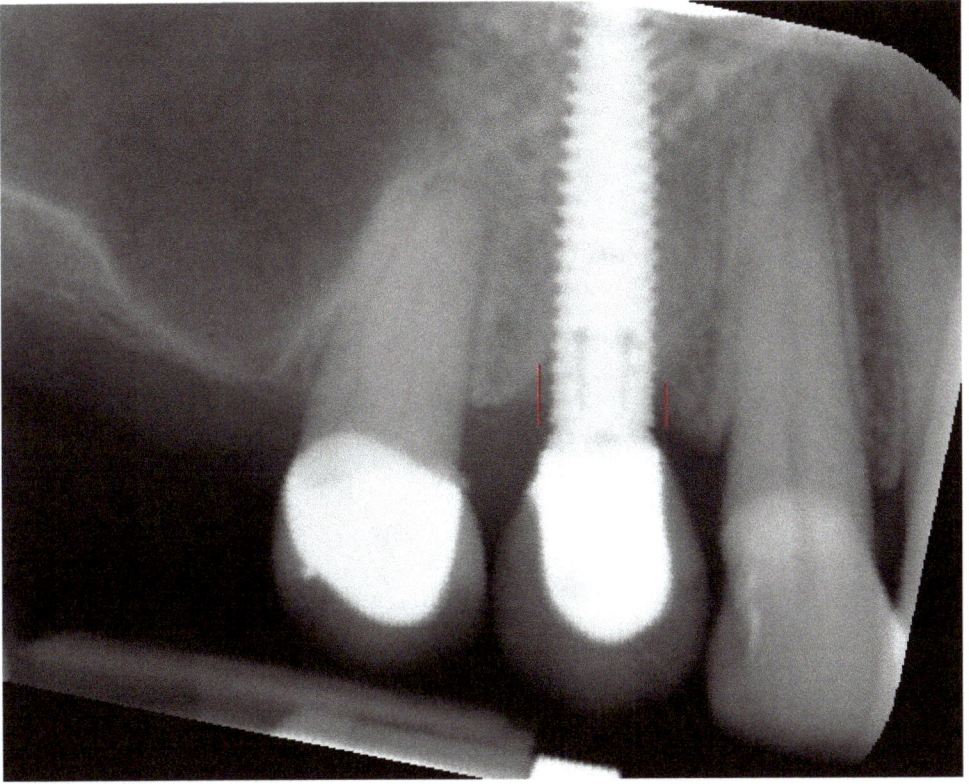

Figure 2. Measuring of marginal bone loss on the radiographic images. Red lines indicate the implant platform to the bottom of the bone loss cavity.

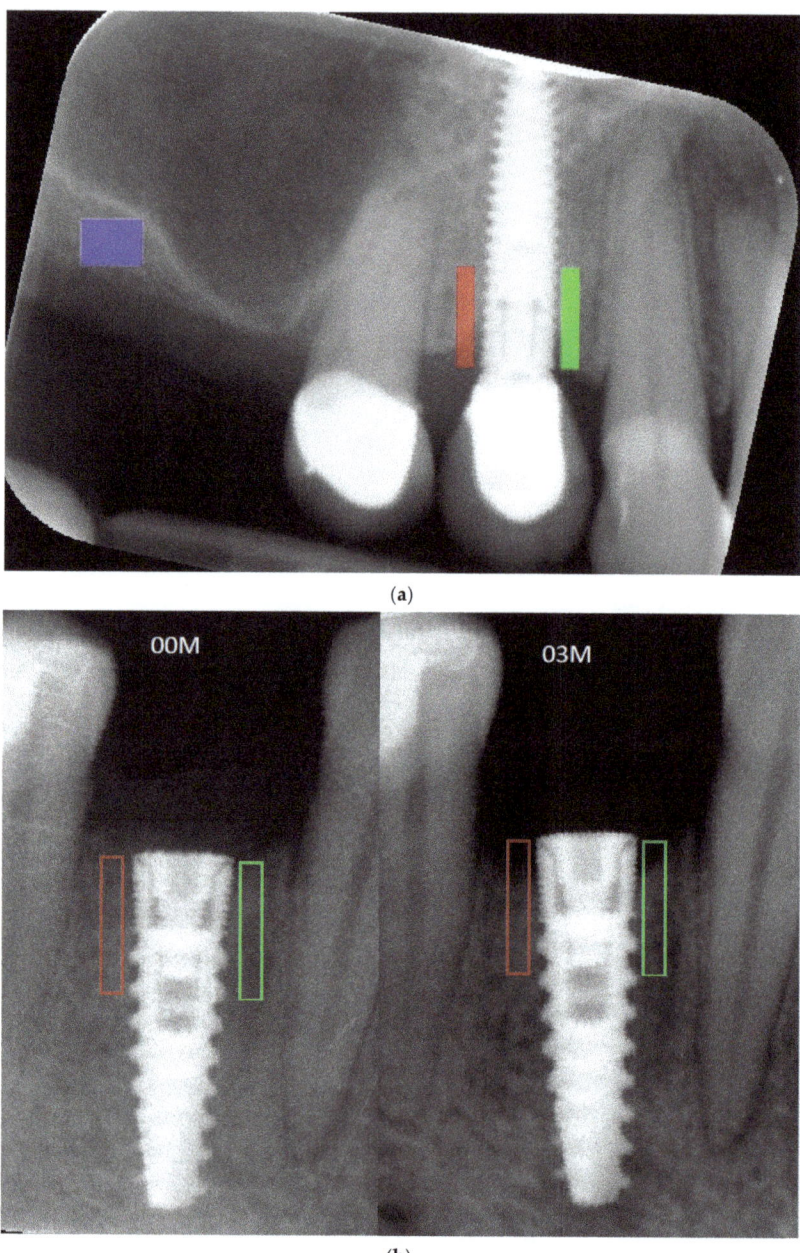

Figure 3. (a) Marking a ROI. ROIs were marked near the implant neck area. Green area—mesial implant neck area; red area—distal implant neck area; blue area—reference bone. Abbreviations: ROI—region of interest. (b) Marking a region of interest on RTG image immediately after inserting the implant and 3 months after the first stage of the healing process. Green area—mesial implant neck area; red area—distal implant neck area. At the bottom of the marked area on the right (03M), it can be noticed that MBL occurred and is analyzed. Abbreviations: MBL—marginal bone loss; 00M—0 months of observation; 03M—3 months of observation.

3. Results

3.1. Marginal Bone Loss Statistical Evaluation

The statistical evaluation revealed that the amount of marginal bone loss was between 0 and 8.05 mm after 3 months of observation; the average MBL for the mandible was 0.29 ± 0.98 mm and for the maxilla was 0.23 ± 0.91 mm, which were both statistically significant at $p < 0.01$. The MBL means for the anterior and posterior parts of the jaw were 0.32 ± 1 mm and 0.22 ± 0.91 mm, respectively, where p was lower than 0.01, which means that that was statistically significant.

3.2. Torque Statistical Evaluation

It was also noticed that when MBL occurred, higher torque was observed in the mandible group (mean 46.77 Ncm $\pm$ 14) than in the maxilla group (mean 40.5 Ncm $\pm$ 11.9), with statistical significance ($p < 0.05$); the torque value during the implantation procedure was between 5 Ncm and 90 Ncm (Table 2).

Table 2. Average values for marginal bone loss and torque. Values are presented for mandible, maxilla, and for anterior and posterior areas of the jaw. Since the p-value is greater than or equal to 0.05, there is no statistically significant relation.

Feature	Marginal Bone Loss	p-Value for MBL	Torque	p-Value for Torque
Mandible	0.29 mm $\pm$ 0.98	$p < 0.01$	42.5 $\pm$ 12.67	$p < 0.01$
Maxilla	0.23 mm $\pm$ 0.91	$p < 0.01$	41.04 $\pm$ 12.7	$p > 0.05$
Anterior	0.32 mm $\pm$ 1	$p < 0.01$	43.15 $\pm$ 11.31	$p < 0.01$
Posterior	0.22 mm $\pm$ 0.91	$p < 0.01$	41.08 $\pm$ 13.07	$p < 0.01$

Abbreviations: p—the probability of obtaining test results at least as extreme as the results actually observed, under the assumption that the null hypothesis is correct.

3.3. Torque Value and Marginal Bone Loss as a Dependency

Marginal bone loss is related to the torque value during the implant placement (CC = 0.06, R^2 = 0.3%, $p < 0.05$). If the torque increases, then MBL occurs more often (Figure 4). The study also showed that the average torque in the group with detected bone loss was higher than in the group without bone loss (42.01 and 40.04, respectively, where p was lower than 0.05, which means that was statistically significant) (Figures 5 and 6).

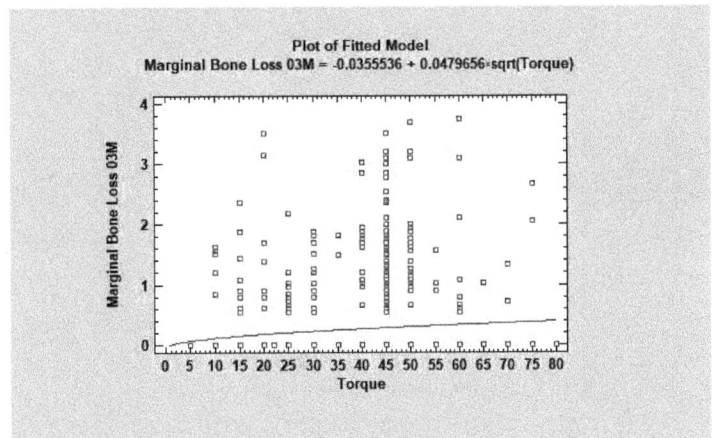

Figure 4. Dependence of marginal bone loss appearance from torque value after the dental implant insertion after 3 months of observation. The greatest number of marginal bone loss samples occurred in implants with a torque value equal to 45 Ncm. The higher the torque, the higher the MBL occurrence (with statistical significance). Abbreviations: MBL—marginal bone loss.

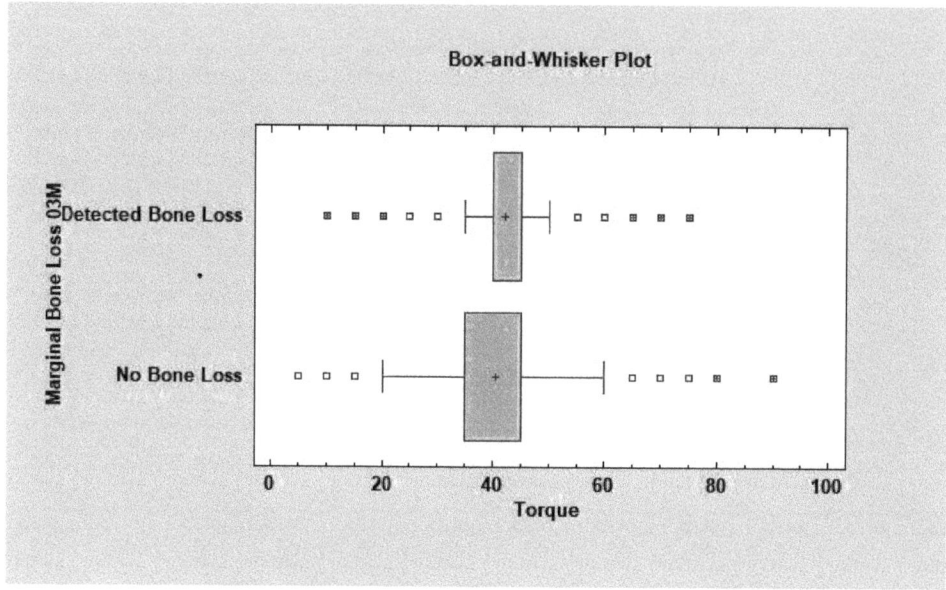

Figure 5. Dependence of average torque to marginal bone loss appearance after 3 months of observation. The mean where marginal bone loss was detected was higher than 42 Ncm. When the torque did not have an influence on MBL, the average torque was 40 Ncm or lower. Abbreviations: MBL—marginal bone loss.

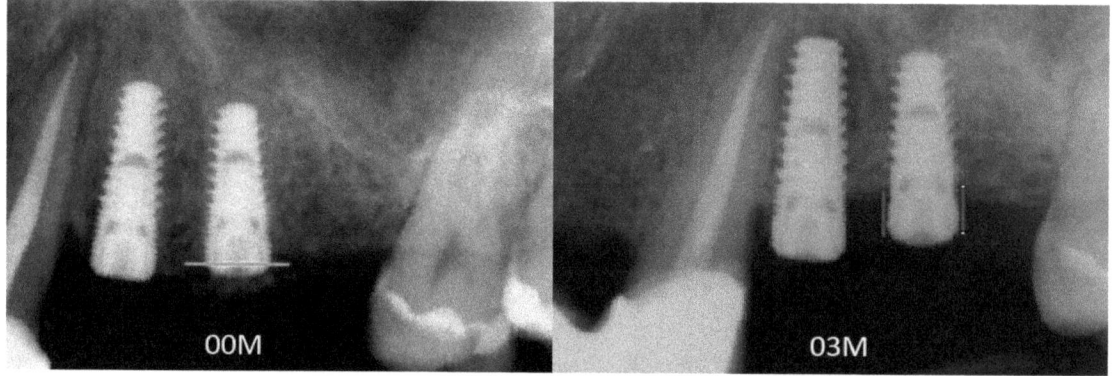

Figure 6. Figure presenting two radiographs. On the left is the radiograph image taken immediately after dental implant placement at 00M. The level of the bone at the beginning of the observation is marked by a green line. On the right is the RTG at 3 months of observation after implant placement. The red lines mark the marginal bone loss in relation to the previous bone level. Abbreviations: RTG—radiograph image; 00M—0 months of observation.

3.4. Implant Placement Region in Jaw

After splitting the implant samples into two groups, the mandible and the maxilla group, the statistical evaluation revealed that marginal bone loss only correlated with torque in the mandible group ($p < 0.01$), even though most samples with MBL in the maxilla group occurred with a torque higher than 40 Ncm (Figure 7). There was no correlation between the groups where augmentation was performed before implant placement ($p > 0.05$).

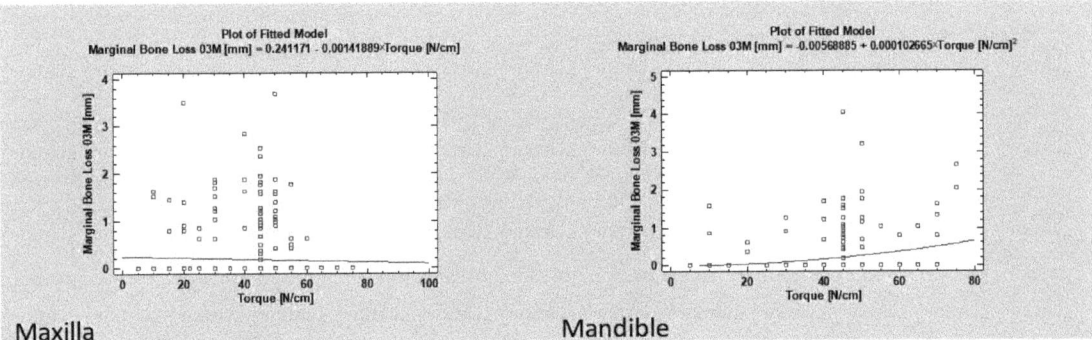

Figure 7. The graph on the left shows the dependence of marginal bone loss from dental implant insertion placement torque in the upper jaw (maxilla). There was no statistically significant difference ($p > 0.05$). The graph on the right presents the dependence of marginal bone loss on dental implant insertion placement torque in the lower jaw (mandible). There was statistical significance ($p < 0.05$).

Not all of the analyzed texture features were statistically significantly related to the marginal bone loss ($p < 0.05$). A p-value lower than 0.05 was observed for the following features after 3 months of observation:

- SumAverg,
- Entropy,
- DifEntr,
- LngREmph,
- ShrtREmph,
- Wavelets 4 and 5.

Texture features where the p-value was higher than 0.05, which means that this is not statistically significant, were:

1. SumOfSqrs,
2. Wavelet 6—was not detected.

As the reference, textural features for the trabecular bone were analyzed. The basal values for SumAverg, Entropy, DifEntr, LngREmph, and ShrtREmph are presented in Table 3.

Table 3. Reference texture feature values. Since the p-value is greater than or equal to 0.05, there is no statistically significant relation.

Texture Feature	Value	p-Value	Reference
SumAverg	63.22 ± 2.32	$p < 0.05$	Trabecular Bone
Entropy	2.70 ± 0.24	$p < 0.05$	Trabecular Bone
DifEntr	1.25 ± 0.12	$p < 0.05$	Trabecular Bone
LngREmph	1.53 ± 0.75	$p < 0.05$	Trabecular Bone
ShrtREmph	0.90 ± 0.05	$p < 0.05$	Trabecular Bone
WavEnLH_s-4	131.03 ± 94.39	$p < 0.05$	Trabecular Bone
WavEnLH_s-5	313.35 ± 213.69	$p < 0.05$	Trabecular Bone
WavEnHH_s-5	42.36 ± 44.35	$p < 0.05$	Trabecular Bone

Abbreviations: p—the probability of obtaining test results at least as extreme as the results actually observed, under the assumption that the null hypothesis is correct.

3.5. SumAverg Changes

The SumAverg for the implant neck area was 64.21 ± 2.9 at 00M. After 3 months, the SumAverg for the implant neck area with MBL was higher than after implantation, presenting 64.35 ± 3.54 and 64.16 ± 3.85, where MBL was not detected, and this was statistically significant ($p < 0.05$). There was no statistical difference between the maxilla and mandible groups ($p > 0.05$).

3.6. Entropy Changes

The Entropy for the implant neck area was 2.58 ± 0.19, and after implantation changed to 2.47 ± 0.21 where MBL was detected and 2.52 ± 0.2 where MBL was not detected, which was statistically significant. Statistically significant ($p < 0.01$) changes were also noticed in the maxilla and mandible groups with MBL (2.58 ± 0.12 changed to 2.52 ± 0.16, $p > 0.05$; and 2.58 ± 0.14 changed to 2.42 ± 0.16, $p < 0.01$, respectively).

3.7. DifEntr Changes

The DifEntr after implantation at 00M near the implant neck area was 1.11 ± 0.16 and changed to 1.01 ± 0.15 with MBL, and to 1.04 ± 0.16 where MBL was not present ($p < 0.05$). The DifEntr in the mandible group with MBL was 1.07 ± 0.15 and changed to 0.95 ± 0.14, which was statistically significant ($p < 0.05$).

3.8. LngREmph Changes

The LngREmph value at 00M was 1.71 ± 0.57 and changed to 2.01 ± 0.55 in the area with MBL, and 1.97 ± 0.75 where MBL did not appear ($p < 0.05$). The LngREmph value in the mandible group changed from 1.74 ± 0.64 to 2.11 ± 0.75 and there was no statistically significant difference ($p > 0.05$).

3.9. ShrtREmph Changes

The ShrtREmph also changed significantly: at 00M it was 0.88 ± 0.05, and after 3 months changed to 0.84 ± 0.05 for the area where MBL appeared and 0.85 ± 0.06 for the implant neck area without MBL. The ShrtREmph in the mandible group where MBL was correlated with MBL changed from 0.88 ± 0.6 to 0.84 ± 0.06, which was not statistically significant ($p > 0.05$).

3.10. Wavelet Decomposition Changes

The value for WavEnLH_s-4 after implantation for the maxilla group was 142.92 ± 111.54 and changed to 118.04 ± 87.24, which was statistically significant ($p < 0.01$). In the mandible group with MBL, the WavEnLH_s-4 changed from 134.35 ± 86.67 to 112.18 ± 116.14, which was statistically significant ($p < 0.05$).

The WavEnLH_s-5 in the mandible group changed from 345.23 ± 203.47 to 212.15 ± 185.22, which was statistically significant ($p < 0.05$). The WavEnHH_s-5 in the mandible group statistically significantly changed from 61.28 ± 65.77 to 35.75 ± 38.44, where the p-value was lower than 0.05 ($p < 0.05$).

Interestingly, the Wavelets 6 disappeared after 3 months of observation in the whole group with marginal bone loss (in the mandible and maxilla groups). The Wavelets 6 were also not detected in the reference trabecular bone. This texture index may be an indicator for cortical bone or changes in structure during the observation (Tables 4–6).

Table 4. Texture feature values at 00M, 03M, and for reference trabecular bone. Since the p-value is greater than or equal to 0.05, there is no statistically significant relation.

Texture Feature	Value at 00M	p-Value 00M	Value at 03M for the Area with MBL	Value at 03M for the Area without MBL	p-Value 03M	Reference Value for Trabecular Bone
SumAverg	64.21 ± 2.9	$p > 0.05$	64.35 ± 3.54	64.16 ± 3.85	$p < 0.05$	63.22 ± 2.32
Entropy	2.58 ± 0.19	$p > 0.05$	2.47 ± 0.21	2.52 ± 0.20	$p < 0.01$	2.70 ± 0.24
DifEntr	1.11 ± 0.16	$p > 0.05$	1.01 ± 0.15	1.04 ± 0.16	$p < 0.01$	1.25 ± 0.12
LngREmph	1.71 ± 0.57	$p > 0.05$	2.01 ± 0.55	1.97 ± 0.75	$p < 0.01$	1.53 ± 0.75
ShrtREmph	0.88 ± 0.05	$p > 0.05$	0.84 ± 0.05	0.85 ± 0.06	$p < 0.01$	0.90 ± 0.05

Abbreviations: 00M—0 months of observation; 03M—3 months of observation, MBL—marginal bone loss; p—the probability of obtaining test results at least as extreme as the results actually observed, under the assumption that the null hypothesis is correct.

Table 5. Texture feature values for mandible and maxilla groups after 3 months.

Texture Feature	Maxilla at 03M with MBL	Maxilla at 03M without MBL	p-Value for Maxilla	Mandible at 03M with	Mandible at 03M without	p-Value for Mandible
SumAverg	64.42 ± 0.91	64.37 ± 1.20	$p > 0.05$	64.76 ± 0.78	64.67 ± 0.89	$p > 0.05$
Entropy	2.52 ± 0.16	2.57 ± 0.14	$p > 0.05$	2.42 ± 0.16	2.50 ± 0.18	$p < 0.01$
DifEntr	1.05 ± 0.16	1.08 ± 0.15	$p > 0.05$	0.95 ± 0.14	1.01 ± 0.15	$p < 0.05$
LngREmph	1.89 ± 0.43	1.84 ± 0.48	$p > 0.05$	2.20 ± 0.68	2.11 ± 0.75	$p > 0.05$
ShrtREmph	0.85 ± 0.05	0.86 ± 0.05	$p > 0.05$	0.83 ± 0.6	0.84 ± 0.06	$p > 0.05$
WavEnLH_s-4	118.04 ± 87.24	122.93 ± 79.40	$p < 0.01$	112.18 ± 116.14	120.90 ± 74.04	$p < 0.05$
WavEnLH_s-5	304.59 ± 208.42	308.534 ± 268.32	$p > 0.05$	212.15 ± 185.22	287.54 ± 209.37	$p < 0.05$
WavEnHH_s-5	73.10 ± 65.97	63.89 ± 66.59	$p > 0.05$	35.75 ± 38.44	63.21 ± 73.00	$p < 0.05$

Abbreviations: 03M—3 months of observation; p—the probability of obtaining test results at least as extreme as the results actually observed, under the assumption that the null hypothesis is correct; MBL—marginal bone loss.

Table 6. Texture feature values for mandible and maxilla groups on the day of surgery.

Texture Feature	Maxilla at 00M before MBL Did Not Occur	Maxilla at 00M before MBL Occurred	Mandible at 00M before MBL Did Not Occur	Mandible at 00M before MBL Occurred
SumAverg	64.14 ± 0.15	64.16 ± 1.22	64.52 ± 0.94	64.71 ± 1.14
Entropy	2.61 ± 0.14	2.58 ± 0.12	2.56 ± 0.14	2.58 ± 0.14
DifEntr	1.15 ± 0.15	1.13 ± 0.12	1.07 ± 0.14	1.07 ± 0.15
LngREmph	1.68 ± 0.41	1.75 ± 0.52	1.77 ± 0.42	1.74 ± 0.64
ShrtREmph	0.88 ± 0.05	0.87 ± 0.05	0.87 ± 0.5	0.88 ± 0.6
WavEnLH_s-4	138.15 ± 94.13	142.92 ± 111.54	133.22 ± 86.73	134.35 ± 86.67
WavEnLH_s-5	331.45 ± 283.28	339.16 ± 300.11	324.12 ± 222.26	345.23 ± 203.47
WavEnHH_s-5	68.31 ± 88.00	69.94 ± 61.29	68.59 ± 75.42	61.28 ± 65.77

Abbreviations: 00M—the day of surgery; p—the probability of obtaining test results at least as extreme as the results actually observed, under the assumption that the null hypothesis is correct. MBL—marginal bone loss.

The research also showed that implant design also has an impact on marginal bone loss near the implant neck. This study compared several design properties: insertion implant level, neck microthreads, body shape, and body threads (thread shape). Apex shape, apex hole, apex groove, and connection type were not taken into account, as in the authors' opinion, these implant features do not have an impact on marginal bone loss in the early period of healing without exposing the implant for oral cavity conditions.

The statistical evaluation showed that MBL in the case of bone-level implants was 0.26 ± 0.97 mm, and for subcrestal implants was 0.09 ± 0.51 mm, which was statistically significant ($p < 0.05$).

Greater MBL occurred near the neck of implants without microthreads (0.31 ± 0.92 mm) than near the implants where microthreads were present (0.25 ± 0.94 mm), and this was statistically significant at $p < 0.05$.

The marginal bone loss for implants without body threads was higher (0.99 ± 0.77 mm) than for the implants where the body threads were V-shaped (0.15 ± 0.64 mm). MBL was also shown in the case of square-, buttress-, and reverse buttress-shaped body threads at 0.28 ± 0.93 mm, 0.67 ± 1.75, and 0.25 ± 0.97 mm, respectively. Statistical significance at $p < 0.05$ was noticed between the reverse buttress and no threads; between square threads and no threads; and between V-shaped threads and no threads.

The research also showed that the MBL in the case of straight-body implants was 0.20 ± 0.49 mm and in the case of tapered implants was 0.25 ± 0.95 mm. There was no statistical significance, as $p > 0.05$ (Table 7).

Taking into account torque as a factor that can lead to MBL, some implant design features were examined depending on the insertion region and the torque used (higher or lower than 45 Ncm). Titanium alloy, the level of implant placement, the presence of microthreads on the implant neck, implant body shape, and also the design of the threads on the implant body were checked.

Table 7. Comparison of marginal bone loss depending on selected implant design features.

Compared Implant Design Feature	MBL	p-Value
Bone-level implant	0.26 ± 0.97 mm	$p < 0.05$
Subcrestal implant	0.09 ± 0.51 mm	
Neck microthreads	0.25 ± 0.94 mm	$p < 0.05$
Without neck microthreads	0.31 ± 0.92 mm	
Without body threads	0.99 ± 0.77 mm	$p < 0.05$
V-shaped threads	0.15 ± 0.64 mm	
Square threads	0.28 ± 0.93 mm	
Buttress threads	0.67 ± 1.75 mm	
Reverse buttress threads	0.25 ± 0.97 mm	

Abbreviations: MBL—marginal bone loss; p—the probability of obtaining test results at least as extreme as the results actually observed, under the assumption that the null hypothesis is correct.

It was noticed that significantly higher MBL occurred in the anterior part of the mandible when the torque was lower than 45 Ncm, where dental implants made of titanium alloy Grade 4 (mean 1.06 ± 0.94 mm) were used. There was no correlation between MBL and titanium alloy in the maxilla samples. In the rest of the samples, titanium alloy was not correlated with MBL due to the localization of the implant or the insertion torque.

The research shows that the level of implant placement has an impact in the case of maxilla and mandible implants. In the anterior of the maxilla, greater MBL was noticed according to the tissue implant level (0.97 ± 0.88 mm) and the smallest MBL was found where subcrestal implants were used (mean 0.24 ± 1.14 mm), but only in cases when the torque was higher than 45 Ncm. In mandible-inserted implants, a subcrestal location had an impact on MBL in cases where the torque was lower than 45 Ncm (mean 1.06 ± 2.14 mm). The level of implant placement had no influence in the maxilla, either for the anterior part with a torque lower than 45 Ncm or the posterior part regardless of the torque used; and for the mandible, the anterior part with a torque higher than 45 Ncm and the posterior part regardless of the torque used.

Higher MBL was noticed in the anterior part of the maxilla when torque higher than 45 Ncm was used for implants without microthreads (mean 0.82 ± 1.76 mm). The presence or absence of neck microthreads in the case of the mandible, the posterior part of the maxilla, and the anterior part of the maxilla with torque lower than 45 Ncm was not correlated with MBL.

The shape of the implant body was not correlated with MBL in the case of maxilla and mandible dental implants regardless of the torque used during the insertions.

The research also showed that in maxilla implants with buttress threads inserted in the anterior part with a torque higher than 45 Ncm, and in the anterior part of the mandible where implants with V-shaped threads on the implant body were inserted with a torque lower than 45 Ncm, the MBL was greater and was statistically significant (mean 2.19 ± 3.34 mm and 1.06 ± 2.24 mm, respectively).

4. Discussion

The question is: Does the torque value of dental implants affect early marginal bone loss after 3 months of healing? There are publications about crestal bone stability claiming that there is no relation between implant torque insertion value and marginal bone loss [17]. In this study, 2196 samples of implant neck areas were analyzed and proved that there is a statistical relationship between a torque higher than 40 Ncm and marginal bone loss after 3 months of healing. Due to the lack of prosthetic loading, it can be declared that high torque during implant insertion is the main surgeon-related factor of MBL near the implant neck after 3 months of healing. Additionally, it was presented that dental implants inserted with a torque higher than 40 Ncm in the lower jaw were more susceptible to marginal bone loss, even though there are studies indicating that there is no correlation between marginal bone loss in the maxilla vs. the mandible [18,19].

The radiological or clinical evaluation of marginal bone loss is not always possible using only visual assessment. Sometimes, changes in the morphological part of the bone or bone substitute materials are not visible. Tomasz Wach et al. and Kozakiewicz et al. show that changes overcome during the healing process can be detected using texture features, already on the level of pixels [12,14,20]. Some of the texture features (inter-pixel relation in the optical density environment) can also be a good indicator of bone structure changes near the implant neck after 3 months of healing.

SumAverg and Entropy change over 3 months. It can be noticed that the decreasing value of SumAverg in cases where MBL was not detected can be a sign that the tissue around the dental implant neck is similar to intact trabecular bone tissue. The increasing value of Entropy also shows that in the group without MBL, the tissue around the dental implant neck after 3 months is more similar to trabecular bone. Referring to the other publications, it can also mean that the texture feature values of tissue near the implant neck after 3 months of healing in the group where MBL was detected approach cortical bone texture feature values [13,14].

The decreasing values of DifEntr and increasing values of LngREmph texture features are further proof that the tissue around the implant neck in the group with marginal bone loss is not similar to the trabecular one. For confirmation, Kozakiewicz et al. also proved that increasing LngREmph texture feature values and decreasing values of DifEntr are one of the signs of corticalization, which is correlated with bone loss [21]. In cases where MBL was detected and was correlated with corticalization, more longitudinal objects were observed (increasing LngREmph) as well as a decrease in chaotic patterns (decreased DifEntr).

Texture feature values that become similar to the reference of cortical bone can be an indicator of MBL. The process called corticalization near the implant neck surface is related to MBL [21]. On the other hand, an increasing value of the Entropy feature can be one of the signs that chaotic patterns have increased. Greater entropy means greater chaos, which can be equal to the decrease in bone structure.

It can be noticed that the values of the texture features in the group where marginal bone loss appeared were similar to the texture features of the reference scale for cortical bone. It is also related to higher torque when placing an implant. This means that higher torque during implant placement may lead to the densification of tissue around the implant neck. Condensed bone can be the first step to cortical bone formation, which is correlated with MBL.

Wavelet decomposition may be a healing process indicator. It can show that the trabecular part of the bone becomes part of the structure surrounding the dental implants. It also indicates the changes of long and small objects: longitudinal or circular shades [14,22]. It was noticed in Wach and Kozakiewicz's study [14] that the higher the scale of wavelet decomposition, the larger the object appears in the texture. The subbands HH and LL indicate circular shades, while LH and HL indicate longitudinal ones. The decrease in wavelets in scale 4 and 5 in subband LH in the mandible group where MBL was detected may be related to the disappearance of bone structure. The disappearance of the decomposition of wavelets in scale 6 in our research was interesting. Our research can lead to the conclusion that the wavelets in scale 6 are an indicator of the healing process that occur later than 3 months post-operation. Wavelets in scale 6 should be observed in the next observation period.

The subcrestal implant level placement looks promising. This study shows that the lowest MBL appeared near this kind of implant. It is likely that the level of implant placement is not the only factor to have an impact on MBL. There are also studies that show that implant level placement does not have an influence on MBL near the implants [6]. MBL before the loading and exposure of the implant may be a result of different stresses of the implant neck.

Implant design features and structural features may also have an impact on marginal bone loss regardless of the torque used or the region of insertion [23,24], or may have preservation influence on the bone around the implants [25]. Taking into consideration that torque was not correlated with marginal bone loss in the case of implants in the maxilla, the research shows a correlation between MBL and implant design in the anterior part of the maxilla where the torque was higher than 45 Ncm. This proves that marginal bone loss in the maxilla is not correlated with a high insertion torque, or high torque along with some other implant feature can result in greater MBL. In the implant samples analyzed in the lower jaw, dental implant design had an insignificant impact on MBL in cases where the torque was lower than 45 Ncm. This is further proof that insertion torque (higher than 45 Ncm) has an impact on MBL near the implant neck after the first 3 months of healing.

One limitation of the study is that the laboratory tests were not checked after 3 months. Another limitation is that the radiograph texture analyses were not compared to the histopathological examination of bone near the implant neck. Clinical marginal bone loss in mm was not carried out because of trauma—the authors checked the marginal bone loss before the second stage of treatment—before exposing the implant. There was also a limited number of samples, as not all patients came back after 3 months of healing and not all of the pictures taken were qualified after visual assessment for analyses. The BMI of the patients was also not taken into account. The research needs further evaluation of other local factors that could have an impact on marginal bone resorption.

5. Conclusions

Marginal bone loss is related to higher torque value during the implant placement procedure (higher than 40 Ncm torque was closely associated with MBL), but only in implants located in the lower jaw. The texture feature values that change over the healing process are closely related to the occurrence of MBL. It can be concluded that there are some texture features that can be used as indicators of problems near the inserted implants. The texture feature values (SumAverg, Entropy, DifEntr, and LngREmph) can indicate the likelihood of MBL occurrence. Haar wavelet decompositions should be observed in the next period of observation. Selected implant design features near the implant neck may have a positive impact on marginal bone, lower early bone loss associated with the neck microthreads and body threads. The level of implant placement also has an effect on early MBL. Additionally, the statistics verified the correlation between the design of the implant, insertion region, and torque, showing that cases where the implants were inserted with higher torque were more vulnerable to MBL near the implant neck in the early period of healing. This study is also the beginning of research into the correlation between texture features near the implant neck on the day of surgery and future bone loss.

Author Contributions: Conceptualization, T.W.; data curation, M.S. and T.W.; formal analysis T.W.; funding acquisition, T.W.; investigation, M.S. and T.W.; methodology, T.W.; resources, T.W.; software T.W.; supervision, G.T.; validation, T.W.; visualization, G.T. and T.W.; writing—original draft, T.W.; writing—review and editing, T.W. and G.T. All authors have read and agreed to the published version of the manuscript.

Funding: This research was funded by the Medical University of Lodz (grant numbers 503/5-061-02/503-51-001-18, 503/5-061-02/503-51-001-17, and 503/5-061-02/503-51-002-18).

Institutional Review Board Statement: The study was conducted according to the guidelines of the Declaration of Helsinki and approved by the Institutional Ethics Committee of the Medical University of Lodz, PL (protocol no. RNN 485/11/KB and date of approval: 14 June 2011).

Informed Consent Statement: Informed consent was obtained from all subjects involved in the study.

Data Availability Statement: The data on which this study is based will be made available upon request at https://www.researchgate.net/profile/Tomasz-Wach, access date 16 October 2022.

Conflicts of Interest: The authors declare no conflict of interest.

References

1. Çankaya, A.B.; Akçay, Ç.; Kahraman, N.; Köseoğlu, B.G. Oral surgical procedures under local anaesthesia in day surgery. *BMC Oral Health* **2018**, *18*, 4–7. [CrossRef] [PubMed]
2. Wach, T.; Kozakiewicz, M. Comparison of two clinical procedures in patient affected with bone deficit in posterior mandible. *Dent. Med. Probl.* **2016**, *53*, 22–28. [CrossRef]
3. Kowalski, J.; Lapinska, B.; Nissan, J.; Lukomska-Szymanska, M. Factors influencing marginal bone loss around dental implants: A narrative review. *Coatings* **2021**, *11*, 865. [CrossRef]
4. Aldahlawi, S.; Demeter, A.; Irinakis, T. The effect of implant placement torque on crestal bone remodeling after 1 year of loading. *Clin. Cosmet. Investig. Dent.* **2018**, *10*, 203–209. [CrossRef]
5. Kwiatek, J.; Jaroń, A.; Trybek, G. Impact of the 25-hydroxycholecalciferol concentration and vitamin d deficiency treatment on changes in the bone level at the implant site during the process of osseointegration: A prospective, randomized, controlled clinical trial. *J. Clin. Med.* **2021**, *10*, 526. [CrossRef]
6. Sargolzaie, N.; Zarch, H.H.; Arab, H.; Koohestani, T.; Ramandi, M.F. Marginal bone loss around crestal or subcrestal dental implants: Prospective clinical study. *J. Korean Assoc. Oral Maxillofac. Surg.* **2022**, *48*, 159–166. [CrossRef]
7. Attanasio, F.; Antonelli, A.; Brancaccio, Y.; Averta, F.; Figliuzzi, M.M.; Fortunato, L.; Giudice, A. Primary Stability of Three Different Osteotomy Techniques in Medullary Bone: An in Vitro Study. *Dent. J.* **2020**, *8*, 21. [CrossRef]
8. Di Domênico, M.B.; Collares, K.F.; Bergoli, C.D.; Dos Santos, M.B.F.; Corazza, P.H.; Özcan, M. Factors related to early marginal bone loss in dental implants—A multicentre observational clinical study. *Appl. Sci.* **2021**, *11*, 11197. [CrossRef]
9. Gehrke, S.A.; Júnior, J.A.; Treichel, T.L.E.; do Prado, T.D.; Dedavid, B.A.; de Aza, P.N. Effects of insertion torque values on the marginal bone loss of dental implants installed in sheep mandibles. *Sci. Rep.* **2022**, *12*, 538. [CrossRef]
10. Raz, P.; Meir, H.; Levartovsky, S.; Sebaoun, A.; Beitlitum, I. Primary Implant Stability Analysis of Different Dental Implant Connections and Designs-An In Vitro Comparative Study. *Materials* **2022**, *15*, 3072. [CrossRef]
11. Kołaciński, M.; Kozakiewicz, M.; Materka, A. Textural entropy as a potential feature for quantitative assessment of jaw bone healing process. *Arch. Med. Sci.* **2015**, *11*, 78–84. [CrossRef]
12. Kozakiewicz, M.; Wach, T. New oral surgery materials for bone reconstruction-a comparison of five bone substitute materials for dentoalveolar augmentation. *Materials* **2020**, *13*, 2935. [CrossRef] [PubMed]
13. Wach, T.; Kozakiewicz, M. Are recent available blended collagen-calcium phosphate better than collagen alone or crystalline calcium phosphate? Radiotextural analysis of a 1-year clinical trial. *Clin. Oral Investig.* **2021**, *25*, 3711–3718. [CrossRef] [PubMed]
14. Wach, T.; Kozakiewicz, M. Fast-versus slow-resorbable calcium phosphate bone substitute materials-texture analysis after 12 months of observation. *Materials* **2020**, *13*, 3854. [CrossRef] [PubMed]
15. Kozakiewicz, M.; Bogusiak, K.; Hanclik, M.; Denkowski, M.; Arkuszewski, P. Noise in subtraction images made from pairs of intraoral radiographs: A comparison between four methods of geometric alignment. *Dentomaxillofacial Radiol.* **2008**, *37*, 40–46. [CrossRef]
16. Szczypiński, P.M.; Strzelecki, M.; Materka, A.; Klepaczko, A. MaZda—A software package for image texture analysis. *Comput. Methods Programs Biomed.* **2009**, *94*, 66–76. [CrossRef]
17. Hof, M.; Pommer, B.; Strbac, G.D.; Vasak, C.; Agis, H.; Zechner, W. Impact of insertion torque and implant neck design on peri-implant bone level: A randomized split-mouth trial. *Clin. Implant Dent. Relat. Res.* **2014**, *16*, 668–674. [CrossRef]
18. Ajanović, M.; Hamzić, A.; Redžepagić, S.; Kamber-Ćesir, A.; Kazazić, L.; Tosum, S. Radiografska procjena gubitka alveolarne kosti oko zubnih implantata u maksili i mandibuli: Jednogodišnje prospektivno kliničko istraživanje. *Acta Stomatol. Croat.* **2015**, *49*, 128–136. [CrossRef]
19. Gheisari, R.; Eatemadi, H.; Alavian, A. Comparison of the Marginal Bone Loss in One-stage versus Two-stage Implant Surgery. *J. Dent.* **2017**, *18*, 272–276.
20. Comparison, L.T.; Beta, T.; Phosphates, T.; Surgery, O. Long Term Comparison of Application of Two Beta—Tricalcium Phosphates in Oral Surgery Porównanie odległych wyników leczenia z zastosowaniem. *Dent. Med. Probl.* **2009**, *46*, 384–388.
21. Kozakiewicz, M.; Skorupska, M. What Does Bone Corticalization around Dental Implants Mean in Light of Ten Years of Follow-Up? *J. Clin. Med.* **2022**, *11*, 3545. [CrossRef] [PubMed]
22. Marcin Kozakiewicz, K.G. Zastosowanie dyskretnej transformacji falkowej do matematycznego opisu radiotekstury kości żuchwy po zabiegach implantologicznych. *Mag. Stomatol.* **2009**, *19*, 90–93.
23. Patil, Y.B.; Asopa, S.J.; Deepa, D.; Goel, A.; Jyoti, D.; Somayaji, N.S.; Sabharwal, R. Influence of Implant Neck Design on Crestal Bone Loss: A Comparative Study. *Niger. J. Surg. Off. Publ. Niger. Surg. Res. Soc.* **2020**, *26*, 22–27.
24. Lovatto, S.T.; Bassani, R.; Sarkis-Onofre, R.; dos Santos, M.B.F. Influence of Different Implant Geometry in Clinical Longevity and Maintenance of Marginal Bone: A Systematic Review. *J. Prosthodont.* **2019**, *28*, e713–e721. [CrossRef]
25. Valderrama, P.; Bornstein, M.M.; Jones, A.A.; Wilson, T.G.; Higginbottom, F.L.; Cochran, D.L. Effects of implant design on marginal bone changes around early loaded, chemically modified, sandblasted Acid-etched-surfaced implants: A histologic analysis in dogs. *J. Periodontol.* **2011**, *82*, 1025–1034. [CrossRef]

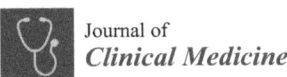

Article

Ultrasound Can Be Usefully Integrated with the Clinical Assessment of Nail and Enthesis Involvement in Psoriasis and Psoriatic Arthritis

Yu-Shin Huang [1], Yu-Huei Huang [2], Chiung-Hung Lin [1,3], Chang-Fu Kuo [1,4,5] and Yun-Ju Huang [1,4,*]

1. School of Medicine, Chang Gung University, Taoyuan City 33305, Taiwan
2. Department of Dermatology, Chang Gung Memorial Hospital, Taoyuan City 33305, Taiwan
3. Department of Thoracic Medicine, Chang Gung Memorial Hospital, Taoyuan City 33305, Taiwan
4. Department of Rheumatology, Allergy and Immunology, Chang Gung Memorial Hospital, Taoyuan City 33305, Taiwan
5. Center for Artificial Intelligence in Medicine, Chang Gung Memorial Hospital, Taoyuan City 33305, Taiwan
* Correspondence: b9502071@cgmh.org.tw; Tel.: +886-3-3281200

Abstract: **Objectives:** This study aimed to examine and compare the findings of nail and enthesis ultrasonography in patients with psoriasis and psoriatic arthritis. **Methods:** We identified 154 patients with psoriatic arthritis and 35 patients with psoriasis who were treated at Chang Gung Memorial Hospital, Taiwan, between September 2018 and January 2019. **Results:** There were significant differences in the Nail Psoriasis Severity Index scores and Glasgow Ultrasound Enthesitis Scoring System scores between patients with psoriasis and those with psoriatic arthritis. B-mode ultrasonography revealed that onychopathic changes were more common in the psoriasis group. The psoriatic arthritis group showed a higher proportion of lower-limb enthesopathy, with significant differences in distal patellar ligament thickness and Achilles tendon thickness. **Conclusion:** The findings of nail ultrasonography were more severe in psoriasis cases, and the ultrasonographic findings of enthesopathy of the lower limb were more severe in cases of psoriatic arthritis.

Keywords: Glasgow Ultrasound Enthesitis Scoring System; nail; psoriasis; psoriatic arthritis; ultrasonography

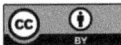

1. Introduction

Psoriatic disease is a noncontagious, multisystem autoimmune disease with predominantly skin and joint involvement [1]. Psoriasis (PsO) manifests with scaly erythematous plaques usually affecting extensor surfaces of the elbows and knees, and sometimes involves other parts of the body [2]. Psoriatic arthritis (PsA) is a chronic multifactorial inflammatory musculoskeletal disease, usually associated with PsO [3]. PsA affects similar diverse organ systems involving the skin, nails, enthesis, and axial and peripheral joints [4]. Diagnosis of PsA is difficult due to variable clinical signs. Nevertheless, classification systems such as the Classification for Psoriatic Arthritis (CASPAR) criteria, and several other screening tools, can facilitate recognition of this disease. Nail dystrophy, including onycholysis, pitting, and hyperkeratosis, is included in the CASPAR criteria [5]. Nail involvement is usually present in psoriatic disease, and the fingernails are more commonly affected than the toenails. In clinical examinations, high-frequency sonography provides valuable information regarding structural changes in the nail unit in PsO patients [6]. These morphostructural changes in PsO and PsA patients include ventral nail plate deposits, increased nail plate thickness, and irregular or completely fused nail plates [7]. Arbault et al. reported that feasibility and reliability were satisfactory for ultrasonography (US) of the nail in PsA [8].

In addition to nail changes, US can accurately detect enthesis involvement, including thickened tendons, hypoechogenicity, bursitis, and bone erosion [9]. The Glasgow Ultrasound Enthesitis Scoring System (GUESS) score is significantly higher in patients with PsO than in healthy controls [10,11]. In addition, entheseal involvement has been reported in asymptomatic patients with PsO, with a high prevalence of subclinical enthesopathy [11]. US may be useful for rheumatologists and dermatologists to identify subclinical PsA based on identification of enthesopathy in the distal interphalangeal (DIP) joint, quadriceps tendon, and the distal and proximal patellar ligament.

In our study, we aimed to establish the status of ultrasound as a valuable tool to evaluate nail changes and enthesopathy in psoriatic patients. This cross-sectional study revealed clinical characteristics and ultrasonographic differences between PsO and PsA in the nails and enthesis.

2. Materials and Methods

2.1. Study Design

This single-centre, cross-sectional study was performed between September 2018 and January 2019 at Chang-Gung Memorial Hospital Linkou branch, Taiwan. The study population consisted of 189 non-consecutive patients comprising 35 with PsO and 154 with PsA (CASPAR criteria) attending the outpatient clinics of the Dermatology and Rheumatology units at Chang-Gung Memorial Hospital. The exclusion criteria were age <18 years, mycosis, trauma and/or local corticosteroid injection within the past 6 weeks at the DIP joints and/or lower-limb entheses. Patients with other causes of hand or leg enthesopathy were also excluded, for example, rheumatoid arthritis, osteoarthritis, or crystalline deposition disease. The study was conducted in accordance with the tenets of the Declaration of Helsinki and local regulations. Ethical approval for the study was obtained from the Chang-Gung Memorial Hospital Local Ethics Committee, and all patients provided informed consent.

The following parameters were included: age, sex ratio, disease duration (years), family history, uveitis, body mass index (BMI), nail PsO, medical treatment including classical disease-modifying antirheumatic drugs (cDMARDs; methotrexate, sulfasalazine, leflunomide, cyclosporine), tumour necrosis factor inhibitor (certolizumab, golimumab, adalimumab, etanercept), interleukin-17 inhibitor (ixekizumab, secukinumab), interleukin-12 and interleukin-23 inhibitor (ustekinumab), and interleukin-23 inhibitor (guselkumab).

2.2. Ultrasound Assessment

Real-time high-resolution US was performed by an experienced rheumatologist using a Siemens ACUSON P300™ US system equipped with a variable-frequency transducer ranging from 6 to 18 MHz (focal range 0.2–3 cm, image field 16 mm), to observe nail anatomy. The parameters for B-mode US examinations were set to maximise the precision of detection. The settings for structures were: full nail structure (18 Hz), superior pole of the patella—quadriceps tendon enthesis (16 Hz), inferior pole of the patella—proximal patellar ligament enthesis (16 Hz), tibial tuberosity—distal patellar ligament enthesis (16 Hz), superior pole of the calcaneus—Achilles tendon enthesis (16 Hz), inferior pole of the calcaneus—plantar aponeurosis enthesis (6 Hz). Definition for abnormal enthesopathy thickness: quadriceps tendon > 6.1 mm, proximal and distal patellar ligament > 4 mm, Achilles tendon > 5.29 mm, plantar aponeurosis > 4.4 mm.

The patient was asked to sit with the forearm in a neutral position over a table, and the nails were scanned in longitudinal and transverse planes. We ensured a sufficient amount of US gel was applied to avoid alteration of nail thickness caused by transducer compression. Fingernails were scanned in grayscale mode with an 18 MHz transducer, to detect morphostructural changes (nail plate thickness, Wortsman's classification, nail bed thickness, hyperechoic spots, nail matrix thickness or loss) [12]. In more detail, nail plate thickness was determined by measuring the distance between the ventral and dorsal nail plates, and nail bed thickness defined as the distance from the ventral nail plate to the dorsal side of the distal phalange 2.5 mm from the proximal nail fold. The following elemental lesions were evaluated by grayscale US assessment according to the Brown University Nail Enthesis Scale (BUNES) preliminary definition of onychopathy (0–90): Wortsman's classification of the nail plate, thickness of the nail bed, hyperechoic spots on the nail bed, and nail matrix loss [7]. The nail plate, nail bed, and nail matrix thickness were measured in millimetres.

Abnormally hypoechoic and/or thickened tendons at the bony attachment, and bony changes including thickness, bursitis, enthesophytes, and erosions, were evaluated by grayscale US assessment at the quadriceps tendon enthesis, proximal patellar ligament enthesis, distal patellar ligament enthesis, Achilles tendon enthesis, and plantar aponeurosis enthesis, according to the GUESS (0–36) preliminary definition of enthesopathy [13].

2.3. Nail Change Assessment

The nail psoriasis severity index (NAPSI) was used for severity grading, which included parameters of the nail matrix (pitting, leuconychia, red spots in the lunula, crumbling) and nail bed (onycholysis, splinter haemorrhage, subungual hyperkeratosis, oil stains).

2.4. Statistical Analysis

Statistical analyses were performed using IBM SPSS Statistics 25.0 for Windows (IBM, Armonk, NY, USA). The results were evaluated using descriptive statistics. Linear correlations were represented using Pearson's correlation coefficient (r). Continuous variables were expressed as the mean ± standard deviation depending on the distribution, and categorical variables were expressed as percentages with the corresponding 95% confidence interval (95% CI). The independent-samples t-test was applied to compare continuous variables, which were expressed as frequencies and crosstabs. Pearson's Chi-square test was applied to compare categorical variables. Associative US features with the presence of nail involvement were also calculated using binary logistic regression analysis, adjusted for other variables. Inferential statistical analysis was conducted at a significance level of 5%, and $p < 0.05$ was taken to indicate statistical significance.

3. Results

3.1. Patient Characteristics

The study population consisted of a total of 189 patients comprising 154 with PsA and 35 with PsO. The characteristics of the study population are presented in Table 1. Nail PsO was observed in 158 of the 189 patients (83.6%).

Table 1. Demographic profile of study population and disease-related data for PsO and PsA patients.

Parameters	All (n = 189)	PsA (n = 154, 81.5%)	PsO (n = 35, 18.5%)	p Value
Age (years), mean ± SD	48.3 ± 14.2	49.3 ± 14.0	43.5 ± 14.6	0.028
Male:female	112:77	90:64	22:13	0.631
Disease duration (years), mean ± SD	12.2 ± 10.9	12.96 ± 11.14	8.83 ± 9.33	0.043
Family history, N (%)	45 (23.8%)	34 (22%)	11 (31.4%)	0.241
Uveitis, N (%)	6 (3.2%)	6 (3.9%)	0 (0%)	0.342
Body mass index (kg/m^2), mean ± SD	27.56 ± 5.272	27.86 ± 5.237	26.24 ± 5.312	0.136
Nail psoriasis, N (%)	158 (83.6%)	126 (82.9%)	32 (91.4%)	0.318
cDMARDs, N %	112 (59%)	97 (63.0%)	15 (42.9%)	0.182
Methotrexate	71 (37.6%)	58 (0.4%)	13 (0.4%)	0.916
Sulfasalazine	50 (26.5%)	49 (31.8%)	1 (2.9%)	0.001
Leflunomide	28 (14.8%)	27 (17.5%)	1 (2.9%)	0.031

Table 1. Cont.

Parameters	All (n = 189)	PsA (n = 154, 81.5%)	PsO (n = 35, 18.5%)	p Value
Cyclosporine	6 (3.2%)	4 (2.6%)	2 (5.7%)	0.318
b-DMARDs, N%	47 (25%)	43 (27.9%)	4 (11.4%)	0.137
TNFi, N %	24 (12.7%)	23 (14.9%)	1 (2.9%)	0.059
Golimumab	2 (1.1%)	2 (1.3%)	0 (0%)	0.506
Adalimumab	16 (8.5%)	16 (10.4%)	0 (0%)	0.050
Etanercept	6 (3.2%)	5 (3.2%)	1 (2.9%)	0.934
IL17i, N %	19 (10%)	18 (11.7%)	1 (2.9%)	0.312
Ixekizumab	2 (1.1%)	2 (1.3%)	0 (0%)	0.506
Secukinumab	18 (9.5%)	17 (11.0%)	1 (2.9%)	0.149
IL12, 23i, N %	6 (3.2%)	4 (2.6%)	2 (5.7%)	0.313
Ustekinumab	6 (3.2%)	4 (2.6%)	2 (5.7%)	0.318
IL23i, N %	1 (0.5%)	1 (0.6%)	0 (0%)	0.639
Guselkumab	1 (0.5%)	0 (0%)	1 (0.6%)	0.638
NAPSI (points), mean ± SD	23.8 ± 23.1	21.4 ± 21.4	33.9 ± 27.5	0.016

PsO, psoriasis; PsA, psoriatic arthritis; n, the number of patients; cDMARD, conventional disease-modifying antirheumatic drugs; bDMARDs, biological disease-modifying antirheumatic drugs; TNFi, tumor necrosis factor inhibitor; IL17i, interleukin 17 inhibitor; IL12, 23i, interleukin 12, 23 inhibitor; IL23i, interleukin 23 inhibitor; GUESS, Glasgow Ultrasound Enthesitis Scoring System; NAPSI, nail psoriasis severity index; BUNES, Brown University Nail Enthesis Scale; SD, standard deviation.

The PsA and PsO groups showed significant differences in mean age (49.3 ± 14.0 vs. 43.5 ± 14.6, respectively; $p = 0.028$), disease duration (12.96 ± 11.14 vs. 8.83 ± 9.33; $p = 0.043$), GUESS value (3.9 ± 2.6 vs. 2.8 ± 1.8; $p = 0.004$), and NAPSI value (21.4 ± 21.4 vs. 33.9 ± 27.5; $p = 0.016$). The PsA and PsO groups showed a modest linear correlation between NAPSI and BUNES scores ($r = 0.365$; $p < 0.0001$). The rates of administration of sulfasalazine, leflunomide, and adalimumab were significantly higher in the PsA group than the PsO group (49 of 154 vs. 1 of 35, respectively; $p = 0.001$; 27 of 154 vs. 1 of 35; $p = 0.031$; 16 of 154 vs. 0 of 35; $p = 0.050$).

3.2. Ultrasonography Findings at Finger Nails

After excluding samples that were not available, 1880 fingernails in the total study population were evaluated: 1530 from the PsA group and 350 from the PsO group.

According to the morphostructural US (Figure 1A–C), there were no significant differences in nail thickness or nail morphometric changes between the PsA and PsO groups (Table 2). Across the total study population, the nail plate thickness was 0.44 ± 0.21 mm, nail bed thickness was 1.78 ± 0.53 mm, and nail matrix thickness was 1.96 ± 0.47 mm. Moreover, 783 of 1880 (41.6%) fingernails showed normal morphometry (Wortsman type 0) and 1097 of 1880 (58.4%) fingernails showed abnormal morphometry (Wortsman types 1–4) in the nail plate. Furthermore, 1355 of the 1880 fingernails showed thickening of the nail bed, 30 (1.6%) showed hyperechoic spots, and 1351 (71.9%) showed nail matrix loss.

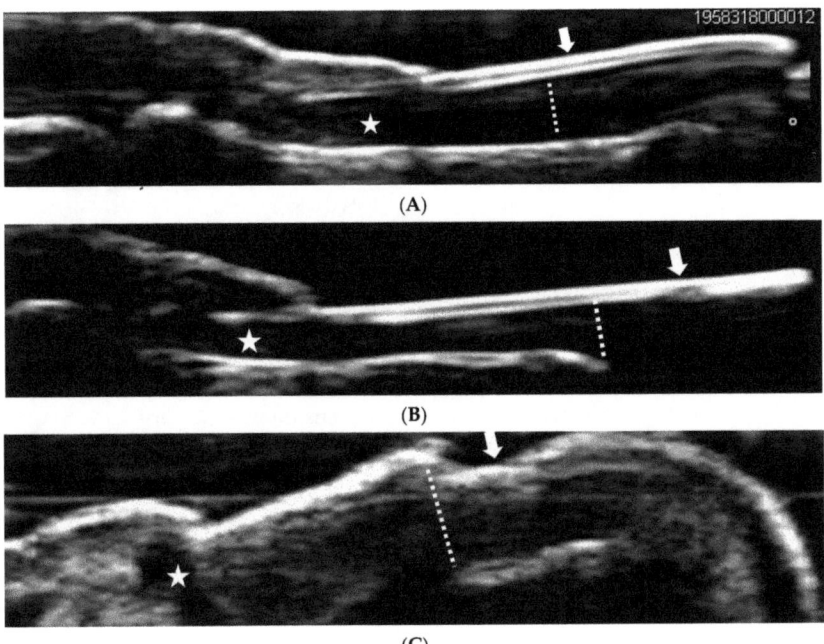

Figure 1. Comparison health control with nail psoriasis. (**A**). Grayscale ultrasonogaphy of the fingernail in a healthy control. Arrow: trilamellar and convex structure of nail plate with two hyperechoic lines, ventral and dorsal, separated by a hypoechoic line. Dashed line: the diameter of the nail bed is thinner in the distal part than the proximal. Asterisk: nail matrix present. (**B**). Grayscale ultrasonography of the fingernail in mild psoriatic nail disease. Arrow: interruption of hyperechoic line and loss of convex structure of nail plate (Wortsmann type II). Dashed line: loss of thinner distal part of nail bed. Asterisk: nail matrix present. (**C**). Grayscale ultrasonography of the fingernail in severe psoriatic nail disease. Arrow: a single and wavy hyperechoic layer losing its normal trilamillar appearance (Wortsmann type IV). Dashed line: thickening of nail bed. Asterisk: loss of normal nail matrix structure.

Table 2. Nail morphometry in ultrasounds.

Parameters	All	PsA (n = 154)	PsO (n = 35)	p Value
BUNES (points), mean ± SD	22.9 ± 8.5	22.6 ± 8.6	24.3 ± 8.3	0.292
Nail plate	1097 (58.4%)	853 (55.8%)	244 (69.7%)	0.276
Normal	783 (41.6%)	677 (44.2%)	106 (30.3%)	0.291
Wortsman type 0	783 (41.6%)	677 (44.2%)	106 (30.3%)	0.291
Abnormal	1097 (58.4%)	853 (55.8%)	244 (69.7%)	0.276
Wortsman type 1	206 (11.0%)	166 (10.8%)	40 (11.4%)	0.355
Wortsman type 2	211 (11.2%)	167 (10.9%)	44 (12.6%)	0.414
Wortsman type 3	84 (4.5%)	65 (4.2%)	19 (5.4%)	0.388
Wortsman type 4	595 (31.6%)	455 (29.7%)	141 (40.3%)	0.279
Nail plate thickness, mean ± SD	0.44 ± 0.21 mm	0.45 ± 0.21 mm	0.40 ± 0.25 mm	0.165
Nail bed	1362 (72.4%)	1083 (70.8%)	279 (79.7%)	0.631

Table 2. Cont.

Parameters	All	PsA (n = 154)	PsO (n = 35)	p Value
Thickness	1355 (72.1%)	1077 (70.4%)	278 (79.4%)	0.604
Hyperechoic spotting	30 (1.6%)	24 (1.6%)	6 (1.7%)	0.670
Nail bed thickness, mean ± SD	1.78 ± 0.53 mm	1.73 ± 0.45 mm	1.98 ± 0.77 mm	0.072
Nail matrix	1351 (71.9%)	1084 (70.8%)	267 (76.3%)	0.551
Loss	1351 (71.9%)	1084 (70.8%)	267 (76.3%)	0.551
Nail matrix thickness, mean ± SD	1.96 ± 0.47 mm	1.94 ± 0.45 mm	2.04 ± 0.54 mm	0.270

PsO, psoriasis; PsA, psoriatic arthritis; n, the number of patients.

The patients with psoriatic disease and clinical fingernail involvement presented onychopathic signs: pitting, leuconychia, crumbling, onycholysis, splinter haemorrhage, subungual hyperkeratosis, and oil stains (Supplementary Table S1). Subungual hyperkeratosis was significantly more common in the PsO group than the PsA group (25.7% vs. 11.7%, respectively; $p = 0.035$), while there were no significant differences in the other subtypes between the two groups.

Binary logistic regression analysis indicated clinical features associated with fingernail thickness (Supplementary Table S2). In particular, NAPSI (OR = 0.977; CI = 0.959–0.995; $p = 0.013$) and GUESS (OR = 1.332; CI = 1.046–1.696; $p = 0.020$) scores were significantly associated with fingernail thickness, independent of age, sex, and BMI.

3.3. Ultrasonographic Findings at the Lower-Limb Enthesis

Multiple sites of enthesopathy were detected with clinical lower-limb involvement in PsA and PsO patients, including quadriceps tendon enthesis, proximal patellar ligament enthesis, distal patellar ligament enthesis, Achilles tendon enthesis, and plantar aponeurosis enthesis (Table 3). US indicated abnormally hypoechoic lesions, thickened tendons at sites of bone attachment, and changes in bones. The ligaments of the lower limbs were thicker in the PsA group than the PsO group, but the differences between the two groups were not significant, except for distal patellar ligament thickness and Achilles tendon thickness, which were significantly greater in patients with PsA than in those with PsO (3.7 ± 0.7 mm vs. 3.4 ± 0.7 mm, respectively; $p = 0.032$; 4.8 ± 1.0 mm vs. 4.5 ± 0.8 mm; $p = 0.044$) (Table 3).

Table 3. GUESS values and tendon thickness of PsA and PsO patients.

Parameters	All (n = 189)	PsA (n = 154)	PsO (n = 35)	p Value
GUESS (points), mean ± SD	3.7 ± 2.5	3.9 ± 2.6	2.8 ± 1.8	0.004
Superior pole of the patella—quadriceps tendon enthesis	75 (39.7%)	64 (41.6%)	11 (31.4%)	0.588
• Quadriceps tendon thickness > 6.1 mm	61 (32.3%)	53 (34.4%)	8 (22.9%)	0.303
Quadriceps tendon thickness (mm), mean ± SD	5.4 ± 1.0 mm	5.4 ± 1.0 mm	5.1 ± 1.1 mm	0.056
• Suprapatellar bursitis	1 (0.5%)	1 (0.6%)	0 (0%)	0.622
• Superior pole of patella erosion	0 (0%)	0 (0%)	0 (0%)	-
• Superior pole of patella enthesophyte	22 (11.6%)	19 (12.3%)	3 (8.6%)	0.159
Inferior pole of the patella—proximal patellar ligament enthesis	130 (68.8%)	104 (67.5%)	26 (74.3%)	0.636
• Patellar ligament thickness > 4 mm	129 (68.3%)	103 (66.9%)	26 (74.3%)	0.626
Proximal patellar ligament thickness (mm), mean ± SD	4.4 ± 0.9 mm	4.5 ± 0.9 mm	4.2 ± 0.8 mm	0.160
• Inferior pole of patella erosion	4 (2.1%)	4 (2.6%)	0 (0%)	0.320
• Inferior pole of patella erosion	4 (2.1%)	4 (2.6%)	0 (0%)	0.320

Table 3. Cont.

Parameters	All (n = 189)	PsA (n = 154)	PsO (n = 35)	p Value
• Inferior pole of patella enthesophyte	2 (1.1%)	1 (0.6%)	1 (2.9%)	0.272
Tibial tuberosity—distal patellar ligament enthesis	94 (49.7%)	82 (53.2%)	12 (34.3%)	0.364
• Patellar ligament thickness > 4 mm	72 (38.1%)	63 (40.9%)	9 (25.7%)	0.140
Distal patellar ligament thickness (mm), mean ± SD	3.6 ± 0.7 mm	3.7 ± 0.7 mm	3.4 ± 0.7 mm	**0.032**
• Infrapatellar bursitis	24 (12.7%)	21 (13.6%)	3 (8.6%)	0.438
• Tibial tuberosity erosion	8 (4.2%)	8 (5.2%)	0 (0%)	0.155
• Tibial tuberosity enthesophyte	9 (4.8%)	9 (5.8%)	0 (0%)	0.319
Superior pole of the calcaneus—Achilles tendon enthesis	95 (50.3%)	79 (51.3%)	16 (45.7%)	0.251
• Achilles tendon thickness > 5.29 mm	69 (36.5%)	57 (37.0%)	12 (34.3%)	0.251
Achilles tendon thickness (mm), mean ± SD	4.8 ± 1.0 mm	4.8 ± 1.0 mm	4.5 ± 0.8 mm	0.044
• Retrocalcaneal bursitis	7 (3.7%)	5 (3.2%)	2 (5.7%)	0.123
• Posterior pole of calcaneus erosion	10 (5.3%)	10 (6.5%)	0 (0%)	0.278
• Posterior pole of calcaneus enthesophyte	39 (20.6%)	35 (22.7%)	4 (11.4%)	0.145
Inferior pole of the calcaneus—plantar aponeurosis enthesis	32 (16.9%)	27 (17.5%)	5 (14.3%)	0.381
Plantar aponeurosis thickness > 4.4 mm	31 (16.4%)	26 (16.9%)	5 (14.3%)	0.416
• Plantar aponeurosis thickness (mm), mean ± SD	3.5 ± 0.7 mm	3.5 ± 0.8 mm	3.4 ± 0.6 mm	0.639
• Inferior pole of calcaneus erosion	1 (0.5%)	1 (0.6%)	0 (0%)	0.622
• Inferior pole of calcaneus enthesophyte	1 (0.5%)	1 (0.6%)	0 (0%)	0.622

PsO, psoriasis; PsA, psoriatic arthritis; n, number of patients; GUESS, Glasgow Ultrasound Enthesitis Scoring System; SD, standard deviation.

3.4. Uniform Score Systems under Different Systemic Therapies

Subgroup analysis was carried out to investigate whether treatments impacted psoriatic nail change and enthesopathy. We selected three uniform score systems (NAPSI, BUNES and GUESS) and defined them as six categorical variables (NAPSI ≥ 20, NPASI < 20, BUNES ≥ 22, BUNES < 22, BUESS ≥ 3, BUNESS < 3). Next, we compared six parameters in relation to psoriatic disease (PsA, PsO) and three subgroup therapies (only cDMARDs, only bDMARDs, and combined therapy). Under Pearson's Chi-square analysis, there were significant differences between high or low GUESS values and PsO or PsA. (p = 0.030). High or low GUESS values also showed significant differences for the three systemic therapies (p = 0.021) (Table 4). Furthermore, for the high or low GUESS parameter, comparisons of cDMARDs versus bDMARDs and bDMARDs versus combined therapy revealed significant differences (p = 0.012, p = 0.007, respectively).

Table 4. NAPSI, BUNES and GUESS values in patients with psoriatic disease receiving systemic therapy.

Parameters	PSO (n = 35)	PSA (n = 154)	p Value	cDMARDs (n = 94)	bDMARDs (n = 29)	Combined Therapy (n = 18)	p Value
High NAPSI (≥20)	21 (60%)	72 (46.8%)	0.157	44 (46.8%)	15 (51.7%)	7 (38.9%)	0.693
Low NAPSI (<20)	14 (40%)	82 (53.2%)	0.157	50 (53.2%)	14 (48.3%)	11 (61.1%)	0.693
High BUNES (≥22)	21 (60%)	74 (48.1%)	0.168	51 (54.3%)	16 (55.2%)	7 (38.9%)	0.416

Table 4. Cont.

Parameters	PSO (n = 35)	PSA (n = 154)	p Value	cDMARDs (n = 94)	bDMARDs (n = 29)	Combined Therapy (n = 18)	p Value
Low BUNES (<22)	13 (37.1%)	78 (50.6%)	0.168	42 (44.7%)	12 (41.4%)	11 (61.1%)	0.416
High GUESS (≥3)	12 (34.3%)	82 (53.2%)	0.030	60 (63.8%)	26 (89.7%)	10 (55.6%)	0.021
Low GUESS (<3)	23 (65.7%)	68 (44.2%)	0.030	31 (33.0%)	3 (10.3%)	8 (44.4%)	0.021

PsO, psoriasis; PsA, psoriatic arthritis; n, number of patients; cDMARDs, only conventional disease-modifying antirheumatic drugs; bDMARDs, only biological disease-modifying antirheumatic drugs; Combined therapy, cDMARDs plus bDMARDs; GUESS, Glasgow Ultrasound Enthesitis Scoring System; NAPSI, nail psoriasis severity index; BUNES, Brown University Nail Enthesis Scale.

4. Discussion

In this study, we used ultrasonography to quantify the severity of enthesopathy affecting nails and lower extremities, aiming to reveal correlations between enthesopathy and subgroups of psoriatic diseases. The prevalence of enthesopathy involvement was demonstrated under designated ultrasound survey. PsA was associated with a higher GUESS value, and nail US was not different between PsO and PsA groups.

In our study population, higher proportions of nail plate, nail bed, and nail matrix abnormalities were seen in patients with PsO than in those with PsA. The mean nail plate thickness was greater in the PsA group, although the difference was not significant. Conversely, the mean nail bed and nail matrix thicknesses were greater in the PsO group, although the differences were not significant (Table 2). However, Naredo et al. reported that nail bed thickness, nail plate thickness, and B-mode scores were significantly higher in the nails of patients with PsO than those with PsA [14]. The nail imaging findings in our study were similar to those of previous studies by Aydin et al. and Idolazzi et al [15,16]. Those studies reported nail involvement in both PsA and PsO, with higher frequencies of structural and inflammatory changes in both groups compared with healthy controls, but no significant differences between the PsA and PsO groups [15,16]. The sample size of the PSO group was small. That may be the reason that that NAPSI value was higher in the PSO group, but no differences in nail morphometry parameters were found between the groups. Numerous surveys have shown a remarkably high frequency of clinically occult musculoskeletal symptoms in psoriasis patients, ultrasound in particular having revealed a high prevalence of subclinical enthesitis and other inflammatory changes. Strategies must recognize and incorporate assessment of community-based psoriasis sufferers with only mild skin disease, as this group is at particular risk of PsA [17].

Among our patients, the GUESS values were significantly higher in the PsA group than the PsO group. A previous study showed that common sites of enthesitis in PsA patients included the insertion of the quadriceps tendon into the patellar bone, insertion of the proximal patellar ligament into the patellar bone, insertion of the distal patellar ligament into the tibial tuberosity, insertion of the Achilles tendon into the calcaneus bone, and insertion of the plantar aponeurosis into the calcaneus bone [18]. Three studies have shown the validity of US for early detection of subclinical enthesopathy in psoriatic diseases [19–21].

In contrast to lesion thickness, the distal patellar ligament and Achilles tendon were significantly thicker in PsA than in PsO (Table 3). Moshrif et al. reported that thickening of the Achilles tendon was the most common sign in patients with enthesitis [22]. In the ULISSE study, Achilles tendon lesion was found to be significantly higher in PsA than in PsO [17]. However, this was contrary to the report by Michelsen et al. indicating no association between clinical and US signs of Achilles enthesitis in PsA [23]. Graceffa et al. reported that thickness of enthesis at the superior pole of the patella was significantly increased in PsA, but not in PsO nor healthy controls [24]. Macchioni et al. also reported that entheseal thickening of the Achilles tendon was significantly greater in PsA than PsO [25].

However, isolated peripheral enthesitis was not significant in most of our study population, except in cases of Achilles tendon thickness and distal patellar ligament thickness.

In our study, the rate of clinical nail abnormalities was higher in the PsO group than the PsA group (32 of 35 (91.4%) vs. 126 of 152 (82.9%), respectively). There were no significant differences between the two groups, except in nail bed subungual hyperkeratosis (Supplementary Table S1). Castellanos-González et al. and Naredo et al. reported that there was a significant correlation between target NAPSI value and evidence of enthesopathy [26]. Our observation that GUESS values were significantly higher in patients with PsO than in healthy controls or those with other dermopathies was consistent with the reports of Gutierrez et al. and Pistone et al. [11,27]. Both of those studies revealed the ability of US to detect signs of subclinical enthesopathy, and demonstrating its value in detecting entheseal changes in psoriatic patients according to GUESS rating.

In the present study, GUESS value was significantly higher in the PsA group than the PsO group on binary logistic regression analysis (OR = 1.332; CI = 1.046–1.696; p = 0.020) (Supplementary Table S2). In addition, there was a modest correlation between GUESS and BUNES scores in the PsA group. Ash et al. reported that enthesopathy and inflammation scores were higher in PsO patients with nail disease than in those without nail disease, or in healthy controls [28]. Furthermore, El Miedany et al. also reported that structural joint damage was significantly associated with onychopathy-defined changes in the trilaminar appearance of the nails, extensor tendon enthesopathy, or enhanced vascularity in the nail bed (OR = 2.30, 95% CI = 1.17–3.69) [29]. Those studies supported the suggestion that clinical evidence of onychopathy may be correlated with enthesopathy in psoriatic patients. Increased GUESS values and/or entheseal thickness are more common in patients with PsA than in those with PsO.

This study had some limitations. First, we did not investigate intraobserver reliability of US features. Second, there was a marked difference in the numbers of patients with PsA (n = 154) and those with PsO (n = 35). Third, we could not discriminate the directionality of the association between nail thickening and skin manifestations of psoriatic disease. Fourth, the sonographer was not blinded to the presence of enthesopathy and nail involvement. Furthermore, the longer duration of PsA might be a suspicious confounding factor in GUESS analysis. We had no data about the subgroups of PsA, the severity of PsA, nor the severity of PsO. Finally, treatment plans and disease activity, including remission, might be important confounding factors.

5. Conclusions

In conclusion, US was valuable for evaluating nail changes and enthesopathy in PsO. We found several quantitative parameters that may be useful in US assessment of psoriatic nails and the entheseal complex. Further US studies of nail and entheseal involvement in psoriatic diseases are required for application in clinical practice.

Supplementary Materials: The following supporting information can be downloaded at: https://www.mdpi.com/article/10.3390/jcm11216296/s1. Table S1: Subtypes of nail psoriasis; Table S2: Independent predictors of fingernail thickness in patients with PsA and PsO.

Author Contributions: Conceptualization, Y.-J.H. and Y.-H.H.; methodology, C.-H.L.; software, Y.-S.H.; validation, C.-H.L., C.-F.K. and Y.-J.H.; formal analysis, Y.-S.H.; investigation, C.-H.L. and Y.-J.H.; resources, Y.-J.H.; data curation, Y.-S.H.; writing—original draft preparation, Y.-S.H.; writing—review and editing, Y.-J.H.; visualization, Y.-S.H.; supervision, C.-F.K.; project administration, Y.-J.H.; funding acquisition, C.-F.K. All authors have read and agreed to the published version of the manuscript.

Funding: This work was partly funded by Grant CLRPG3H0014 at Chang Gung Memorial Hospital, Taiwan

Institutional Review Board Statement: The study was conducted in accordance with the tenets of the Declaration of Helsinki and local regulations. Ethical approval for the study was obtained from the Chang-Gung Memorial Hospital Local Ethics Committee.

Informed Consent Statement: All patients provided informed consent.

Data Availability Statement: Restrictions apply to the availability of these data. Data was obtained from Chang Gung Memorial Hospital and are available from the authors with the permission of Chang Gung Memorial Hospital.

Acknowledgments: The authors would like to acknowledge the support of the Division of Rheumatology, Allergy and Immunology, Chang Gung Memorial Hospital, Taoyuan, Taiwan.

Conflicts of Interest: The authors declare no conflict of interest.

References

1. Kim, W.B.; Jerome, D.; Yeung, J. Diagnosis and management of psoriasis. *Can. Fam. Physician* **2017**, *63*, 278–285. [PubMed]
2. Zlatkovic-Svenda, M.; Kerimovic-Morina, D.; Stojanovic, R.M. Psoriatic arthritis classification criteria: Moll and Wright, ESSG and CASPAR—A comparative study. *Acta Reumatol. Port.* **2013**, *38*, 172–178. [PubMed]
3. Gladman, D.D. Psoriatic arthritis. *Dermatol. Ther.* **2004**, *17*, 350–363. [CrossRef] [PubMed]
4. Ritchlin, C.T.; Colbert, R.A.; Gladman, D.D. Psoriatic Arthritis. *N. Engl. J. Med.* **2017**, *376*, 957–970. [CrossRef]
5. Taylor, W.; Gladman, D.; Helliwell, P.; Marchesoni, A.; Mease, P.; Mielants, H. Classification criteria for psoriatic arthritis: Development of new criteria from a large international study. *Arthritis Rheum.* **2006**, *54*, 2665–2673. [CrossRef]
6. Marina, M.E.; Solomon, C.; Bolboaca, S.D.; Bocsa, C.; Mihu, C.M.; Tătaru, A.D. High-frequency sonography in the evaluation of nail psoriasis. *Med. Ultrason.* **2016**, *18*, 312–317. [CrossRef]
7. Cunha, J.S.; Qureshi, A.A.; Reginato, A.M. Nail Enthesis Ultrasound in Psoriasis and Psoriatic Arthritis: A Report from the 2016 GRAPPA Annual Meeting. *J. Rheumatol.* **2017**, *44*, 688–690. [CrossRef]
8. Arbault, A.; Devilliers, H.; Laroche, D.; Cayot, A.; Vabres, P.; Maillefert, J.F.; Ornetti, P. Reliability, validity and feasibility of nail ultrasonography in psoriatic arthritis. *Jt. Bone Spine* **2016**, *83*, 539–544. [CrossRef]
9. Grassi, W.; Gutierrez, M. Psoriatic arthritis: Need for ultrasound in everyday clinical practice. *J. Rheumatol. Suppl.* **2012**, *89*, 39–43. [CrossRef]
10. Gisondi, P.; Tinazzi, I.; El-Dalati, G.; Gallo, M.; Biasi, D.; Barbara, L.M.; Girolomoni, G. Lower limb enthesopathy in patients with psoriasis without clinical signs of arthropathy: A hospital-based case-control study. *Ann. Rheum. Dis.* **2008**, *67*, 26–30. [CrossRef]
11. Gutierrez, M.; Filippucci, E.; De Angelis, R.; Salaffi, F.; Filosa, G.; Ruta, S.; Bertolazzi, C.; Grassi, W. Subclinical entheseal involvement in patients with psoriasis: An ultrasound study. *Semin. Arthritis Rheum.* **2011**, *40*, 407–412. [CrossRef] [PubMed]
12. Wortsman, X.; Jemec, G.B. Ultrasound imaging of nails. *Dermatol. Clin.* **2006**, *24*, 323–328. [CrossRef]
13. Balint, P.V.; Kane, D.; Wilson, H.; McInnes, I.B.; Sturrock, R.D. Ultrasonography of entheseal insertions in the lower limb in spondyloarthropathy. *Ann. Rheum. Dis.* **2002**, *61*, 905–910. [CrossRef] [PubMed]
14. Naredo, E.; Janta, I.; Baniandrés-Rodríguez, O.; Valor, L.; Hinojosa, M.; Bello, N.; Serrano, B.; Garrido, J. To what extend is nail ultrasound discriminative between psoriasis, psoriatic arthritis and healthy subjects? *Rheumatol. Int.* **2019**, *39*, 697–705. [CrossRef] [PubMed]
15. Aydin, S.Z.; Castillo-Gallego, C.; Ash, Z.R.; Marzo-Ortega, H.; Emery, P.; Wakefield, R.J.; Wittmann, M.; McGonagle, D. Ultrasonographic assessment of nail in psoriatic disease shows a link between onychopathy and distal interphalangeal joint extensor tendon enthesopathy. *Dermatology* **2012**, *225*, 231–235. [CrossRef]
16. Idolazzi, L.; Gisondi, P.; Fassio, A.; Viapiana, O.; Giollo, A.; Rossini, M.; Girolomoni, G.; Gatti, D. Ultrasonography of the nail unit reveals quantitative and qualitative alterations in patients with psoriasis and psoriatic arthritis. *Med. Ultrason.* **2018**, *20*, 177–184. [CrossRef]
17. Savage, L.; Tinazzi, I.; Zabotti, A.; Laws, P.M.; Wittmann, M.; McGonagle, D. Defining Pre-Clinical Psoriatic Arthritis in an Integrated Dermato-Rheumatology Environment. *J. Clin. Med.* **2020**, *9*, 3262. [CrossRef]
18. Raposo, I.; Torres, T. Nail psoriasis as a predictor of the development of psoriatic arthritis. *Actas Dermo-Sifiliogr.* **2015**, *106*, 452–457. [CrossRef]
19. Galluzzo, E.; Lischi, D.M.; Taglione, E.; Lombardini, F.; Pasero, G.; Perri, G.; Riente, L. Sonographic analysis of the ankle in patients with psoriatic arthritis. *Scand. J. Rheumatol.* **2000**, *29*, 52–55.
20. De Filippis, L.G.; Caliri, A.; Lo Gullo, R.; Bartolone, S.; Miceli, G.; Cannavò, S.P.; Borgia, F.; Basile, G.; Aloisi, G.; Zimbaro, G.; et al. Ultrasonography in the early diagnosis of psoriasis-associated enthesopathy. *Int. J. Tissue React.* **2005**, *27*, 159–162.
21. Hussein, S.; Elhefny, A.; Abdurrahman, M.; Aziz, N. Early detection of subclinical lower limb enthesopathy by ultrasonography in patients with psoriasis: Relation to disease severity. *Egypt. Rheumatol.* **2021**, *43*, 153–157. [CrossRef]
22. Moshrif, A.; Mosallam, A.; Mohamed, E.E.; Gouda, W.; Doma, M. Subclinical enthesopathy in patients with psoriasis and its association with other disease parameters: A power Doppler ultrasonographic study. *Eur. J. Rheumatol.* **2017**, *4*, 24–28. [CrossRef] [PubMed]
23. Michelsen, B.; Diamantopoulos, A.P.; Soldal, D.M.; Hammer, H.B.; Kavanaugh, A.; Haugeberg, G. Achilles enthesitis defined by ultrasound is not associated with clinical enthesitis in patients with psoriatic arthritis. *RMD Open* **2017**, *3*, e000486. [CrossRef] [PubMed]
24. Graceffa, D.; Bonifati, C.; Lora, V.; Saraceni, P.L.; De Felice, C.; Chimenti, M.S.; Perricone, R.; Morrone, A. Ultrasound assessment of enthesis thickness in psoriasis and psoriatic arthritis: A cross-sectional study. *Indian J. Dermatol. Venereol. Leprol.* **2019**, *85*, 175–181.

25. Macchioni, P.; Salvarani, C.; Possemato, N.; Gutierrez, M.; Grassi, W.; Gasparini, S.; Perricone, C.; Perrotta, F.M.; Grembiale, R.D.; Bruno, C.; et al. Ultrasonographic and Clinical Assessment of Peripheral Enthesitis in Patients with Psoriatic Arthritis, Psoriasis, and Fibromyalgia Syndrome: The ULISSE Study. *J. Rheumatol.* **2019**, *46*, 904–911. [CrossRef]
26. Castellanos-González, M.; Joven, B.E.; Sánchez, J.; Andrés-Esteban, E.M.; Vanaclocha-Sebastián, F.; Romero, P.O.; Díaz, R.R. Nail involvement can predict enthesopathy in patients with psoriasis. *J. Dtsch. Dermatol. Ges.* **2016**, *14*, 1102–1107. [CrossRef]
27. Pistone, G.; La Vecchia, M.; Pistone, A.; Bongiorno, M.R. Achilles tendon ultrasonography may detect early features of psoriatic arthropathy in patients with cutaneous psoriasis. *Br. J. Dermatol.* **2014**, *171*, 1220–1222. [CrossRef]
28. Ash, Z.R.; Tinazzi, I.; Gallego, C.C.; Kwok, C.; Wilson, C.; Goodfield, M.; Gisondi, P.; Tan, A.L.; Marzo-Ortega, H.; Emery, P.; et al. Psoriasis patients with nail disease have a greater magnitude of underlying systemic subclinical enthesopathy than those with normal nails. *Ann. Rheum. Dis.* **2012**, *71*, 553–556. [CrossRef]
29. El Miedany, Y.; El Gaafary, M.; Youssef, S.; Ahmed, I.; Nasr, A. Tailored approach to early psoriatic arthritis patients: Clinical and ultrasonographic predictors for structural joint damage. *Clin. Rheumatol.* **2015**, *34*, 307–313. [CrossRef]

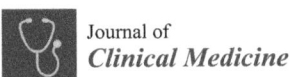

Article

Significance of Temporal Muscle Thickness in Chronic Subdural Hematoma

Daniel Dubinski [1,*], Sae-Yeon Won [1], Bedjan Behmanesh [1], Daniel Cantré [2], Isabell Mattes [1], Svorad Trnovec [1], Peter Baumgarten [3], Patrick Schuss [4], Thomas M. Freiman [1] and Florian Gessler [1]

1. Department of Neurosurgery, Rostock University Medical Center, 18057 Rostock, Germany
2. Institute of Diagnostic and Interventional Radiology, Pediatric Radiology and Neuroradiology, Rostock University Medical Center, 18057 Rostock, Germany
3. Department of Neurosurgery, University Hospital, Schiller University Jena, 07747 Jena, Germany
4. Department of Neurosurgery, Unfallkrankenhaus Berlin, 12683 Berlin, Germany
* Correspondence: danieldubinski@gmail.com; Tel.: +49-381-494-6439

Abstract: Background: Reduced temporal muscle thickness (TMT) was verified as an independent negative prognostic parameter for outcome in brain tumor patients. Independent thereof, chronic subdural hematoma (CSDH) is a neurosurgical condition with high recurrence rates and unreliable risk models for poor outcome. Since sarcopenia was associated with poor outcome, we investigated the possible role of TMT and the clinical course of CSDH patients. Methods: This investigation is a single-center retrospective study on patients with CSDH. We analyzed the radiological and clinical data sets of 171 patients with surgically treated CSDH at a University Hospital from 2017 to 2020. Results: Our analysis showed a significant association between low-volume TMT and increased hematoma volume ($p < 0.001$), poor outcome at discharge ($p < 0.001$), and reduced performance status at 3 months ($p < 0.002$). Conclusion: TMT may represent an objective prognostic parameter and assist the identification of vulnerable CSDH patients.

Keywords: temporal muscle thickness; sarcopenia; chronic subdural hematoma; recurrence; outcome; risk factors

1. Introduction

Chronic subdural hematoma (CSDH) is the most common neurosurgical condition, and with the increasing age of the Western population, the incidence of CSDH is expected to further increase in the near future [1]. To date, the major challenges in the management of CSDH is the difficult prognostication of outcome and high recurrence with reported rates of up to 40% [2]. Predictive models remain inconsistent and have not been routinely translated into clinical practice [3]. On the other hand, the loss of skeletal muscle mass (sarcopenia) was recently introduced as an objective parameter for outcome in hospitalized older patients [4]. Sarcopenia is usually verified through muscle function tests such as the gait speed test and the grip strength test [5,6]. However, measuring muscle function with the abovementioned techniques often cannot be performed in CSDH patients because of the frequently present disturbances of consciousness and/or hemiparesis. However, an alternative evaluation of muscle mass and function was recently shown through the association of radiologically measured temporal muscle thickness (TMT) and outcome in brain tumor patients [7–9]. Further, CT scans (computed tomography) are routinely performed on CSDH patients, and TMT measurement is easy and rapid to implement. We therefore investigated TMT as an alternative method to evaluate muscle mass and investigated its role as an objective parameter for CSDH outcome.

2. Materials and Methods

2.1. Patients and Data Collection

All patients admitted to the neurosurgical department of the authors' institution between August 2017 and June 2020 with the diagnosis of a CSDH were included in the analysis. The inclusion criteria were: (1) chronic subdural hematoma diagnosed by CT or MRI scan and (2) patients aged 18 years and above. The patient characteristics and medical data were collected using the institutional electronic database. For this retrospective analysis, ethical approval was obtained from the Ethics Committee of the University Medicine Rostock, Germany (identification number: A 2021-0112). As a non-interventional monocentric study, patient consent was waived. The exclusion criteria were lack of radiological data or hospital discharge in less than 24 h after admission. The investigated medical record parameters included: age at admission, sex, GCS at admission, anticoagulation status, preexisting conditions, symptoms at admission, radiological parameters such as hematoma diameter and midline shift, clinical course, and status at discharge and at 3 months after operation.

2.2. Image Analysis

Preoperative, postoperative, and follow-up CT scans were analyzed with PACS software Jivex® v5.2 (VISUS Technology Transfer GmbH, Bochum, Germany). Image analysis was performed by two neurosurgeons (D.D. and S.Y.-W.) that were blinded to the patients' medical data. A representative analysis is displayed in Figure 1. TMT was measured on the left and on the right side separately in each patient and each side was summed up and divided by two, resulting in a mean TMT per patient. The TMT side showed no statistical difference. High-volume TMT was defined as mean of 6–9 mm and low-volume TMT as 1–5 mm.

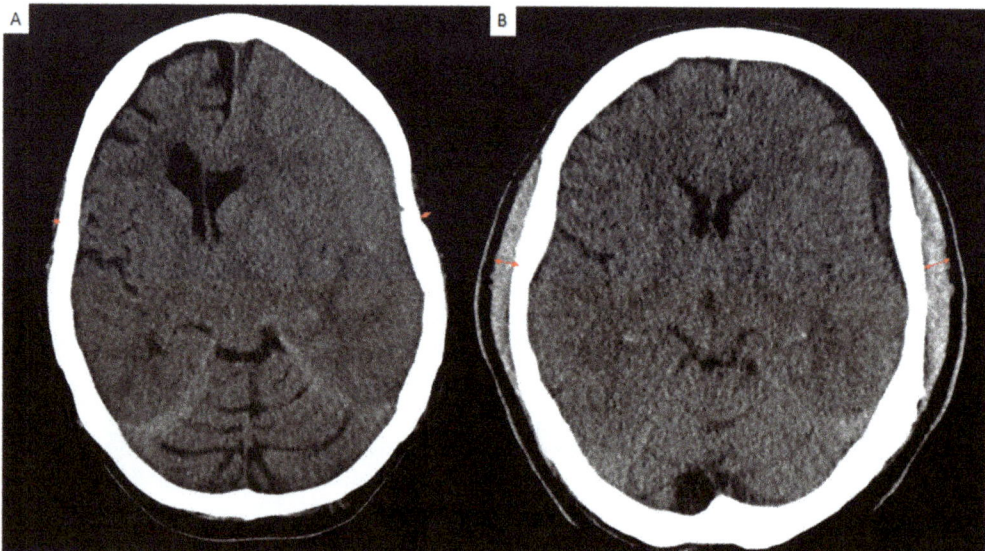

Figure 1. Representative case for the assessment of temporalis muscle thickness (TMT) on cranial CT scan shown in red arrows. (**A**) TMT measurement on axial CT scan image of a patient with low-volume TMT (bilateral mean TMT = 2.3 mm) and (**B**) a patient with a high-volume TMT on axial CT scan analysis (bilateral mean TMT = 8.1 mm).

2.3. Surgical Treatment

Unless there was a known history of cephalosporin allergy, all patients received a perioperative intravenous cefazolin (2 g) prophylaxis for evacuation. A closed subdural drainage system after evacuation was implanted in all cases. A postoperative CT scan was obtained prior to drain removal. Prophylactic low molecular weight heparin was started after 24 h in all patients. In cases with preoperative anticoagulation, the anticoagulant was re-administered not earlier than postoperative day 7. Recurrence was defined as the accumulation of chronic subdural fluid requiring re-operation. A second surgery performed during the same hospitalization was not considered as a recurrence.

2.4. Study Design

The present analysis is a retrospective, single center study of patients with CSDH. The aim of the study was to observe patients' TMT on preoperative CT scans and to correlate the TMT volume with patient outcomes.

2.5. Statistics

The data analysis was performed with IBM SPSS Statistics version 23.0 (SPSS Inc., IBM Corp, Armonk, NY, USA). For the patient characteristics, descriptive statistics were used. Fisher's exact test was used for the comparison of categorical variables between the cohorts. For continuous parameters, the Wilcoxon/Mann–Whitney test was used. Bivariable and multi-variable logistic regression models were used to find correlations with TMT. The multivariable logistic regression analysis included variables with a p-value of less than or equal to 0.05 in the bivariable regression. A p-value < 0.05 was considered to determine statistical significance. To assess the impact of the variables, odds ratios (ORs) with 95% confidence intervals (CIs) were calculated. Results with $p \leq 0.05$ were considered statistically relevant.

3. Results

3.1. Participant Characteristics

A total of 173 CSDH patients were analyzed. Two patients were excluded due to lack of radiological data, therefore a total of 171 CSDH patients were included in the final analysis. The mean TMT was 5 mm (IQR 3–9). The average age was 74.5 (IQR: 63–82) and 115 (67%) of the patients were male. The median GCS at admission was 15 (IQR: 14–15) and 96 patients (56%) received anticoagulation at admission. In terms of preexisting conditions, 112 patients presented with a history of hypertension (71%), 39 with atrial fibrillation (23%), 47 with diabetes mellitus (27%), 77 with coronary heart disease (45%), and 21 with dementia (12%). The symptoms at admission were headache in 59 cases (35%), confusion in 35 (20%), impaired consciousness in 40 (23%), nausea in 16 (9%), hemiparesis in 119 (70%), and seizure in 9 (5%). On initial axial CT scan, the maximal hematoma width was 18.4mm (IQR: 12–25) and the median width was 3.5mm (IQR: 4–6). The median midline shift was 6mm (IQR: 2–9). A total of five patients had postoperative seizures, six patients had early (<7 postoperative days) seizures (4%), four patients late (>7 postoperative days) seizures (3%), and one patient had status epilepticus (1%). Recurrence was seen in 56 patients (33%) and the modified Rankin scale at 3 months was 1.5 (IQR: 0.5–3) (Table 1).

Table 1. Demographics, management, and surgical data. IQR: Inter quartile range; GCS: Glasgow Coma Score; mRS: Modified rankin scale.

Patient Characteristics	(n = 171)
Sex	
male, n (%)	115 (67)
Age, median (IQR)	74.5 (63–82)
GCS at admission, median (IQR)	15 (14–15)
Anticoagulation, n (%)	96 (56)
Preexisting conditions	

Table 1. *Cont.*

Patient Characteristics	(n = 171)
Hypertension, n (%)	122 (71)
Atrial fibrillation, n (%)	39 (23)
Diabetes mellitus, n (%)	47 (27)
Coronary heart disease, n (%)	77 (45)
Dementia, n (%)	21 (12)
Symptoms at admission	
Headache, n (%)	59 (35)
Confusion, n (%)	35 (20)
Impaired consciousness, n (%)	40 (23)
Nausea, n (%)	16 (9)
Hemiparesis, n (%)	119 (70)
Seizure, n (%)	9 (5)
Radiological parameters	
Hematoma median, mm (IQR)	18.4 (12–25)
Midline-shift, median, mm (IQR)	6 (2–9)
Postoperative seizures	
Early seizure (<7 d), n (%)	6 (4)
Late seizure (>7 d), n (%)	4 (3)
Status epilepticus, n (%)	1 (1)
Status at discharge	
GCS at discharge, median (IQR)	15 (15–15)
mRS at discharge, median (IQR)	2 (1–3)
Recurrence, n (%)	56 (33)
Outcome	
mRS3 months, median (IQR)	1.5 (0.5–3)

3.2. Characteristics and Admission Status in CSDH According to Temporal Muscle Thickness

In our uni- and multivariate analysis, male patients showed an association with low-volume TMT (59% of patients with low-volume TMT were male vs. 76% in the high-volume TMT cohort; $p = 0.022$). Furthermore, uni- and multivariate analysis showed a significant association between low-volume TMT and increased age (median age of 79 in the low volume TMT cohort vs. 70 years in the high-volume TMT cohort; $p = 0.001$). The GCS at admission as well as the anticoagulation status were not significantly associated with TMT volume ($p = 1$ for GCS and $p = 0.089$ for anticoagulation status). (Table 2)

3.3. Preexisting Conditions and Temporal Muscle Thickness in Patients with CSDH

In our analysis, atrial fibrillation, diabetes mellitus, and coronary heart disease showed no significant association with TMT volume ($p = 1$; $p = 0.606$ and $p = 0.760$, respectively) (Table 3). However, in uni- but not multivariate analysis, 78% of the patients with low-volume TMT had a history of hypertension vs. 51% of patients with high-volume TMT ($p = 0.043$ in univariate and $p = 0.102$ in multivariate analysis). Furthermore, in the univariate analysis, patients with low-volume TMT showed a history of dementia in 20% vs. 3% in patients with high-volume TMT ($p = 0.001$ for univariate). Multivariate analysis showed approximating significance with $p = 0.05$.

Table 2. Univariate analysis of juxtaposed characteristics according to TMT volume in CSDH. Abbreviations: OR: odds ratio, IQR: interquartile range, GCS: Glasgow Coma Scale, CRP: C-reactive protein.

Patient Characteristics (n = 171)	Mean TMT		Univariate		
	Low Volume n = 91	High Volume n = 80	OR	95% CI	p-Value
Sex					
male, n (%)	54 (59.3)	61 (76.3)	0.5	0.23–0.88	0.022
Age, median (IQR)	79 (71–84)	70 (56–79)	-	4.58–13.42	0.000
GCS at admission, median (IQR)	15 (14–15)	15 (14–15)	-	−0.44–0.44	1
Anticoagulation, n (%)	57 (62.6)	39 (48.8)	1.8	0.96–3.25	0.089
Preexisting conditions					
Hypertension, n (%)	71 (78)	51 (63.8)	2	1.03–4.00	0.043
Atrial fibrillation, n (%)	21 (23.1)	18 (22.5)	1	0.51–2.12	1
Diabetes mellitus, n (%)	27 (29.7)	20 (25.0)	1.3	0.64–2.50	0.606
Coronary heart disease, n (%)	42 (46.2)	35 (43.8)	1.1	0.60–2.02	0.760
Dementia, n (%)	18 (19.8)	3 (3.8)	6.3	1.79–22.39	0.001
Symptoms at admission					
Headache, n (%)	24 (26.4)	35 (43.8)	0.5	0.24–0.88	0.023
Confusion, n (%)	33 (36.3)	12 (15.0)	3.2	1.53–6.81	0.001
Impaired consciousness, n (%)	20 (22.0)	20 (25.0)	0.9	0.42–1.72	0.718
Nausea, n (%)	3 (3.3)	13 (16.3)	0.2	0.10–0.64	0.004
Hemiparesis, n (%)	39 (42.9)	40 (50.0)	0.8	0.41–1.37	0.361
Seizure, n (%)	5 (5.5)	4 (5.0)	1.1	0.29–4.26	1
Radiological parameters					
Hematoma median, mm (IQR)	20 (13–25)	17 (11–25)	1.5	0.49–5.1	0.019
Midline-shift, median, mm (IQR)	6 (2–8)	6 (2–11)	-	−1.44–1.44	1
Postoperative seizures					
Early seizure (<7 d), n (%)	2 (2.2)	4 (5.0)	0.4	0.08–40	0.420
Late seizure (>7 d), n (%)	3 (3.3)	1 (1.3)	2.7	0.27–26.43	0.623
Status epilepticus, n (%)	1 (1.1)	0 (0)	-	-	1
Status at discharge					
GCS at discharge, median (IQR)	15 (15–15)	15 (15–15)	-	−0.13–0.13	1
mRS at discharge, median (IQR)	2 (1–3)	1 (0.75–2)	-	0.58–1.42	0.001
Recurrence, n (%)	27 (29.7)	29 (36.3)	0.7	0.39–1.41	0.415
Outcome					
mRS3 months, median (IQR)	2 (1–4)	1 (0–2)	-	0.36–1.63	0.002

3.4. Symptoms at Admission and Temporal Muscle Thickness in Patients with CSDH

In the univariate analysis, headache as the leading symptom was significantly associated with low-volume TMT (26% in the low-volume TMT cohort vs. 35% in high-volume TMT, $p = 0.023$). Furthermore, confusion was present in 36% of patients with low-volume TMT vs. 15% in the high-volume cohort, which was statistically significant ($p = 0.001$). Nausea was present in 3% of the low-volume TMT vs. 16% in the high-volume TMT cohort, an association that is also statistically significant in univariate analysis ($p = 0.004$). Impaired consciousness, hemiparesis, and seizures were not significantly associated with patients' TMT volume. Multivariate analysis only confirmed a significant association for nausea ($p = 0.054$).

3.5. Association of Radiological Parameters and TMT in Patients with CSDH

The median hemorrhage diameter in patients with low-volume TMT was 20 mm (IQR 13–25) vs. 17 mm (IQR 11–25) in patients with high-volume TMT, which showed a statistical significance in the univariate ($p = 0.019$) and multivariate analysis ($p = 0.012$). On the other hand, the midline shift was not statistically associated with patients' TMT volume ($p = 1$).

Table 3. Uni- and multivariate analysis of juxtaposed characteristics according to TMT volume in CSDH. Abbreviations: OR: odds ratio, IQR: interquartile range, GCS: Glasgow Coma Scale, CRP: C-reactive protein.

Patient Characteristics (n = 171)	Mean TMT		Univariate			Multivariate		
	1–5 mm N = 91	6–9 mm N = 80	OR	95% CI	p-Value	OR	95% CI	p-Value
Sex								
Male, n (%)	54 (59.3)	61 (76.3)	0.5	0.23–0.88	0.022	2.8	1.31–6.05	0.008
Age, median (IQR)	79 (71–84)	70 (56–79)	-	4.58–13.42	0.001			
Preexisting conditions								
Hypertension, n (%)	71 (78.0)	51 (63.8)	2	1.03–4.00	0.043	0.5	0.25–1.14	0.102
Dementia, n (%)	18 (19.8)	3 (3.8)	6.3	1.79–22.39	0.001	0.3	0.07–1.0	0.050
Symptoms at admission								
Headache, n (%)	24 (26.4)	35 (43.8)	0.5	0.24–0.88	0.023	1.7	0.78–3.58	0.183
Confusion, n (%)	33 (36.3)	12 (15.0)	3.2	1.53–6.81	0.001	0.5	0.21–1.21	0.124
Nausea, n (%)	3 (3.3)	13 (16.3)	0.2	0.10–0.64	0.004	4.1	1.0–17.43	0.054
Radiological parameters								
Hematoma median, mm (IQR)	20 (13–25)	17 (11–25)	1.5	0.49–5.1	0.019	8.1	0.26–0.61	0.012
Outcome								
mRS3 months, median (IQR)	2 (1–4)	1 (0–2)	-	0.36–1.63	0.002	0.2	0.58–1.36	0.613

3.6. Postoperative Seizures and Temporal Muscle Thickness in Patients with CSDH

Neither early nor postoperative seizures were statistically associated with patients' temporal muscle thickness: $p = 0.420$ for early and $p = 0.623$ for late postoperative seizures. Status epilepticus was observed in only one patient among the analyzed cohort and was therefore not statistically significant ($p = 1$).

3.7. Clinical Outcome and Temporal Muscle Thickness in Patients with CSDH

The GCS at discharge showed no significant association with patients' TMT volume, with 15 in both groups ($p = 1$). However, mRS showed a significant association ($p = 0.001$) with a median mRS of 2 (IQR 1–3) in the low-volume TMT cohort vs. 1 in the high-volume TMT cohort (IQR: 0.75–2). This statistical significance was not observed in the multivariate analysis. Regarding the CSDH recurrence, no significant association was observed in the analyzed cohort: 27% in patients with low-volume TMT vs. 29% with high-volume TMT ($p = 0.415$). Furthermore, the 3-month follow-up confirmed better mRS status in the high-volume TMT cohort (1 vs. 2 in the low-volume cohort). This statistical significance could not be replicated in multivariate analysis.

4. Discussion

This study investigates the value of TMT volume on conventional preoperative CT scans preformed on patients with CSDH. The major finding is the significant association of low-volume TMT and increased hematoma volume as well as decreased outcome status at 3 months. The findings of this study suggest that TMT may represent an objective parameter with prognostic value, novel for CSDH patients.

Frailty and sarcopenia are emerging as (substantially overlapping) parameters that are gaining recent scientific attention since both showed an association with a wide range of ageing outcomes and were shown to be predictive for mortality and morbidity in the elderly [10]. In the case of frailty, recent studies argued for the incorporation of frailty assessment into risk models for mortality and outcome in elderly patients with CSDH [11]. Sarcopenia, on the other hand, has been shown to be a negative prognostic factor for the outcome of brain tumor patients, although the underlying pathophysiology remains unclear. Among the discussed hypotheses were the association of TMT with general physical fitness, insufficient nutrition status, or inflammatory processes [12]. A possible crossover of this finding to CSDH patients is unexamined at this time.

In terms of TMT as a general physical fitness parameter, several studies confirmed the reliability of sarcopenia as a useful assessment instrument in older trauma patients. Tanabe et al. could show an association of sarcopenia and increased 1-year mortality in older trauma patients [13]. However, in their analysis, a different muscle group (masseter) as well as distinct measuring techniques were used. Our results are in line with the available literature, but extend the applicability to the CSDH disease pattern.

Patients' nutritional status is certainly of significant importance for postoperative outcome in CSDH patients. Scaretti et al. recently showed that reduced nutritional status analyzed via Mini Nutritional Assessment (MNA) in 178 CSDH patients was a strong predictor of poor clinical outcome after hematoma evacuation [14]. Our analysis confirms the previously mentioned negative association between reduced nutritional status and poor outcome as our cohort with a low-volume TMT showed similarly poor clinical outcome. Furthermore, in their multivariate analysis of SAH patients, Katsuki et al. confirmed TMT as a prognostic factor in older patients. Similar results were seen in ischemic stroke patients [15–17]. Our findings add CSDH as a common neurosurgical condition to the list of previous publications on the prognostic value of TMT in intracranial hematoma patients.

With regard to the possible interaction between inflammatory processes and TMT volume, several studies highlighted the possible component of inflammation in the formation and maintenance of CSDH. Local inflammatory cells including neutrophils, lymphocytes, monocytes, and eosinophils have been observed on the outer CSDH membrane [18]. Inflammation regulates muscle protein metabolism and is known to be associated with a chronic state of slightly increased plasma levels of pro-inflammatory mediators, such as tumor necrosis factor α (TNFα), interleukin 6 (IL-6), and C-reactive protein (CRP) [19]. Whether sarcopenia as a possible consequence of chronic inflammation in CSDH has its rationale and influences hematoma membrane formation and maintenance remains speculative at this time since our analysis did not show a significant impact on recurrence rates.

Another interesting finding of our study is the significant association of TMT and dementia. The loss of muscle mass is known to be associated with brain atrophy in Alzheimer's disease (AD), and skeletal muscle mass is proportionately reduced in patients with dementia compared to those with mild cognitive impairment [20]. Our analysis confirms this aspect, as patients with reduced TMT volume (hence, reduced muscle mass) had significantly more often dementia as a subsidiary diagnosis.

Furthermore, several studies could show that protocols for automatic geriatrician consultation in trauma patients 70 years and older resulted in improved advanced care planning and increased multidisciplinary care. In the ICU, advanced care planning reduces readmission and length of stay [21]. In summary, the major possible benefit of implementing TMT values in clinical routine should be the early identification of vulnerable CSDH patients that are at high risk of poor outcome.

5. Limitations

Although our analysis shows the value of TMT in a sizable cohort of CSDH patients, our study faces some limitations. Firstly, after stratification by hematoma volume, our cohort showed a significant age difference, which could influence outcome. However, previous studies could not show a significant association between patients' age and TMT volume [22]. Further, we performed multivariable statistical approaches to consider this effect. The statistically significant overrepresentation of the male sex in CSDH is a known phenomenon that should therefore not present a clinically relevant bias [23]. Secondly, the retrospective analysis of TMT prohibited the evaluation of anatomical–functional relationships. Furthermore, patients' blood type was previously described as a significant risk factor for rebleeding in acute SDH and SAH patients [24–26]. Due to the lack of patients' blood type, we could not include this parameter in our analysis, but stress the necessity for future studies. Furthermore, postoperative pneumocephalus following CSDH evacuation has been found to be a risk factor for re-accumulation, and we did not analyze the incidence of pneumocephalus. Future studies should investigate its role in CSDH recurrence. Even though recent studies have shown a direct correlation between TMT and sarcopenia, a generalization in terms of sarcopenia remains to be proven in future studies [27,28]. As this is a retrospective observational study, confounding, selection bias, and uncontrolled statistical error risk cannot be excluded. Hence, further prospective randomized trials with large cohorts are necessary to validate our findings.

6. Conclusions

The results described in this study could pave the way for the implementation of TMT measurement for the assessment of sarcopenia in CSDH and therefore identify vulnerable patients with the opportunity of postoperative follow-up optimization.

Author Contributions: D.D. collected the data and wrote the first draft. F.G. supervised the manuscript. All authors supplied additional information, edited the manuscript, and contributed to the critical review and revision of the manuscript. All authors have read and agreed to the published version of the manuscript.

Funding: This research received no external funding.

Institutional Review Board Statement: The study was conducted according to the guidelines of the Declaration of Helsinki, and approved by the Ethics Committee of the University Medicine Rostock, Germany (identification number: A 2021-0112).

Informed Consent Statement: Not applicable.

Data Availability Statement: The data presented in this study are available on request from the corresponding author.

Acknowledgments: D.D. is a recipient of Novartis Foundation graduate fellowship and FORUN in therapeutic research.

Conflicts of Interest: D.D. received financial support from Novartis, Fresenius, Inovitro and Novocure. None of the stated financial support conflicts with the interest of this study.

References

1. Bounajem, M.T.; Campbell, R.A.; Denorme, F.; Grandhi, R. Paradigms in chronic subdural hematoma pathophysiology: Current treatments and new directions. *J. Trauma Acute Care Surg.* **2021**, *91*, e134–e141. [CrossRef] [PubMed]
2. Feghali, J.; Yang, W.; Huang, J. Updates in Chronic Subdural Hematoma: Epidemiology, Etiology, Pathogenesis, Treatment, and Outcome. *World Neurosurg.* **2020**, *141*, 339–345. [CrossRef] [PubMed]
3. Won, S.Y.; Dubinski, D.; Eibach, M.; Gessler, F.; Herrmann, E.; Keil, F.; Seifert, V.; Konczalla, J.; Behmanesh, B. External validation and modification of the Oslo grading system for prediction of postoperative recurrence of chronic subdural hematoma. *Neurosurg. Rev.* **2021**, *44*, 961–970. [CrossRef]
4. Strasser, E.M.; Draskovits, T.; Praschak, M.; Quittan, M.; Graf, A. Association between ultrasound measurements of muscle thickness, pennation angle, echogenicity and skeletal muscle strength in the elderly. *Age* **2013**, *35*, 2377–2388. [CrossRef] [PubMed]
5. Cruz-Jentoft, A.J.; Bahat, G.; Bauer, J.; Boirie, Y.; Bruyère, O.; Cederholm, T.; Cooper, C.; Landi, F.; Rolland, Y.; Sayer, A.A.; et al. Sarcopenia: Revised European consensus on definition and diagnosis. *Age Ageing* **2019**, *48*, 16–31. [CrossRef]
6. Chen, L.K.; Woo, J.; Assantachai, P.; Auyeung, T.W.; Chou, M.Y.; Iijima, K.; Jang, H.C.; Kang, L.; Kim, M.; Kim, S.; et al. Asian Working Group for Sarcopenia: 2019 Consensus Update on Sarcopenia Diagnosis and Treatment. *J. Am. Med. Dir. Assoc.* **2020**, *21*, 300–307.e2. [CrossRef] [PubMed]
7. Furtner, J.; Genbrugge, E.; Gorlia, T.; Bendszus, M.; Nowosielski, M.; Golfinopoulos, V.; Weller, M.; Van Den Bent, M.J.; Wick, W.; Preusser, M. Temporal muscle thickness is an independent prognostic marker in patients with progressive glioblastoma: Translational imaging analysis of the EORTC 26101 trial. *Neuro-Oncol.* **2019**, *21*, 1587–1594. [CrossRef] [PubMed]
8. Furtner, J.; Weller, M.; Weber, M.; Gorlia, T.; Nabors, B.; Reardon, D.A.; Tonn, J.C.; Stupp, R.; Preusser, M. Temporal Muscle Thickness as a Prognostic Marker in Patients with Newly Diagnosed Glioblastoma: Translational Imaging Analysis of the CENTRIC EORTC 26071-22072 and CORE Trials. *Clin. Cancer Res.* **2022**, *28*, 129–136. [CrossRef]
9. Yan, O.Y.; Teng, H.B.; Fu, S.N.; Chen, Y.Z.; Liu, F. Temporal Muscle Thickness is an Independent Prognostic Biomarker in Patients with Glioma: Analysis of 261 Cases. *Cancer Manag. Res.* **2021**, *13*, 6621. [CrossRef]
10. Dodds, R.; Sayer, A.A. Sarcopenia and frailty: New challenges for clinical practice. *Clin. Med.* **2016**, *16*, 455. [CrossRef]
11. Hernández-Durán, S.; Behme, D.; Rohde, V.; von der Brelie, C. A matter of frailty: The modified Subdural Hematoma in the Elderly (mSHE) score. *Neurosurg. Rev.* **2022**, *45*, 701. [CrossRef] [PubMed]

12. Furtner, J.; Berghoff, A.S.; Schöpf, V.; Reumann, R.; Pascher, B.; Woitek, R.; Asenbaum, U.; Pelster, S.; Leitner, J.; Widhalm, G.; et al. Temporal muscle thickness is an independent prognostic marker in melanoma patients with newly diagnosed brain metastases. *J. Neurooncol.* **2018**, *140*, 173–178. [CrossRef] [PubMed]
13. Tanabe, C.; Reed, M.J.; Pham, T.N.; Penn, K.; Bentov, I.; Kaplan, S.J. Association of Brain Atrophy and Masseter Sarcopenia With 1-Year Mortality in Older Trauma Patients. *JAMA Surg.* **2019**, *154*, 716. [CrossRef] [PubMed]
14. Scerrati, A.; Pangallo, G.; Dughiero, M.; Mongardi, L.; Ricciardi, L.; Lofrese, G.; Dones, F.; Cavallo, M.A.; De Bonis, P. Influence of nutritional status on the clinical outcome of patients with chronic subdural hematoma: A prospective multicenter clinical study. *Nutr. Neurosci.* **2022**, *25*, 1756–1763. [CrossRef]
15. Katsuki, M.; Suzuki, Y.; Kunitoki, K.; Sato, Y.; Sasaki, K.; Mashiyama, S.; Matsuoka, R.; Allen, E.; Saimaru, H.; Sugawara, R.; et al. Temporal Muscle as an Indicator of Sarcopenia is Independently Associated with Hunt and Kosnik Grade on Admission and the Modified Rankin Scale Score at 6 Months of Patients with Subarachnoid Hemorrhage Treated by Endovascular Coiling. *World Neurosurg.* **2020**, *137*, e526–e534. [CrossRef]
16. Katsuki, M.; Kakizawa, Y.; Nishikawa, A.; Yamamoto, Y.; Uchiyama, T.; Agata, M.; Wada, N.; Kawamura, S.; Koh, A. Temporal Muscle and Stroke—A Narrative Review on Current Meaning and Clinical Applications of Temporal Muscle Thickness, Area, and Volume. *Nutrients* **2022**, *14*, 687. [CrossRef]
17. Katsuki, M.; Kakizawa, Y.; Nishikawa, A.; Yamamoto, Y.; Uchiyama, T. Temporal muscle thickness and area are an independent prognostic factors in patients aged 75 or younger with aneurysmal subarachnoid hemorrhage treated by clipping. *Surg. Neurol. Int.* **2021**, *12*, 151. [CrossRef]
18. Edlmann, E.; Giorgi-Coll, S.; Whitfield, P.C.; Carpenter, K.L.H.; Hutchinson, P.J. Pathophysiology of chronic subdural haematoma: Inflammation, angiogenesis and implications for pharmacotherapy. *J. Neuroinflammation* **2017**, *14*, 108. [CrossRef]
19. Dalle, S.; Rossmeislova, L.; Koppo, K. The Role of Inflammation in Age-Related Sarcopenia. *Front. Physiol.* **2017**, *8*, 1045. [CrossRef]
20. Cho, J.; Park, M.; Moon, W.J.; Han, S.H.; Moon, Y. Sarcopenia in patients with dementia: Correlation of temporalis muscle thickness with appendicular muscle mass. *Neurol. Sci.* **2022**, *43*, 3089–3095. [CrossRef]
21. Khandelwal, N.; Kross, E.K.; Engelberg, R.A.; Coe, N.B.; Long, A.C.; Curtis, J.R. Estimating the effect of palliative care interventions and advance care planning on ICU utilization: A systematic review. *Crit. Care Med.* **2015**, *43*, 1102–1111. [CrossRef] [PubMed]
22. Katsuki, M.; Narita, N.; Sasaki, K.; Sato, Y.; Suzuki, Y.; Mashiyama, S.; Tominaga, T. Standard values for temporal muscle thickness in the Japanese population who undergo brain check-up by magnetic resonance imaging. *Surg. Neurol. Int.* **2021**, *12*, 67. [CrossRef] [PubMed]
23. Kanat, A.; Kayaci, S.; Yazar, U.; Kazdal, H.; Terzi, Y. Chronic subdural hematoma in adults: Why does it occur more often in males than females? Influence of patient's sexual gender on occurrence. *J. Neurosurg. Sci.* **2010**, *54*, 99–103.
24. Dubinski, D.; Won, S.Y.; Behmanesh, B.; Brawanski, N.; Geisen, C.; Seifert, V.; Senft, C.; Konczalla, J. The clinical relevance of ABO blood type in 100 patients with acute subdural hematoma. *PLoS ONE* **2018**, *13*, e0204331. [CrossRef] [PubMed]
25. Dubinski, D.; Won, S.Y.; Konczalla, J.; Mersmann, J.; Geisen, C.; Herrmann, E.; Seifert, V.; Senft, C. The Role of ABO Blood Group in Cerebral Vasospasm, Associated Intracranial Hemorrhage, and Delayed Cerebral Ischemia in 470 Patients with Subarachnoid Hemorrhage. *World Neurosurg.* **2017**, *97*, 532–537. [CrossRef] [PubMed]
26. Dubinski, D.; Won, S.Y.; Behmanesh, B.; Kashefiolasl, S.; Geisen, C.; Seifert, V.; Senft, C.; Konczalla, J. Influence of ABO blood type on the outcome after non-aneurysmal subarachnoid hemorrhage. *Acta Neurochir.* **2018**, *160*, 761–766. [CrossRef] [PubMed]
27. Nozoe, M.; Kubo, H.; Kanai, M.; Yamamoto, M.; Okakita, M.; Suzuki, H.; Shimada, S.; Mase, K. Reliability and validity of measuring temporal muscle thickness as the evaluation of sarcopenia risk and the relationship with functional outcome in older patients with acute stroke. *Clin. Neurol. Neurosurg.* **2021**, *201*, 106444. [CrossRef]
28. Lee, B.; Bae, Y.J.; Jeong, W.J.; Kim, H.; Choi, B.S.; Kim, J.H. Temporalis muscle thickness as an indicator of sarcopenia predicts progression-free survival in head and neck squamous cell carcinoma. *Sci. Rep.* **2021**, *11*, 19717. [CrossRef]

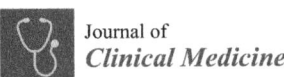

Article

A New Role for Epidurography: A Simple Method for Assessing the Adequacy of Decompression during Percutaneous Plasma Disc Decompression

Ho Young Gil [1], Wonseok Seo [1], Gyu Bin Choi [1], Eunji Ha [1], Taekwang Kim [1], Jungyul Ryu [2], Jae Hyung Kim [2] and Jong Bum Choi [1,*]

[1] Department of Anesthesiology and Pain Medicine, Ajou University School of Medicine, Suwon 16499, Republic of Korea
[2] Department of Anesthesiology and Pain Medicine, Dongtan Sacred Heart Hospital, Hallym University School of Medicine, Hwaseong 18450, Republic of Korea
* Correspondence: romeojb@naver.com; Tel.: +82-31-219-5571

Abstract: Percutaneous plasma disc decompression (PPDD) is a minimally invasive treatment for discogenic low back pain and herniated disc-related symptoms. However, there are no known outcome predictive variables during the procedure. The purpose of this study was to evaluate and validate epidurography as an intra-procedure outcome predictor. We retrospectively enrolled 60 consecutive patients who did not respond to conventional treatments. In the next stage of treatment, PPDD was performed, and the epidurography was conducted before and after the PPDD. We analyzed the relationship between epidurographic improvement and the success rate. The Numerical Rating Scale and the Oswestry Disability Index were used to assess pain and functional capacity, respectively, before the procedure and 1 month after the procedure. The pain reduction and the success rate in the epidurographic improvement group were significantly higher than in the epidurographic non-improvement group. Both the Numerical Rating Scale and the Oswestry Disability Index scores were significantly reduced in both groups, but there was no significant difference in Oswestry Disability Index scores. This study's results showed that PPDD is an effective treatment method. We also suggested that epidurography may be a potential outcome predictor for ensuring successful outcomes and determining the endpoint of the procedure.

Keywords: decompression; discogenic low back pain; epidurography; intervertebral disc displacement; low back pain; lumbar radicular pain; nucleoplasty; outcome; percutaneous plasma disc decompression

1. Introduction

Low back pain is very common and affects 80% of individuals at some point in their lives [1,2]. According to one study, about 40% of chronic low back pain is caused by discogenic back pain, and most discogenic back pain is caused by disc prolapse or degenerative disc disease. Although these are common findings in asymptomatic patients, provocative discography has been used to distinguish between a painful disc and a nonpainful disc [3].

Management of chronic discogenic low back pain includes noninvasive conservative treatments, such as medications, physical therapy, behavior management, psychotherapy, and invasive surgical approaches. In a recent meta-analysis, it was argued that surgical treatment is not superior to non-surgical treatment as a treatment for chronic low back pain [4]. In addition, the range of indications for surgery is extremely small; it includes the paralysis of functionally important muscles and cauda equina syndrome, but not most patients with disc herniations.

Percutaneous plasma disc decompression (PPDD) was approved in the USA by the Food and Drug Administration (FDA) as a minimally invasive technique for discogenic

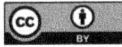

back pain in 2000 [5]. It is possible to reduce intradiscal pressures and disc volume through ablation and coagulation (Coblation® technique) using bipolar radiofrequency energy to remove disc material [6]. PPDD is a minimally invasive procedure with few complications, and its effects on long-term pain reduction and functional improvement have been previously demonstrated [7].

To evaluate the success of the procedure, standardized pain measuring tools—e.g., a visual analog scale (VAS); numerical rating scale (NRS); and standardized assessments of functional capacity in spinal mobility deficit caused by back pain, such as the Oswestry Disability Index (ODI)—were used. In addition, several imaging modalities, such as plain radiography, computed tomography (CT), and magnetic resonance imaging (MRI), were used to evaluate the success of the procedure. However, these modalities are expensive, do not offer real-time assessment during the intra-procedure period, and may take longer to show changes in disc volume. Moreover, their results do not always coincide with the patients' symptoms [8].

Although there are studies on variables that can predict and evaluate the success of PPDD before and after the procedure, there is no study on intra-procedure outcome predictive variables [6,9]. In order to increase the PPDD success rate, the physician's technique to accurately place the needle on the target disc is required. However, since the process of decompression is made by the manufactured guideline, outcome predictive variables that enable real-time assessment during the procedure are still required [10–12].

When disc protrusion occurs in the epidural space, the contrast medium does not spread well on the epidurography. Consequently, epidurography was used during percutaneous epidural neuroplasty and spinal surgery to confirm the success of the procedure [13,14].

We speculated that PPDD would reduce the disc volume, ensuring the epidural space and resulting in the improvement of epidurography. Thus, the purpose of this study was to evaluate and validate epidurography as an intra-procedure outcome predictor by correlating the change in epidurography with the change in the pain and functional score after PPDD.

2. Materials and Methods

2.1. Patients

This retrospective observational study was approved by the Institutional Review Board of Ajou University Hospital of Korea (IRB No. AJIRB-MED-MDB-19-409) in November 2019. The requirement for informed consent was waived because of the retrospective case-control nature of the study.

From January 2017 to December 2019, we retrospectively enrolled 60 consecutive patients with low back pain, with or without leg radicular pain (NRS $\geq$ 4), who did not respond to physical therapy, medications, and epidural steroid injections [15]. As the next step of treatment, PPDD was performed. The diagnosis was based on the patient's symptoms, neurological examination, and imaging studies. Inclusion criteria were: (1) age between 20 and 80 years old, (2) low back pain with or without leg radicular pain, (3) unresponsiveness to conservative therapy for more than three months, (4) MRI evidence of contained disc protrusion, (5) preservation of a disc height of $\geq$50%, (6) accurate identification of the symptomatic disc level prior to the procedure, (7) discography only if the physician is not sure about the treating level of the lumbar disc, and (8) PPDD with insertion of a wire-type epidural catheter. Exclusion criteria were: (1) disc height < 50%, (2) evidence of sequestration disc, (3) moderate/severe spinal stenosis, (4) previously operated segments, (5) spinal instability, (6) loss of follow-up, (7) inability to evaluate the outcome of PPDD because of other severe diseases, such as cancer, infection, and fracture, and (8) incomplete medical records. Patients were regularly followed up until 1 month after PPDD.

2.2. Percutaneous Plasma Disc Decompression

PPDD was performed on an outpatient basis by a pain physician with more than 10 years of experience in the field. (Figure 1). A prophylactic dose of 1 g cefazolin was administered intravenously 1 h prior to the procedure. If necessary, discography was performed prior to PPDD. The patient was placed in a prone position under sterile conditions. The involved disc space was localized under fluoroscopic guidance, and the soft tissues were infiltrated with local anesthetics.

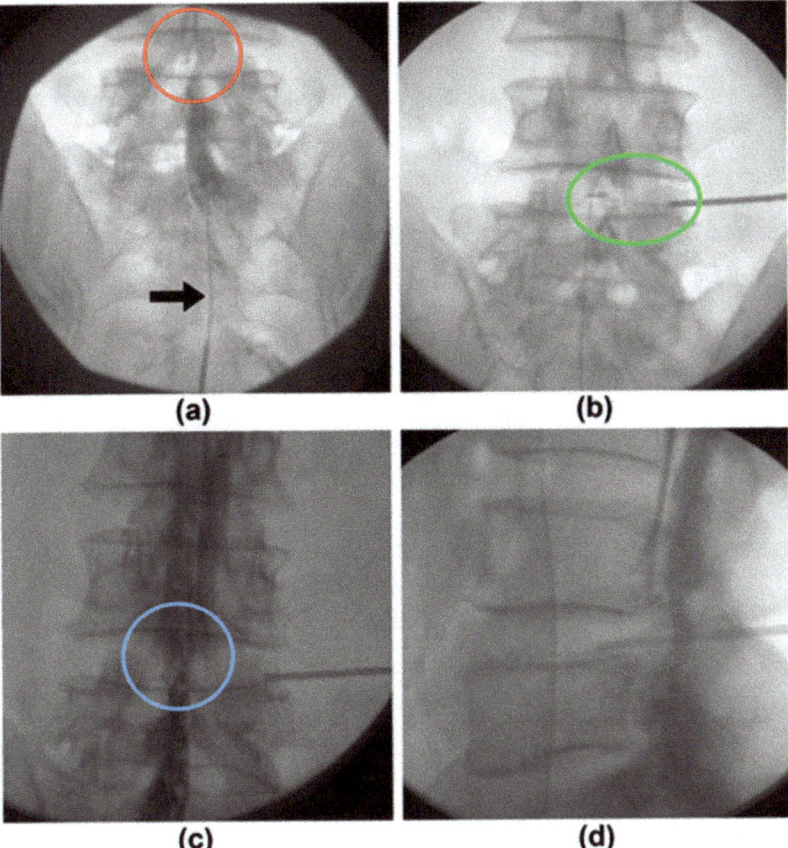

Figure 1. (a) Fluoroscopic anterior-posterior view of the pre-percutaneous plasma disc decompression (pre-PPDD). The filling defect was present at lumbar 4/5 disc level. (b) Fluoroscopic anterior-posterior view of the during-PPDD. (c) Fluoroscopic anterior-posterior view of the post-PPDD. The resolution of filling defect was verified. (d) Fluoroscopic lateral view of the post-PPDD. The 17-gauge spinal cannula was positioned at the junction of the annulus and nucleus Arrow, ABEL catheter; Red circle, the contrast media does not spread well above the involved disc level; Green circle, the into-LB was situated 6 o'clock position within the nucleus; Blue circle, the contrast media sufficiently spread above the involved disc level.

A 17-gauge spinal cannula was introduced into the disc using the Kambin's triangle approach. The Kambin's triangle was formed by the path of the spinal nerve, upper border of the lower vertebral body, and anterior border of the superior articular process of the low vertebra.

After the cannula was positioned at the junction of the annulus and nucleus, the stylet was removed from the cannula, and the into-LB (intocare Co., Ltd., Yangju, Republic of Korea) was placed into the spinal cannula and advanced until its tip was approximately 5 mm beyond the tip of the spinal cannula. At this point, the active portion of the into-LB was situated beyond the inner layer of the annulus and within the nucleus. A total of 6 channels were created at the 2, 4, 6, 8, 10, and 12 o'clock positions. After the withdrawal of the into-LB, 2 mL of 0.3% mepivacaine was injected into the PPDD tract, but not intradiscally. The skin puncture site was then closed with a suture or Steri-Strips.

2.3. Epidurography

Before the PPDD, a wire-type epidural catheter, ABEL catheter (GS Medical, Cheongwon, Republic of Korea), was inserted via the sacral hiatus toward the anterior epidural space of the involved disc level under fluoroscopic guidance. After confirming the position of the wire-type epidural catheter, 5 cc of a nonionic contrast medium (Iopamiro 300 inj.; Bracco Imaging Korea, Ltd., Seoul, Republic of Korea) was injected (Figure 1a), and the physician assessed and recorded whether the contrast media spread above the involved disc level. In addition, the physician tried to insert the catheter upward past the involved disc level and recorded whether it was possible. After PPDD, a second epidurography was conducted to assess any changes in epidural spreading (Figure 1c,d). Then, the physician tried to insert the catheter more proximally again and recorded whether it was possible after PPDD, and finally the catheter was carefully removed.

2.4. Post-Procedure Care

All the patients were observed for 2–4 h postoperatively for any development of neurological deficit or other procedure-related complications. Before discharge, we provided patients with post-procedure precautions and information about rehabilitation treatment [16]. For the first 3 days, the patients were allowed to walk, stand, and sit for up to 10–20 min at a time, but the patients were instructed not to perform any lifting or bending activity during this period. No driving was allowed for the first 2 days. Return to sedentary or light work was permitted 3–4 days following PPDD. Lifting was limited to 3–4 kg during the first 2 weeks, and all the patients were prescribed 500 mg of oral cefadroxil bid for 5 days.

2.5. Evaluation of Outcome Variables

Each patient's epidurograms (pre- and post-PPDD anteroposterior, lateral views) were analyzed by two pain physicians, who were not involved in the procedures and were only aware of the spinal level to be investigated. The analysis of the epidurograms was categorized as "improvement" or "no improvement." Epidurographic improvement was defined as post-PPDD contrast media extending above the involved disc level in the anteroposterior view, although it did not extend above the involved disc level in pre-PPDD contrast media (Figure 1a,c). Epidurographic non-improvement was defined as no improvement in post-PPDD epidurograms. When the analyses differed, a third physician assessed the epidurograms, and a consensus was reached. After analysis of the fluoroscopic images, we divided the patients who underwent PPDD into two groups. The first, Group I, was defined as demonstrating an improvement in the epidurogram. The second, Group N, was defined as demonstrating no improvement in the epidurogram.

The patient's degree of pain was measured using a standardized 11-point (0–10) NRS and evaluated by a well-trained physician at baseline 1 month after PPDD. The severity of pain was scored from 0 to 10, where "0" represented no pain and "10" represented the worst pain. The patients were encouraged to express their feelings regarding the pain.

The ODI was used to assess the patients' degree of dysfunction. The ODI assessments were performed at baseline 1 month after PPDD. The ODI is a 10-item questionnaire used globally to functionally assess patients with low back pain. However, in this study, we used the 9-item Korean version of the ODI, which excludes the assessment of sexual function, for cultural reasons [17].

A successful treatment after 1 month was defined as over a 50% reduction in the NRS score post-PPDD. Further, we analyzed the relationship between epidurographic improvement and the success rate.

2.6. Statistical Analysis

When estimating the sample size by the pilot study, the total sample size was 28 patients when the significance level was 0.0500 and the power was 0.8 in the Chi-square test. However, since the number of patients is small and if w (Phi) is corrected, a suitable total sample size of 60 was obtained. The patients' demographic data were analyzed using the Student's t-test, Chi-square test, and Mann–Whitney U test. A Wilcoxon signed-rank test was used to determine the difference in NRS and ODI scores before and after PPDD. The relationship between epidurographic improvement and the success rate was analyzed using the Chi-square test.

3. Results

The demographic data are shown in Table 1. There was no significant difference between group I and group N. Changes in the NRS and ODI scores were analyzed before and 1 month after PPDD. Both NRS and ODI scores were significantly reduced in both groups. The NRS scores were significantly reduced between the groups, but there was no significant difference in ODI (Table 2). However, the success rate in group I was significantly higher than in group N (Table 3, $p < 0.001$).

Table 1. Demographic data.

Variable	Improvement Group (n = 39)	Non-Improvement Group (n = 21)	p-Value
Sex			0.725 [a]
Male	20 (51.28%)	9 (42.86%)	
Female	19 (48.72%)	12 (57.14%)	
Age, years			0.981 [b]
Mean ± SD	58.51 ± 16.27	58.61 ± 15.60	
Height, cm			0.433 [c]
Mean ± SD	164.08 ± 7.67	165.57 ± 6.82	
Weight, kg			0.053 [b]
Mean ± SD	67.79 ± 11.29	62.27 ± 8.15	

[a] Chi-squared test was used. [b] Student t-test was used. [c] Mann–Whitney test was used.

Table 2. Comparison of NRS score and ODI score before and after PPDD.

Variable	Before	After	Difference	† p-Value
NRS				
Group I	7.56 ± 1.63	3.18 ± 1.76	4.38 ± 20.9	<0.001 [a]
Group N	6.43 ± 1.16	4.71 ± 1.27	1.70 ± 1.19	<0.001 [b]
‡ p-Value	0.005 [d]	0.001 [d]	<0.001 [d]	
ODI				
Group I	39.44 ± 11.43	25.38 ± 11.43	14.05 ± 14.12	<0.001 [b]
Group N	40.71 ± 12.10	32.62 ± 13.84	8.10 ± 7.66	<0.001 [a]
‡ p-Value	0.692 [d]	0.059 [c]	0.368 [d]	

[a] Paired samples t-test was used. [b] Wilcoxon signed-rank test was used. [c] Independent samples t-test was used. [d] Wilcoxon rank sum test. † p-Value, difference in each groups. ‡ p-Value, difference between the two groups. PPDD, percutaneous plasma disc decompression; NRS, Numerical Rating Scale score; ODI, Oswestry Disability Index score; Group I, Improvement Group; Group N, Non-Improvement Group.

Table 3. Comparison of success rate between Group I and Group N.

	Group I	Group N	p-Value
Success rate	29/39 (74.36%)	3/21 (14.29%)	<0.001 [a]

[a] Chi-square test was used.

4. Discussion

In this study, we found that PPDD is effective in reducing pain and improving functional capacity in patients who have chronic discogenic low back pain and herniated lumbar disc-related symptoms, regardless of the groups. Our results were similar to those of previous studies [7]. Although there were no significant differences in improvement of functional capacity between the two groups, the pain reduction and success rate were significantly higher in the epidurographic improvement group (Group I) than in the epidurographic non-improvement (Group N). Based on the results of this study, intra-procedure epidurography is a useful real-time assessment method for predicting successful PPDD outcomes, as well as a reliable determinant of the endpoint of the procedure.

PPDD mechanisms on the intervertebral discs have been well established [18]. PPDD shows its effect by down-regulating local inflammatory mediators, reducing disc size, and initiating the repair process. Ren et al. [19] found that PPDD effectively degraded phospholipase A2 (PLA2) activity. PLA2 activity is closely associated with intervertebral disc degeneration, intervertebral disc herniation, radicular pain, and lumbar discogenic pain. It is considered the rate-limiting enzyme in the inflammatory cascade reaction. They suggest that when intervertebral disc degeneration occurs, PLA2 is activated by various proinflammatory mediators, such as interleukin-1, tumor necrosis factor-α, and interleukin-6, which are secreted by the degenerative intervertebral disc. Interleukin-1, especially, is an important pathophysiologic factor in painful disc disorders [20].

The disc volume reduction effect of PPDD has been demonstrated in several studies [8,21]. Chen et al. [21] in a human cadaveric study showed that PPDD reduced intradiscal pressures significantly, especially in younger, healthy discs as compared to degenerative discs. Consequently, PPDD can alleviate nerve root compression and discogenic low back pain. Kasch et al. [22] evaluated this effect using 7.1 Tesla ultrahigh-field MRI in porcine discs. They showed volume reductions of 0.114 (SD: 0.054) mL, or 14.72% (thoracic) and 0.093 (SD: 0.081) mL, or 11.61% (thoracolumbar) compared with the placebo group.

Numerous studies have found favorable results with PPDD in the treatment of discogenic low back pain and herniated lumbar disc, especially contained disc protrusion [6,7,10,12,18,23–31]. The success rate of substantial pain relief post-PPDD varies from 6.3% to 84% [5,24,32,33]. Most studies have reported a success rate of >50%. Sharps and Isaac [11] showed the efficacy of PPDD. Overall 79% of 49 patients had a minimum of 2-points reduction on a VAS. Liliang et al. [9] reported that 21 patients (21/31, 67.7%) experienced substantial pain relief for an average period of 10 months (4–17 months). Furthermore, they reported that positive discography results prior to PPDD could improve and predict the success rate of the procedure, among other variables, such as age, sex, body mass index, hyper-intensity zone, Modic change, and spinal instability. In a systemic review and meta-analysis study, PPDD reduced VAS scores in the long term (24 months) and improved ODI scores. In addition, the review suggested that PPDD is a more effective, low-complication, and minimally invasive procedure compared to other treatments [7]. In two long-term follow-up studies conducted in China, PPDD was shown to be effective for pain relief and function improvement for 2–3 years. However, there is no significant difference between the 3- and 5-year postoperative VAS and ODI scores, and excellent or good patient satisfaction was 87.9% at 1 week, 72.4% at 1 year, 67.7% at 3 years, and 63.4% at 5 years [19,34].

The safety and efficacy of the PPDD procedure using Coblation® technology have been analyzed. PPDD achieved a volumetric reduction of the disc tissues without overt thermal or structural damage to adjacent tissues [35]. Lee et al. [36] showed that PPDD does not rely on heat for tissue removal, and, therefore, does not introduce excessive heat that causes tissue damage in the disc. The temperature during PPDD is typically 40 °C to 70 °C, and the total reduction of thermal influence was 5 mm from the tip [35,37]. In a porcine model, the coblation channel had a clear coagulation boundary of the nucleus pulposus. In addition, there was no evidence of direct mechanical or thermal damage to the annulus and endplate, and neural elements of the spinal cord and nerve roots at the level of the procedure were observed in the histologic examination [38].

In addition to the pain and functional scores, there are various methods to verify the success of PPDD. Radiological imaging studies, including plain radiography, CT, and MRI have been used [8,22], and there are also studies that have evaluated the PPDD outcome by thermography [39,40]. The thermal difference and pain scores were improved after PPDD, but there was no significant correlation [40]. However, these methods do not provide detailed information and are expensive. Moreover, they are not available for real-time assessment in the procedure room; thus, a simple and quick intra-procedure morphological assessment of the adequacy of decompression is still required.

Traditionally, epidurography during epidural steroid injections provided safe and accurate therapeutic injection [41–43]. It is a simple, quick, real-time, less expensive, and relatively safe method. In addition, epidurography is used to determine the degree of epidural adhesion. Although advanced technology, including CT and MRI, have made significant advances in the diagnosis of epidural fibrosis, it is believed that epidural adhesions are best diagnosed by epidurography [44]. Notably, epidurography correlated with the success of the percutaneous epidural neuroplasty, severity of pain, relief of pain, and patient satisfaction [13,45]. Moreover, it is used to assess the adequacy of decompression during spinal surgery, which is very similar to this study [14].

In this study, we applied the advantages of epidurography to the decompression effect of a disc by PPDD. Before PPDD, we observed that the contrast media did not extend above the involved disc level. After PPDD, when the disc was decompressed, we observed that the contrast media extended above the involved disc level. Moreover, the wire-type epidural catheter, which had not been passed before, was passed in some cases. We assumed that the partial removal of the nucleus pulposus by radiofrequency energy ensured the epidural space. Similar to other studies' results on the efficacy of epidurography mentioned above, our study showed that the high success rate of PPDD is correlated with an improvement in epidurography. Based on our results, intra-procedure epidurography may be a reliable method for ensuring adequate decompression of the disc. Therefore, it is expected that the patient's outcomes can be improved by using intra-procedure epidurography in addition to the existing manufacturer guidelines during PPDD.

Our findings need to be interpreted within the limitations of the study. First, this study was retrospective and had a relatively small sample size. Second, we could not analyze the difference in disc volume change by MRI before and after PPDD because of the cost implications. Third, the different proportions of type and severity of disc herniation between the two groups, which may affect the success rate of the procedure, were not evaluated on MRI. Fourth, epidural adhesion was not evaluated. A herniated disc may cause inflammation within the epidural space, and it can also make epidural adhesion that affects contrast media spreading. Fifth, the observation periods were relatively short. A randomized, controlled, double-blind, long-term follow-up study should be conducted to support the finding of this study.

This study's results showed that PPDD is an effective treatment method for patients with chronic discogenic low back pain and herniated lumbar disc-related symptoms. We also suggested that intra-procedure epidurography may be a potential PPDD outcome predictor for ensuring successful outcomes and determining the endpoint of the procedure.

Author Contributions: Conceptualization, J.B.C.; Methodology, J.B.C. and H.Y.G.; Investigation, W.S. and G.B.C.; Data Curation, E.H. and T.K.; Writing—Original Draft Preparation, H.Y.G.; Writing—Review & Editing, H.Y.G.; Supervision, J.H.K. and J.B.C.; Formal analysis, J.R.; Visualization, J.R.; Validation, J.H.K. All authors have read and agreed to the published version of the manuscript.

Funding: This research received no external funding.

Institutional Review Board Statement: This retrospective observational study was conducted according to the guidelines of the Declaration of Helsinki and was approved by the Institutional Review Board of Ajou University Hospital of Korea (IRB No. AJIRB-MED-MDB-19-409) in November 2019.

Informed Consent Statement: The requirement for informed consent was waived because of the retrospective case-control nature of the study.

Data Availability Statement: The study's data are available on request from the corresponding author.

Conflicts of Interest: The authors declare no conflict of interest.

References

1. Schmidt, C.O.; Raspe, H.; Pfingsten, M.; Hasenbring, M.; Basler, H.D.; Eich, W.; Kohlmann, T. Back pain in the German adult population: Prevalence, severity, and sociodemographic correlates in a multiregional survey. *Spine* **2007**, *32*, 2005–2011. [CrossRef] [PubMed]
2. Ren, D.J.; Liu, X.M.; Du, S.Y.; Sun, T.S.; Zhang, Z.C.; Li, F. Percutaneous nucleoplasty using coblation technique for the treatment of chronic nonspecific low back pain: 5-year follow-up results. *Chin. Med. J.* **2015**, *128*, 1893–1897. [CrossRef] [PubMed]
3. Schwarzer, A.C.; Aprill, C.N.; Derby, R.; Fortin, J.; Kine, G.; Bogduk, N. The prevalence and clinical features of internal disc disruption in patients with chronic low back pain. *Spine* **1995**, *20*, 1878–1883. [CrossRef]
4. Wang, X.; Wanyan, P.; Tian, J.H.; Hu, L. Meta-analysis of randomized trials comparing fusion surgery to non-surgical treatment for discogenic chronic low back pain. *J. Back Musculoskelet. Rehabil.* **2015**, *28*, 621–627. [CrossRef]
5. Gerges, F.J.; Lipsitz, S.R.; Nedeljkovic, S.S. A systematic review on the effectiveness of the Nucleoplasty™ procedure for discogenic pain. *Pain Physician* **2010**, *13*, 117–132.
6. Lee, D.Y.; Jeong, S.T.; Oh, J.Y.; Kim, D.H. Nucleoplasty: Percutaneous plasma disc decompression for the treatment of lumbar disc herniation. *J. Korean Soc. Spine Surg.* **2017**, *24*, 129–137. [CrossRef]
7. Eichen, P.M.; Achilles, N.; Konig, V.; Mosges, R.; Hellmich, M.; Himpe, B.; Kirchner, R. Nucleoplasty, a minimally invasive procedure for disc decompression: A systematic review and meta-analysis of published clinical studies. *Pain Physician* **2014**, *17*, E149–E173.
8. Bonaldi, G.; Baruzzi, F.; Facchinetti, A.; Fachinetti, P.; Lunghi, S. Plasma radio-frequency-based diskectomy for treatment of cervical herniated nucleus pulposus: Feasibility, safety, and preliminary clinical results. *AJNR Am. J. Neuroradiol.* **2006**, *27*, 2104–2111. [PubMed]
9. Liliang, P.C.; Lu, K.; Liang, C.L.; Chen, Y.W.; Tsai, Y.D.; Tu, Y.K. Nucleoplasty for treating lumbar disk degenerative low back pain: An outcome prediction analysis. *J. Pain Res.* **2016**, *9*, 893–898. [CrossRef]
10. Kallas, J.L.; Godoy, B.L.; Andraus, C.F.; Carvalho, F.G.; Andraus, M.E. Nucleoplasty as a therapeutic option for lumbar disc degeneration related pain: A retrospective study of 396 cases. *Arq. Neuro-Psiquiatr.* **2013**, *71*, 46–50. [CrossRef]
11. Sharps, L.S.; Isaac, Z. Percutaneous disc decompression using nucleoplasty. *Pain Physician* **2002**, *5*, 121–126. [CrossRef]
12. Singh, V.; Piryani, C.; Liao, K.; Nieschulz, S. Percutaneous disc decompression using coblation (nucleoplasty) in the treatment of chronic discogenic pain. *Pain Physician* **2002**, *5*, 250–259. [CrossRef]
13. Kim, J.H.; Jung, H.J.; Nahm, F.S.; Lee, P.B. Does improvement in epidurography following percutaneous epidural neuroplasty correspond to patient outcome? *Pain Pract.* **2015**, *15*, 407–413. [CrossRef] [PubMed]
14. Hejazi, N.; Witzmann, A.; Hassler, W. Intraoperative cervical epidurography: A simple modality for assessing the adequacy of decompression during anterior cervical procedures. *J. Neurosurg.* **2003**, *98*, 96–99. [CrossRef] [PubMed]
15. Manchikanti, L.; Staats, P.S.; Nampiaparampil, D.E.; Hirsch, J.A. What is the role of epidural injections in the treatment of lumbar discogenic pain: A systematic review of comparative analysis with fusion. *Korean J. Pain* **2015**, *28*, 75–87. [CrossRef] [PubMed]
16. Puentedura, E.J.; Brooksby, C.L.; Wallmann, H.W.; Landers, M.R. Rehabilitation following lumbosacral percutaneous nucleoplasty: A case report. *J. Orthop. Sport. Phys. Ther.* **2010**, *40*, 214–224. [CrossRef]
17. Kim, D.Y.; Lee, S.H.; Lee, H.Y.; Lee, H.J.; Chang, S.B.; Chung, S.K.; Kim, H.J. Validation of the Korean version of the oswestry disability index. *Spine* **2005**, *30*, E123–E127. [CrossRef] [PubMed]
18. Kumar, N.S.; Shah, S.M.; Tan, B.W.; Juned, S.; Yao, K. Discogenic axial back pain: Is there a role for nucleoplasty? *Asian Spine J.* **2013**, *7*, 314–321. [CrossRef]
19. Ren, D.; Zhang, Z.; Sun, T.; Li, F. Effect of percutaneous nucleoplasty with coblation on phospholipase A2 activity in the intervertebral disks of an animal model of intervertebral disk degeneration: A randomized controlled trial. *J. Orthop. Surg. Res.* **2015**, *10*, 38. [CrossRef]
20. O'Neill, C.W.; Liu, J.J.; Leibenberg, E.; Hu, S.S.; Deviren, V.; Tay, B.K.; Chin, C.T.; Lotz, J.C. Percutaneous plasma decompression alters cytokine expression in injured porcine intervertebral discs. *Spine J.* **2004**, *4*, 88–98. [CrossRef]
21. Chen, Y.C.; Lee, S.H.; Chen, D. Intradiscal pressure study of percutaneous disc decompression with nucleoplasty in human cadavers. *Spine* **2003**, *28*, 661–665. [CrossRef] [PubMed]
22. Kasch, R.; Mensel, B.; Schmidt, F.; Drescher, W.; Pfuhl, R.; Ruetten, S.; Merk, H.R.; Kayser, R. Percutaneous disc decompression with nucleoplasty-volumetry of the nucleus pulposus using ultrahigh-field MRI. *PLoS ONE* **2012**, *7*, e41497. [CrossRef] [PubMed]
23. Bokov, A.; Skorodumov, A.; Isrelov, A.; Stupak, Y.; Kukarin, A. Differential treatment of nerve root compression pain caused by lumbar disc herniation applying nucleoplasty. *Pain Physician* **2010**, *13*, 469–480. [CrossRef] [PubMed]
24. Mirzai, H.; Tekin, I.; Yaman, O.; Bursali, A. The results of nucleoplasty in patients with lumbar herniated disc: A prospective clinical study of 52 consecutive patients. *Spine J.* **2007**, *7*, 88–92. [CrossRef] [PubMed]

25. Gerszten, P.C.; Welch, W.C.; King, J.T., Jr. Quality of life assessment in patients undergoing nucleoplasty-based percutaneous discectomy. *J. Neurosurg. Spine* **2006**, *4*, 36–42. [CrossRef]
26. Manchikanti, L.; Falco, F.J.; Benyamin, R.M.; Caraway, D.L.; Deer, T.R.; Singh, V.; Hameed, H.; Hirsch, J.A. An update of the systematic assessment of mechanical lumbar disc decompression with nucleoplasty. *Pain Physician* **2013**, *16*, SE25–SE54. [CrossRef]
27. Cesaroni, A.; Nardi, P.V. Plasma disc decompression for contained cervical disc herniation: A randomized, controlled trial. *Eur. Spine J.* **2010**, *19*, 477–486. [CrossRef]
28. Gerszten, P.C.; Smuck, M.; Rathmell, J.P.; Simopoulos, T.T.; Bhagia, S.M.; Mocek, C.K.; Crabtree, T.; Bloch, D.A.; Group, S.S. Plasma disc decompression compared with fluoroscopy-guided transforaminal epidural steroid injections for symptomatic contained lumbar disc herniation: A prospective, randomized, controlled trial. *J. Neurosurg. Spine* **2010**, *12*, 357–371. [CrossRef]
29. Nikoobakht, M.; Yekanineajd, M.S.; Pakpour, A.H.; Gerszten, P.C.; Kasch, R. Plasma disc decompression compared to physiotherapy for symptomatic contained lumbar disc herniation: A prospective randomized controlled trial. *Neurol. Neurochir. Pol.* **2016**, *50*, 24–30. [CrossRef]
30. Karaman, H.; Tufek, A.; Olmez Kavak, G.; Yildirim, Z.B.; Temel, V.; Celik, F.; Akdemir, M.S.; Kaya, S. Effectiveness of nucleoplasty applied for chronic radicular pain. *Med. Sci. Monit.* **2011**, *17*, CR461–CR466. [CrossRef]
31. Sim, S.E.; Ko, E.S.; Kim, D.K.; Kim, H.K.; Kim, Y.C.; Shin, H.Y. The results of cervical nucleoplasty in patients with cervical disc disorder: A retrospective clinical study of 22 patients. *Korean J. Pain* **2011**, *24*, 36–43. [CrossRef] [PubMed]
32. Cincu, R.; Lorente Fde, A.; Gomez, J.; Eiras, J.; Agrawal, A. One decade follow up after nucleoplasty in the management of degenerative disc disease causing low back pain and radiculopathy. *Asian J. Neurosurg.* **2015**, *10*, 21–25. [CrossRef] [PubMed]
33. Cohen, S.P.; Williams, S.; Kurihara, C.; Griffith, S.; Larkin, T.M. Nucleoplasty with or without intradiscal electrothermal therapy (IDET) as a treatment for lumbar herniated disc. *J. Spinal Disord. Tech.* **2005**, *18*, S119–S124. [CrossRef] [PubMed]
34. Zhu, H.; Zhou, X.Z.; Cheng, M.H.; Shen, Y.X.; Dong, Q.R. The efficacy of coblation nucleoplasty for protrusion of lumbar intervertebral disc at a two-year follow-up. *Int. Orthop.* **2011**, *35*, 1677–1682. [CrossRef]
35. Stalder, K.; Woloszko, J.; Brown, I.; Smith, C. Repetitive plasma discharges in saline solutions. *J. Appl. Phys. Lett.* **2001**, *79*, 4503–4505. [CrossRef]
36. Lee, M.S.; Cooper, G.; Lutz, G.E.; Doty, S.B. Histologic characterization of coblation nucleoplasty performed on sheep intervertebral discs. *Pain Physician* **2003**, *6*, 439–442.
37. Wullems, J.A.; Halim, W.; van der Weegen, W. Current evidence of percutaneous nucleoplasty for the cervical herniated disk: A systematic review. *Pain Pract.* **2014**, *14*, 559–569. [CrossRef]
38. Chen, Y.C.; Lee, S.H.; Saenz, Y.; Lehman, N.L. Histologic findings of disc, end plate and neural elements after coblation of nucleus pulposus: An experimental nucleoplasty study. *Spine J.* **2003**, *3*, 466–470. [CrossRef]
39. Kim, T.Y.; Jeon, B.C.; Lee, H.D.; Seo, S.W. Retrospective outcome evaluation of cervical chemonucleolysis with digital infrared thermographic imaging. *J. Korean Neurosurg. Soc.* **1999**, *28*, 48–54.
40. Kim, D.H.; Kim, Y.S.; Shin, S.J.; Kang, H.; Kim, S.; Shin, H.Y. Retrospective outcome evaluation of cervical nucleoplasty using digital infrared thermographic imaging. *Neurospine* **2019**, *16*, 325–331. [CrossRef]
41. Johnson, B.A.; Schellhas, K.P.; Pollei, S.R. Epidurography and therapeutic epidural injections: Technical considerations and experience with 5334 cases. *AJNR Am. J. Neuroradiol.* **1999**, *20*, 697–705. [PubMed]
42. Gupta, R.; Singh, S.; Kaur, S.; Singh, K.; Aujla, K. Correlation between epidurographic contrast flow patterns and clinical effectiveness in chronic lumbar discogenic radicular pain treated with epidural steroid injections via different approaches. *Korean J. Pain* **2014**, *27*, 353–359. [CrossRef]
43. Hong, J.H. An analysis of pattern of transforaminal epidurography. *Korean J. Pain* **2006**, *19*, 175–180. [CrossRef]
44. Manchikanti, L.; Bakhit, C.E. Percutaneous lysis of epidural adhesions. *Pain Physician* **2000**, *3*, 46–64. [CrossRef] [PubMed]
45. Jo, D.H.; Jang, S. The correlation between caudal epidurogram and low back pain. *Korean J. Pain* **2012**, *25*, 22–27. [CrossRef] [PubMed]

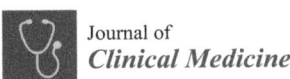

Article

Exploring the Importance of Corticalization Occurring in Alveolar Bone Surrounding a Dental Implant

Marcin Kozakiewicz * and Tomasz Wach

Department of Maxillofacial Surgery, Medical University of Lodz, 113 Żeromskiego Str., 90-549 Lodz, Poland
* Correspondence: marcin.kozakiewicz@umed.lodz.pl; Tel.: +48-42-6393422

Abstract: Several measures describing the transformation of trabecular bone to cortical bone on the basis of analysis of intraoral radiographs are known (including bone index or corticalization index, CI). At the same time, it has been noted that after functional loading of dental implants such transformations occur in the bone directly adjacent to the fixture. Intuitively, it seems that this is a process conducive to the long-term maintenance of dental implants and certainly necessary when immediate loading is applied. The authors examined the relationship of implant design features to marginal bone loss (MBL) and the intensity of corticalization over a 10-year period of functional loading. This study is a general description of the phenomenon of peri-implant bone corticalization and an attempt to interpret this phenomenon to achieve success of implant treatment in the long term. Corticalization significantly increased over the first 5-year functional loading (CI from 200 ± 146 initially to 282 ± 182, $p < 0.001$) and maintained a high level (CI = 261 ± 168) in the 10-year study relative to the reference bone (149 ± 178). MBL significantly increased throughout the follow-up period—5 years: 0.83 ± 1.26 mm ($p < 0.001$), 10 years: 1.48 ± 2.01 mm ($p < 0.001$). MBL and radiographic bone structure (CI) were evaluated in relation to intraosseous implant design features and prosthetic work performed. In the scope of the study, it can be concluded that the phenomenon of peri-implant jawbone corticalization seems an unfavorable condition for the future fate of bone-anchored implants, but it requires further research to fully explain the significance of this phenomenon.

Keywords: dental implants; long-term results; long-term success; marginal bone loss; functional loading; intra-oral radiographs; radiomics; texture analysis; corticalization; bone remodeling

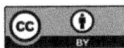

1. Introduction

The use of dental implants is the primary method of replacing missing teeth. Nowadays, it is very widely modified [1–3] and applied from simple oral surgery [4] to very advanced craniomaxillofacial procedures [5–8]. This implant treatment has good long-term results, but still some implants are lost.

It has long been noted that bone apposition and remodeling processes occur around dental implants. Direct evidence of these phenomena is provided by dental implants removed after many years of their functional load [9]. Retrieval and histological analysis of dental implants for fracture or other reasons (such as orthodontic, psychological, esthetic, and hygienic reasons) [10] is able to explain the corticalization phenomenon induced by implants. Most of the present histological studies on human specimens find compact, lamellar bone with many Haversian systems and osteons near the implant surface with increased bone-implant contact (BIC) up to 60–90% in 7–8 years mean duration of functional loading [11–31]. It is also worth summarizing two well-known truths on the basis of these studies. First, loaded implants presented an average of 10% higher BIC when compared with unloaded ones. Second, approx. 10–12% higher BIC is reported for immediately loaded dental implants [32–35]. In loaded implants, transverse collagen fibers of the bone are more abundant, while in unloaded implants, these collagen fibers in bone tended to run in a more longitudinal way. Peri-implant bone is particularly thickened around the top of the threads [36]. Rougher surfaces have approx. a 10% higher area of bone apposition than machined surfaces. However, the Scandinavians, having introduced implants with a machined surface in the 1970s, still believe that these implants have superiority over implants with a moderately rough surface [37]. Multiple remodeled regions representing many remodeling cycles over the years are found in peri-implant bone. Ongoing apposition and resorption phenomena were present inside the threads. The osteocyte number is higher near loaded versus unloaded implants [10].

Moreover, it was already reported [38] that loading was able to stimulate bone remodeling at the interface, that a higher percentage of lamellar bone was found in loaded implants and more osteoblasts and osteoclasts were found in those loaded implants. The implant loading seemed to determine differences in the distribution of the bone collagen fibers too [14,39,40]. The transverse collagen fibers were mainly located at the lower flank of the threads, where compressive loads exerted their effects. Transverse collagen fibers have been described as the fibers most able to resist compressive loads, and this fact can explain their higher quantity in loaded than unloaded implants. A lower mineral density was present in the peri-implant bone around unloaded implants [41]. The loading forces direction could have determined a higher mineralization of the osseous tissue located in the coronal side of the threads when compared to that in an apical location [42].

The above-mentioned observations are probably so pronounced in the jaws because the bone appositional index here is one of the highest in the human body [43]. It is higher than in the iliac bone, femur or vertebrae. This process leads to the osseointegration of the dental implants firstly but later probably is responsible for the corticalization. The remodeling and the superimposition of new osteons on the older ones is found too [44].

Knowing that crestal bone is the basis for dental implants to function as intended [45,46], it seems that other factors such as gingival pocket, biotype, width of keratinized gingival zone, color and translucency of soft tissues [47–49] are secondary. In recent years, there seems to be a growing interest in the phenomenon of corticalization [50–52]. It has been hypothesized that almost no bone loss can be expected after bone remodeling over the implant neck [53]. It will be interesting to see whether the corticalization phenomenon affects the height of the bone supporting the implant. The question arises as to how this process is related to vertical bone loss and how it relates to the long-term success of implant treatment. For this, analysis of the microstructure of the bone surrounding the implant is needed [54], and the key place is the bone adjacent to the implant neck [55,56].

Fine bone morphology can be registered using microcomputed tomography as well as even using 3-tesla magnetic-resonance imaging (MRI) [57]. Magnetic resonance tomography instruments that trigger a field of 7 tesla have also been available for several years and are being used to analyze bone microstructure [58]. However, a series of limitations of these advanced technologies should be highlighted. In daily clinical practice, it is standard practice to use intraoral radiographs [59–64] or pantomographic radiographs [65–68] to analyze the condition of the peri-implant jawbone. Cone-beam tomographs [69] are used much less frequently. The cost of a 7-tesla scanner is not inconsiderable. There is little availability of this newly developed technology. There are no developed sequences for peri-implant jawbone imaging. Metal components such dental implants and parts of prosthetic work can create artifacts in MRI images and interfere with the diagnostic process, not to mention advanced studies of the bone structure at the implant wall [70], and most importantly, MRI is used to study the cancellous bone, not the structure of the cortical bone [71–75]. This is still a matter of the future [76], and for now, one can rely on imaging studies with the use of intraoral, periapical radiographs [77,78] for the reasons cited above.

The suspected long-term disadvantage of corticalization [79] is based on bone index (BI) analysis. There are some doubts about the specificity of this measure in detecting corticalization [80]. It seems that this measure does not discriminate very strongly between homogeneous dark areas (crestal bone loss) and homogeneous bright areas (corticalization of trabecular bone). Another inconvenience is the need to use the inverse of the bone index, i.e., 1/BI. Next, it is known that 1/BI is highest in bone loss regions, significantly lower in cortical bone and lowest significantly at the site of trabecular bone [80].

The aim of this study was to determine whether corticalization (basing on the corticalization index) in long-term follow-up is a negative phenomenon for the fate of dental implants.

2. Materials and Methods

The collected material is the result of prospective acquisition of radiological data during the clinical course of oral implantological treatment of patients with missing teeth in the maxillary and mandibular region. Inclusion criteria: at least 18 years of age, bleeding on gingival probing < 20%, probing depth ≤ 3 mm, good oral hygiene, regular follow-ups, following doctor's orders. Exclusion criteria: uncontrolled internal co-morbidity (diabetes mellitus, thyroid dishormonoses, rheumatoid disease and other immunodeficiencies), a history of oral radiation therapy, past or current use of cytostatic drugs, soft tissue augmentation, low quality or lack of follow-up radiographs. General health was confirmed via anamnesis and evaluation of body mass index (BMI) using a serum test of thyrotropin, calcium and triglycerides (the way to describe their general condition, i.e., emanation of the health status on entry to the study). Finally, clinical and radiological data of 911 persons were included in this study.

The dental implants were inserted by one dentist (M.K.) according to the protocols recommended by the manufacturers. A total of 22 types of dental implant were used in this study: AB Dental Devices I5 (www.ab-dent.com (accessed on 21 July 2022), Ashdod, Israel) 102 pieces, ADIN Dental Implants Touareg (www.adin-implants.com (accessed on 21 July 2022), Afula, Israel) 89 pieces, Alpha Bio ARRP (www.alpha-bio.net (accessed on 21 July 2022), Petah-Tikva, Israel) 14 pieces, Alpha Bio ATI (www.alpha-bio.net (accessed on 21 July 2022), Petah-Tikva, Israel) 139 pieces, Alpha Bio DFI (www.alpha-bio.netv (accessed on 21 July 2022), Petah-Tikva, Israel) 43 pieces, Alpha Bio OCI (www.alpha-bio.net (accessed on 21 July 2022), Petah-Tikva, Israel) 28 pieces, Alpha Bio SFB (www.alpha-bio.net (accessed on 21 July 2022), Petah-Tikva, Israel) 62 pieces, Alpha Bio SPI (www.alpha-bio.net (accessed on 21 July 2022), Petah-Tikva, Israel) 448 pieces, Argon K3pro Rapid (www.argon-dental.de (accessed on 21 July 2022), Bingen am Rhein, Germany) 182 pieces, Bego Semados RI (www.bego-implantology.com (accessed on 21 July 2022), Bremen, Germany) 12 pieces, Dentium Super Line (www.dentium.com (accessed on 21 July 2022), Gyeonggi-do, South Korea) 38 pieces, Friadent Ankylos C/X (www.dentsplysirona.com (accessed on 21 July 2022), Warszawa, Poland) 14 pieces, Implant Direct InterActive (www.implantdirect.com (accessed on 21 July 2022), Thousand Oaks, United States of America) 139 pieces, Implant Direct Legacy 3 (www.implantdirect.com (accessed on 21 July 2022), Thousand Oaks, United States of America) 48 pieces, MIS BioCom M4 (www.mis-implants.com (accessed on 21 July 2022), Bar-Lev Industrial Park, Israel) 8 pieces, MIS C1 (www.mis-implants.com (accessed on 21 July 2022), Bar-Lev Industrial Park, Israel) 307 pieces, MIS Seven (www.mis-implants.com (accessed on 21 July 2022), Bar-Lev Industrial Park, Israel) 921 pieces, MIS UNO One Piece (www.mis-implants.com (accessed on 21 July 2022), Bar-Lev Industrial Park, Israel) 40 pieces, Osstem Implant Company GS III (www.en.osstem.com (accessed on 21 July 2022), Seoul, South Korea) 15 pieces, SGS Dental P7N (www.sgs-dental.com (accessed on 21 July 2022), Schaan, Liechtenstein) 12 pieces, TBR Implanté (www.tbr.dental (accessed on 21 July 2022), Toulouse, France) 6 pieces, and Wolf Dental Conical Screw-Type (www.wolf-dental.com (accessed on 21 July 2022), Osnabrück, Germany) 31 pieces. The total number of introduced dental implants was 2700 pieces. The appearance of the tested implants is shown in Figure 1.

All implants were loaded late, i.e., min. 3 months after the implants were placed in the bone. Standardized intraoral radiographs [81] were taken immediately before prosthetic restoration (initial radiograph), 5 and 10 years later. Focus X-ray apparatus (Instrumental Dental, Tuusula, Finland) was set to the constant technical parameters: exposure time 0.1 s, voltage in the lamp 70 kV and current 7 mA. An intraoral parallel technique was used. To ensure an identical relative position of the implant, an X-ray tube and radiation detector and a set of RINN XCP rings and holders were utilized (Dentsply International Inc., Cheung Sha Wan, Hong Kong, China) with a silicone bite index. The video part of the system was a recording plate with a photosensitive storage surface (Digora Optime digital radiography system—Soredex, Tuusula, Finland [61]). Immediately after the X-ray exposure, the storage phosphor plate was placed in a scanner that reads radiographic information (the image size was 476 × 620 pixels; the pixel size was 70 μm × 70 μm). A computer coupled with the scanner processed, presented and archived acquired images. Patients included in the study were followed by a single dentist during the entire period. The average marginal bone loss (MBL) of the alveolar crest after osseointegration (initial) at 5 and 10 years of functional loading was measured. In addition, the bone texture features at these time periods were calculated. The influence of factors related to implant design (Table 1) was evaluated.

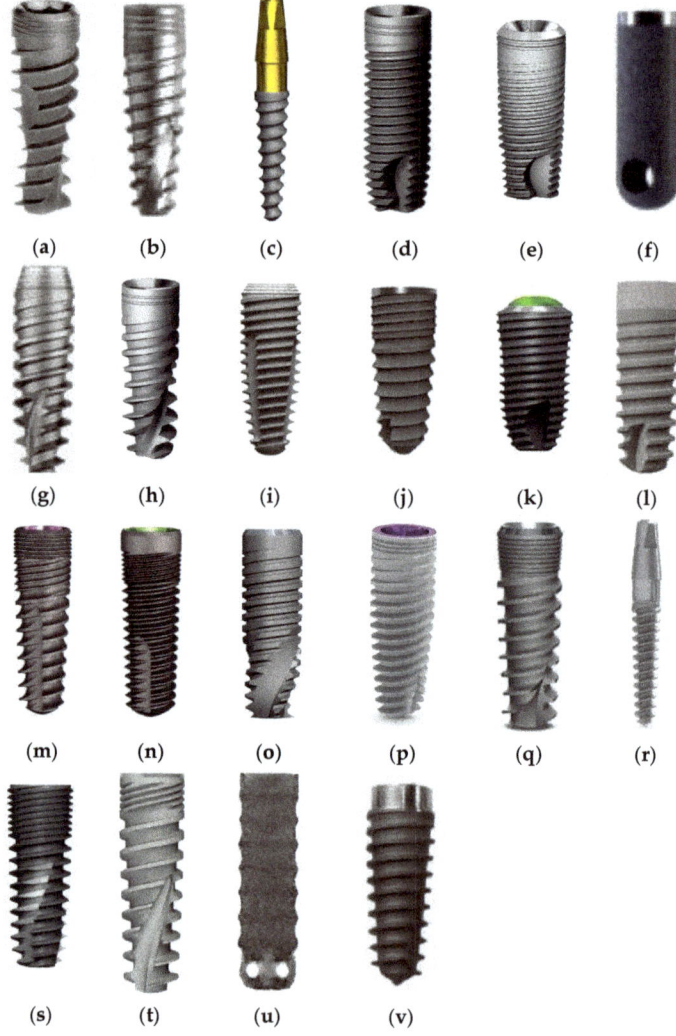

Figure 1. The appearance of the dental implants compared in this study, in alphabetical order: (**a**) AB Dental Devices I5; (**b**) ADIN Dental Implants Touareg; (**c**) Alpha Bio ARRP; (**d**) Alpha Bio ATI; (**e**) Alpha

Bio DFI; (**f**) Alpha Bio OCI; (**g**) Alpha Bio SFB; (**h**) Alpha Bio SPI; (**i**) Argon Medical Productions K3pro Rapid; (**j**) Bego Semados RI; (**k**) Dentium Super Line; (**l**) Friadent Ankylos C/X; (**m**) Implant Direct InterActive; (**n**) Implant Direct Legacy 3; (**o**) MIS BioCom M4; (**p**) MIS C1; (**q**) MIS Seven; (**r**) MIS UNO One Piece; (**s**) Osstem Implant Company GS III; (**t**) SGS Dental P7N; (**u**) TBR Implanté; (**v**) Wolf Dental Conical Screw-Type.

Table 1. Design features of dental implant used in this study (www.spotimplant.com/en/ (access on 21 July 2022)). Alphabetical order of the implant names.

Manufacturer Implant Type	Titanium Alloy	Level	Connection Type	Connection Shape	Neck Shape	Neck Micro-threads	Body Shape	Body Threads	Apex Shape	Apex Hole	Apex Groove
AB Dental Devices I5	Grade 5	Bone Level	Internal	Hexagon	Straight	No	Tapered	Square	Flat	No Hole	Yes
ADIN Dental Implants Touareg	Grade 5	Bone Level	Internal	Hexagon	Straight	Yes	Tapered	Square	Flat	No Hole	Yes
Alpha Bio ARRP	Grade 5	Tissue Level	Custom	One Piece Abutment	Straight	No	Tapered	Reverse Buttress	Cone	No Hole	No
Alpha Bio ATI	Grade 5	Bone Level	Internal	Hexagon	Straight	Yes	Straight	Square	Flat	No Hole	Yes
Alpha Bio DFI	Grade 5	Bone Level	Internal	Hexagon	Straight	Yes	Tapered	Square	Flat	No Hole	Yes
Alpha Bio OCI	Grade 5	Bone Level	Internal	Hexagon	Straight	No	Straight	No Threads	Dome	Round	No
Alpha Bio SFB	Grade 5	Bone Level	Internal	Hexagon	Straight	No	Tapered	V Shaped	Flat	No Hole	Yes
Alpha Bio SPI	Grade 5	Bone Level	Internal	Hexagon	Straight	Yes	Tapered	Square	Flat	No Hole	Yes
Argon Medical Prod. K3pro Rapid	Grade 4	Subcrestal	Internal	Conical	Straight	Yes	Tapered	V Shaped	Dome	No Hole	Yes
Bego Semados RI	Grade 4	Bone Level	Internal	Hexagon	Straight	Yes	Tapered	Reverse Buttress	Cone	No Hole	Yes
Dentium Super Line	Grade 5	Bone Level	Internal	Conical	Straight	No	Tapered	Buttress	Dome	No Hole	Yes
Friadent Ankylos C/X	Grade 4	Subcrestal	Internal	Conical	Straight	No	Tapered	V Shaped	Dome	No Hole	Yes
Implant Direct InterActive	Grade 5	Bone Level	Internal	Conical	Straight	Yes	Tapered	Reverse Buttress	Dome	No Hole	Yes
Implant Direct Legacy 3	Grade 5	Bone Level	Internal	Hexagon	Straight	Yes	Tapered	Reverse Buttress	Dome	No Hole	Yes
MIS BioCom M4	Grade 5	Bone Level	Internal	Hexagon	Straight	No	Straight	V Shaped	Flat	No Hole	Yes
MIS C1	Grade 5	Bone Level	Internal	Conical	Straight	Yes	Tapered	Reverse Buttress	Dome	No Hole	Yes
MIS Seven	Grade 5	Bone Level	Internal	Hexagon	Straight	Yes	Tapered	Reverse Buttress	Dome	No Hole	Yes
MIS UNO One Piece	Grade 5	Tissue Level	Custom	One Piece Abutment	Straight	No	Tapered	Square	Dome	No Hole	Yes
Osstem Implant Company GS III	Grade 5	Bone Level	Internal	Conical	Straight	Yes	Tapered	V Shaped	Dome	No Hole	Yes
SGS Dental P7N	Grade 5	Bone Level	Internal	Hexagon	Straight	Yes	Tapered	V Shaped	Flat	No Hole	Yes
TBR Implanté	Grade 5	Bone Level	Internal	Octagon	Straight	No	Straight	No Threads	Flat	Round	Yes
Wolf Dental Conical Screw-Type	Grade 4	Bone Level	Internal	Hexagon	Straight	No	Tapered	V Shaped	Cone	No Hole	Yes

In the radiographs obtained in this way, a region of interest (ROI) was established in the area of bone near the implant neck (Figure 2, green). The second ROI was established in an image of intact bone distant from the dental implant (it was referent bone, yellow). The surface area of each ROI was 1500 pixels squared.

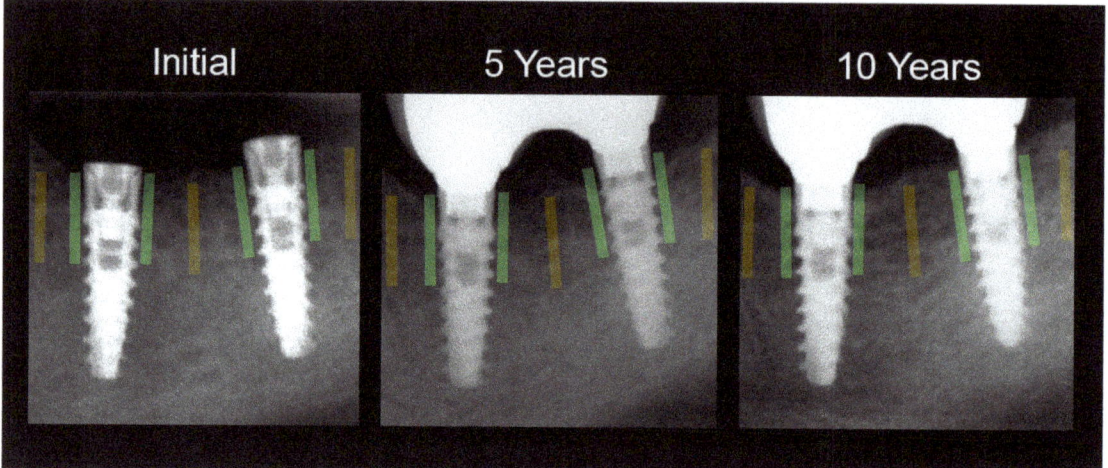

Figure 2. Image data acquisition method for texture analysis in intraoral radiographs. ROIs highlighted in yellow are sites in the alveolar crest distant from the dental implants (reference). ROIs marked in green are sites examined along the neck portion of the implants and represent, respectively: radiographs taken immediately prior to prosthetic work—initial ROI; radiographs taken after five years of functional loading—5 years ROI; radiographs taken after ten years of functional loading—10 years ROI. The data extracted from these ROIs were later analyzed in freeware MaZda 4.6 [79,80,82] and used to calculate the corticalization index.

Radiologically recorded peri-implant bone structure was studied via digital texture analysis using the corticalization index previously proposed [80] as version 1 (CI). It consists of the product of a measure that evaluates the number of long series of pixels of similar optical density with the mean optical density of the studied site (in the numerator) and the magnitude of the chaotic arrangement of the texture pattern, i.e., differential entropy (in the denominator).

The texture of X-ray images was analyzed in MaZda 4.6 freeware invented by the University of Technology in Lodz [82] to test measures of corticalization in the per-implant environment of trabecular bone (representing original bone before implant-dependent alterations) and soft tissue (representing product of marginal bone loss). MaZda provides both first-order (mean optical density) and second-order (differential entropy: DifEntr, long-run emphasis moment: LngREmph) data. Due to the fact that the second-order data are given for four directions in the image and in the present study the authors do not wish to search for directional features, the arithmetic mean of these four primary data was included for further analysis. The regions of interest (ROIs) were normalized ($\mu \pm 3\sigma$) to share the same mean (μ) and standard deviation (σ) of optical density within the ROI. To eliminate noise [83] further, worked on data were reduced to 6 bits. For analysis in a co-occurrences matrix, a spacing of 5 pixels was chosen. In the formulas that follow, $p(i)$ is a normalized histogram vector (i.e., histogram whose entries are divided by the total number of pixels in ROI), $i = 1, 2, \ldots, N_g$, and N_g denotes the number of optical density levels. The mean optical density feature (only a first order feature) was calculated as below:

$$\text{Mean Optical Density} = \sum_{i=1}^{Ng} ip(i) \qquad (1)$$

Second order features:

$$\text{DifEntr} = -\sum_{i=1}^{Ng} p_{x-y}(i)\log\left(p_{x-y}(i)\right) \qquad (2)$$

where Σ is the sum, N_g is the number of levels of optical density in the radiograph, i and j are the optical density of pixels 5 pixels distant one from another, p is the probability and log is the common logarithm [54]. The differential entropy calculated in this way is a measure of the overall scatter of bone structure elements in a radiograph. Its high values are typical for cancellous bone [64,84–86]. Next, the last primary texture feature was calculated:

$$\text{LngREmph} = \frac{\sum_{i=1}^{Ng}\sum_{k=1}^{Nr} k^2 p(i,k)}{\sum_{i=1}^{Ng}\sum_{k=1}^{Nr} p(i,k)} \qquad (3)$$

where Σ is the sum, N_r is the number of series of pixels with density level i and length k, N_g is the number of levels for image optical density, N_r is the number of pixel in the series and p is the probability [87,88]. This texture feature describes thick, uniformly dense, radio-opaque bone structures in intra-oral radiograph images [84,86].

The equations for mean optical density, DifEntr and LngREmph were subsequently used for the corticalization index (CI) construction [80]:

$$\text{LngREmph} = \frac{\sum_{i=1}^{Ng}\sum_{k=1}^{Nr} k^2 p(i,k)}{\sum_{i=1}^{Ng}\sum_{k=1}^{Nr} p(i,k)} \qquad (4)$$

Statistical analysis includes feature distribution evaluation, mean (t-test) or median (W-test) comparison, analysis of regression and one-way analysis of variance or the Kruskal-Wallis test as no-normal distribution or between-group variance indicated significant differences in investigated groups. Detected differences or relationships were assumed to be statistically significant when $p < 0.05$. Statgraphics Centurion version 18.1.12 (StatPoint Technologies, Warrenton, VA, USA) was used for statistical analyses.

3. Results

In the implantological material collected, it was found at baseline (initial) that 86.7% of the implants were not affected by marginal bone loss at all and 13.3% of the implants had some degree of bone loss (in this subgroup the MBL was 1.93 ± 1.85 mm). After 5 years, bone loss was not present in 54.4% of the implants, and bone loss was noted in 43.6% of the implants (in this subgroup the MBL was 1.91 ± 1.26 mm). At the final point of the study, i.e., after 10 years of functional loading, there was zero bone loss in 44.4% of implants, while 55.6% were affected to some degree by marginal bone loss (in this subgroup the MBL was 2.67 ± 2.04 mm).

A sequential, significant increase in the CI in peri-implant bone was observed from the initial study (i.e., just after functional loading) to five years ($p < 0.001$). Subsequently, a slight decrease in the CI was noted at the ten-year study ($p < 0.05$), but the CI is significantly higher than on the day functional loading began. When analyzing MBL, it was found to progress statistically significantly throughout the study with high significance ($p < 0.001$). When examining the relationship between CI and MBL, it was noticed that the two variables were associated with each other from five years after the functional loading of the dental implants, i.e., at the fifth year: CC = 0.11, R^2 = 1.2%, $p < 0.001$, and at the tenth year: CC = 0.12, R^2 = 1.4%, $p < 0.01$. MBL was directly proportionally related with an increase in the CI (Table 2 and Figure 3).

Table 2. The progressive increase in the difference in bone structure of implant-loaded versus reference cancellous bone and the observed relationship with marginal bone loss.

Region of Interest/Period	Corticalization Index	Marginal Bone Loss [mm]	Simple Regression
Reference Cancellous Bone	149 ± 178	0.00 ± 0.00	n.a.
Initial Peri-Implant Observation	200 ± 146	0.25 ± 0.94	n.s.
5 Years Peri-Implant Observation	282 ± 182	0.83 ± 1.26	CC = 0.11; R^2 = 1.2%; $p < 0.001$
10 Years Peri-Implant Observation	261 ± 168	1.48 ± 2.01	CC = 0.12; R^2 = 1,4%; $p < 0.01$

Abbreviations: n.a.—not applicable; n.s.—no statistical significance; CC—correlation coefficient: R^2—coefficient of determination.

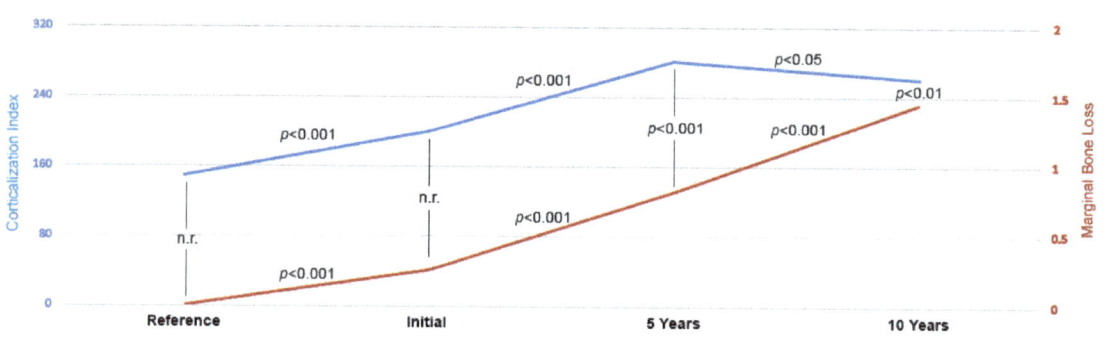

Figure 3. The results of peri-implant bone corticalization assessment (corticalization index, blue line, data without a unit) and marginal bone loss (red line, data in millimeters). There was a statistically significant increase in the values of both variables at each stage of the study. Moreover, it was noted that there was a directly proportional relationship of marginal bone loss with the progression of corticalization at 5 years and 10 years of functional loading of the implants. Abbreviations: n.r.—no relationship.

It is important to evaluate corticalization in relation to basic epidemiological data. Hence, the relationship with gender, smoking, location, etc. is shown below (Table 3).

Sex, pre-prosthetic surgical augmentation procedures and surgical technique for augmentation are not a differentiating factor for the study population at any stage of the survey. In contrast, the opposite is true of localization. For smokers with implants put in the mandible or posterior part of the dental arch, corticalization is higher than in the smoker group (excluding 5-year observation) with implants in the maxilla or posterior dental arch, throughout the study period. The association of increasing weight, height and BMI (as well as serum calcium levels) in patients with a decreasing corticalization index can be seen. On the other hand, increasing age (but no relation found in 10-year investigation) and thyrotropin levels in the patients studied are accompanied by an increasing corticalization index (Figure 4).

The results obtained for the different types of implants that remained under long-term follow-up are shown below (Figure 5). They are arranged in all four graphs from the implant type with the lowest peri-implant bone corticalization to the highest corticalization (for both CI and MBL). It is noticeable that MBL does not correspond directly to CI values for individual implants. Therefore, further analyses were performed in groups organized differently, i.e., according to the features of the implant designs (Table 4) and the prosthetic restoration used (Table 5).

Table 3. Presentation of included population. Assessment of the impact of baseline epidemiological data on the corticalization index observed in peri-implant bone.

Clinical Feature	Option/Value of the Feature	Corticalization Index		
		Initial	5 Years	10 Years
Sex	Female	205 ± 169	279 ± 176	263 ± 151
	Male	194 ± 114	285 ± 190	260 ± 190
Tobacco Smoking	Non-Smoker	200 ± 152 [L]	283 ± 185	257 ± 166 [L]
	Smoker	203 ± 91 [H]	272 ± 155	301 ± 184 [H]
Jaw	Maxilla	175 ± 108 [L]	239 ± 151 [L]	223 ± 148 [L]
	Mandible	190 ± 179 [H]	336 ± 203 [H]	302 ± 179 [H]
Localization in Dental Arch	Anterior	166 ± 92 [L]	247 ± 163 [L]	226 ± 162 [L]
	Posterior	212 ± 174 [H]	295 ± 188 [H]	273 ± 169 [H]
Jawbone Status	Augmented	220 ± 210	267 ± 164	263 ± 142
	Intact	193 ± 116	286 ± 188	261 ± 176
Augmentation Technique	Implant Neck Bone Chips	236 ± 269	292 ± 187	271 ± 133
	Implant Neck Bone Substitute	183 ± 107	210 ± 138	280 ± 211
	Bone Substitute Sinus Lift	210 ± 143	248 ± 138	252 ± 135
Age	47 ± 13 years	Direct Relation *	Direct Relation *	No Relation
Patient Height	1.70 ± 0.09 m	No Relation	No Relation	Inverse Relation *
Patient Weight	75 ± 19 Kg	No Relation	Inverse Relation *	Inverse Relation *
Body Mass Index	26 ± 4	No Relation	Inverse Relation *	Inverse Relation *
Serum Thyrotropin	1.73 ± 1.07 mU/L	Direct Relation *	Direct Relation *	Direct Relation *
Total Serum Calcium	2.39 ± 0.61 mmol/dL	Inverse Relation *	Inverse Relation *	Inverse Relation *
Serum Triglycerides	1.24 ± 0.57 mmol/L	Direct Relation *	No Relation	No Relation

[H] value higher than in other implant design options within observation period ($p < 0.05$); [L] value lower than in other implant design options within observation period ($p < 0.05$); * means significant relationship ($p < 0.05$) between corticalization index and the clinical quantitative (i.e., numerical) feature.

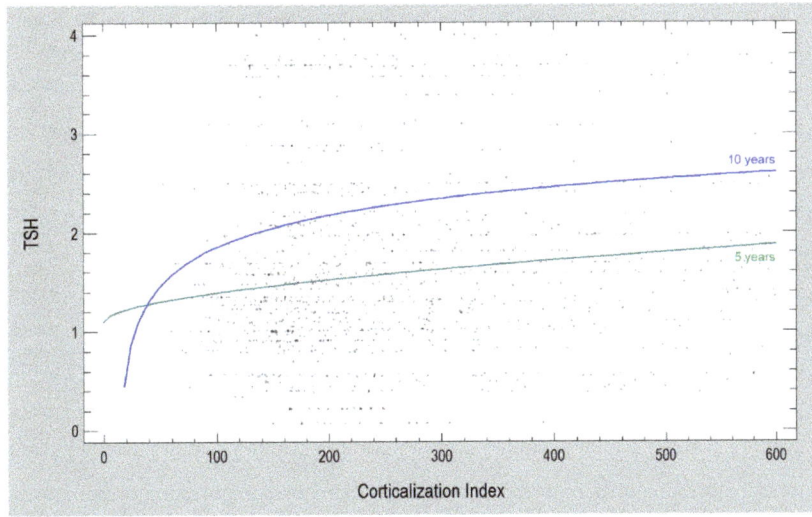

Figure 4. An example of the relationship found between patients' general condition (TSH: thyrotropin serum level in mU/L) and the corticalization index. Both relationships are statistically significant ($p < 0.05$).

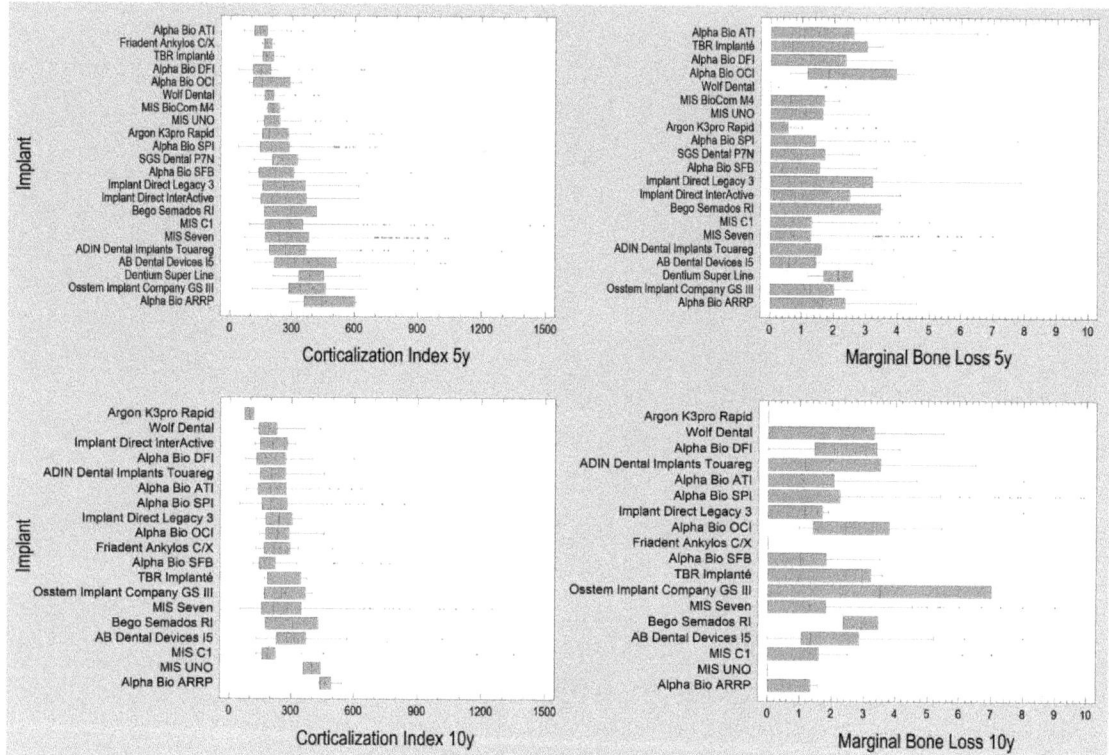

Figure 5. The results obtained for the types of dental implants studied. The charts on the left show the results of the corticalization evaluation (five and ten years). The results here are arranged from lowest mean (**top**) to highest mean (**bottom**). On the right are the results of marginal bone loss arranged in the same order as for corticalization—it can be seen that bone loss does not absolutely correspond to corticalization.

Table 4. Peri-implant bone feature observed among examined implant designs groups.

Design Parameter	Option	Feature	Initial	5 Years	10 Years
Titanium Alloy $n = 2196$	Grade 4	MBL	$0.00^{\,L}$	$0.00^{\,L}$	0.00
		CI	$184^{\,H}$	$179^{\,L}$	189
	Grade 5	MBL	$0.00^{\,H}$	$0.00^{\,H}$	0.91
		CI	$163^{\,L}$	$225^{\,H}$	209
Immersion Level $n = 2196$	Subcrestal	MBL	$0.00^{\,L}$	$0.00^{\,L}$	$0.00^{\,L}$
		CI	$198^{\,H}$	181	$201^{\,L}$
	Bone Level	MBL	0.00	0.00	$0.97^{\,H}$
		CI	$163^{\,L}$	224	$205^{\,L}$
	Tissue Level	MBL	$0.00^{\,H}$	$1.24^{\,H}$	0.00
		CI	154	222	$439^{\,H}$
Connection Type $n = 2196$	Internal	MBL	$0.00^{\,L}$	$0.00^{\,L}$	0.91
		CI	167	221	$205^{\,L}$
	Custom	MBL	$0.00^{\,H}$	$1.24^{\,H}$	0.00
		CI	154	222	$439^{\,H}$

Table 4. Cont.

Design Parameter	Option	Feature	Initial	5 Years	10 Years
Connection Shape $n = 2196$	Conical	MBL	0.00	0.00	0.00
		CI	202 [H]	225	200 [L]
	Internal Hexagon	MBL	0.00	0.00	0.97
		CI	151 [L]	220	205 [L]
	Internal Octagon	MBL	0.00	0.67	2.91
		CI	205	168	268
	One Piece Abutm	MBL	0.00	1.24	0.00
		CI	154	222	439 [H]
Head Microthreads $n = 2196$	Yes	MBL	0.00	0.00 [L]	0.73 [L]
		CI	170 [H]	221	201
	No	MBL	0.00	0.61 [H]	1.15 [H]
		CI	158 [L]	222	227
Body Shape $n = 2196$	Tapered	MBL	0.00	0.00 [L]	0.85
		CI	167	226 [H]	206
	Straight	MBL	0.00	1.33 [H]	1.15
		CI	172	147 [L]	206
Body Threads $n = 1760$	Butteress	MBL	0.00	2.15 [H]	n.a.
		CI	190	383 [H]	n.a
	Reverse Butteress	MBL	0.00 [L]	0.00 [L]	0.79 [L]
		CI	171 [H]	239 [H]	213
	V Shape	MBL	0.00 [L]	0.00 [L]	0.00 [L]
		CI	174 [H]	197 [L]	184
	Square	MBL	0.00 [L]	0.00 [L]	0.91 [L]
		CI	150 [L]	201 [L]	211
	No Threads	MBL	0.30 [H]	1.54 [H]	2.57 [H]
		CI	190	164 [L]	232
Apex Shape $n = 2196$	Cone	MBL	0.00	0.00	0.00
		CI	122 [L]	199	193
	Dome	MBL	0.00	0.00	0.79
		CI	174 [H]	230 [H]	213
	Flat	MBL	0.00	0.45 [H]	1.21
		CI	148	103 [L]	201
Apex Hole $n = 1447$	Round	MBL	0.00 [L]	1.54 [H]	2.57 [H]
		CI	190	164 [L]	232
	No or other	MBL	0.30 [H]	0.00 [L]	0.79 [L]
		CI	167	221 [H]	206
Apex Groove $n = 2196$	Yes	MBL	0.00 [L]	0.00 [L]	0.79 [L]
		CI	167	220	105
	No	MBL	0.00 [H]	1.66 [H]	2.00 [H]
		CI	154	297	258

[H] value higher than in other implant design options within observation period ($p < 0.05$); [L] value lower than in other implant design options within observation period ($p < 0.05$); n—number of evaluated dental implants; MBL—marginal bone loss is given as median due to non-normal distribution in mm; CI—corticalization index is given as median due to non-normal distribution.

In the group of implants made of grade 5 titanium alloy, lower corticalization was noted in the initial period, which increased significantly at 5 years. A higher MBL occurred in the later observation periods. Throughout the observation period, implants inserted subcrestally have the lowest MBL. However, surprisingly, during the initial period, the lowest bone loss is accompanied by the highest level of corticalization. These differences disappear at the five-year follow-up period, and then at the ten-year follow-up period the relationships reverse—the lowest corticalization is with subcrestally inserted implants as also the MBL is the lowest. One-piece implants (i.e., of the "Custom" connection type contrary to internal connection) were characterized by higher MBL up to and including the fifth year of observation. This is not followed by the CI value. Evaluating the connection shape, it could be seen that corticalization is greatest with one-piece implants (i.e., without a socket for the abutment), but this does not go hand in hand with the MBL value at five and ten years. When the implants do not have a haed microthread, higher MBL values are recorded with them. CI values are also elevated, but statistically insignificant. The shape of the implant body has no effect on corticalization and marginal loss at either the initial or the 10-year follow-up period. It was only noted that in the fifth year of functional loading there was less corticalization and more bone loss with tapered implants. The lowest MBL and highest CI were noted in implants with a V shape and reverse butteress thread. The lowest bone loss supported by an increased CI occurred with flat apex implants. Only increasing bone loss over time was observed in implants with apex groove. This was not followed by increasing CI values.

Table 5. The prosthetic works examined in this study.

Prosthetic	n	Feature	Initial	5 Years	10 Years
Single Crown	734	MBL	0.00 [H]	0.00	0.91
		CI	153 [L]	196 [L]	186 [L]
Splinted Crowns	794	MBL	0.00	0.00	1.20 [H]
		CI	198	224	227 [H]
Bridge	576	MBL	0.00 [L]	0.00 [L]	0.00 [L]
		CI	172 [H]	251 [H]	215
Overdenture	160	MBL	0.00	0.49 [H]	0.00 [L]
		CI	185 [H]	392 [H]	239 [H]
Platform Switching	509	MBL	0.00	0.00	1.06
		CI	155 [L]	197 [L]	200

[H] value higher than in other prosthetic solutions ($p < 0.05$); [L] value lower than in other prosthetic solutions ($p < 0.05$); n—number of evaluated dental implants; MBL—marginal bone loss is given as median due to non-normal distribution in mm; CI—corticalization index is given as median due to non-normal distribution.

Platform switching induces less corticalization of peri-implant bone, as do single-crown restorations. Such restorations have low MBLs, but the lowest MBLs are found in cases of bridges. Implant-supported bridges initially have a high CI, but at 10-year follow-up, corticalization is already lower than in splinted crowns and overdentures.

4. Discussion

The healing process and osseointegration in dental implants is a dynamic phenomenon. When an implant is installed, the next surgical procedure causes some marginal bone loss [89]. Within the initial healing phase, the recruitment and migration of osteoprogenitor cells to the surface of the implant occurs. During the secondary healing phase, new bone is apposited. Next, the peri-implant bone is reabsorbed and replaced with a new viable bone, i.e., remodeling is featured [32–35,44,89]. In cases of successful treatment, this reaction reaches a balance with the patient's body, and only in disequilibrium does the MBL increase, thereby damaging peri-implant bone [90]. Pinpointing what underlies this dysfunction is crucial for current dental implantology.

In a long-term study [91], assessment of corticalization in peri-implant bone was performed only visually (Figure 2 in Buser's study) and described in the 10-year data as "well-corticalized". In the current state of development of image analysis methods, a much more precise description can be obtained [82,92]. However, this is a high-quality study, and the authors collected results depicting the corticalization phenomenon. This can be seen in the radiological figures, e.g., Figure 9 in Ref. [91], where MBL is preceded in the bone by a pronounced disappearance of trabeculation and an increase in bone density. However, the authors did not point out the corticalization. Similarly, this is seen in Figure 5 in Albrektsson's publication [93]. Today, the phenomenon of bone density increase can be analyzed qualitatively and, of course, in relation to the MBL [44,45]. Similar interesting illustrative material can be found in another 10-year follow-up study [37] where there are clear features of severe peri-implant bone corticalization in their Figure 1b. Unfortunately, the corticalization term is not used at all by the authors. This is probably due to the purpose of the paper and the lack of publications analyzing bone texture at dental implants in detail. One can also find a publication based on radiographic material, which does not include a single X-ray in the text [94]. In this case, it is impossible to determine what the authors faced in their study. The second issue is the use of simple quantitative measures (they do not describe the internal state of the bone), e.g., the percentage of implant surface remaining in contact with the jawbone (bone-to-implant contact, BIC) or the amount of marginal bone loss from the alveolar crest (MBL). Intuitively, it seems that bone quality (structure testing) is important in the long-term maintenance of dental implants [95].

Corticalization (and associated marginal bone loss) related with the type of implant used is not easy to interpret but is definitely the result of the aforementioned balance and bone remodeling. It probably depends on the type of implant, but implant selection is not random. It depends on the bone conditions and the possibility of using prosthetic solutions in a given implantological system, which correspond to a given dento-gnathic status. Finally, certainly, it depends on the dentist's preferences for using a particular implant system. The results presented here are derived from these many influencing factors, but this is a typical situation in everyday clinical work and hence worth considering and trying to understand.

It is now known from everyday clinical work that implant treatment is very long term or even over a lifetime [96]. It seems that the changes in peri-implant bone structure observed at this time are not a simple projection of the occlusal load in the bone [40], but a complex modulation of osteoimmunological activity [97–99]. Recently, it has been noticed that mechanotransduction may promote the alteration of bone marrow monocyte activation. Thus, occlusal force may modulate the osteoimmunity in peri-implant bone [100]. In addition, there is a synergy between mechanical loading and the signaling pathway for macrophage function, which is related to the αM integrin controlling the activity of the mechanosensitive ion channel Piezo1 [101] and the genetically determined bone reaction [102]. Further confirmation of an osteoimmodulatory mechanism, rather than a simple loading reaction, in peri-implant bone remodeling is the positive role of topically applied bisphosphonates in reducing MBL [103–105]. In the near future, a biological analysis approach combining genomic with clinical data including bone structure will be able to explain the mechanism of corticalization [102].

The arrangement of implant types from causing the least peri-implant bone corticalization at 5 and 10 years to the implant causing the most corticalization does not reflect the same arrangement of implant types relative to marginal bone loss (Figure 5). Thus, the relationship is not a simple one of the type given implant = defined bone loss, and yet, this would be supported by the corticalization index value. However, when considering all 2700 implants, the association of corticalization with marginal bone loss is statistically highly significant ($p < 0.001$). Therefore, the study material here was divided differently (see Table 4). The names of the implants were discarded, and the design features were taken, and thus, the implants were combined into groups with common design features.

It is interesting to note that one-piece implants are not associated with the smallest MBLs, despite not having a micro-gap or the possibility of bacterial contamination in the gingival sulcus and junctional epithelium [106]. Perhaps this is due to the fact that these implants are narrower than two-part implants and can be used in a narrower alveolar crest. Probably, the smaller volume of the bone base is prone to atrophy due to limited bone vascularization and mechanical reasons even though there is no contamination from the microgap. On the other hand, it is not surprising that implants inserted subcrestally have low MBL and low corticalization values [107]. Considering the 10-year follow-up period, these 2 characteristics indicate a good prognosis for subcrestal implants. Prosthetic work placed on such implants leaves adequate biological space for good marginal periodontal function [108], and there is certainly more bone around them from the start than if one-piece implants are used. This ensures permanent maintenance of the peri-implant bone level [109]. When considering the significance of the micro-thread implant neck, it should be noted that the MBL observed in this study is slightly lower than in studies known from the literature [110,111]. At the same time, these studies here confirmed the effectiveness of micro-thread use in minimizing MBL over a 10-year period of functional loading. However, there was no significant change in the peri-implant jawbone cortication of micro-thread implants. The interaction of thread parameters has a significant influence on the peak compressive and tensile strains at the cancellous as well cortical bone. Body-related parameters are more effective on the peak compressive strain at the cortical interface only [112]. The results of this work here seem to confirm these results from the numerical analysis. CI and MBL proceed independently of the implant body, or in other words, alternative further features determine corticalization and marginal bone loss (general health, osteopenia, sarcopenia, dietary supplements taken, drug or behavioral weight loss, details of prosthetic work, occlusion, parafunctions, history of prosthetic repairs, additional dental treatment, saliva composition and active protein content, overactive tongue, etc.). The high MBL (and disparate CI results) observed with rounded apex hole implants seems to be more related to the fact that they are cylindrical implants without threads and with no modifications in the neck area rather than to the effect of the apex hole on the condition of the neck peri-implant bone.

Single crowns do not cause bone structure changes around the implants on which they are set. At the same time, they characterize low marginal bone loss. In cases loaded with bridges, lower measures of corticalization and lower MBL were noted at 5 years than in overdentures and compared to splinted crowns at 10 years. In the case of works using switching platforms, it was noted that corticalization values are always lower than in works without prosthetic platform switching. No differences were noted in terms of MBL. Among the multitude of implant design features and series of prosthetic solutions considered, it should be noted that the lowest long-term bone loss was observed in cases of implant loading with bridges. In contrast, the highest MBL was recorded in cases of splinted crowns. These changes were accompanied by corresponding CI values (higher in high MBL and lower in low MBL). Surprisingly, platform switching was not noted to affect MBL, but there was a significantly lower CI with such implants. However, MBL in the platform-switched prosthetic was lower than total MBL at the 10-year follow-up.

Marginal bone loss has been postulated to have a multi-factorial etiology [113] and can be considered to occur early or late in the lifetime of an implant. It is certain that within the first year after placement, MBL observed is a consequence of bone remodeling subsequent to surgical and prosthetic work [56] as well early loading challenges undertaken by an implant and its associated prosthesis [113,114]. It has been known for a long time that smoking as well as previous history of periodontitis are associated with peri-implantitis and may represent risk factors for this disease [115]. Given the role of adaptive bone remodeling, corticalization may be influenced by infection as a barrier for oral microflora invasion. Over the longer term, the cumulative effect of chronic etiological factors that are immunological, environmental, patient-related factors such as motivation, smoking, para- or disfunctions, infection and inflammation, as well the influence of the surgeon or prosthodontist can affect the increase of corticalization and bone loss in long-term observation [113,114,116,117]. Due to the poorly studied phenomenon of corticalization in dental implantology, the authors speculate that the phenomenon of increased bone structure density itself may be heterogeneous. They would not be surprised if it turns out that some specific form of corticalization or the degree of its severity may be prognostically favorable, while another form may be unfavorable, as appears to be the case after this study.

Corticalization index increasing with age (although observed in 5-year follow-up), rising TSH levels and decreasing serum calcium levels seem to support the negative significance of the peri-implant bone corticalization phenomenon. These selected markers similarly behave with the progression of the aging process [118,119]. In this regard, the matter of interpreting the observed phenomenon in bone is not clear. Only a narrow fragment of possible systemic effects on bone has been examined. However, it is a contribution to further interesting research.

The conclusions of this work cannot be radical. The suspicion of corticalization as an unfavorable predictor for the development of marginal bone loss is based on several hundred implants observed over a 10-year period. This, unfortunately, confirms previous suspicions [79]. Undoubtedly, to establish more certain relationships [120–122], studies should be conducted on a larger number of implants. This kind of research is prompted by the relationship noted here between low MBL and surprisingly high CI with V shape and reverse butteress threaded implants. Multicenter studies are also needed. Different surgical and prosthetic protocols are worth testing. Both authors of this study believe that other (easier and widely available) techniques for assessing the corticalization phenomenon in peri-implant bone should also be tried.

5. Conclusions

In the scope of the study, it can be concluded that the phenomenon of peri-implant jawbone corticalization clearly seems to be a condition that is unfavorable for the future fate of bone-anchored implants.

Author Contributions: Conceptualization, M.K.; data curation, T.W.; formal analysis, T.W.; funding acquisition, M.K.; investigation, T.W.; methodology, T.W.; resources, T.W.; software, T.W.; supervision, M.K.; validation, T.W.; visualization, M.K. and T.W.; writing—original draft, M.K.; writing—review and editing, T.W. All authors have read and agreed to the published version of the manuscript.

Funding: This research was funded by the Medical University of Lodz (grant numbers 503/5-061-02/503-51-001-18, 503/5-061-02/503-51-001-17, and 503/5-061-02/503-51-002-18).

Institutional Review Board Statement: The study was conducted according to the guidelines of the Declaration of Helsinki and approved by the Institutional Ethics Committee of the Medical University of Lodz, PL (protocol no. RNN 485/11/KB and date of approval: 14 June 2011).

Informed Consent Statement: Informed consent was obtained from all subjects involved in the study.

Data Availability Statement: The data on which this study is based will be made available upon request at https://www.researchgate.net/profile/Marcin-Kozakiewicz (accessed on 22 October 2022).

Conflicts of Interest: The authors declare no conflict of interest.

References

1. Chęcińska, K.; Chęciński, M.; Sikora, M.; Nowak, Z.; Karwan, S.; Chlubek, D. The Effect of Zirconium Dioxide (ZrO$_2$) Nanoparticles Addition on the Mechanical Parameters of Polymethyl Methacrylate (PMMA): A Systematic Review and Meta-Analysis of Experimental Studies. *Polymers* **2022**, *14*, 1047. [CrossRef] [PubMed]
2. Pokrowiecki, R.; Szałaj, U.; Fudala, D.; Zaręba, T.; Wojnarowicz, J.; Łojkowski, W.; Tyski, S.; Dowgierd, K.; Mielczarek, A. Dental Implant Healing Screws as Temporary Oral Drug Delivery Systems for Decrease of Infections in the Area of the Head and Neck. *Int. J. Nanomed.* **2022**, *17*, 1679–1693. [CrossRef]
3. Hadzik, J.; Kubasiewicz-Ross, P.; Simka, W.; Gębarowski, T.; Barg, E.; Cieśla-Niechwiadowicz, A.; Szajna, A.T.; Szajna, E.; Gedrange, T.; Kozakiewicz, M.; et al. Fractal Dimension and Texture Analysis in the Assessment of Experimental Laser-Induced Periodic Surface Structures (LIPSS) Dental Implant Surface—In Vitro Study Preliminary Report. *Materials* **2022**, *15*, 2713. [CrossRef] [PubMed]
4. Wach, T.; Kozakiewicz, M. Comparison of Two Clinical Procedures in Patient Affected with Bone Deficit in Posterior Mandible. *Dent. Med. Probl.* **2016**, *53*, 22–28. [CrossRef]
5. Dowgierd, K.; Borowiec, M.; Kozakiewicz, M. Bone changes on lateral cephalograms and CBCT during treatment of maxillary narrowing using palatal osteodistraction with bone-anchored appliances. *J. Cranio-Maxillofac. Surg.* **2018**, *46*, 2069–2081. [CrossRef] [PubMed]

6. Dowgierd, K.; Lipowicz, A.; Kulesa-Mrowiecka, M.; Wolański, W.; Linek, P.; Myśliwiec, A. Efficacy of immediate physiotherapy after surgical release of zygomatico-coronoid ankylosis in a young child: A case report. *Physiother. Theory Pract.* **2022**, *38*, 3187–3193. [CrossRef] [PubMed]
7. Dowgierd, K.; Pokrowiecki, R.; Borowiec, M.; Sokolowska, Z.; Dowgierd, M.; Wos, J.; Kozakiewicz, M.; Krakowczyk, Ł. Protocol and Evaluation of 3D-Planned Microsurgical and Dental Implant Reconstruction of Maxillary Cleft Critical Size Defects in Adolescents and Young Adults. *J. Clin. Med.* **2021**, *10*, 2267. [CrossRef] [PubMed]
8. Michalak, P.; Wyszyńska-Pawelec, G.; Szuta, M.; Hajto-Bryk, J.; Zapała, J.; Zarzecka, J.K. Fractures of the Craniofacial Skeleton in the Elderly: Retrospective Studies. *Int. J. Environ. Res. Public Health* **2021**, *18*, 11219. [CrossRef]
9. Iezzi, G.; Pecora, G.; Scarano, A.; Perrotti, V.; Piattelli, A. Immediately loaded screw implant retrieved after a 12-year loading period: A histologic and histomorphometric case report. *J. Osseointegration* **2009**, *1*, 54–59. [CrossRef]
10. Tumedei, M.; Piattelli, A.; Degidi, M.; Mangano, C.; Iezzi, G. A Narrative Review of the Histological and Histomorphometrical Evaluation of the Peri-Implant Bone in Loaded and Unloaded Dental Implants. A 30-Year Experience (1988–2018). *Int. J. Environ. Res. Public Health* **2020**, *17*, 2088. [CrossRef]
11. Yonezawa, D.; Piattelli, A.; Favero, R.; Ferri, M.; Iezzi, G.; Botticelli, D. Bone Healing at Functionally Loaded and Unloaded Screw-Shaped Implants Supporting Single Crowns: A Histomorphometric Study in Humans. *Int. J. Oral Maxillofac. Implant.* **2018**, *33*, 181–187. [CrossRef] [PubMed]
12. Mangano, F.G.; Pires, J.T.; Shibli, J.A.; Mijiritsky, E.; Iezzi, G.; Piattelli, A.; Mangano, C. Early Bone Response to Dual Acid-Etched and Machined Dental Implants Placed in the Posterior Maxilla: A Histologic and Histomorphometric Human Study. *Implant Dent.* **2017**, *26*, 24–29. [CrossRef]
13. Mangano, C.; Piattelli, A.; Mortellaro, C.; Mangano, F.; Perrotti, V.; Iezzi, G. Evaluation of Peri-Implant Bone Response in Implants Retrieved for Fracture After More Than 20 Years of Loading: A Case Series. *J. Oral Implantol.* **2015**, *41*, 414–418. [CrossRef] [PubMed]
14. Traini, T.; Mangano, C.; Perrotti, V.; Caputi, S.; Coelho, P.; Piattelli, A.; Iezzi, G. Human bone reactions around implants with adverse interfacial bone strain over 20 years. *J. Biomed. Mater. Res. Part B Appl. Biomater.* **2014**, *102*, 1342–1352. [CrossRef]
15. Piattelli, A.; Artese, L.; Penitente, E.; Iaculli, F.; Degidi, M.; Mangano, C.; Shibli, J.A.; Coelho, P.G.; Perrotti, V.; Iezzi, G. Osteocyte density in the peri-implant bone of implants retrieved after different time periods (4 weeks to 27 years). *J. Biomed. Mater. Res. Part B Appl. Biomater.* **2014**, *102*, 239–243. [CrossRef] [PubMed]
16. Iezzi, G.; Piattelli, A.; Mangano, C.; Shibli, J.A.; Vantaggiato, G.; Frosecchi, M.; Di Chiara, C.; Perrotti, V. Peri-implant bone tissues around retrieved human implants after time periods longer than 5 years: A retrospective histologic and histomorphometric evaluation of 8 cases. *Odontology* **2014**, *102*, 116–121. [CrossRef] [PubMed]
17. Mangano, C.; Piattelli, A.; Mangano, F.; Rustichelli, F.; Shibli, J.A.; Iezzi, G.; Giuliani, A. Histological and synchrotron radiation-based computed microtomography study of 2 human-retrieved direct laser metal formed titanium implants. *Implant Dent.* **2013**, *22*, 175–181. [CrossRef] [PubMed]
18. Mangano, C.; Perrotti, V.; Raspanti, M.; Mangano, F.; Luongo, R.; Piattelli, A.; Iezzi, G. Human Dental Implants with a Sandblasted, Acid-Etched Surface Retrieved After 5 and 10 Years: A Light and Scanning Electron Microscopy Evaluation of Two Cases. *Int. J. Oral Maxillofac. Implant.* **2013**, *28*, 917–920. [CrossRef]
19. Iezzi, G.; Degidi, M.; Shibli, J.; Vantaggiato, G.; Piattelli, A.; Perrotti, V. Bone Response to Dental Implants After a 3- to 10-Year Loading Period: A Histologic and Histomorphometric Report of Four Cases. *Int. J. Periodontics Restor. Dent.* **2013**, *33*, 755–761. [CrossRef]
20. Iezzi, G.; Degidi, M.; Piattelli, A.; Shibli, J.A.; Perrotti, V. A Histological and Histomorphometrical Evaluation of Retrieved Human Implants with a Wettable, Highly Hydrophilic, Hierarchically Microstructured Surface: A retrospective analysis of 14 implants. *Implant Dent.* **2013**, *22*, 138–142. [CrossRef]
21. Iezzi, G.; Vantaggiato, G.; Shibli, J.A.; Fiera, E.; Falco, A.; Piattelli, A.; Perrotti, V. Machined and sandblasted human dental implants retrieved after 5 years: A histologic and histomorphometric analysis of three cases. *Quintessence Int.* **2012**, *43*, 287–292. [PubMed]
22. Degidi, M.; Perrotti, V.; Piattelli, A.; Iezzi, G. Mineralized bone-implant contact and implant stability quotient in 16 human implants retrieved after early healing periods: A histologic and histomorphometric evaluation. *Int. J. Oral Maxillofac. Implant.* **2010**, *25*, 45–48.
23. Shibli, J.A.; Mangano, C.; D'Avila, S.; Piattelli, A.; Pecora, G.E.; Mangano, F.; Onuma, T.; Cardoso, L.A.; Ferrari, D.S.; Aguiar, K.C.; et al. Influence of direct laser fabrication implant topography on type IV bone: A histomorphometric study in humans. *J. Biomed. Mater. Res. Part A* **2010**, *93*, 607–614. [CrossRef]
24. Shibli, J.A.; Grassi, S.; Piattelli, A.; Pecora, G.E.; Ferrari, D.S.; Onuma, T.; D'Avila, S.; Coelho, P.G.; Barros, R.; Iezzi, G. Histomorphometric Evaluation of Bioceramic Molecular Impregnated and Dual Acid-Etched Implant Surfaces in the Human Posterior Maxilla. *Clin. Implant Dent. Relat. Res.* **2010**, *12*, 281–288. [CrossRef] [PubMed]
25. Vantaggiato, G.; Iezzi, G.; Fiera, E.; Perrotti, V.; Piattelli, A. Histologic and Histomorphometric Report of Three Immediately Loaded Screw Implants Retrieved from Man After a Three-Year Loading Period. *Implant Dent.* **2008**, *17*, 192–199. [CrossRef] [PubMed]
26. Di Stefano, D.; Iezzi, G.; Scarano, A.; Perrotti, V.; Piattelli, A. Immediately Loaded Blade Implant Retrieved from a Man After a 20-year Loading Period: A Histologic and Histomorphometric Case Report. *J. Oral Implantol.* **2006**, *32*, 171–176. [CrossRef]

27. Romanos, G.E.; Testori, T.; Degidi, M.; Piattelli, A. Histologic and Histomorphometric Findings from Retrieved, Immediately Occlusally Loaded Implants in Humans. *J. Periodontol.* **2005**, *76*, 1823–1832. [CrossRef]
28. Degidi, M.; Scarano, A.; Iezzi, G.; Piattelli, A. Histologic and Histomorphometric Analysis of an Immediately Loaded Implant Retrieved from Man after 14 Months of Loading. *J. Long-Term Eff. Med. Implant.* **2005**, *15*, 489–498. [CrossRef]
29. Degidi, M.; Petrone, G.; Iezzi, G.; Piattelli, A. Histologic evaluation of a human immediately loaded titanium implant with a porous anodized surface. *Clin. Implant Dent. Relat. Res.* **2002**, *4*, 110–114. [CrossRef]
30. Piattelli, A.; Scarano, A.; Piattelli, M.; Bertolai, R.; Panzoni, E. Histologic Aspects of the Bone and Soft Tissues Surrounding Three Titanium Non-Submerged Plasma-Sprayed Implants Retrieved at Autopsy: A Case Report. *J. Periodontol.* **1997**, *68*, 694–700. [CrossRef]
31. Trisi, P.; Quaranta, M.; Emanuelli, M.; Piattelli, A. A Light Microscopy, Scanning Electron Microscopy, and Laser Scanning Microscopy Analysis of Retrieved Blade Implants After 7 to 20 Years of Clinical Function. A Report of 3 Cases. *J. Periodontol.* **1993**, *64*, 374–378. [CrossRef] [PubMed]
32. Shibli, J.A.; Mangano, C.; Mangano, F.; Rodrigues, J.A.; Cassoni, A.; Bechara, K.; Ferreia, J.D.B.; Dottore, A.M.; Iezzi, G.; Piattelli, A. Bone-to-Implant Contact Around Immediately Loaded Direct Laser Metal-Forming Transitional Implants in Human Posterior Maxilla. *J. Periodontol.* **2013**, *84*, 732–737. [CrossRef] [PubMed]
33. Degidi, M.; Piattelli, A.; Shibli, J.A.; Perrotti, V.; Iezzi, G. Early bone formation around immediately restored implants with and without occlusal contact: A human histologic and histomorphometric evaluation. Case report. *Int. J. Oral Maxillofac. Implant.* **2009**, *24*, 734–739.
34. Degidi, M.; Piattelli, A.; Shibli, J.A.; Perrotti, V.; Iezzi, G. Bone formation around immediately loaded and submerged dental implants with a modified sandblasted and acid-etched surface after 4 and 8 weeks: A human histologic and histomorphometric analysis. *Int. J. Oral Maxillofac. Implant.* **2009**, *24*, 896–901.
35. Degidi, M.; Scarano, A.; Petrone, G.; Piattelli, A. Histologic Analysis of Clinically Retrieved Immediately Loaded Titanium Implants: A Report of 11 Cases. *Clin. Implant Dent. Relat. Res.* **2003**, *5*, 89–94. [CrossRef]
36. Piattelli, A.; Trisi, P.; Romasco, N.; Emanuelli, M. Histologic analysis of a screw implant retrieved from man: Influence of early loading and primary stability. *J. Oral Implantol.* **1993**, *19*, 303–306.
37. Rasperini, G.; Siciliano, V.I.; Cafiero, C.; Salvi, G.E.; Blasi, A.; Aglietta, M. Crestal Bone Changes at Teeth and Implants in Periodontally Healthy and Periodontally Compromised Patients. A 10-Year Comparative Case-Series Study. *J. Periodontol.* **2014**, *85*, e152–e159. [CrossRef]
38. Degidi, M.; Scarano, A.; Iezzi, G.; Piattelli, A. Histologic Analysis of an Immediately Loaded Implant Retrieved after 2 Months. *J. Oral Implantol.* **2005**, *31*, 247–254. [CrossRef]
39. Traini, T.; Pecora, G.; Iezzi, G.; Piattelli, A. Preferred Collagen Fiber Orientation in Human Peri-implant Bone After a Short- and Long-term Loading Period: A Case Report. *J. Oral Implantol.* **2006**, *32*, 177–181. [CrossRef]
40. Traini, T.; Degidi, M.; Caputi, S.; Strocchi, R.; Di Iorio, D.; Piattelli, A. Collagen Fiber Orientation in Human Peri-Implant Bone Around Immediately Loaded and Unloaded Titanium Dental Implants. *J. Periodontol.* **2005**, *76*, 83–89. [CrossRef]
41. Traini, T.; Degidi, M.; Iezzi, G.; Artese, L.; Piattelli, A. Comparative evaluation of the peri-implant bone tissue mineral density around unloaded titanium dental implants. *J. Dent.* **2007**, *35*, 84–92. [CrossRef] [PubMed]
42. Gandolfi, M.G.; Zamparini, F.; Iezzi, G.; Degidi, M.; Botticelli, D.; Piattelli, A.; Prati, C. Microchemical and Micromorphologic ESEM-EDX Analysis of Bone Mineralization at the Thread Interface in Human Dental Implants Retrieved for Mechanical Complications after 2 Months to 17 Years. *Int. J. Periodontics Restor. Dent.* **2018**, *38*, 431–441. [CrossRef] [PubMed]
43. Tam, C.; Harrison, J.; Reed, R.; Cruickshank, B. Bone apposition rate as an index of bone metabolism. *Metabolism* **1978**, *27*, 143–150. [CrossRef]
44. Pazzaglia, U.E.; Congiu, T.; Marchese, M.; Spagnuolo, F.; Quacci, D. Morphometry and Patterns of Lamellar Bone in Human Haversian Systems. *Anat. Rec. Adv. Integr. Anat. Evol. Biol.* **2012**, *295*, 1421–1429. [CrossRef]
45. Kungsadalpipob, K.; Supanimitkul, K.; Manopattanasoontorn, S.; Sophon, N.; Tangsathian, T.; Arunyanak, S.P. The lack of keratinized mucosa is associated with poor peri-implant tissue health: A cross-sectional study. *Int. J. Implant Dent.* **2020**, *6*, 28. [CrossRef]
46. Albrektsson, T.; Brånemark, P.-I.; Hansson, H.-A.; Lindström, J. Osseointegrated Titanium Implants: Requirements for Ensuring a Long-Lasting, Direct Bone-to-Implant Anchorage in Man. *Acta Orthop. Scand.* **1981**, *52*, 155–170. [CrossRef] [PubMed]
47. Brånemark, P.; Adell, R.; Albrektsson, T.; Lekholm, U.; Lundkvist, S.; Rockler, B. Osseointegrated titanium fixtures in the treatment of edentulousness. *Biomaterials* **1983**, *4*, 25–28. [CrossRef]
48. Linkevicius, T.; Puisys, A.; Linkeviciene, L.; Peciuliene, V.; Schlee, M. Crestal Bone Stability around Implants with Horizontally Matching Connection after Soft Tissue Thickening: A Prospective Clinical Trial. *Clin. Implant Dent. Relat. Res.* **2015**, *17*, 497–508. [CrossRef]
49. Vlachodimou, E.; Fragkioudakis, I.; Vouros, I. Is There an Association between the Gingival Phenotype and the Width of Keratinized Gingiva? A Systematic Review. *Dent. J.* **2021**, *9*, 34. [CrossRef]
50. Baer, R.A.; Nölken, R.; Colic, S.; Heydecke, G.; Mirzakhanian, C.; Behneke, A.; Behneke, N.; Gottesman, E.; Ottria, L.; Pozzi, A.; et al. Immediately provisionalized tapered conical connection implants for single-tooth restorations in the maxillary esthetic zone: A 5-year prospective single-cohort multicenter analysis. *Clin. Oral Investig.* **2022**, *26*, 3593–3604. [CrossRef]

51. Kinaia, B.M.; Shah, M.; Neely, A.L.; Goodis, H.E. Crestal Bone Level Changes Around Immediately Placed Implants: A Systematic Review and Meta-Analyses With at Least 12 Months' Follow-Up After Functional Loading. *J. Periodontol.* **2014**, *85*, 1537–1548. [CrossRef] [PubMed]
52. Linkevicius, T.; Linkevicius, R.; Gineviciute, E.; Alkimavicius, J.; Mazeikiene, A.; Linkeviciene, L. The influence of new immediate tissue level abutment on crestal bone stability of subcrestally placed implants: A 1-year randomized controlled clinical trial. *Clin. Implant Dent. Relat. Res.* **2021**, *23*, 259–269. [CrossRef] [PubMed]
53. Linkevicius, T.; Puisys, A.; Linkevicius, R.; Alkimavicius, J.; Gineviciute, E.; Linkeviciene, L. The influence of submerged healing abutment or subcrestal implant placement on soft tissue thickness and crestal bone stability. A 2-year randomized clinical trial. *Clin. Implant Dent. Relat. Res.* **2020**, *22*, 497–506. [CrossRef] [PubMed]
54. Kołaciński, M.; Kozakiewicz, M.; Materka, A. Textural entropy as a potential feature for quantitative assessment of jaw bone healing process. *Arch. Med. Sci.* **2015**, *11*, 78–84. [CrossRef] [PubMed]
55. Dewan, H.; Robaian, A.; Divakar, D.D.; Hegde, S.M.R.; Shankar, S.M.; Poojari, B. Levels of peri-implant sulcular fluid levels of soluble urokinase plasminogen activator receptor and TNF-α among cigarette smokers and non-smokers with peri-implantitis. *Technol. Health Care* **2022**. *epub ahead of print*. [CrossRef]
56. Naveau, A.; Shinmyouzu, K.; Moore, C.; Avivi-Arber, L.; Jokerst, J.; Koka, S. Etiology and Measurement of Peri-Implant Crestal Bone Loss (CBL). *J. Clin. Med.* **2019**, *8*, 166. [CrossRef]
57. Bohner, L.; Tortamano, P.; Meier, N.; Gremse, F.; Kleinheinz, J.; Hanisch, M. Trabecular Bone Assessment Using Magnetic-Resonance Imaging: A Pilot Study. *Int. J. Environ. Res. Public Health* **2020**, *17*, 9282. [CrossRef]
58. Guenoun, D.; Fouré, A.; Pithioux, M.; Guis, S.; Le Corroller, T.; Mattei, J.-P.; Pauly, V.; Guye, M.; Bernard, M.; Chabrand, P.; et al. Correlative Analysis of Vertebral Trabecular Bone Microarchitecture and Mechanical Properties: A Combined Ultra-High Field (7 Tesla) MRI and Biomechanical Investigation. *Spine* **2017**, *42*, E1165–E1172. [CrossRef]
59. Hadrowicz, J.; Hadrowicz, P.; Gesing, A.; Kozakiewicz, M. Age dependent alteration in bone surrounding dental implant. *Dent. Med. Probl.* **2014**, *51*, 27–34.
60. Hadrowicz, P.; Hadrowicz, J.; Kozakiewicz, M.; Gesing, A. Assessment of Parathyroid Hormone Serum Level as a Predictor for Bone Condition Around Dental Implants. *Int. J. Oral Maxillofac. Implant.* **2017**, *32*, e207–e212. [CrossRef]
61. Kozakiewicz, M.; Szyszkowski, A. Evaluation of selected prognostic factors in dental implant treatment–two-year follow-up. *Dent. Med. Probl.* **2014**, *51*, 439–447.
62. Różyło-Kalinowska, I. Digital radiography density measurements in differentiation between periapical granulomas and radicular cysts. *Med. Sci. Monit.* **2007**, *13* (Suppl. 1), 129–136. [PubMed]
63. Szyszkowski, A.; Kozakiewicz, M. Effect of Implant-Abutment Connection Type on Bone Around Dental Implants in Long-Term Observation: Internal cone versus internal hex. *Implant Dent.* **2019**, *28*, 430–436. [CrossRef] [PubMed]
64. Wach, T.; Kozakiewicz, M. Are recent available blended collagen-calcium phosphate better than collagen alone or crystalline calcium phosphate? Radiotextural analysis of a 1-year clinical trial. *Clin. Oral Investig.* **2021**, *25*, 3711–3718. [CrossRef] [PubMed]
65. Grocholewicz, K.; Janiszewska-Olszowska, J.; Aniko-Włodarczyk, M.; Preuss, O.; Trybek, G.; Sobolewska, E.; Lipski, M. Panoramic radiographs and quantitative ultrasound of the radius and phalanx III to assess bone mineral status in postmenopausal women. *BMC Oral Health* **2018**, *18*, 127. [CrossRef] [PubMed]
66. Bayrakdar, I.S.; Orhan, K.; Çelik, Ö.; Bilgir, E.; Sağlam, H.; Kaplan, F.A.; Görür, S.A.; Odabaş, A.; Aslan, A.F.; Różyło-Kalinowska, I. A U-Net Approach to Apical Lesion Segmentation on Panoramic Radiographs. *BioMed Res. Int.* **2022**, *2022*, 7035367. [CrossRef] [PubMed]
67. Bilgir, E.; Bayrakdar, I.; Çelik, Ö.; Orhan, K.; Akkoca, F.; Sağlam, H.; Odabaş, A.; Aslan, A.F.; Ozcetin, C.; Kıllı, M.; et al. An artificial intelligence approach to automatic tooth detection and numbering in panoramic radiographs. *BMC Med. Imaging* **2021**, *21*, 124. [CrossRef] [PubMed]
68. Srebrzyńska-Witek, A.; Koszowski, R.; Różyło-Kalinowska, I. Relationship between anterior mandibular bone thickness and the angulation of incisors and canines—A CBCT study. *Clin. Oral Investig.* **2018**, *22*, 1567–1578. [CrossRef]
69. Moshfeghi, M.; Safi, Y.; Różyło-Kalinowska, I.; Gandomi, S. Does the size of an object containing dental implant affect the expression of artifacts in cone beam computed tomography imaging? *Head Face Med.* **2022**, *18*, 20. [CrossRef]
70. Bohner, L.; Hanisch, M.; Sesma, N.; Blanck-Lubarsch, M.; Kleinheinz, J. Artifacts in magnetic resonance imaging caused by dental materials: A systematic review. *Dentomaxillofacial Radiol.* **2022**, *51*, 20210450. [CrossRef]
71. Chang, G.; Honig, S.; Liu, Y.; Chen, C.; Chu, K.K.; Rajapakse, C.S.; Egol, K.; Xia, D.; Saha, P.K.; Regatte, R.R. 7 Tesla MRI of bone microarchitecture discriminates between women without and with fragility fractures who do not differ by bone mineral density. *J. Bone Miner. Metab.* **2015**, *33*, 285–293. [CrossRef]
72. Guenoun, D.; Pithioux, M.; Souplet, J.-C.; Guis, S.; Le Corroller, T.; Fouré, A.; Pauly, V.; Mattei, J.-P.; Bernard, M.; Guye, M.; et al. Assessment of proximal femur microarchitecture using ultra-high field MRI at 7 Tesla. *Diagn. Interv. Imaging* **2020**, *101*, 45–53. [CrossRef]
73. Krug, R.; Carballido-Gamio, J.; Banerjee, S.; Burghardt, A.J.; Link, T.M.; Majumdar, S. In vivo ultra-high-field magnetic resonance imaging of trabecular bone microarchitecture at 7 T. *J. Magn. Reson. Imaging* **2008**, *27*, 854–859. [CrossRef] [PubMed]
74. Rajapakse, C.S.; Magland, J.; Zhang, X.H.; Liu, X.S.; Wehrli, S.L.; Guo, X.E.; Wehrli, F.W. Implications of noise and resolution on mechanical properties of trabecular bone estimated by image-based finite-element analysis. *J. Orthop. Res.* **2009**, *27*, 1263–1271. [CrossRef] [PubMed]

75. Rajapakse, C.S.; Kobe, E.; Batzdorf, A.S.; Hast, M.W.; Wehrli, F.W. Accuracy of MRI-based finite element assessment of distal tibia compared to mechanical testing. *Bone* **2018**, *108*, 71–78. [CrossRef]
76. Seifert, A.C.; Wehrli, F.W. Solid-State Quantitative ^{1}H and ^{31}P MRI of Cortical Bone in Humans. *Curr. Osteoporos. Rep.* **2016**, *14*, 77–86. [CrossRef]
77. Dudek, D.; Kozakiewicz, M. Szerokość beleczek kostnych w szczęce i żuchwie człowieka na podstawie cyfrowych radiologicznych zdjęć wewnąrzustnych [Bone trabecula width in the human maxilla and mandible based on digital intraoral radiographs]. *Mag. Stomatol.* **2012**, *236*, 77–80.
78. Rózyło-Kalinowska, I.; Michalska, A.; Burdan, F. Optimization of analysis of skeletal ossification of laboratory animals by means of digital radiography software options. *Ann. Univ. Mariae Curie-Sklodowska* **2003**, *58*, 95–100.
79. Kozakiewicz, M.; Skorupska, M.; Wach, T. What Does Bone Corticalization around Dental Implants Mean in Light of Ten Years of Follow-Up? *J. Clin. Med.* **2022**, *11*, 3545. [CrossRef]
80. Kozakiewicz, M. Measures of Corticalization. *J. Clin. Med.* **2022**, *11*, 5463. [CrossRef]
81. Kozakiewicz, M.; Wilamski, M. Technika standaryzacji wewnątrzustnych zdjęć rentgenowskich [Standardization technique for intraoral radiographs]. *Czas. Stomatol.* **1999**, *52*, 673–677.
82. Szczypiński, P.M.; Strzelecki, M.; Materka, A.; Klepaczko, A. MaZda–The Software Package for Textural Analysis of Biomedical Images. In *Computers in Medical Activity*; Advances in Intelligent and Soft Computing; Springer: Berlin/Heidelberg, Germany, 2009; Volume 65, pp. 73–84.
83. Kozakiewicz, M.; Bogusiak, K.; Hanclik, M.; Denkowski, M.; Arkuszewski, P. Noise in subtraction images made from pairs of intraoral radiographs: A comparison between four methods of geometric alignment. *Dentomaxillofacial Radiol.* **2008**, *37*, 40–46. [CrossRef] [PubMed]
84. Kozakiewicz, M.; Szymor, P.; Wach, T. Influence of General Mineral Condition on Collagen-Guided Alveolar Crest Augmentation. *Materials* **2020**, *13*, 3649. [CrossRef] [PubMed]
85. Kozakiewicz, M.; Wach, T. New Oral Surgery Materials for Bone Reconstruction—A Comparison of Five Bone Substitute Materials for Dentoalveolar Augmentation. *Materials* **2020**, *13*, 2935. [CrossRef]
86. Wach, T.; Kozakiewicz, M. Fast-Versus Slow-Resorbable Calcium Phosphate Bone Substitute Materials—Texture Analysis after 12 Months of Observation. *Materials* **2020**, *13*, 3854. [CrossRef]
87. Haralick, R.M. Statistical and structural approaches to texture. *Proc. IEEE* **1979**, *67*, 786–804. [CrossRef]
88. Materka, A.; Strzelecki, M. *Texture Analysis Methods–A Review, COST B11 Report*. Presented at MC Meeting and Workshop, Brussels, Belgium, 25 June 1998; Technical University of Lodz: Lodz, Poland, 1998.
89. Eriksson, R.A.; Albrektsson, T.; Magnusson, B. Assessment of Bone Viability After Heat Trauma: A Histological, Histochemical and Vital Microscopic Study in the Rabbit. *Scand. J. Plast. Reconstr. Surg.* **1984**, *18*, 261–268. [CrossRef] [PubMed]
90. Albrektsson, T.; Dahlin, C.; Jemt, T.; Sennerby, L.; Turri, A.; Wennerberg, A. Is Marginal Bone Loss around Oral Implants the Result of a Provoked Foreign Body Reaction? *Clin. Implant. Dent. Relat. Res.* **2014**, *16*, 155–165. [CrossRef]
91. Buser, D.; Janner, S.F.M.; Wittneben, J.-G.; Brägger, U.; Ramseier, C.A.; Salvi, G.E. 10-Year Survival and Success Rates of 511 Titanium Implants with a Sandblasted and Acid-Etched Surface: A Retrospective Study in 303 Partially Edentulous Patients. *Clin. Implant. Dent. Relat. Res.* **2012**, *14*, 839–851. [CrossRef]
92. Szczypinski, P.M.; Klepaczko, A.; Kociolek, M. QMaZda—Software tools for image analysis and pattern recognition. In Proceedings of the 2017 Signal Processing: Algorithms, Architectures, Arrangements, and Applications (SPA), Poznan, Poland, 20–22 September 2017; pp. 217–221. [CrossRef]
93. Albrektsson, T.; Tengvall, P.; Amengual-Peñafiel, L.; Coli, P.; Kotsakis, G.; Cochran, D.L. Implications of considering peri-implant bone loss a disease, a narrative review. *Clin. Implant Dent. Relat. Res.* **2022**, *24*, 532–543. [CrossRef]
94. Roccuzzo, M.; De Angelis, N.; Bonino, L.; Aglietta, M. Ten-year results of a three-arm prospective cohort study on implants in periodontally compromised patients. Part 1: Implant loss and radiographic bone loss. *Clin. Oral Implant. Res.* **2010**, *21*, 490–496. [CrossRef]
95. Pandey, C.; Rokaya, D.; Bhattarai, B.P. Contemporary Concepts in Osseointegration of Dental Implants: A Review. *BioMed Res. Int.* **2022**, *2022*, 6170452. [CrossRef] [PubMed]
96. Papaspyridakos, P.; Chen, C.-J.; Singh, M.; Weber, H.-P.; Gallucci, G.O. Success criteria in implant dentistry: A systematic review. *J. Dent. Res.* **2012**, *91*, 242–248. [CrossRef] [PubMed]
97. Amengual-Peñafiel, L.; Córdova, L.A.; Jara-Sepúlveda, M.C.; Brañes-Aroca, M.; Marchesani-Carrasco, F.; Cartes-Velásquez, R. Osteoimmunology drives dental implant osseointegration: A new paradigm for implant dentistry. *Jpn. Dent. Sci. Rev.* **2021**, *57*, 12–19. [CrossRef] [PubMed]
98. Chen, Z.; Wu, C.; Xiao, Y. Convergence of Osteoimmunology and Immunomodulation for the Development and Assessment of Bone Biomaterials. In *The Immune Response to Implanted Materials and Devices*; Corradetti, B., Ed.; Springer: Cham, Switzerland, 2017. [CrossRef]
99. Negrescu, A.-M.; Cimpean, A. The State of the Art and Prospects for Osteoimmunomodulatory Biomaterials. *Materials* **2021**, *14*, 1357. [CrossRef] [PubMed]
100. Lin, W.; Li, Q.; Zhang, D.; Zhang, X.; Qi, X.; Wang, Q.; Chen, Y.; Liu, C.; Li, H.; Zhang, S.; et al. Mapping the immune microenvironment for mandibular alveolar bone homeostasis at single-cell resolution. *Bone Res.* **2021**, *9*, 17. [CrossRef]

101. Atcha, H.; Meli, V.S.; Davis, C.T.; Brumm, K.T.; Anis, S.; Chin, J.; Jiang, K.; Pathak, M.M.; Liu, W.F. Crosstalk Between CD11b and Piezo1 Mediates Macrophage Responses to Mechanical Cues. *Front. Immunol.* **2021**, *12*, 689397. [CrossRef]
102. Refai, A.K.; Cochran, D.L. Harnessing Omics Sciences and Biotechnologies in Understanding Osseointegration—Personalized Dental Implant Therapy. *Int. J. Oral Maxillofac. Implant.* **2020**, *35*, e27–e39. [CrossRef]
103. Tengvall, P.; Skoglund, B.; Askendal, A.; Aspenberg, P. Surface immobilized bisphosphonate improves stainless-steel screw fixation in rats. *Biomaterials* **2004**, *25*, 2133–2138. [CrossRef]
104. Abtahi, J.; Henefalk, G.; Aspenberg, P. Impact of a zoledronate coating on early post-surgical implant stability and marginal bone resorption in the maxilla—A Split-Mouth Randomized Clinical Trial. *Clin. Oral Implant. Res.* **2019**, *30*, 49–58. [CrossRef]
105. Abtahi, J.; Henefalk, G.; Aspenberg, P. Randomised trial of bisphosphonate-coated dental implants: Radiographic follow-up after five years of loading. *Int. J. Oral Maxillofac. Surg.* **2016**, *45*, 1564–1569. [CrossRef]
106. Kim, J.-J.; Lee, J.-H.; Kim, J.C.; Lee, J.-B.; Yeo, I.-S.L. Biological Responses to the Transitional Area of Dental Implants: Material- and Structure-Dependent Responses of Peri-Implant Tissue to Abutments. *Materials* **2020**, *13*, 72. [CrossRef] [PubMed]
107. Palacios-Garzón, N.; Velasco-Ortega, E.; López-López, J. Bone Loss in Implants Placed at Subcrestal and Crestal Level: A Systematic Review and Meta-Analysis. *Materials* **2019**, *12*, 154. [CrossRef] [PubMed]
108. Piattelli, A.; Vrespa, G.; Petrone, G.; Iezzi, G.; Annibali, S.; Scarano, A. Role of the Microgap Between Implant and Abutment: A Retrospective Histologic Evaluation in Monkeys. *J. Periodontol.* **2003**, *74*, 346–352. [CrossRef] [PubMed]
109. Linkevicius, T.; Apse, P.; Grybauskas, S.; Puisys, A. The influence of soft tissue thickness on crestal bone changes around implants: A 1-year prospective controlled clinical trial. *Int. J. Oral Maxillofac. Implant.* **2009**, *24*, 712–719.
110. Aslroosta, H.; Akbari, S.; Naddafpour, N.; Adnaninia, S.T.; Khorsand, A.; Esfahani, N.N. Effect of microthread design on the preservation of marginal bone around immediately placed implants: A 5-years prospective cohort study. *BMC Oral Health* **2021**, *21*, 541. [CrossRef] [PubMed]
111. Covani, U.; Chiappe, G.; Bosco, M.; Orlando, B.; Quaranta, A.; Barone, A. A 10-Year Evaluation of Implants Placed in Fresh Extraction Sockets: A Prospective Cohort Study. *J. Periodontol.* **2012**, *83*, 1226–1234. [CrossRef] [PubMed]
112. Sheikhan, E.; Kadkhodazadeh, M.; Amid, R.; Lafzi, A. Interactive Effects of Five Dental Implant Design Parameters on the Peak Strains at the Interfacial Bone: A Finite Element Study. *Int. J. Oral Maxillofac. Implant.* **2022**, *37*, 302–310. [CrossRef]
113. Bryant, S.R. Oral Implant Outcomes Predicted by Age- and Site-Specific Aspects of Bone Condition. Ph.D. Thesis, University of Toronto, Toronto, ON, Canada, 2001.
114. Linkevicius, T.; Puisys, A.; Vindasiute, E.; Linkeviciene, L.; Apse, P. Does residual cement around implant-supported restorations cause peri-implant disease? A retrospective case analysis. *Clin. Oral Implant. Res.* **2013**, *24*, 1179–1184. [CrossRef]
115. Carcuac, O.; Jansson, L. Peri-implantitis in a specialist clinic of periodontology. Clinical features and risk indicators. *Swed. Dent. J.* **2010**, *34*, 53–61.
116. Roos-Jansåker, A.-M. Long time follow up of implant therapy and treatment of peri-implantitis. *Swed. Dent. J. Suppl.* **2007**, *188*, 7–66.
117. Fransson, C.; Lekholm, U.; Jemt, T.; Berglundh, T. Prevalence of subjects with progressive bone loss at implants. *Clin. Oral Implant. Res.* **2005**, *16*, 440–446. [CrossRef] [PubMed]
118. Gesing, A. The thyroid gland and the process of aging. *Thyroid Res.* **2015**, *8*, A8. [CrossRef]
119. Biondi, B.; Cooper, D.S. The Clinical Significance of Subclinical Thyroid Dysfunction. *Endocr. Rev.* **2008**, *29*, 76–131. [CrossRef] [PubMed]
120. Borowska, M.; Bębas, E.; Szarmach, J.; Oczeretko, E. Multifractal characterization of healing process after bone loss. *Biomed. Signal Process. Control* **2019**, *52*, 179–186. [CrossRef]
121. Borowska, M.; Szarmach, J.; Oczeretko, E. Fractal texture analysis of the healing process after bone loss. *Comput. Med. Imaging Graph.* **2015**, *46*, 191–196. [CrossRef]
122. Pociask, E.; Nurzynska, K.; Obuchowicz, R.; Bałon, P.; Uryga, D.; Strzelecki, M.; Izworski, A.; Piórkowski, A. Differential Diagnosis of Cysts and Granulomas Supported by Texture Analysis of Intraoral Radiographs. *Sensors* **2021**, *21*, 7481. [CrossRef]

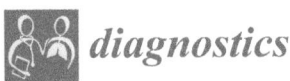

Article

Diagnostics Using the Change-of-Direction and Acceleration Test (CODAT) of the Biomechanical Patterns Associated with Knee Injury in Female Futsal Players: A Cross-Sectional Analytical Study

Loreto Ferrández-Laliena [1], Lucía Vicente-Pina [1], Rocío Sánchez-Rodríguez [1], Eva Orantes-González [2], José Heredia-Jimenez [3], María Orosia Lucha-López [1,*], César Hidalgo-García [1,*] and José Miguel Tricás-Moreno [1]

[1] Unidad de Investigación en Fisioterapia, Spin off Centro Clínico OMT-E Fisioterapia SLP, Universidad de Zaragoza, Domingo Miral s/n, 50009 Zaragoza, Spain
[2] Department of Sports and Computer Science, Faculty of Physical Education and Sports, University of Pablo de Olavide, 41013 Sevilla, Spain
[3] Department of Physical Education and Sports, Faculty of Education, Economy & Technology, University of Granada, 51001 Ceuta, Spain
* Correspondence: orolucha@unizar.es (M.O.L.-L.); hidalgo@unizar.es (C.H.-G.); Tel.: +34-626-480-131 (M.O.L.-L.)

Abstract: The primary aim of this study was to identify kinematic differences at initial contact between female futsal players with and without previous knee injury, using a functional motor pattern test. The secondary aim was to determine kinematic differences between the dominant and non-dominant limb in the whole group, using the same test. A cross-sectional study was performed in 16 female futsal players allocated into two groups: eight females with a previous knee injury, i.e., affected by the valgus collapse mechanism without surgical intervention, and eight with no previous injury. The evaluation protocol included the change-of-direction and acceleration test (CODAT). One registration was made for each lower limb, i.e., the dominant (the preferred kicking limb) and non-dominant limb. A 3D motion capture system (Qualisys AB, Göteborg, Sweden) was used to analyze the kinematics. The Cohen's d effect sizes between the groups demonstrated a strong effect size towards more physiological positions in the non-injured group in the following kinematics in the dominant limb: hip adduction (Cohen's d = 0.82), hip internal rotation (Cohen's d = 0.88), and ipsilateral pelvis rotation (Cohen's d = 1.06). The t-test for the dominant and non-dominant limb in the whole group showed the following differences in knee valgus: dominant limb (9.02 ± 7.31 degrees) and non-dominant limb (1.27 ± 9.05 degrees) (p = 0.049). Conclusions: The players with no previous history of knee injury had a more physiological position for avoiding the valgus collapse mechanism in the hip adduction and internal rotation, and in the pelvis rotation in the dominant limb. All the players showed more knee valgus in the dominant limb, which is the limb at greater risk of injury.

Keywords: knee injury; kinematics; soccer; sports; anterior cruciate ligament; prevention; physiotherapy; CODAT

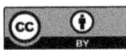

1. Introduction

Knee injury incidence is one of the most frequent in soccer, reaching values of 0.7 injuries per 1000 h of exposure [1]. With respect to knee ligament injuries, the anterior cruciate ligament (ACL) is the most common injury, reaching an incidence of 0.45 per 1000 h of exposure, and is also the most common reason for players requiring medical leave of more than 120 days [1,2]. Previous studies have reported that female soccer players have a risk of sustaining ACL injuries that is two or three times higher than the equivalent risk in males [3–5], and is usually caused by a non-contact mechanism [6,7], while in men the cause is a direct impact of external force [3,8].

Non-contact mechanisms causing ACL injury are due to a failure in biomechanical patterns, which include a lack of control in proprioceptive and neuromuscular activation [9]. Moreover, it is conditioned by non-modifiable risk factors, such as anatomical [10,11] and hormonal factors [12]. Prospective studies have found that most ACL injuries were caused during dynamic high-intensity stabilization situations such as landings and changes of direction or decelerations, activities that are very common in the defensive roles of pressing/tracking actions in sports [13,14]. In addition, the pressing pattern is one of the most frequent, due to the unexpected stimulus of the opponent and the match context situations [13].

A recent study by DiPaolo et al. [15] showed a compilation of the main biomechanical risk factor thresholds from prospective video analysis studies, which explain the "perfect loading storm" that defines ACL injury mechanisms [6,15,16], valgus collapse being the main biomechanical risk factor related to ACL injury. Arundale et al. [17] explained "valgus collapse" as the combination of hip adduction and internal rotation, and knee abduction. Valgus collapse causes a medial pivoting of the femur on the tibia plateau and compression on the lateral side of the knee. Therefore, an increase in medial yawing of the joint puts the ACL fibres at maximal tension [11,18].

In addition, before the ACL injury appears, on average 48 milliseconds after the initial contact, other kinematics faults have been observed [6,19]. During change-of-direction tasks, at the initial contact phase, the female players who sustained ACL injury showed less trunk, hip, and knee flexion [5,6]. Consequently, this could be related to higher vertical ground reaction forces during impact stabilization. An extended position avoids the load damping of limb joints, which causes an increase in anterior tibial shear forces, potentially resulting in higher strain in the ACL [20]. Zebis et al. [5] indicated a risk reduction of 44% per each increase in 10° of hip flexion at this phase [5]. In addition, studies have considered greater hip and knee rotation movement during change-of-direction tasks as risks of ACL injury [5,21]. Research shows that knee internal rotation at initial contact is significantly related with ACL injury risk, with a 13% increased risk per 1° increase in knee internal rotation. Knee internal rotation was related to higher hip internal rotation during a change-of-direction task, which was considered as a risky movement in terms of non-contact mechanisms causing ACL injury [16,21,22]. Internal hip rotation promotes a displacement of the ground reaction force vector, which is focused medial and posterior on the tibial plateau during the impact. Increased ACL load is caused by the resultant relative anterior and lateral shear of the tibia [16,23,24].

Latest research has studied the incidence ratio based on limb dominance, related to the fact that in futsal the ball determinates the biomechanical pattern [25]. Studies explain that the dominant limb (DL) usually has a higher injury incidence ratio than the non-dominant limb (NDL) [2,25]. During kicking, each limb plays a different role: the DL usually impacts the ball, while the NDL performs a stabilization function to provide a foundation for the kicking task [25]. These different activity profiles influence the load on each limb during kicking, a task that takes place many times during each training session or match [13,26]. This imbalance in loading between the two limbs influences the kinematic response of the limbs to the rest of the tasks in the match, especially in tasks such as changes of direction. Changes of directions have been identified as task related to a high risk of ACL injury.

Most previous studies have analysed the implications of the biomechanical risks factors between two groups, injured and non-injured players [5,27], the former category including injured players who have suffered an ACL injury. Thus, in this group, surgery could have modified the biomechanical patterns. Currently no studies have used as a sample injured players who have already suffered a knee injury based on the valgus collapse mechanism, causing damage to the ACL or another joint structure with the same injury mechanism, which has been treated without surgical intervention. We hypothesized that female futsal players with previous knee injury based on the valgus collapse mechanism, without surgical intervention, had kinematic patterns similar to those identified as risk patterns for ACL injury, in a change-of-direction task. Therefore, this study aimed to identify kinematic differences at initial contact between female futsal players with and without previous knee injury, in a motor pattern test including change of direction, stabilization, and acceleration. A secondary aim was to determine the kinematic differences between the DL and NDL for the whole group, in the same tasks.

2. Materials and Methods

2.1. Study Design

This study has a cross-sectional design. The allocation ratio was [1:1] between two groups. Allocation depended on clinical history: previous knee injury (KI) involving the valgus collapse mechanism without surgical intervention (injury group), or no injury (control group). The Research Ethics Committee of Community of Aragón approved this study (code PI20/127), which observed the ethical principles of the Declaration of Helsinki (64th WMA General Assembly, Fortaleza, Brazil, October 2013) [28].

2.2. Sample Size

The sample size was calculated based on the outcomes of previous studies [19,29]. The main variable used for sample size calculation was dynamic knee valgus at the first contact. The sample size was calculated with the GRANMO 7.12 calculator (Institut Municipal d'Investigació Mèdica, Barcelona, Spain) (https://www.imim.es/ofertadeserveis/software-public/granmo/, accessed on 1 November 2021), with an alpha risk of 0.05, a beta risk of 0.20, and the two-side test. We used a common standard deviation of 5.1 degrees [29] and a minimum expected difference of 8.4 degrees [19], estimating a follow-up loss of 20%. A total sample of 16 subjects (8 per group) was obtained.

2.3. Participants

The president of the Real Federación de Fútbol de Ceuta was contacted regarding participation in the study. He contacted all the national female futsal players registered in the federation, of whom 16 volunteered to participate in the study. The average age was 23.4 + 5.03 years and the average height was 1.62 ± 0.06 m. They had an active national futsal licence, and they had attended futsal training for more than 4 h per week for at least 4 months. Players were excluded if they had had an injury incompatible with regular training in the past 4 months. All the players gave written informed consent prior to their participation in the study.

2.4. Procedure

The first part of the evaluation was a survey to collect the individual clinical history of each participant. The data from the clinical history were used to allocate the subjects into the KI or control group. All players who had suffered a knee injury involving the valgus collapse non-contact mechanism, without surgical intervention, were included in the KI group [16,17,30]. The recorded information included age, height, weight, knee injury history, lower limb dominance, injury mechanism, medical diagnosis, pain region, time to recovery, treatment received, possible relapse, and futsal level league at the time the injury occurred. Eight players were allocated to each group.

The data collection was conducted in one session. Before the test procedure, a short mobility and warm-up activity was carried out.

The evaluation protocol included the functional change-of-direction and acceleration test (CODAT) [31,32]. This was conducted for each lower limb dominant (DL) and non-dominant (NDL). Limb dominance criteria was defined as the preferred kicking limb [25]. A 3D motion capture system (Qualisys AB, Göteborg, Sweden) was used to analyze the kinematics of change of direction with a full body model marker set without head and upper extremities. Twenty-six reflective markers were placed with adhesive tape on the players' skin on both sides of the lower limbs and trunk. The palpation of the reflective markers was carried out following anatomical references. A force plate (Optima HPS464508-

2000, AMTI, Watertown, MA, USA) was used to record the maximal torque of the ground reaction force during the initial contact phase.

The 26 markers were placed to make a static picture. The locations were at the first and fifth metatarsal head, second metatarsophalangeal, medial and lateral malleolus, large posterior surface of calcaneus, lateral and medial femoral epicondyle, anterior and posterior superior iliac spine, acromioclavicular joints, inferior scapula angle, and thoracic spinous process of T3 and T12. In addition, a cluster with four markers was placed in the lateral of the shank and thigh of both limbs. Finally, another cluster with three markers was fixed to the lateral part of the pelvic girdle on both sides. After calibration in order for the computer to recognize precisely the situation of the cameras and all the markers to create a static record for the CODAT test performance, the malleolus, epicondyles, posterior superior iliac spine, and acromioclavicular joint markers were removed from the player to avoid interference with the maximal speed task. The set-up of the markers was in line with the recommendations of Codamotion system protocols (Charnwood Dynamics Ltd., Leicestershire, UK).

The reflective marker locations were registered through 12 infrared high-speed cameras at a rate of 250 Hz. The calibration of the space was conducted with a wand (with a length of 751.1 mm) before each data collection and the standard deviations of the wand's length measurements were below 0.5 mm. Visual3D software (C-Motion Inc., Germantown, MD, USA) was used to analyze the change-of-direction task (Figure 1).

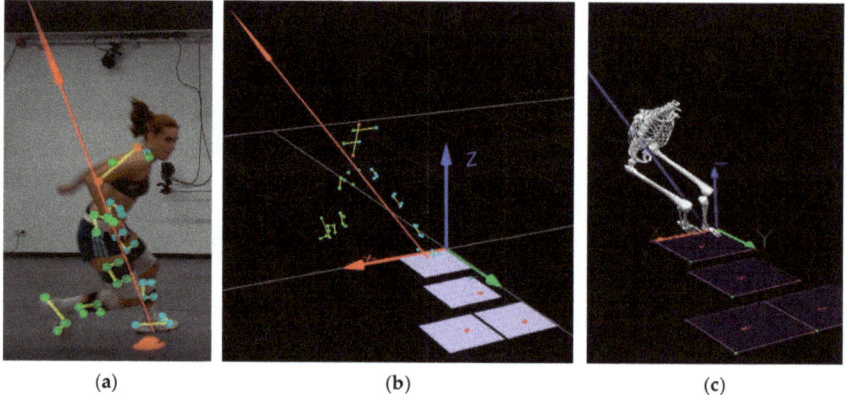

Figure 1. Capture moment of kinematic data during CODAT test: (**a**) Capture moment from a 2D camera that shows the player's task; (**b**) Signal from 12 infrared high-speed cameras being processed with Visual3D software; (**c**) Final avatar processed by Virtual 3D software.

Players carried out the CODAT test (Figure 2). This is a specific test that combines a sprint mechanism with the stabilization and acceleration needed for a change of direction. It involves placing a high load onto the knee in a similar way to tasks performed during training or a match [31–33]. Moreover, most injuries involving non-contact mechanisms occur in defensive roles, so we performed the CODAT test without a ball to recreate the defensive role during the match [13]. The CODAT test integrates a four-diagonal change-of-direction task, two of 45° and the other two of 90°, mixed with 3-m sprints and followed by a 10-m sprint. All the tests were performed at maximal speed. Prior research has observed that the average time of each sprint in soccer is 2 s and that the average distance is 10 m, which agrees with the maximal distance in the CODAT test [31]. Moreover, a 3-m sprint allows for a complete gait cycle before the change-of-direction task.

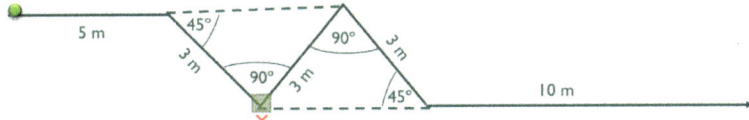

Figure 2. CODAT test diagram. The initial point of the test is drawn with a green ball. The green square shows the location of the force plate. The red cross identifies the change-of-direction task that was recorded with the 3D motion capture system.

2.5. Outcome Variables

Since the risk of ACL injury is highest during the initial contact phase, only the moment of the maximal ground reaction torque forces at the initial contact phase in the 90° change of direction was analysed [34] (Figure 2).

Mean and standard deviation (in degrees) of the flexion/extension, adduction/abduction and internal/external rotation of the trunk, pelvis, hip, and knee were computed for the DL and NDL. For the variables in the sagittal plane projection angle (*x*-axis), positive values (>0) refer to flexion, and negative values (<0) refer to extension. In the frontal plane projection angle (*y*-axis), positive values (>0) refer to trunk inclination towards the non-supporting limb side (contralateral), contralateral pelvic tilt, hip abduction, and knee varus; and negative values (<0) refer to the trunk inclination towards the supporting limb side (ipsilateral), ipsilateral pelvic tilt, hip adduction, and knee valgus. In the transversal plane projection angle (*z*-axis), positive values (>0) refer to the non-supporting limb side, contralateral trunk rotation, contralateral pelvis rotation, and hip and knee internal rotation; and negative values (<0) refer to ipsilateral trunk displacement, ipsilateral pelvis rotation, and hip and knee external rotation.

2.6. Data Analysis

Data were analysed with SPSS software v.25 (SPSS Inc., Chicago, IL, USA). Normality was determined by the Kolmogorov–Smirnov test. To determine the differences in the kinematic angles between the KI and control groups, independent *t*-tests were used to compare the means. Furthermore, to determinate the differences in the kinematic angles between the DL and NDL, independent *t*-tests analysis was developed without distinguishing between players with and without injury. The level of statistical significance was set at $p < 0.05$. The effect size of the kinematic angles between the groups and limbs was determined using *Cohen's d*. The following values were used to distinguish the levels of the effect size: 1 to 0.8 (strong effect size); 0.8 to 0.5 (moderate effect size); and 0.5 to 0.0 (less or no effect size).

3. Results

Eight players were allocated to each of the two groups, KI and control. The KI players had suffered a previous knee injury involving the valgus collapse mechanism, treated without surgical intervention, four of them in their DL and the rest in their NDL.

The independent *t*-test revealed that there were no significant differences between the groups in any kinematic parameters. However, strong *Cohen's d* effect sizes, above 0.8, between the groups were found in the hip adduction, hip rotation, and pelvis rotation in the dominant limb (Table 1). The KI group had higher hip adduction than the control group (14.15 ± 4.64 degrees versus 10.69 ± 4.92 degrees in the control group) (*Cohen's d* = 0.82). The KI group presented a hip internal rotation of 1.26 ± 14.68 degrees, versus 11.55 ± 14.29 degrees of hip external rotation in the control group (*Cohen's d* = 0.88). The KI group showed a contralateral pelvis rotation of 6.11 ± 8.21 degrees, versus 1.35 ± 5.67 degrees of ipsilateral pelvis rotation in the control group (*Cohen's d* = 1.06) (Table 1).

The analysis based on limb dominance taking both groups together was significant only for the knee valgus variable. Knee valgus was higher in the DL (9.02 ± 7.31 degrees versus 1.27 ± 9.05 degrees in the NDL) ($p < 0.05$), with a strong effect size (*Cohen's d* = 0.94) (Table 2). All the other variables showed similar values between the DL and NDL.

Table 1. Comparative analysis of the kinematic outcomes between KI and control groups in DL and NDL.

	Dominant Limb					Non-Dominant Limb				
	KI Mean ± SD	Control Mean ± SD	p-Value	Cohen's d	CI (95%)	KI Mean ± SD	Control Mean ± SD	p-Value	Cohen's d	CI (95%)
Knee Flexion (°) (+flexion/−extension)	29.64 ± 9.74	29.60 ± 9.87	0.994	0.00	(−10.93–11.01)	26.54 ± 20.44	35.50 ± 12.21	0.314	0.53	(−27.44–9.52)
Pelvis Flexion (°) (+flexion/−extension)	10.30 ± 10.24	13.38 ± 12.71	0.618	0.27	(−16.09–9.93)	12.93 ± 17.19	13.44 ± 10.69	0.945	0.04	(−16.10–15.22)
Trunk Flexion (°) (+flexion/−extension)	11.66 ± 4.70	12.22 ± 13.42	0.934	0.06	(−15.07–13.93)	14.04 ± 18.84	11.41 ± 12.87	0.754	0.16	(−15.15–20.41)
Knee Valgus (°) (+varus/−valgus)	−10.58 ± 5.64	−8.87 ± 8.45	0.657	0.24	(−15.79–(−5.36))	−0.15 ± 10.99	−2.87 ± 8.01	0.59	0.28	(−9.57–3.83)
Hip Adduction (°) (+abduction/−adduction)	−14.15 ± 4.64	−10.69 ± 4.92	0.184	0.82 **	(−8.84–1.87)	−14.02 ± 15.00	−15.82 ± 13.36	0.810	0.12	(−14.02–17.60)
Pelvis tilt (°) (+contralateral/−ipsilateral)	−6.24 ± 9.31	−10.57 ± 8.02	0.350	0.50	(−14.85–2.36)	−7.67 ± 8.82	−2.28 ± 15.77	0.439	0.42	(−15.47–10.90)
Trunk displacement (°) (+contralateral/−ipsilateral)	−12.23 ± 8.97	−12.05 ± 14.30	0.977	0.01	(−20.53–(−3.94))	−14.18 ± 9.66	−8.27 ± 10.98	0.292	0.57	(−17.44–0.91)
Knee rotation (°) (+internal/−external)	6.36 ± 10.74	1.85 ± 9.30	0.399	0.45	(−3.57–16.29)	5.53 ± 8.20	4.99 ± 4.82	0.877	0.08	(−4.25–6.21)
Hip rotation (°) (+internal/−external)	1.26 ± 14.68	−11.55 ± 14.29	0.111	0.88 **	(−12.31–14.84)	−8.97 ± 11.74	−1.17 ± 12.65	0.314	0.64	(−11.75–9.40)
Pelvis rotation (°) (+contralateral/−ipsilateral)	6.11 ± 8.21	−1.35 ± 5.67	0.059	1.06 **	(−13.70–1.48)	1.82 ± 14.01	8.52 ± 11.71	0.331	0.52	(−18.31–1.27)
Trunk rotation (°) (+contralateral/−ipsilateral)	3.22 ± 9.29	7.81 ± 12.90	0.450	0.41	(−11.81–5.38)	1.62 ± 9.96	5.89 ± 10.12	0.426	0.42	(−14.35–2.57)

** Effect size strong to excellent d > 0.8.

Table 2. Comparative analysis of the kinematic outcomes between the DL and the NDL in the whole group.

	DL	NDL			
	Mean ± SD	Mean ± SD	p-Value	Cohen's d	CI (95%)
Knee Flexion (°) (+flexion/−extension)	31.12 ± 10.93	32.62 ± 16.84	0.757	0.11	(−9.33–6.48)
Hip Flexion (°) (+flexion/−extension)	46.85 ± 37.07	41.98 ± 21.01	0.559	0.16	(−8.92–9.74)
Pelvis Flexion (°) (+flexion/−extension)	13.92 ± 13.50	15.35 ± 15.66	0.706	0.10	(−8.41–14.96)
Trunk Flexion (°) (+flexion/−extension)	10.66 ± 13.16	10.25 ± 17.67	0.926	0.03	(−11.61–8.62)
Knee Valgus (°) (+varus/−valgus)	−9.02 ± 7.31	−1.27 ± 9.05	0.049 *	0.94 **	(−15.46–(−0.04))
Hip Adduction (°) (+abduction/−adduction)	−13.04 ± 5.64	−14.85 ± 13.20	0.624	0.18	(−5.90–9.52)
Pelvis tilt (°) (+contralateral/−ipsilateral)	−9.23 ± 8.76	−5.62 ± 12.85	0.449	0.33	(−14.85–2.36)
Trunk displacement (°) (+contralateral/−ipsilateral)	−12.47 ± 11.37	−11.35 ± 10.20	0.826	0.10	(−11.66–9.70)
Knee rotation (°) (+internal/−external)	4.36 ± 9.70	5.11 ± 6.17	0.809	0.09	(−3.57–16.29)
Hip rotation (°) (+internal/−external)	−5.92 ± 14.98	−4.94 ± 12.05	0.847	0.07	(−11.66–9.70)
Pelvis rotation (°) (+contralateral/−ipsilateral)	2.08 ± 7.47	5.72 ± 12.47	0.391	0.35	(−5.15–12.43)
Trunk rotation (°) (+contralateral/−ipsilateral)	4.96 ± 11.20	2.99 ± 10.25	0.606	0.18	(−9.92–5.99)

* Statistical significance $p < 0.05$/** Effect size strong to excellent $d > 0.8$.

4. Discussion

The main purpose of this study was to investigate kinematic differences at initial contact between female futsal players with and without previous knee injury, in a motor-pattern test including change of direction, stabilization, and acceleration. None of the variables showed significant differences between female futsal players with and without previous knee injury. However, a strong effect size between groups was obtained in some kinematics in the DL. With respect to the secondary aim of this study, to determine kinematic differences between the DL and NDL for the whole group, only knee valgus was significantly higher in the DL.

Knee valgus was significantly higher in the DL (9.02 ± 7.31 degrees) than in the NDL (1.27 ± 9.05 degrees) (p = 0.049) in the whole group. As other studies have explained, the ACL usually breaks at an average of 13 degrees of knee valgus at initial contact and 22 degrees of knee valgus at the moment of injury, 48 milliseconds after the initial contact [6]. In our findings, the KI and control players were near to these values at initial contact in the DL, without significant differences between them (KI: 10.58 ± 5.64 degrees; control group: 8.87 ± 8.45). However, in the NDL, the values were much lower (KI: 0.15 ± 10.99 degrees; control group: 2.87 ± 8.01). Knee valgus is one of most relevant risk factors in ACL non-contact injury mechanisms, and 88% to 100% of the knee injuries in female soccer are induced by non-contact mechanisms [6,7]. As observed in the pivot shift test, during a valgus knee movement, the femur moves medially relative to the tibia, which causes the lateral condyle to slide into the medial side. These movements cause medial yawing of the knee that increases the ACL load. If the load on the ACL is too high, it might break and cause subluxation of the tibia, usually at around 30 degrees of knee flexion that reduces in deeper flexion [24,35]. Recently, Di Paolo et al. [36] and Collings et al. [37] have verified that higher knee valgus values in different tasks were associated with future noncontact ACL injury in elite female soccer players. Our results showed a higher ACL injury risk position in the DL than in the NDL. DeLang et al. [25], in their meta-analysis, explain that soccer players are more likely to suffer injuries in their DL regardless of their playing level or gender. This is due to two main reasons. Firstly, there is neuromuscular fatigue in the DL as a result of the maximal effort involved in the kicking activity and the high-intensity stabilization actions. In futsal, the DL also accumulates more burden than the NDL. Futsal is a sport with changes of intensity and direction each 3.3 s on average. Therefore, 26% of the match is played at high intensity [26]. This fact produces fatigue in both limbs, but the dominant one is also the kicking leg. Studies explain that players receive the ball twice a minute on average, and 84% of this is with the DL [25,38]. In this way, the DL accumulates fatigue relative to the intensity of the game with additional fatigue due to the maximal effort of kicking. Secondly, there are intrinsic (capability, comfortability, or awareness) and extrinsic factors (opponent position or game situation) that make it necessary to use the DL as the stabilization limb, and it may not be used to these actions [25]. Furthermore, most ACL injuries occur in defensive "pressing/tackling" or offensive duel "tackling" situations. These are high-speed actions and are driven by the match conditions, in which player does not have enough time to decide on the use of the DL or NDL. These forced actions are the most likely to result in injury. In contrast, both groups presented better knee valgus values in the NDL; this might be due to better neuromuscular control in this limb, since it is more used to the stabilization task.

"Valgus collapse" has been defined as the combination of hip adduction, hip internal rotation, and knee abduction. In the current study, in the DL, the limb which had a level of knee valgus near to the injury risk threshold, the KI players had more hip adduction than the control players in the change-of-direction task (*Cohen's d*: 0.82). This was explained by the fact that when the KI players carried out a task that promoted high knee valgus values, their stabilization pattern was pathological, as explained by what is described in the literature as the "perfect storm" of ACL injury mechanism [15,16,19]. These results agree with previous research, such as the study by Dix et al. [39], who verified that players who suffered ACL injury had a higher "valgus collapse", a combination of knee valgus, hip adduction, and internal hip rotation, during preseason testing, before ACL injury. The authors noted significant differences between injured and non-injured players only in the hip adduction variable. This study developed prospective data collection in national female soccer players, comparing initial kinematic values in a change-of-direction task of 90° between groups. Therefore, the hypothesis of our KI group performing a kinematic pattern similar to the ACL injury pattern is confirmed.

Hip and knee internal rotation are involved in knee valgus definition, as explained in video analysis research [6,14,40]. In the current study, both groups had knee internal rotation at the evaluation moment, but the KI players had hip internal rotation in contrast to control players who developed hip external rotation (*Cohen's d*: 0.88). Hip internal rotation, combined with hip adduction and knee abduction, increases structural stress on the ACL due to its anatomical situation from the front internal tibial surface to the back external femur condyle [11,39,41]. Therefore, if the hip internal rotation range of movement is increased, the strain fibres are at maximum stress and are broken easily. At the same time, increases in knee abduction and hip adduction cause medial displacement of the center of mass [24,39,41], and the joining of both conditions facilitates ACL risk injury. As is explained by Lucarno et al. [6] in their systematic video analysis, 80% of the non-contact ACL injuries that occurred during matches in female players in six of the top leagues in the Federation International of Football Association (FIFA) Women's World Ranking were associated with hip internal rotation movement. Koga et al. show the same result in female players of other sports, such as basketball or handball. Our results showed that the KI players had a greater hip internal rotation range of motion than the control players, in agreement with previous research. Furthermore, hip internal rotation might be the result of weakness in the hip external rotation muscles., especially the gluteus maximus, which becomes weak due to accumulated fatigue. Fatigue could be the result of carrying out many functions at the same time. As strong external rotation is an important factor in avoiding knee valgus, we can say that it is a protective factor of ACL injury involving non-contact mechanisms. In fact, our control players showed hip external rotation in the DL during the change-of-direction task.

All the players in our study, in both the KI and control groups, had a contralateral trunk rotation from the supporting limb. Many authors have demonstrated that if the contralateral trunk rotation increases, the knee valgus increases too, raising the risk of ACL injury [6,14,16,42]. As Della Villa et al. [14] shows in their research, 53% of the players with ACL injuries had contralateral trunk rotation at the moment of injury, especially during pressing and landing tasks. As Lloyd et al. [16] explain in their "perfect storm" definition of ACL injury mechanisms, contralateral rotation causes a medial displacement of the center of mass, which increases the loading on the medial knee compartment. However, no prior authors have studied the influence of pelvic rotation. In our study, the KI players performed a contralateral pelvic rotation following the trunk motion direction. On the contrary, members the control group in whom contralateral trunk rotation existed realized an ipsilateral pelvic rotation to the DL (*Cohen's d*: 1.06). This might be a balance mechanism to counteract the opposite trunk rotation, and to decelerate the medial velocities suffered by the knee as a result of the trunk rotation movement [43]. It would be interesting to develop studies to explore this hypothesis in the future.

Limitations

This study is limited by the relatively small sample size and by the cross-sectional design conducted in a single geographic location; thus, any causality can be referred to the relationship in the relevant results. Due to the study design, it was not possible to state whether the worst kinematic patterns observed in the KI group were present before the knee injury, making the injury more likely to occur, or whether they existed as a result of the disfunctions induced by the injury. A future larger cohort and prospective studies might support our findings and develop new analysis in pelvic kinematics. However, the current findings may be relevant for the development of specific preventive training in female soccer players. The preventive training should be based on intensive neuromuscular training to avoid fatigue of the muscles, especially of the DL, and in the reinforcement of the hip external rotation muscles.

5. Conclusions

The current study found kinematic differences at initial contact between female futsal players with and without previous knee injury, in a motor pattern test. The players with no previous history of knee injury had a more physiological position to avoid the valgus collapse mechanism in hip adduction and internal rotation, and in the pelvis rotation, in the dominant limb. The players with previous injury had a kinematic pattern closer to those related to LCA injury, which might have existed before the injury, making it more likely to occur, or as a result of the disfunctions induced by the injury. All the players showed more knee valgus in their dominant limb, which is the limb with a greater risk of injury, revealing the clinical relevance of neuromuscular stabilization training for this limb.

Author Contributions: Conceptualization, L.F.-L. and J.M.T.-M.; methodology, L.F.-L., L.V.-P. and R.S.-R.; formal analysis, L.F.-L. and M.O.L.-L.; investigation, L.F.-L., L.V.-P., E.O.-G. and J.H.-J.; data curation, E.O.-G. and J.H.-J.; writing—original draft preparation, L.F.-L., M.O.L.-L., E.O.-G. and C.H.-G.; writing—review and editing, L.F.-L., M.O.L.-L., E.O.-G. and C.H.-G.; visualization, L.F.-L., L.V.-P. and R.S.-R.; project administration, J.M.T.-M. and L.F.-L.; resources, E.O.-G. and J.H.-J.; supervision, J.M.T.-M. and J.H.-J. All authors have read and agreed to the published version of the manuscript.

Funding: This research received no external funding.

Institutional Review Board Statement: The study was conducted in accordance with the Declaration of Helsinki, and approved by the Research Ethics Committee of Community of Aragón (protocol code PI20/127; date of approval: 18 March 2020).

Informed Consent Statement: Informed consent was obtained from all the subjects involved in the study. Written informed consent was obtained from the subject in Figure 1.

Data Availability Statement: The datasets presented in this study are available on request from the corresponding author. All data covered by this study are included in this manuscript.

Acknowledgments: The authors thank the volunteer subjects for their altruistic participation.

Conflicts of Interest: The authors declare no conflict of interest.

References

1. Ruiz-Pérez, I.; López-Valenciano, A.; Jiménez-Loaisa, A.; Elvira, J.L.L.; de Ste Croix, M.; Ayala, F. Injury incidence, characteristics and burden among female sub-elite futsal players: A prospective study with three-year follow-up. *PeerJ* **2019**, *7*, e7989. [CrossRef]
2. Olivares-Jabalera, J.; Fílter-Ruger, A.; Dos'Santos, T.; Afonso, J.; della Villa, F.; Morente-Sánchez, J.; Soto-Hermoso, V.M.; Requena, B. Exercise-Based Training Strategies to Reduce the Incidence or Mitigate the Risk Factors of Anterior Cruciate Ligament Injury in Adult Football (Soccer) Players: A Systematic Review. *Int. J. Environ. Res. Public Health* **2021**, *18*, 13351. [CrossRef]
3. Larruskain, J.; Lekue, J.A.; Diaz, N.; Odriozola, A.; Gil, S.M. A comparison of injuries in elite male and female football players: A five-season prospective study. *Scand. J. Med. Sci. Sports* **2018**, *28*, 237–245. [CrossRef]
4. Waldén, M.; Hägglund, M.; Werner, J.; Ekstrand, J. The epidemiology of anterior cruciate ligament injury in football (soccer): A review of the literature from a gender-related perspective. *Knee Surg. Sport. Traumatol. Arthrosc.* **2011**, *19*, 3–10. [CrossRef] [PubMed]
5. Zebis, M.K.; Aagaard, P.; Andersen, L.L.; Hölmich, P.; Clausen, M.B.; Brandt, M.; Husted, R.S.; Lauridsen, H.B.; Curtis, D.J.; Bencke, J. First-time anterior cruciate ligament injury in adolescent female elite athletes: A prospective cohort study to identify modifiable risk factors. *Knee Surg. Sport. Traumatol. Arthrosc.* **2022**, *30*, 1341–1351. [CrossRef] [PubMed]
6. Lucarno, S.; Zago, M.; Buckthorpe, M.; Grassi, A.; Tosarelli, F.; Smith, R.; Della Villa, F. Systematic Video Analysis of Anterior Cruciate Ligament Injuries in Professional Female Soccer Players. *Am. J. Sports Med.* **2021**, *49*, 1794–1802. [CrossRef] [PubMed]
7. Agustín, R.M.-S.; Medina-Mirapeix, F.; Esteban-Catalán, A.; Escriche-Escuder, A.; Sánchez-Barbadora, M.; Benítez-Martínez, J.C. Epidemiology of Injuries in First Division Spanish Women's Soccer Players. *Int. J. Environ. Res. Public Health* **2021**, *18*, 3009. [CrossRef] [PubMed]

8. Montalvo, A.M.; Schneider, D.K.; Silva, P.L.; Yut, L.; Webster, K.E.; Riley, M.A.; Kiefer, A.W.; Doherty-Restrepo, J.L.; Myer, G.D. 'What's my risk of sustaining an ACL injury while playing football (soccer)?' A systematic review with meta-analysis. *Br. J. Sports Med.* **2019**, *53*, 1333–1340. [CrossRef]
9. Montalvo, A.M.; Schneider, D.K.; Webster, K.E.; Yut, L.; Galloway, M.T.; Heidt, R.S.; Kaeding, C.C.; Kremcheck, T.E.; Magnussen, R.A.; Parikh, S.N.; et al. Anterior Cruciate Ligament Injury Risk in Sport: A Systematic Review and Meta-Analysis of Injury Incidence by Sex and Sport Classification. *J. Athl. Train.* **2019**, *54*, 472–482. [CrossRef]
10. Staeubli, H.-U.; Adam, O.; Becker, W.; Burgkart, R. Anterior Cruciate Ligament and Intercondylar Notch in the Coronal Oblique Plane: Anatomy Complemented by Magnetic Resonance Imaging in Cruciate Ligament–Intact Knees. *Arthrosc. J. Arthrosc. Relat. Surg.* **1999**, *15*, 349–359. [CrossRef]
11. Navacchia, A.; Bates, N.A.; Schilaty, N.D.; Krych, A.J.; Hewett, T.E. Knee Abduction and Internal Rotation Moments Increase ACL Force During Landing Through the Posterior Slope of the Tibia. *J. Orthop. Res.* **2019**, *37*, 1730–1742. [CrossRef]
12. Griffin, L.; Albohm, M.; Arendt, E.; Bahr, R.; Beynnon, B.; DeMaio, M.; Dick, R.; Engebretsen, L.; Garrett, W.; Hannafin, J.; et al. Update on ACL Injury Prevention: Theoretical and Practical Considerations: A Review of the Hunt Valley II Meeting. *Febr. Am. J. Sport. Med.* **2006**, *34*, 1512–1532. [CrossRef] [PubMed]
13. Brophy, R.H.; Stepan, J.G.; Silvers, H.J.; Mandelbaum, B.R. Defending Puts the Anterior Cruciate Ligament at Risk During Soccer: A Gender-Based Analysis. *Sports Health* **2015**, *7*, 244–249. [CrossRef] [PubMed]
14. Della Villa, F.; Buckthorpe, M.; Grassi, A.; Nabiuzzi, A.; Tosarelli, F.; Zaffagnini, S.; Della Villa, S. Systematic video analysis of ACL injuries in professional male football (soccer): Injury mechanisms, situational patterns and biomechanics study on 134 consecutive cases. *Br. J. Sports Med.* **2020**, *54*, 1423–1432. [CrossRef]
15. Di Paolo, S.; Bragonzoni, L.; Della Villa, F.; Grassi, A.; Zaffagnini, S. Do healthy athletes exhibit at-risk biomechanics for anterior cruciate ligament injury during pivoting movements? *Sports Biomech.* **2022**, 1–14. [CrossRef] [PubMed]
16. Lloyd, D. The future of in-field sports biomechanics: Wearables plus modelling compute real-time in vivo tissue loading to prevent and repair musculoskeletal injuries. *Sports Biomech.* **2021**, 1–29. [CrossRef]
17. Arundale, A.J.H.; Silvers-Granelli, H.J.; Marmon, A.; Zarzycki, R.; Dix, C.; Snyder-Mackler, L. Changes in biomechanical knee injury risk factors across two collegiate soccer seasons using the 11+ prevention program. *Scand. J. Med. Sci. Sports* **2018**, *28*, 2592–2603. [CrossRef]
18. Ishida, T.; Koshino, Y.; Yamanaka, M.; Ueno, R.; Taniguchi, S.; Ino, T.; Kasahara, S.; Samukawa, M.; Tohyama, H. Larger hip external rotation motion is associated with larger knee abduction and internal rotation motions during a drop vertical jump. *Sports Biomech.* **2021**, 1–15. [CrossRef]
19. Hewett, T.E.; Myer, G.D.; Ford, K.R.; Heidt, R.S., Jr.; Colosimo, A.J.; McLean, S.G.; Van Den Bogert, A.J.; Paterno, M.V.; Succop, P. Biomechanical Measures of Neuromuscular Control and Valgus Loading of the Knee Predict Anterior Cruciate Ligament Injury Risk in Female Athletes: A Prospective Study. *Am. J. Sports Med.* **2005**, *33*, 492–501. [CrossRef]
20. Hearn, D.W.; Frank, B.S.; Padua, D.A. Use of double leg injury screening to assess single leg biomechanical risk variables. *Phys. Ther. Sport* **2021**, *47*, 40–45. [CrossRef]
21. Nishizawa, K.; Hashimoto, T.; Hakukawa, S.; Nagura, T.; Otani, T.; Harato, K. Effects of foot progression angle on kinematics and kinetics of a cutting movement. *J. Exp. Orthop.* **2022**, *9*, 11. [CrossRef] [PubMed]
22. Kiapour, A.M.; Demetropoulos, C.K.; Kiapour, A.; Quatman, C.E.; Wordeman, S.C.; Goel, V.K.; Hewett, T.E. Strain Response of the Anterior Cruciate Ligament to Uniplanar and Multiplanar Loads During Simulated Landings: Implications for Injury Mechanism. *Am. J. Sports Med.* **2016**, *44*, 2087–2096. [CrossRef] [PubMed]
23. Ueno, R.; Navacchia, A.; Schilaty, N.D.; Myer, G.D.; Hewett, T.E.; Bates, N.A. Anterior Cruciate Ligament Loading Increases with Pivot-Shift Mechanism during Asymmetrical Drop Vertical Jump in Female Athletes. *Orthop. J. Sports Med.* **2021**, *9*, 2325967121989095. [CrossRef] [PubMed]
24. Wilczyński, B.; Zorena, K.; Ślęzak, D. Dynamic Knee Valgus in Single-Leg Movement Tasks. Potentially Modifiable Factors and Exercise Training Options. A Literature Review. *Int. J. Environ. Res. Public Health* **2020**, *17*, 8208. [CrossRef]
25. DeLang, M.D.; Salamh, P.A.; Farooq, A.; Tabben, M.; Whiteley, R.; van Dyk, N.; Chamari, K. The dominant leg is more likely to get injured in soccer players: Systematic review and meta-analysis. *Biol. Sport* **2021**, *38*, 397–435. [CrossRef]
26. Dogramaci, S.N.; Watsford, M.L.; Murphy, A.J. Time-Motion Analysis of International and National Level Futsal. *J. Strength Cond. Res.* **2011**, *25*, 646–651. [CrossRef]
27. Nilstad, A.; Petushek, E.; Mok, K.-M.; Bahr, R.; Krosshaug, T. Kiss goodbye to the 'kissing knees': No association between frontal plane inward knee motion and risk of future non-contact ACL injury in elite female athletes. *Sports Biomech.* **2021**, *22*, 65–79. [CrossRef]
28. World Medical Association. World Medical Association Declaration of Helsinki: Ethical principles for medical research involving human subjects. *JAMA* **2013**, *310*, 2191–2194. [CrossRef] [PubMed]
29. Ho, K.-Y.; Murata, A. Asymmetries in Dynamic Valgus Index after Anterior Cruciate Ligament Reconstruction: A Proof-of-Concept Study. *Int. J. Environ. Res. Public Health* **2021**, *18*, 7047. [CrossRef]
30. Aoki, A.; Kubota, S.; Morinaga, K.; Zheng, N.N.; Wang, S.S.; Gamada, K. Detection of knee wobbling as a screen to identify athletes who may be at high risk for ACL injury. *Int. Biomech.* **2021**, *8*, 30–41. [CrossRef]

31. Lockie, R.G.; Schultz, A.B.; Callaghan, S.J.; Jeffriess, M.D.; Berry, S.P. Reliability and Validity of a New Test of Change-of-Direction Speed for Field-Based Sports: The Change-of-Direction and Acceleration Test (CODAT). *J. Sports Sci. Med.* **2013**, *12*, 88–96. [PubMed]
32. Nimphius, S.; Callaghan, S.J.; Bezodis, N.E.; Lockie, R.G.; Sciences, H.; Sports, A.; Kingdom, U. Change of Direction and Agility Tests: Challenging Our Current Measures of Performance. *Strength Cond. J.* **2018**, *40*, 26–38. [CrossRef]
33. Dos'Santos, T.; Thomas, C.; Comfort, P.; Jones, P.A. The Effect of Training Interventions on Change of Direction Biomechanics Associated with Increased Anterior Cruciate Ligament Loading: A Scoping Review. *Sports Med.* **2019**, *49*, 1837–1859. [CrossRef] [PubMed]
34. Nedergaard, N.J.; Dalbø, S.; Petersen, S.V.; Zebis, M.K.; Bencke, J. Biomechanical and neuromuscular comparison of single- and multi-planar jump tests and a side-cutting maneuver: Implications for ACL injury risk assessment. *Knee* **2020**, *27*, 324–333. [CrossRef]
35. Quatman, C.E.; Hewett, T.E. The anterior cruciate ligament injury controversy: Is "valgus collapse" a sex-specific mechanism? What is the inciting event in non-contact acl injury? *Br. J. Sports Med.* **2009**, *43*, 328–335. [CrossRef]
36. Di Paolo, S.; Zaffagnini, S.; Tosarelli, F.; Aggio, F.; Bragonzoni, L.; Grassi, A.; Della Villa, F. A 2D qualitative movement assessment of a deceleration task detects football players with high knee joint loading. *Knee Surg. Sport. Traumatol. Arthrosc.* **2021**, *29*, 4032–4040. [CrossRef] [PubMed]
37. Collings, T.J.; Diamond, L.E.; Barrett, R.O.D.S.; Timmins, R.G.; Hickey, J.T.; DU Moulin, W.S.; Williams, M.D.; Beerworth, K.A.; Bourne, M.N. Strength and Biomechanical Risk Factors for Noncontact ACL Injury in Elite Female Footballers: A Prospective Study. *Med. Sci. Sports Exerc.* **2022**, *54*, 1242–1251. [CrossRef]
38. Castagna, C.; D'Ottavio, S.; Vera, J.G.; Álvarez, J.C.B. Match demands of professional Futsal: A case study. *J. Sci. Med. Sport* **2009**, *12*, 490–494. [CrossRef]
39. Dix, C.; Arundale, A.; Silvers-Granelli, H.; Marmon, A.; Zarzycki, R.; Snyder-Mackler, L. Biomechanical measures during two sport-specific tasks differentiate between soccer players who go on to anterior cruciate ligament injury and those who do not: A prospective cohort analysis. *Int. J. Sports Phys. Ther.* **2020**, *15*, 928–935. [CrossRef]
40. Krosshaug, T.; Slauterbeck, J.R.; Engebretsen, L.; Bahr, R. Biomechanical analysis of anterior cruciate ligament injury mechanisms: Three-dimensional motion reconstruction from video sequences. *Scand. J. Med. Sci. Sports* **2007**, *17*, 508–519. [CrossRef]
41. Taylor, J.B.; Ford, K.R.; Nguyen, A.-D.; Shultz, S.J. Biomechanical Comparison of Single- and Double-Leg Jump Landings in the Sagittal and Frontal Plane. *Orthop. J. Sports Med.* **2016**, *4*, 2325967116655158. [CrossRef] [PubMed]
42. Dempsey, A.R.; Lloyd, D.G.; Elliott, B.C.; Steele, J.R.; Munro, B.J.; Russo, K.A. The Effect of Technique Change on Knee Loads during Sidestep Cutting. *Med. Sci. Sports Exerc.* **2007**, *39*, 1765–1773. [CrossRef] [PubMed]
43. Critchley, M.L.; Davis, D.J.; Keener, M.M.; Layer, J.S.; Wilson, M.A.; Zhu, Q.; Dai, B. The effects of mid-flight whole-body and trunk rotation on landing mechanics: Implications for anterior cruciate ligament injuries. *Sports Biomech.* **2019**, *19*, 421–437. [CrossRef] [PubMed]

Disclaimer/Publisher's Note: The statements, opinions and data contained in all publications are solely those of the individual author(s) and contributor(s) and not of MDPI and/or the editor(s). MDPI and/or the editor(s) disclaim responsibility for any injury to people or property resulting from any ideas, methods, instructions or products referred to in the content.

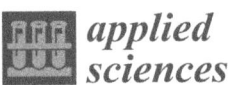

Article

Comfort and Support Values Provided by Different Pillow Materials for Individuals with Forward Head Posture

Ceyhun Türkmen [1,*], Serdar Yılmaz Esen [2], Zafer Erden [2] and Tülin Düger [2]

[1] Department of Ergotherapy, Faculty of Health Sciences, Çankırı Karatekin University, Çankırı 18100, Türkiye
[2] Faculty of Physical Therapy and Rehabilitation, Hacettepe University, Ankara 06230, Türkiye
* Correspondence: ceyhunturkmen@karatekin.edu.tr; Tel.: +90-376-2131702

Abstract: Based on the pressure distributions in the head, neck, and upper body and the spine support values, this study aims to recommend the most suitable pillow for those with forward head posture (FHP) according to different sleeping positions. This descriptive cross-sectional study recruited thirty healthy 18- to 55-year-old men and women with body mass indexes of less than 30 kg/m^2. Participants tried five different pillows (viscose, fiber, cotton, goose feather, and wool) on a medium-firm hybrid mattress at room temperature with a humidity of 45–55%. Participants tried the pillows first in the supine position, then side-lying, and finally in the prone position. A pressure-mapping system was utilized to measure the pressure distributions of the head and shoulder areas in millimeters of mercury (mmHg) and the amount of support provided by the pillow to these regions in square centimeters (cm^2). When the comfort and support parameters of different pillow materials were compared among all participants, for the supine position, Pillow B and Pillow E provided higher head comfort ($p < 0.001$), while Pillow A and Pillow E provided higher shoulder support ($p = 0.044$). In the side-lying position, Pillow B provided higher head comfort ($p < 0.001$) and Pillow C ($p = 0.003$) higher shoulder comfort. In the prone position, Pillow B and Pillow E provided higher head comfort ($p < 0.001$), while Pillow E also provided higher shoulder support ($p = 0.002$). This study showed pillow materials affect the spine comfort and support of the participants, and these values may vary according to different spinal alignments, such as FHP. According to the preferred sleeping position, the pillow material that supports the spine and its comfort and support values may also change.

Keywords: ergonomic assessment; head-down tilt; household equipment; sleeping habit; sleep quality

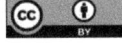

1. Introduction

People can perform their duties in a sitting position at a desk, standing, or walking, depending on their occupation. Today, 75 percent of workers do their jobs sitting down [1]. This rate can go up to 90 percent for software developers, 80.7 percent for accountants, and 80.3 percent for insurance sales representatives [2]. In modern working life, the behavior of employees working in a static position and long-term inactivity may cause them to adopt distorted body postures and thus cause musculoskeletal disorders. Many factors, such as sleeping with the head elevated too high, using the computer for a long time, and weakness in the back muscles, also cause this. Postural disorders and spinal diseases may accompany these changes [3]. A pillow can provide enough head and neck support to help people maintain normal neck and thoracic curvature. A comfy sleeping pillow has been shown in studies to assist with relaxing the neck muscles, enabling sleep, and effectively relieving pain in the neck, shoulders, back, and head [4].

Research on the support and comfort of human contact surfaces has addressed different points. Yu-Chi et al. concluded that choosing the right combination of mattress pad thickness and firmness is important for achieving optimum sleep posture and improving physiological measures during sleep [5]. Another study suggests the mattress material plays a crucial role in reducing pressure during sleep, and memory foam and latex foam mattresses may be more suitable for people who want to relieve pressure points during sleep, especially in the supine and prone positions [6]. A different study examining mattress pressure values indicated the pressure distribution across the interface of the body and support surface is a significant factor in determining sleep quality. The study found uneven pressure distribution could cause poor sleep quality, characterized by reduced deep sleep and increased sleep fragmentation. Consequently, mattresses with even pressure distribution might be more effective in promoting better sleep quality for those seeking to improve their sleeping experience [7]. In addition to studies examining the pressure distribution of mattresses, studies on pillows have also been carried out. Lei et al. suggested many factors should be considered, including the person's height, BMI, sleeping position, and the distance between the neck and the mattress, to determine the appropriate pillow height for optimum ergonomic support during sleep. Therefore, personalized pillow height recommendations based on these factors may be more effective in promoting healthy sleep and preventing neck pain and other musculoskeletal disorders [8]. Based on the findings of another study, it can be concluded that the use of a body pillow during sleep can have several benefits, such as improving sleeping posture, reducing the number of positional shifts, and increasing the amount of deep sleep. Since deep sleep is essential for physical and mental health, body pillows can be considered a useful tool for individuals who experience discomfort while sleeping or desire to enhance the quality of their sleep [9]. While previous studies have provided valuable insights, it is hypothesized that the material type of the pillow may also impact the level of support, leading equally to improved pressure distribution and improve proprioception.

In current research on pillows, assessments can be made subjectively or objectively. Subjective evaluations are made by completing an evaluation form based on the person's self-report after the sleep test. In this evaluation form, the amount of comfort and support the person receives from the pillow is questioned. Although this method directly reveals one's own thoughts, it has poor reproducibility, the results can be easily manipulated, it takes a long time to be done, and it is not suitable for complex experiments [10]. Objective assessments can be made by analyzing body pressure distributions [11], EMG signals [12], and anthropometric characteristics [13]. According to the results of the studies, the evaluation method performed with body pressure distributions is the most effective method [3,14]. This may be because body pressure distribution can respond quickly to materials used, support arrangements, human weight, or lying positions.

Long-term high pressure applied to specific portions of the human body has been demonstrated in studies to have an effect on the human central nervous, blood circulation, and endocrine systems [15–17]. Furthermore, due to variances in subcutaneous tissue and tissue architecture, certain areas of the human body are extremely sensitive to pressure. In terms of ergonomics, the human body's pressure perception can be separated into dull and sensitive sections. Dull portions can handle higher pressures, but sensitive parts can only feel comfortable at low pressures. As a result, one of the primary goals in choosing a pillow should be to reduce pressure on sensitive points [18,19].

Although it has been claimed that the pillow's primary function is to optimize head and neck posture, there has been little research on its effectiveness in terms of head and neck posture [20]. A third of our lives are spent sleeping, during which the spine is out of our cognitive control. Pillows, as a result, serve a crucial function in maintaining proper head and neck posture and can alter muscle activity [21]. The position of the head and neck has a significant impact on sleep quality. It has been noted that while sleeping, cervical control decreases, putting undue strain on spinal tissues. During this time, symptoms, such as neck and shoulder pain, tension headaches, and muscle stiffness, diminish sleep quality [22]. As a result, there is an urgent need to research how alternative pillow materials might properly support the cervical spine, hence reducing neck pain and improving sleep quality [23].

Forward head posture (FHP) is the anterior cervical spine alignment; it is also known as "text neck," "scholar's neck," "wearies neck," and "reading neck." One of the most frequent postural issues is FHP, which is a bad habitual cervical posture. FHP is significantly linked to a variety of musculoskeletal diseases, including neck pain, suboccipital trigger points, headache, restricted neck movement, and functional impairment of the neck and thorax. A lack of established back muscle strength as well as nutritional deficiencies, such as calcium deficiency, all contribute to this postural condition. Age is associated with decreased cervical ROM, thoracic kyphosis with greater cervical flexion, and forward head posture with larger deficits in cervical rotation and flexion ROM [24]. This sagittal plane cervical spine dislocation is distinguished by the position of the head anterior to the vertical line running through the lateral malleolus. This postural aberration is distinguished by an increase in upper cervical extension and lower cervical flexion, which might result in compensatory responses, such as thoracic kyphosis and rounded shoulders. These structural changes result in muscular tension imbalances, altered muscle strength and morphology, diminished cervical spine and thorax mobility and function, and altered muscle recruitment around the neck and back. These biomechanical changes could affect the stresses on the neck and back musculoskeletal structure during functional activity and various resting positions, including sleeping postures [25].

Scientific evidence suggests head postural changes affect the development and persistence of neck pain [26]. Kiatkulanusorn et al. argued pillows or mattresses specifically designed for people with FHP could reduce muscle fatigue and potential musculoskeletal pain in patients with FHP [25]; therefore, it should be one of the main factors in choosing an ergonomically correct pillow. In addition, the cervical muscles play an important role in the control of neck posture. During sleep, the ideal pillow should support and maintain good spinal alignment while minimizing biological stress on the musculoskeletal system. Consequently, maintaining horizontal alignment of the spine in the side position while utilizing the most suitable pillow is essential. In addition, a good support cushion should reduce the activity of the neck and back muscles, encourage symmetrical activation of the bilateral muscles, and provide a pleasant feeling of relaxation [27,28]. The reduced ability of these muscles to maintain the upright posture of the cervical spine may indicate their endurance is impaired, and they are unable to maintain cervical lordosis. Because various studies frequently report a significant association between weak neck muscles, poor posture, and the experience of neck pain and because a pillow can reduce pain and disability, individuals with a forward head posture may have different pillow needs [29,30].

Pillow comfort research is relatively new, and the factors affecting the selection of the right pillow are still unclear. For example, it is not correct to accept the head and neck regions as a whole and accept comfort and support demands as similar. Because the position of the head in relation to the height varies in normal head posture, the comfort or support properties of the pillow may be affected. Due to differences in head posture, the comfort and support demands of the head and neck areas in contact with the pillow will also vary [31]. There is consensus among researchers that supporting the natural lordotic curve of the cervical spine is necessary to achieve longer periods of deep sleep [27]. In addition, a pillow can improve sleep quality by cooling the head, lowering body temperature, reducing sweating, or slowing the heart rate during sleep. However, the evidence to support these claims is currently limited. It has been claimed by pillow manufacturers that many design-related pillow parameters are effective in improving sleep quality and reducing neck pain. However, most of these recommendations are based on personal experience [22,32].

There is no consensus on the most effective pillow, despite several prior studies focused on developing and evaluating neck support pillows with the goals of minimizing awakening symptoms, offering relaxation, and guaranteeing a proper resting position. Available on the market are numerous pillows with various shapes, fillings, and materials. To choose the best pillow, it is necessary to consider a number of criteria, including pillow designs (such as shapes and height) and the material used. A cushion should provide a proper alignment position angle and the least amount of muscular activation to prevent unneeded physiological stress [33,34]. The void in the literature must be filled by an objective presentation of these cushion measures. Based on the pressure distribution in the head, neck, and upper body and the spine support values, this study aims to recommend the most suitable pillow for those with forward head positions according to different sleeping positions. Two factors were used to evaluate the recommended pillows: comfort and support.

2. Materials and Methods

2.1. Participants

This descriptive cross-sectional study recruited healthy 18- to 55-years-old men and women with a body mass index (BMI) of less than 30 kg/m^2. Exclusion criteria included a history of neck pain, carpal tunnel syndrome, a shoulder joint lesion in the past three months, cervical spine trauma, inflammatory or viral illnesses of the spine, spinal surgery, or congenital spinal deformities. All experimental procedures in this study were approved by the Human Ethics Committee of Çankırı Karatekin University (approval number: 19/01/2023-30). Study protocol was registered with the United States National Library Trial Registry (ClinicalTrials.gov Identifer: NCT05707715) There is FHP if the imaginary line between the tragus of the ear and the middle of the shoulder is not on the same line when viewed from the side. Additionally, the horizontal distance between those two vertical lines indicates the severity of FHP (Figure 1). The level of FHP is classified as mild or severe based on the horizontal length. To analyze at least 15 participants and thus obtain a good estimate of the mean effect, the participants were divided into two groups according to their median values. This value was close to the 2.5 cm value accepted in another study [35]. The slight FHP is accepted to be lower than 2.8 cm, and the severe FHP is greater than 2.8 cm. Thirty participants (15 with mild and 15 with severe FHP) were included in the study. The following is some basic information about the subjects: age 25 ± 2, height 172.1 ± 4.3 cm, and weight 60.2 ± 4.2 kg for men; for women, age 25 ± 2 years, height 161.1 ± 3.1 cm, and weight 51.4 ± 2.8 kg. The Pittsburgh Sleep Quality Index was used to measure the current sleep quality of the participants [36], and the International Physical Activity Questionnaire was used to measure the level of physical activity, which is one of the possible factors that can change their sleep habits [37]. Sleeping pillows with five different materials (cotton, fiber, wool, viscose, and goose feather), which are the most preferred on the market, were chosen as examples. Analyses were carried out between November and December 2022 at the ASO Technopark Campus in Ankara. The shapes and basic parameters of the pillows are shown in Table 1 and Figure 2.

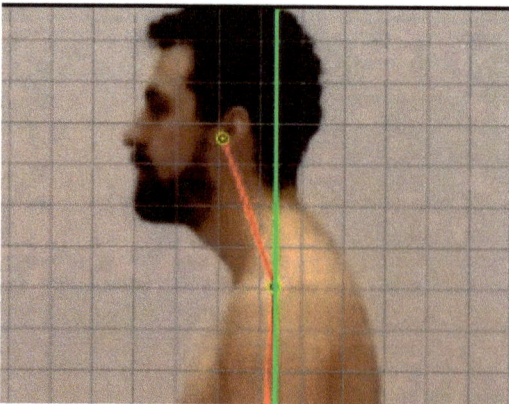

Figure 1. Forward head posture measurement.

Table 1. Structural features of pillow designs.

Pillow Designs	Fabric Type	Pillow Stuffing	Weight	Size (cm)
Pillow A (Viscose)	35% Viscose, 65% Polyester	50 DNS Polyurethane Viscose	800 gr.	$57 \times 37 \times 10$
Pillow B (Fiber)	100% Cotton	100% Microgel	1000 gr.	$50 \times 70 \times 19$
Pillow C (Cotton)	100% Cotton	100% Cotton	1000 gr.	$50 \times 70 \times 16$
Pillow D (Wool)	100% Cotton	100% Wool	900 gr.	$50 \times 70 \times 15$
Pillow E (Goose feather)	100% Cotton	70% Goose jowl feather, 30% Goose back feather	1150 gr.	$50 \times 70 \times 16$

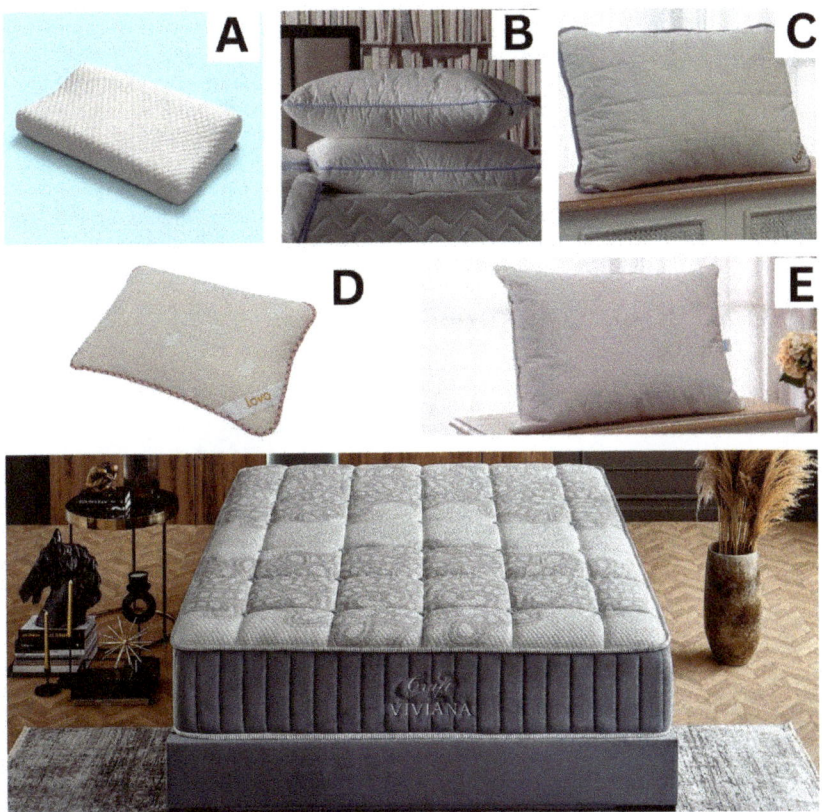

Figure 2. Mattress and pillows used in the research. (**A**). Viscose pillow, (**B**). Fiber pillow, (**C**). Cotton pillow, (**D**). Wool pillow, (**E**). Goose feather pillow).

2.2. Determination of Forward Head Posture

The postures of the participants were evaluated with the PostureScreen mobile application. According to the results of the lateral posture analysis obtained from the application, a tilt above 2.8 cm was accepted as severe forward head posture. To assess forward head posture, participants were asked to stand at a distance of 3.5 m with their feet 30 cm apart. The participants' postures were analyzed using a high-resolution camera positioned 1.5 meters away. Relevant reference points were determined manually based on the image obtained with the tablet camera. The measurements were made automatically by the PostureScreen mobile application after the reference points were placed, and the vertical lines of the 13 parameters as well as the means of deviation from the middle and middle part were displayed. Next, the analysis results were obtained in PDF file format [38]. Overall, the stance was analyzed from the region above to the region below. The app was able to detect changes in selected variables, including sagittal and coronal plane translations and angulations, with intraclass correlation coefficients (ICCs) reaching 0.84 [39].

2.3. Comfort and Support Assessment

A pressure mapping system (X3 SENSOR PX 100:64.160.02, X-Sensor®, Calgary, AB, Canada) was utilized to measure the pressure distributions of the head and shoulder areas in millimeters of mercury (mmHg) and the amount of support provided by the pillow to these regions in square centimeters (cm^2). The pressure-mapping system used has a sensing area of 81.3×203.2 cm ($32'' \times 80''$) and provides high-resolution sensing (1.27 cm or 0.5'') using 10,240 sensing points with an accuracy of ±2 mmHg. It is calibrated to measure values between 5 and 200 mmHg. For the purpose of our study, the pressure-mapping system was positioned under the pillow, and the patients were asked to lie on the mapping system once in supine, side-lying, and prone positions. Pressure distribution was recorded for 1 minute for each lying position. The purpose of these measurements was to describe the pressure distribution created by the participants in the pillow and the supported areas as well as to find the differences that may occur between the pillows. A lower average pressure measured by the device was defined as indicating "higher comfort", while greater contact between the head area and the pillow was considered to indicate "better support" (Figure 3).

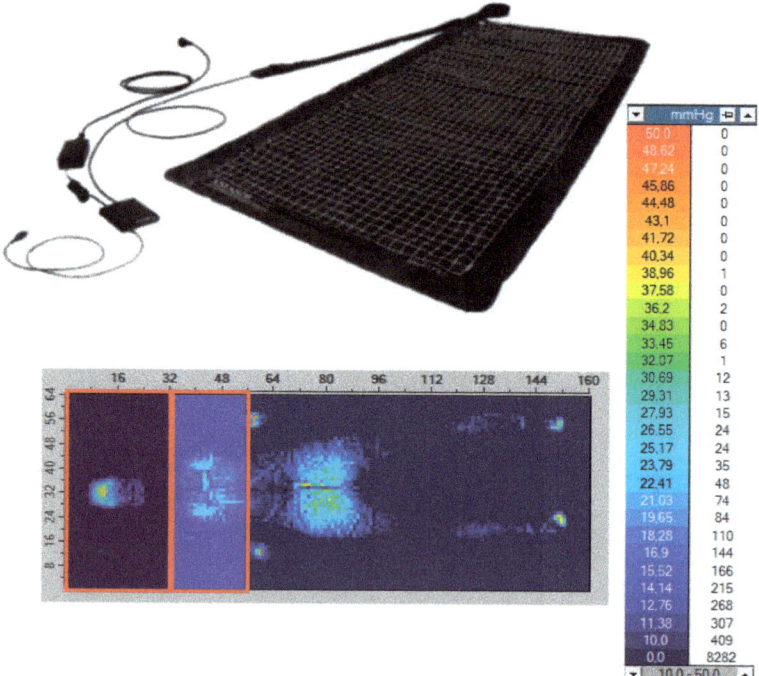

Figure 3. Pressure-mapping blanket (**upper** panel) and pressure distribution map (**lower** panel). Upper panel: The X3 R&D Mattress System is a full body pressure mapping blanket used to accurately test mattresses and mattress components. This blanket consists of 10,240 sensing points. The ComfortMap image shows how well a mattress conforms to a patient's body, and the curve illustrates pressure distribution. For analyzing the pressure distribution, pressure was measured in mmHg and recorded from each sensing point for each participant in each group.

2.4. Experimental Procedure

Participants tried five different pillows on a medium-firm hybrid mattress at room temperature with a humidity of 45–55%. Participants tried the pillows first in the supine position, then side-lying, and finally in the prone position. While trying the pillows, the researchers instructed the participants to relax and then take deep breaths with their eyes closed. Evaluation of body pressure distribution was initiated after participants had inhaled and exhaled at least five times. The participants were advised to retain their arms on both sides of their bodies while lying supine. The participants were allowed to bend their knees while lying on their right side in the side-lying position. Data on the distribution of body pressure in the head and neck were gathered. To decrease tiredness, a two-minute rest interval was provided during the position transfer. To reduce the impact of continuous testing on subjective evaluation, subjects were allowed to get up and move around for 5 min between pillow tests.

2.5. Sample Size

"We used G*Power 3.0.1 (Franz Faul, University of Kiel, Kiel, Germany) to determine the required sample size. With an alpha of 0.05, power of 0.80, effect size of 0.86, and two tails, the software predicted a sample size of 28 (14 per group) based on the means and standard deviations from the pilot study. To account for a 10% dropout rate, we expanded the sample size to 32."

2.6. Statistical Analysis

For continuous variables, mean and standard deviations were computed, and for categorical variables, percentage frequency distributions were computed. The mean and standard deviation were utilized in the descriptive analysis. The Shapiro–Wilk test was performed to determine the normality of the quantitative data. Based on these findings, the Friedman test and various post-hoc comparisons (Bonferroni adjustments) were utilized to compare the five different pillow variables as needed. The "chi-square" test and the "Student's t test" were used to compare the mild and severe FHP groups. p values less than 0.05 were considered statistically significant. SPSS 28.0 (IBM SPSS Inc., Armonk, NY, USA) was used for all statistical analyses.

3. Results

Between January and February 2023, 112 participants were screened, and 34 met the eligibility criteria, entered the study, and were allocated to the mild (17) and severe (17) FHP groups. Four of the participants were excluded because they could not complete the pillow assessment for sensor device or time-related reasons. As a result, the data from these four participants were not included in the analysis. Table 2 shows the distribution of the participants based on the severity of FHP and the similarity between the groups regarding the baseline demographic and clinical characteristics.

In the supine position, Pillow D ($p = 0.011$) provided better head comfort in participants with mild FHP, while Pillow C ($p = 0.045$) and Pillow E ($p = 0.046$) provided better head support. There was no difference between the groups in the rest of the support and comfort parameters of the head and shoulder region ($p > 0.05$). In the side-lying position, the support and comfort values provided by the pillows did not differ between the groups separated according to the FHP degree ($p > 0.05$). In the prone position, the support values provided to the shoulder-upper back region were higher for the A ($p = 0.040$) and D ($p = 0.022$) pillows for individuals with a mild FHP group. There was no difference between the groups in the rest of the support and comfort parameters of the head and shoulder region ($p > 0.05$) (Table 3).

Table 2. Demographic, physical, and psychosocial characteristics of individuals with FHP.

Features	FHP< 2.8 cm (n = 15)	FHP ≥ 2.8cm (n = 15)	p
Gender (n(%)) Female Male	11 4	8 7	0.450 [a]
Age	30.00 ± 7.72	30.60 ± 8.26	0.867 [b]
BMI	23.99 ± 3.12	22.84 ± 3.08	0.714 [b]
Physical Activity Level (IPAQ)	1491 ± 1007	1626 ± 675	0.279 [b]
Pittsburg Sleep Quality Index	5.67 ± 2.80	5.62 ± 2.10	0.959 [b]
Head Anterior Tilt (cm)	1.70 ± 0.77	4.01 ± 0.70	>0.00 [b]

[a] Chi square test, [b] Student's t test. FHP: forward head posture, BMI: body mass index, IPAQ: International Physical Activity Questionnaire, cm: centimeter.

When the comfort and support parameters of pillow materials were compared among all participants, Pillow B and Pillow E provided higher head comfort ($p < 0.001$), while Pillow E also provided higher shoulder support ($p = 0.044$) in the supine position. In other parameters, there was no difference between the pillows ($p > 0.05$). In the side-lying position, Pillow B provided higher head comfort ($p < 0.001$) and Pillow A ($p = 0.003$) higher head support. There was no difference between the pillows in other parameters ($p > 0.05$). In the prone position, Pillow B and Pillow E provided higher head comfort ($p < 0.001$), while Pillow E also provided higher shoulder support ($p = 0.002$). There was no difference between the pillows in other parameters ($p > 0.05$) (Table 4). Pairwise comparisons of pillows with the help of post-hoc tests are also shown in Figure 4.

Table 3. Comfort and support values provided by different pillow designs according to the severity of FHP.

Pillow Designs		FHP < 2.8 cm (n = 15)		FHP ≥ 2.8 cm (n = 15)		p	
Supine Position		Head	Shoulder-Upper Back	Head	Shoulder-Upper Back	Head	Shoulder-Upper Back
Pillow A (Viscose)	Comfort (mmHg)	18.69 ± 2.11	18.44 ± 1.81	19.29 ± 2.06	18.47 ± 2.22	0.445	0.976
	Support (cm²)	308 ± 87	1083 ± 201	301 ± 125	1055 ± 236	0.872	0.731
Pillow B (Fiber)	Comfort (mmHg)	14.65 ± 0.88	18.15 ± 1.84	15.90 ± 2.59	18.72 ± 2.12	0.087	0.438
	Support (cm²)	363 ± 146	1197 ± 226	287 ± 157	1106 ± 262	0.182	0.321
Pillow C (Cotton)	Comfort (mmHg)	16.24 ± 1.46	18.46 ± 1.42	17.52 ± 3.02	18.53 ± 1.72	0.150	0.897
	Support (cm²)	383 ± 164	1148 ± 176	266 ± 140	1150 ± 221	0.045 *	0.980
Pillow D (Wool)	Comfort (mmHg)	16.38 ± 1.20	18.88 ± 1.86	17.59 ± 1.22	18.92 ± 2.26	0.011 *	0.952
	Support (cm²)	392 ± 164	1164 ± 300	288 ± 168	1096 ± 252	0.098	0.509
Pillow E (Goose feather)	Comfort (mmHg)	15.44 ± 1.27	19.18 ± 1.39	16.16 ± 1.20	18.76 ± 1.81	0.289	0.489
	Support (cm²)	427 ± 172	121 ± 225	308 ± 138	1158 ± 231	0.046 *	0.515
Side-lying Position		Head	Shoulder-upper back	Head	Shoulder-upper back	Head	Shoulder-upper back
Pillow A (Viscose)	Comfort (mmHg)	17.58 ± 1.63	22.96 ± 1.93	17.94 ± 2.01	23.13 ± 2.27	0.593	0.824
	Support (cm²)	232 ± 93	1444 ± 258	211 ± 98	1346 ± 270	0.552	0.318
Pillow B (Fiber)	Comfort (mmHg)	15.05 ± 2.42	23.19 ± 1.83	14.71 ± 1.31	23.27 ± 2.49	0.638	0.922
	Support (cm²)	185 ± 101	1548 ± 323	155 ± 65	1399 ± 285	0.349	0.192
Pillow C (Cotton)	Comfort (mmHg)	16.39 ± 2.14	23.44 ± 2.17	16.69 ± 2.66	23.66 ± 2.83	0.741	0.814
	Support (cm²)	167 ± 77	1495 ± 240	153 ± 63	1396 ± 262	0.606	0.291
Pillow D (Wool)	Comfort (mmHg)	16.69 ± 2.66	23.53 ± 2.18	16.89 ± 2.08	22.94 ± 2.58	0.439	0.507
	Support (cm²)	192 ± 85	1491 ± 332	176 ± 81	1383 ± 268	0.605	0.339
Pillow E (Goose feather)	Comfort (mmHg)	16.37 ± 2.39	23.47 ± 1.75	15.65 ± 1.92	23.78 ± 2.66	0.375	0.703
	Support (cm²)	184 ± 100	1555 ± 395	173 ± 46	1383 ± 244	0.707	0.162

Table 3. Cont.

Pillow Designs		FHP < 2.8 cm (n = 15)		FHP ≥ 2.8 cm (n = 15)		p	
Supine Position		Head	Shoulder-Upper Back	Head	Shoulder-Upper Back	Head	Shoulder-Upper Back
Prone Position							
Pillow A (Viscose)	Comfort (mmHg)	18.82 ± 1.77	20.25 ± 2.05	18.45 ± 2.71	19.38 ± 2.73	0.654	0.328
	Support (cm^2)	430 ± 187	1001 ± 291	488 ± 219	788 ± 247	0.444	0.040 *
Pillow B (Fiber)	Comfort (mmHg)	14.86 ± 1.42	20.73 ± 2.64	14.64 ± 0.90	19.04 ± 2.64	0.619	0.092
	Support (cm^2)	403 ± 194	1011 ± 301	499 ± 279	845 ± 167	0.286	0.073
Pillow C (Cotton)	Comfort (mmHg)	16.77 ± 1.77	20.97 ± 2.19	16.36 ± 1.40	19.18 ± 2.84	0.492	0.064
	Support (cm^2)	411 ± 144	991 ± 237	498 ± 268	908 ± 193	0.279	0.299
Pillow D (Wool)	Comfort (mmHg)	17.24 ± 1.72	20.31 ± 2.84	17.55 ± 2.28	20.04 ± 2.46	0.683	0.789
	Support (cm^2)	480 ± 185	970 ± 245	490 ± 269	776 ± 189	0.908	0.022 *
Pillow E (Goose feather)	Comfort (mmHg)	16.23 ± 1.35	21.67 ± 2.44	15.43 ± 1.33	20.09 ± 2.36	0.116	0.083
	Support (cm^2)	461 ± 167	1031 ± 225	442 ± 214	913 ± 214	0.792	0.154

p: Student's t test, FHP: forward head posture, * statistically significant difference.

Table 4. Comparison of comfort and support values provided to individuals with FHP by different pillow designs.

Pillow Designs	FHP (n = 30)						
	Head				Shoulder and Upper Back		
Supine Position	Comfort (mmHg)	p	Support (cm²)	p	Comfort (mmHg)	p	Support (cm²)	p
Pillow A (Viscose)	18.98 ± 2.07 [L]	<0.001 *	304 ± 106	0.948	18.46 ± 1.99	0.455	1069 ± 216 [L]	0.044 *
Pillow B (Fiber)	15.28 ± 2.00 [H]		325 ± 154		18.43 ± 1.97		1151 ± 245	
Pillow C (Cotton)	16.88 ± 2.42 [L]		325 ± 161		18.50 ± 1.55		1149 ± 196	
Pillow D (Wool)	16.99 ± 1.34 [L]		340 ± 171		18.90 ± 2.03		1130 ± 274 [L]	
Pillow E (Goose feather)	15.80 ± 1.80 [H]		368 ± 164		18.97 ± 1.60		1186 ± 226 [H]	
Side-lying Position								
Pillow A (Viscose)	17.76 ± 1.81 [L]	<0.001 *	221 ± 95 [H]	0.003 *	23.05 ± 2.07	0.336	1395 ± 264	0.201
Pillow B (Fiber)	14.88 ± 1.92 [H]		170 ± 85		23.23 ± 2.14		1473 ± 309	
Pillow C (Cotton)	16.54 ± 2.38 [L]		160 ± 70 [L]		23.55 ± 2.48		1445 ± 252	
Pillow D (Wool)	17.18 ± 2.04 [L]		184 ± 82		23.24 ± 2.37		1437 ± 301	
Pillow E (Goose feather)	16.01 ± 2.16		179 ± 77		23.63 ± 2.22		1469 ± 334	
Prone Position								
Pillow A (Viscose)	18.63 ± 2.26 [L]	<0.001 *	459 ± 202	0.960	19.81 ± 2.41	0.076	894 ± 286 [L]	0.002*
Pillow B (Fiber)	14.75 ± 1.18 [H]		451 ± 241		19.89 ± 2.79		928 ± 254	
Pillow C (Cotton)	16.57 ± 1.58 [L]		454 ± 216		20.07 ± 2.65		950 ± 217	
Pillow D (Wool)	17.40 ± 1.99 [L]		485 ± 227		20.17 ± 2.61		873 ± 236 [L]	
Pillow E (Goose feather)	15.83 ± 1.38 [H]		452 ± 189		20.88 ± 2.49		972 ± 224 [H]	

p: Friedman test. [H]: Higher profile pillow compared to pairwise comparisons using Bonferroni correction. [L]: Lower profile pillow compared to pairwise comparisons using Bonferroni correction. FHP: forward head posture, * statistically significant difference.

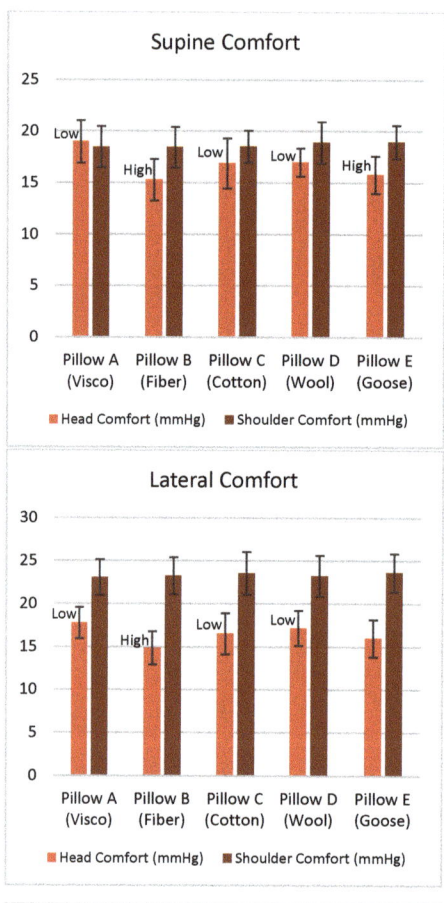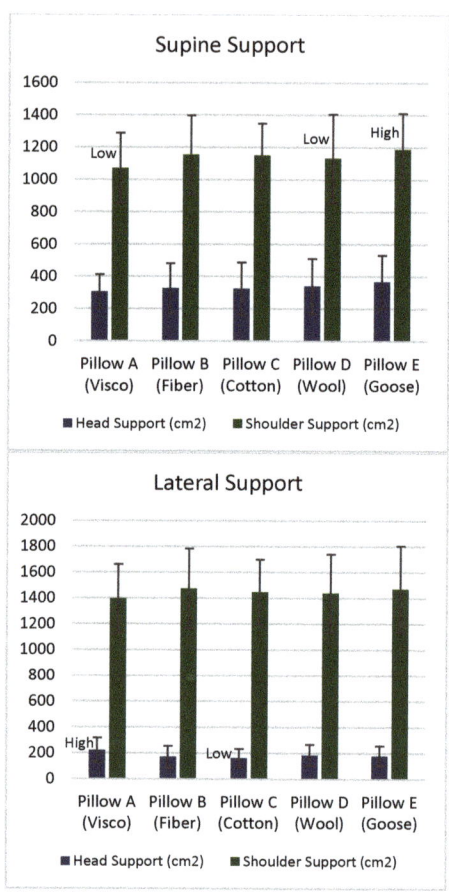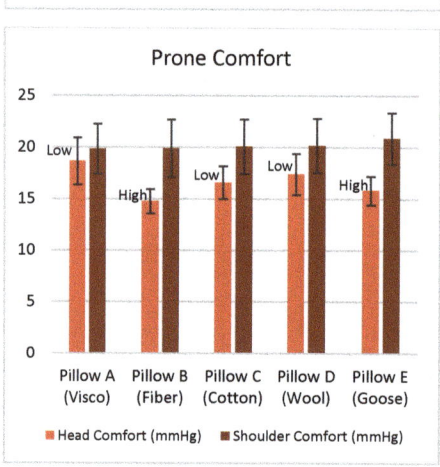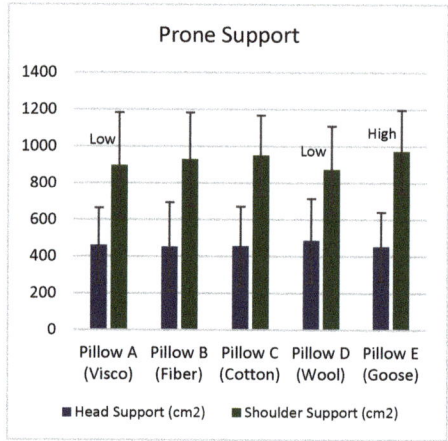

Figure 4. Graphical representation of the comfort and support values provided to individuals with FHP by different pillow designs.

4. Discussion

The higher comfort and better support of the pillow are often used to reduce stress on the body while sleeping. An efficient pillow eliminates unwanted muscle activation, improves spinal support, enhances proprioception, and reduces segmental pressure. Unfortunately, the effects of various pillow materials on the neck and upper back regions of individuals with FHP is still unknown. Our study revealed five main findings. First, in the supine position, Pillow D, made of wool material, provided more head comfort in mild FHP, while Pillow C made of cotton material, and Pillow E made of goose down material, provided more head support in mild FHP. Second, in the prone position, Pillow A, made of viscose material, and Pillow D, made of wool material, provided more upper back support in mild FHP. Thirdly, in the supine position, Pillow B, made of fiber material, and Pillow E, made of goose down material, provided higher levels of head comfort, while Pillow E, made of goose feathers, provided better upper back support. Fourth, in the side-lying position, Pillow B, made of fiber material, provides a higher level of head comfort, while Pillow A, made of cotton material, had better head support. Finally, in the prone position, Pillow B and Pillow E made of fiber and goose down, respectively, provided higher levels of head comfort, while Pillow E, made of goose down, provided better back support. According to our study findings, the comfort and support values provided by different pillow materials may differ according to the posture of the head. In addition, the pillows made of goose down in the supine position provided higher head comfort and better back support than other pillows, the fiber pillow in the side-lying position increased the head comfort, the cotton pillow increased the head support, and the goose down pillows provided higher comfort and better support in the prone position.

Four of the pillows (Pillow B, C, D, and E) we investigated in the studies on comfort and support levels of pillows were classified as "traditional", "standard", or "regular" pillows, while the pillow made of viscose material (Pillow A) was classified as contour-type, ergonomic, or orthopedic. Our first and second findings were related to the fact that the comfort and support levels provided by pillows may vary with the severity of FHP. Previous studies examining the relationship of pillow materials to the cervical spine have generally investigated muscle activations in this region. Fazli et al. showed the ergonomic latex pillow changed the craniovertebral angle and increased the endurance of the neck extensor muscles, unlike traditional pillows [30]. In another study, it was shown all the different pillow designs cause unwanted superficial muscle activation and are not suitable for individuals with FHP [25,40]. Even though these studies that look at how the pillow affects the spine have objective data, there are still indirect ways to measure the health of the spine. Regarding sleep quality and symptoms, pillow shape was the primary cause of the three major sleeping symptoms (head tiredness, neck fatigue, and shoulder pain) that affected sleep quality [41]. Therefore, it can be stated the design of a pillow's shape for each body part (head, neck, and shoulders) is the most significant component for best comfort. Radwan et al. showed moderate evidence that a contoured pillow design containing memory foam or latex material can improve sleep quality and spinal alignment and reduce sleep-related neck pain. In our study, the support and comfort levels provided to the spine by Pillow A, which is contour designed and produced from viscose material, remained not extremely higher than those provided by conventional pillows. This result may have occurred because the spinal alignments in individuals with FHP are different from normal posture [32]. As a result, Pillow A, produced from contour designed viscose material, is insufficient in terms of head comfort and back support for individuals with FHP. Among the traditional pillow materials, we can say Pillow E, produced from goose feather material, is the most suitable pillow for sleeping on the back and in the prone position, while Pillow B, produced from fiber material, is the most suitable pillow for the side-lying position.

According to the other results of our study, effective pillow materials may differ according to sleeping position. There are many pillow parameters that affect sleep comfort and quality. Pillow height influences spinal alignment, activation of cervical muscles, subjective comfort, and overall pressures in the cervical and cranial regions. This variable was standardized by choosing pillows of almost the same height in our study [42,43]. The shape of a pillow is a very important element in pillow design as it contributes to the amount of neck support and the overall comfort level of the wearer. The sleeping position can also determine the most suitable pillow shape for each user. In studies examining the effect of contour pillow design on sleep quality, Gordon et al. analyzed five different pillows similar to our study and found contour pillows, such as Pillow A, provided higher sleep quality and pillow comfort than other traditional feather pillows [44]. Cai and Chen similarly examined an experimentally designed "U-shaped" contour pillow to measure various items related to sleep quality and showed this pillow was effective in increasing rapid eye movement (REM) sleep duration and sleep quality score. These findings suggest contour pillows provide deeper and better-quality sleep [45]. Our study results showed that contrary to the studies mentioned, the support and comfort data provided by the viscose pillow to the spine were lower than those provided by the traditional pillows. Another important element of the pillow is the material. It was concluded that sleep quality, neck comfort, and waking symptoms varied greatly depending on which pillow was used [44]. The effect of pillow materials on the human body has been investigated before. Fazli et al. demonstrated the ergonomic latex pillow increases functional capacity in patients with cervical spondylosis using self-reported subjective methods, such as the Neck Disability Index and the Numerical Pain Rating Scale [46]. Gordon et al. reported the use of latex pillows for 28 days will lead to an increase in quality of life and cervical spine joint opening compared to the use of traditional pillows in patients who wake up at night due to cervical pain. This study was also supported subjectively by the self-report method or by objective measures, such as range of motion, which could not measure the comfort and support value provided by the pillow [47]. Vanti et al. showed that when individuals with nonspecific neck pain regularly used a spring pillow for four weeks, their head and neck pain were significantly reduced. Similarly, these measurements were carried out with indirect outcome measures, such as the Neck Disability Index [48]. Since the objective measurement method used in our study was measured with pressure sensors, independent of the participant's feedback, there was no need for an average evaluation period of four weeks, such as other studies. The comfort and support values investigated in previous studies were subjectively obtained from the participants by the self-reporting method [39]. We used the Visual Analog Scale to measure pillow comfort subjectively. In a prior study, orthopedic pillows were found to be more comfortable than traditional pillows when evaluated with the VAS [49]. However, our study is unique in that we utilized objective measures to evaluate the comfort and support properties of pillow materials and their association with cervical spine disorders. Our study is the first to use objective outcome measures for comfort and support values of pillow materials and to examine their relationship with cervical spine disorders.

Our study is the first to use objective measures to look at how comfortable and supportive different pillow materials are and how they relate to problems with the neck and spine. Similar to our study, other studies were conducted to measure the support and comfort values of pillows with the help of pressure sensors; however, these studies did not evaluate the pillow material. Kim et al. investigated the comfort values provided by different pillow shapes with the help of a pressure mat and showed the contour designed pillow reduced the pressure values in the occipital region [50]. Ren et al. investigated the pressure values provided by four different pillows, whose heights vary between 11 and 17 cm, with the help of a pressure mat and stated the height of the pillow with the least pressure on the head is 11 cm [28].

Study Limitations

Firstly, the study's sample size could have been larger, which is the first limitation. Participants were evaluated in a state of completely relaxed rest, rather than during actual sleep, limiting the clinical application of these findings to asymptomatic adults. Additionally, only a medium-firm hybrid mattress was used, and while conventional pillows were of similar height, the viscose pillow's height differed due to production standards, which is another limitation. Sleep health includes both subjective and objective parameters, and although the study objectively demonstrated spine-related comfort and support parameters, these data alone cannot explain sleep quality and comfort levels. Future studies should include subjective outcome measurements taken from individuals using the self-report method to support the results. Despite having clear exclusion criteria, we did not ask the participants about ear diseases or breathing problems, which could affect their posture and sleep, indicating another limitation of the study.

5. Conclusions

This study showed pillow materials affect the spine comfort and support of the participants, and these values may vary according to different spinal alignments, such as FHP. According to the preferred sleeping position, the pillow material that supports the spine and increases its comfort will also change. This study revealed the pillows that support the spine of the individual and provide comfort objectively. These results can be blended with the preferences and feedback of the people about the pillow in future studies and may help in choosing a personalized pillow.

Author Contributions: Conceptualization, C.T. and T.D.; methodology, C.T., T.D. and S.Y.E.; formal analysis, C.T. and Z.E.; investigation, C.T., S.Y.E. and T.D.; data curation, C.T., Z.E. and S.Y.E.; writing—original draft preparation, C.T. and S.Y.E.; writing—review and editing, T.D. and Z.E. All authors have read and agreed to the published version of the manuscript.

Funding: This research received no external funding.

Institutional Review Board Statement: The study was conducted in accordance with the Declaration of Helsinki and approved by the Ethics Committee at Çankırı Karatekin University (Approval number: 19/01/2023-30).

Informed Consent Statement: Informed consent was obtained from all subjects involved in the study.

Data Availability Statement: Data is unavailable due to privacy or ethical restrictions.

Acknowledgments: This work was supported by the Doganlar Holding.

Conflicts of Interest: The authors have no conflicts of interest to declare regarding this study.

References

1. Hartvigsen, J.; Leboeuf-Yde, C.; Lings, S.; Corder, E.H. Is sitting-while-at-work associated with low back pain? A systematic, critical literature review. *Scand. J. Public Health* **2000**, *28*, 230. [CrossRef]
2. Dubey, N.; Dubey, G.; Tripathi, H.; Naqvi, Z.A. Ergonomics for desk job workers-an overview. *Int. J. Health Sci. Res.* **2019**, *9*, 257–266.
3. Li, Y.; Wu, J.; Lu, C.; Tang, Z.; Li, C. Pillow Support Model with Partitioned Matching Based on Body Pressure Distribution Matrix. *Healthcare* **2021**, *9*, 571. [CrossRef]
4. Vaz, G.; Roussouly, P.; Berthonnaud, E.; Dimnet, J. Sagittal morphology and equilibrium of pelvis and spine. *Eur. Spine J.* **2001**, *11*, 80–87. [CrossRef] [PubMed]
5. Yu-Chi, L.; Chih-Yun, L.; Mao-Jiun, W. Better combination of thickness and hardness of mattress topper for supine sleeping posture: A physiological measurements evaluation. *Int. J. Ind. Ergon.* **2020**, *78*, 102979. [CrossRef]
6. Low, F.-Z.; Chua, M.C.-H.; Lim, P.-Y.; Yeow, C.-H. Effects of Mattress Material on Body Pressure Profiles in Different Sleeping Postures. *J. Chiropr. Med.* **2017**, *16*, 1–9. [CrossRef] [PubMed]
7. Chen, Z.; Li, Y.; Liu, R.; Gao, D.; Chen, Q.; Hu, Z.; Guo, J. Effects of Interface Pressure Distribution on Human Sleep Quality. *PLoS ONE* **2014**, *9*, e99969. [CrossRef] [PubMed]
8. Lei, J.-X.; Yang, P.-F.; Yang, A.-L.; Gong, Y.-F.; Shang, P.; Yuan, X.-C. Ergonomic Consideration in Pillow Height Determinants and Evaluation. *Healthcare* **2021**, *9*, 1333. [CrossRef]
9. Park, I.; Suzuki, C.; Suzuki, Y.; Kawana, F.; Yajima, K.; Fukusumi, S.; Satoh, M. Effects of Body Pillow Use on Sleeping Posture and Sleep Architecture in Healthy Young Adults. *Sleep Med. Res.* **2021**, *12*, 57–63. [CrossRef]
10. Wu, J.; Yuan, H.; Li, X. A novel method for comfort assessment in a supine sleep position using three-dimensional scanning technology. *Int. J. Ind. Ergon.* **2018**, *67*, 104–113. [CrossRef]
11. Andreoni, G.; Santambrogio, G.C.; Rabuffetti, M.; Pedotti, A. Method for the analysis of posture and interface pressure of car drivers. *Appl. Ergon.* **2002**, *33*, 511–522. [CrossRef] [PubMed]

12. Porter, J.; Gyi, D.; Tait, H.A. Interface pressure data and the prediction of driver discomfort in road trials. *Appl. Ergon.* **2003**, *34*, 207–214. [CrossRef]
13. Le, P.; Rose, J.; Knapik, G.; Marras, W.S. Objective classification of vehicle seat discomfort. *Ergonomics* **2014**, *57*, 536–544. [CrossRef] [PubMed]
14. de Looze, M.P.; Kuijt-Evers, L.F.; van Dieën, J. Sitting comfort and discomfort and the relationships with objective measures. *Ergonomics* **2003**, *46*, 985–997. [CrossRef]
15. Tanaka, S.; Midorikawa, T.; Tokura, H. Effects of pressure exerted on the skin by elastic cord on the core temperature, body weight loss and salivary secretion rate at 35 °C. *Eur. J. Appl. Physiol.* **2005**, *96*, 471–476. [CrossRef] [PubMed]
16. Jeong, J.-R.; Kim, H.-E. Effects of skin pressure by an all-in-one undergarment on core temperature and the secretion of urinary melatonin. *Biol. Rhythm. Res.* **2009**, *40*, 317–324. [CrossRef]
17. Miyatsuji, A.; Matsumoto, T.; Mitarai, S.; Kotabe, T.; Takeshima, T.; Watanuki, S. Effects of Clothing Pressure Caused by Different Types of Brassieres on Autonomic Nervous System Activity Evaluated by Heart Rate Variability Power Spectral Analysis. *J. Physiol. Anthr. Appl. Hum. Sci.* **2002**, *21*, 67–74. [CrossRef]
18. Zhong, S.; Shen, L.; Zhou, L.; Guan, Z. Predict human body indentation lying on a spring mattress using a neural network approach. *Proc. Inst. Mech. Eng. Part H: J. Eng. Med.* **2014**, *228*, 787–799. [CrossRef]
19. Leilnahari, K.; Fatouraee, N.; Khodalotfi, M.; Sadeghein, M.A.; Kashani, Y.A. Spine alignment in men during lateral sleep position: Experimental study and modeling. *Biomed. Eng. Online* **2011**, *10*, 103. [CrossRef]
20. Huysmans, T.; Haex, B.; De Wilde, T.; Van Audekercke, R.; Sloten, J.V.; Van der Perre, G. A 3D active shape model for the evaluation of the alignment of the spine during sleeping. *Gait Posture* **2006**, *24*, 54–61. [CrossRef]
21. Ambrogio, N.; Cuttiford, J.; Lineker, S.; Li, L. A comparison of three types of neck support in fibromyalgia patients. *Arthritis Rheum.* **1998**, *11*, 405–410. [CrossRef] [PubMed]
22. Radwan, A.; Fess, P.; James, D.; Murphy, J.; Myers, J.; Rooney, M.; Taylor, J.; Torii, A. Effect of different mattress designs on promoting sleep quality, pain reduction, and spinal alignment in adults with or without back pain; systematic review of controlled trials. *Sleep Health* **2015**, *1*, 257–267. [CrossRef] [PubMed]
23. Hoy, D.; Protani, M.; De, R.; Buchbinder, R. The epidemiology of neck pain. *Best Pract. Res. Clin. Rheumatol.* **2010**, *24*, 783–792. [CrossRef]
24. Worlikar, A.N.; Shah, M.R. Incidence of forward head posture and associated problems in desktop users. *Int. J. Health Sci. Res.* **2019**, *9*, 96–100.
25. Kiatkulanusorn, S.; Suato, B.P.; Werasirirat, P. Analysis of neck and back muscle activity during the application of various pillow designs in patients with forward head posture. *J. Back Musculoskelet. Rehabil.* **2021**, *34*, 431–439. [CrossRef] [PubMed]
26. Diab, A.A.; Moustafa, I. The efficacy of forward head correction on nerve root function and pain in cervical spondylotic radiculopathy: A randomized trial. *Clin. Rehabil.* **2011**, *26*, 351–361. [CrossRef] [PubMed]
27. Liu, S.-F.; Lee, Y.-L.; Liang, J.-C. Shape design of an optimal comfortable pillow based on the analytic hierarchy process method. *J. Chiropr. Med.* **2011**, *10*, 229–239. [CrossRef] [PubMed]
28. Ren, S.; Wong, D.W.-C.; Yang, H.; Zhou, Y.; Lin, J.; Zhang, M. Effect of pillow height on the biomechanics of the head-neck complex: Investigation of the cranio-cervical pressure and cervical spine alignment. *PeerJ* **2016**, *4*, e2397. [CrossRef]
29. Silverman, J.L.; Rodriquez, A.A.; Agre, J.C. Quantitative cervical flexor strength in healthy subjects and in subjects with mechanical neck pain. *Arch. Phys. Med. Rehabil.* **1991**, *72*, 679–681.
30. Fazli, F.; Farahmand, B.; Azadinia, F.; Amiri, A. The Effect of Ergonomic Latex Pillow on Head and Neck Posture and Muscle Endurance in Patients With Cervical Spondylosis: A Randomized Controlled Trial. *J. Chiropr. Med.* **2019**, *18*, 155–162. [CrossRef]
31. Wong, D.W.-C.; Wang, Y.; Lin, J.; Tan, Q.; Chen, T.L.-W.; Zhang, M. Sleeping mattress determinants and evaluation: A biomechanical review and critique. *PeerJ* **2019**, *7*, e6364. [CrossRef] [PubMed]
32. Radwan, A.; Ashton, N.; Gates, T.; Kilmer, A.; VanFleet, M. Effect of different pillow designs on promoting sleep comfort, quality, & spinal alignment: A systematic review. *Eur. J. Integr. Med.* **2020**, *42*, 101269. [CrossRef]
33. Gordon, S.J.; Grimmer, K.; Trott, P. Pillow use: The behaviour of cervical pain, sleep quality and pillow comfort in side sleepers. *Man. Ther.* **2009**, *14*, 671–678. [CrossRef]
34. Gordon, S.J.; Grimmer-Somers, K.A.; Trott, P.H. A randomized, comparative trial: Does pillow type alter cervico-thoracic spinal posture when side lying? *J. Multidiscip. Healthc.* **2011**, *4*, 321–327. [CrossRef] [PubMed]
35. Gu, S.-Y.; Hwangbo, G.; Lee, J.-H. Relationship between position sense and reposition errors according to the degree of upper crossed syndrome. *J. Phys. Ther. Sci.* **2016**, *28*, 438–441. [CrossRef]
36. Buysse, D.J.; Reynolds, C.F., III; Monk, T.H.; Berman, S.R.; Kupfer, D.J. The Pittsburgh sleep quality index: A new instrument for psychiatric practice and research. *Psychiatry Res.* **1989**, *28*, 193–213. [CrossRef] [PubMed]
37. Saglam, M.; Arikan, H.; Savci, S.; Inal-Ince, D.; Bosnak-Guclu, M.; Karabulut, E.; Tokgozoglu, L. International Physical Activity Questionnaire: Reliability and Validity of the Turkish Version. *Percept. Mot. Ski.* **2010**, *111*, 278–284. [CrossRef] [PubMed]
38. Iacob, S.M.P.; Chisnoiu, A.M.P.; Lascu, L.M.P.; Berar, A.M.P.; Studnicska, D.M.; Fluerasu, M.I.P. Is PostureScreen®Mobile app an accurate tool for dentists to evaluate the correlation between malocclusion and posture? *Cranio* **2020**, *38*, 233–239. [CrossRef] [PubMed]
39. Szucs, K.A.; Brown, E.V.D. Rater reliability and construct validity of a mobile application for posture analysis. *J. Phys. Ther. Sci.* **2018**, *30*, 31–36. [CrossRef] [PubMed]

40. Kiatkulanusorn, S.; Luangpon, N.; Tudpor, K. Increased upper and lower trapezius muscle activities during rest in side-lying position in young adults with forward head posture. *Indian J. Physiother. Occup. Ther.* **2020**, *14*, 271–276.
41. Son, J.; Jung, S.; Song, H.; Kim, J.; Bang, S.; Bahn, S. A Survey of Koreans on Sleep Habits and Sleeping Symptoms Relating to Pillow Comfort and Support. *Int. J. Environ. Res. Public Health* **2020**, *17*, 302. [CrossRef]
42. Kim, H.C.; Jun, H.S.; Kim, J.H.; Ahn, J.H.; Chang, I.B.; Song, J.H.; Oh, J.K. The Effect of Different Pillow Heights on the Parameters of Cervicothoracic Spine Segments. *Korean J. Spine* **2015**, *12*, 135–138. [CrossRef]
43. Sacco, I.C.; Pereira, I.L.; Dinato, R.C.; Silva, V.C.; Friso, B.; Viterbo, S.F. The Effect of Pillow Height on Muscle Activity of the Neck and Mid-Upper Back and Patient Perception of Comfort. *J. Manip. Physiol. Ther.* **2015**, *38*, 375–381. [CrossRef]
44. Gordon, S.J.; Grimmer-Somers, K. Your Pillow May Not Guarantee a Good Night's Sleep or Symptom-Free Waking. *Physiother. Can.* **2011**, *63*, 183–190. [CrossRef] [PubMed]
45. Cai, D.; Chen, H.-L. Ergonomic approach for pillow concept design. *Appl. Ergon.* **2016**, *52*, 142–150. [CrossRef] [PubMed]
46. Fazli, F.; Farahmand, B.; Azadinia, F.; Amiri, A. A preliminary study: The effect of ergonomic latex pillow on pain and dis-ability in patients with cervical spondylosis. *Med. J. Islam Repub. Iran.* **2018**, *32*, 81. [CrossRef]
47. Gordon, S.J.; Grimmer, K.A.; Buttner, P. Pillow preferences of people with neck pain and known spinal degeneration: A pilot randomized controlled trial. *Eur. J. Phys. Rehabil. Med.* **2020**, *55*, 783–791. [CrossRef]
48. Vanti, C.; Banchelli, F.; Marino, C.; Puccetti, A.; Guccione, A.A.; Pillastrini, P. Effectiveness of a "spring pillow" versus ed-ucation in chronic nonspecific neck pain: A randomized controlled trial. *Phys. Ther.* **2019**, *99*, 1177–1188. [CrossRef]
49. Jeon, M.Y.; Jeong, H.; Lee, S.; Choi, W.; Park, J.H.; Tak, S.J.; Choi, D.H.; Yim, J. Improving the Quality of Sleep with an Optimal Pillow: A Randomized, Comparative Study. *Tohoku J. Exp. Med.* **2014**, *233*, 183–188. [CrossRef] [PubMed]
50. Kim, J.H.; Won, B.H.; Sim, W.S.; Jang, K.S. Biomechanical Effectiveness and Anthropometric Design Aspects of 3-dimensional Contoured Pillow. *J. Ergon. Soc. Korea* **2016**, *35*, 503–517. [CrossRef]

Disclaimer/Publisher's Note: The statements, opinions and data contained in all publications are solely those of the individual author(s) and contributor(s) and not of MDPI and/or the editor(s). MDPI and/or the editor(s) disclaim responsibility for any injury to people or property resulting from any ideas, methods, instructions or products referred to in the content.

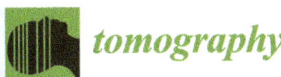

Article

The Efficacy of CT Temporal Subtraction Images for Fibrodysplasia Ossificans Progressiva

Mami Iima [1,2,*], Ryo Sakamoto [1], Takahide Kakigi [1], Akira Yamamoto [1,3], Bungo Otsuki [4], Yuji Nakamoto [1], Junya Toguchida [4,5] and Shuichi Matsuda [4]

1. Department of Diagnostic Imaging and Nuclear Medicine, Graduate School of Medicine, Kyoto University, 54 Shogoin-Kawaharacho, Sakyo-ku, Kyoto 606-8507, Japan
2. Institute for Advancement of Clinical and Translational Science (iACT), Kyoto University Hospital, 54 Shogoin-Kawaharacho, Sakyo-ku, Kyoto 606-8507, Japan
3. Medical Education Center, Kyoto University, Yoshida Konoe-cho, Sakyo-ku, Kyoto 606-8501, Japan
4. Department of Orthopaedic Surgery, Graduate School of Medicine, Kyoto University, 54 Shogoin-Kawaharacho, Sakyo-ku, Kyoto 606-8507, Japan
5. Department of Fundamental Cell Technology, Center for iPS Cell Research and Application, Kyoto University, 53 Shogoin-Kawahara-cho, Sakyo-ku, Kyoto 606-8507, Japan
* Correspondence: mamiiima@kuhp.kyoto-u.ac.jp

Abstract: Purpose: To evaluate the usefulness of CT temporal subtraction (TS) images for detecting emerging or growing ectopic bone lesions in fibrodysplasia ossificans progressiva (FOP). Materials and Methods: Four patients with FOP were retrospectively included in this study. TS images were produced by subtracting previously registered CT images from the current images. Two residents and two board-certified radiologists independently interpreted a pair of current and previous CT images for each subject with or without TS images. Changes in the visibility of the lesion, the usefulness of TS images for lesions with TS images, and the interpreter's confidence level in their interpretation of each scan were assessed on a semiquantitative 5-point scale (0–4). The Wilcoxon signed-rank test was used to compare the evaluated scores between datasets with and without TS images. Results: The number of growing lesions tended to be larger than that of the emerging lesions in all cases. A higher sensitivity was found in residents and radiologists using TS compared to those not using TS. For all residents and radiologists, the dataset with TS tended to have more false-positive scans than the dataset without TS. All the interpreters recognized TS as useful, and confidence levels when using TS tended to be lower or the same as when not using TS for two residents and one radiologist. Conclusions: TS improved the sensitivity of all interpreters in detecting emerging or growing ectopic bone lesions in patients with FOP. TS could be applied further, including the areas of systematic bone disease.

Keywords: fibrodysplasia ossificans progressive; bone; computed tomography; image processing; computer-assisted

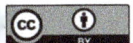

1. Introduction

Fibrodysplasia ossificans progressiva (FOP) is a very rare genetic disorder that causes systemic and progressive ossification in various fibrous tissues such as muscles, tendons, and ligaments throughout the body, often preceded by an episode of painful soft tissue swellings called flare-ups. This leads to a reduced range of motion and ankylosis of limb joints, and reduced mobility and deformity of the trunk [1]. Over the course of their lives, patients develop a second skeleton, resulting in the growing risk of immobility and early death arising from infectious diseases, thoracic insufficiency, and traumatic falls [2].

Plain X-rays, ultrasound, MRI, and CT scans are used at different stages of FOP, and CT is most frequently used for monitoring patients with FOP [3]. MRI is superior to ultrasound for evaluating edema in the early stages of an FOP flare-up, and the early detection of perosseous lesions can also be assessed using MRI [4].

Although the analog method for radiographic assessment of ectopic bone in FOP has been proposed and the strong correlation of ectopic bone lesions with ectopic bone volumes has been demonstrated [5], the evaluation of ectopic bone lesions from radiographs at various anatomic locations cannot be easily performed, which restricts the applicability of this approach in clinical practice.

CT images are more effective than plain radiographs for evaluating ectopic bone lesions of FOP [4], and the sensitivity of whole-body computed tomography (WBCT) is higher than dual-energy X-ray absorptiometry (DXA) for evaluating disease progression in patients with FOP [6]. However, as FOP lesions can arise in any part of the body, evaluating all of the individual lesions in detail takes more time and effort as the number of lesions increases.

Thus, there is a need for a new method that can easily capture image findings and will be useful for the evaluation of disease progression and treatment response in FOP [4].

A temporal subtraction (TS) technique has been developed to subtract a previous image from the current scan using medical images taken at two different points in a time series [7–14]. TS images obtained using an advanced nonrigid image registration algorithm, termed large deformation diffeomorphic metric mapping (LDDMM), have been found useful for detecting various lesions such as lung nodules [9], bone metastases [12,14], and cerebral infarctions [13]. The TS image technique is considered beneficial for analyzing focal temporal changes, especially in ectopic ossification diseases such as FOP, which require a detailed evaluation of lesions occurring in any part of the whole body. Thus, the purpose of this study was to evaluate the usefulness of TS images in the detection of emerging or growing ectopic bone lesions in patients with FOP.

2. Materials and Methods

2.1. Study Population

This retrospective study was approved by our institutional review board and included four patients (16, 18, 25, and 55 years old, three male and one female) diagnosed with FOP. CT scans were performed between 1 March 2016 and 31 December 2019. One patient's images were selected for interpreters to practice evaluating TS images and were thus not included in the analysis. Out of the remaining three patients, two were scanned three times and one was scanned four times using CT (Aquilion PRIME, Aquilion ONE Vision Edition, Canon Medical Systems, Otawara, Japan). The CT images were reconstructed with a slice thickness of 1 mm using a soft-tissue kernel (FC13). The interval of the scans was 201 ± 59 days (mean and standard deviation).

2.2. Generation of TS Images

The TS images were generated using a dedicated workstation: Vitrea SURE Subtraction Time Lapse Ortho (Canon Medical Systems, Otawara, Japan). In brief, following the nonrigid registration of the previous and current CT images using LDDMM, TS images were produced by subtracting the previously registered CT images from the current CT images in each interval. Thus, seven datasets of TS images (two patients for 2 intervals and one patient for 3 intervals) were generated and evaluated by interpreters (Table 1).

The detailed process for obtaining TS images is described in a previous report [14].

2.3. Searching Ectopic Bone Lesions

Two residents (M.K. and E.N.) with 1–2 months' experience interpreting CT images and two board-certified radiologists (M.I. and T.K.) with more than ten years of experience independently interpreted a pair of current and previous CT images for each subject with and without TS images in the axial orientation. All interpreters were familiarized with TS images by reading two datasets of TS images from one patient prior to the study evaluation; the practice readings were not included in the analysis. The interpreters were allowed to change the window level and window width. They were informed of the patient's age and sex and that the patient had FOP, and they were blinded to all other clinical data.

Image interpretation was conducted twice for each image dataset, with and without TS images. The order of the datasets was randomized. One resident and one radiologist interpreted first without TS images and then with TS images, and vice versa for the other resident and radiologist. An interval of more than 30 days was set between the two reading sessions to minimize the memory effect.

They were asked to identify newly emerging or growing ectopic bone lesions in each interval. Ectopic bone lesions were defined as hyper intense lesions (over 200 H.U., approximately) outside or adjacent to normal skeletal bone, such as in the subcutaneous regions, muscles, and skeletal joints; the evaluation range was from the first thoracic spine level to that of ischial tuberosity. Emerging lesions were those that did not exist in the previous image, but appeared in the current image; growing lesions were those that existed in the previous image and were enlarged in the current image.

The other board-certified radiologist (R.S.), with more than ten years of experience, reviewed the CT images to evaluate the emerging or growing ectopic bone lesions between the two serial scans, and these evaluations were defined as the reference standards. R.S. then judged all of the lesions detected by the interpreters as identical or not identical to the reference standards.

2.4. Evaluation of TS Images

The following three surveys were conducted, and evaluation items were scored on a 5-point scale:

- Survey 1: The visibility of lesion changes on a per-lesion basis (0, difficult to see; 1, slightly difficult to see; 2, neither hard nor easy to see; 3, slightly easy to see; 4, easy to see).
- Survey 2: The usefulness of TS images to identify lesions on a per-lesion basis (0, useless; 1, not very useful; 2, somewhat useful; 3, very useful; 4, extremely useful).
- Survey 3: The confidence level of the interpreter in their interpretation of each scan (0, very low; 1, low; 2, moderate; 3, high; 4, very high).

The reading time of each session was also recorded.

2.5. Statistical Analysis

Lesion-based sensitivity and false-positive rates per scan were estimated.

The Wilcoxon signed-rank test was used to assess differences in the scores of survey 1 and survey 3 between the datasets with and without TS images. The statistical analysis was performed using MedCalc version 20.211 (MedCalc, Mariakerke, Belgium).

3. Results

The number of emerging and growing lesions as the reference standard is described in Table 1. The number of growing lesions tended to be greater than the number of emerging lesions in all cases.

Table 1. The number of emerging and growing lesions for each case and their intervals.

	Interval 1		Interval 2		Interval 3		
	Emerging	Growing	Emerging	Growing	Emerging	Growing	
Case A	0	6	0	5	n/a	n/a	
Case B	0	2	0	3	n/a	n/a	
Case C	4	4	4	6	4	5	
Total	4	12	4	14	4	5	43

Cases A and B had two scans each, and Case C had three scans at follow-up.

TS images were successfully generated in all cases. The processing time used in this study was approximately 30 min per case.

The diagnostic performance in detecting newly ectopic bone lesions is shown in Table 2. The detection sensitivity of both residents and radiologists tended to be greater when using TS compared to when not using TS. The false-positive rates per scan tended to increase when using TS for both residents and radiologists.

Table 2. The diagnostic performance in detecting newly ectopic bone lesions without and with TS.

		Resident A	Resident B	Radiologist A	Radiologist B
Sensitivity (%)	Without TS	25.6	14.0	16.3	20.9
	With TS	51.2	30.2	41.9	46.5
Number of false-positive cases	Without TS	0	0	2	0
	With TS	7	3	1	1

Table 3 shows the scores for the visibility of new lesions (survey 1), the usefulness of TS images for identifying lesions (survey 2), the confidence levels of the interpreters in their interpretation for each scan (survey 3), and the reading time for each interpreter. The scores of survey 1 were comparable for all interpreters. In survey 2, all interpreters recognized TS as useful, and the radiologists tended to find TS more useful than the residents. The confidence levels for most interpreters tended to be the same or decreased when using TS compared to when not using TS, except for the confidence level of radiologist A, which was significantly higher when using TS.

Table 3. The scores for each survey and the reading times.

		Resident A	Resident B	Radiologist A	Radiologist B
Survey 1	Without TS	2 (0–4)	2 (0–3)	2 (0–4)	4 (0–4)
	With TS	1.5 (0–4)	2 (1–3)	2 (1–4)	4 (3–4)
Survey 2		3 (0–4)	3 (1–4)	4 (0–4)	4 (1–4)
Survey 3	Without TS	3 (1–3)	0 (0–2)	2 (1–3)	4 (4–4)
	With TS	2 (2–4)	0 (0–2)	3 (3–4) *	3 (1–4)
Reading time	Without TS	718 ± 266	1543 ± 477	814 ± 162	429 ± 160
	With TS	1920 ± 876	891 ± 258	780 ± 211	437 ± 161

Survey 1: Visibility of new lesions (0, difficult to see; 1, slightly difficult to see; 2, neither hard nor easy to see; 3, slightly easy to see; 4, easy to see). Survey 2: Usefulness of TS images for identifying lesions (0, useless; 1, not very useful; 2, somewhat useful; 3, very useful; 4, extremely useful). Survey 3: Confidence level of the interpreter in their interpretation of each scan (0, very low; 1, low; 2, moderate; 3, high; 4, very high) on a 5-point scale. Median values with ranges are shown for each survey. Reading times are demonstrated as means with standard deviations. * Significant difference ($p = 0.02$).

The reading times decreased when using TS compared to when not using TS for all interpreters, except for resident A (Table 3).

Representative Cases

Representative cases are shown in Figures 1 and 2. Both cases showed better detectability of emerging or growing ossifications when using TS compared to when not using TS.

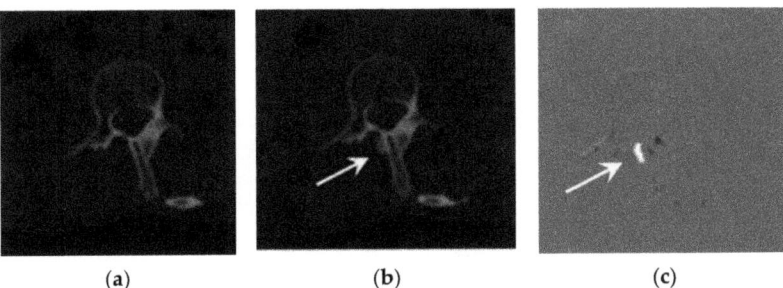

Figure 1. Example of an emerging lesion. CT images of a 25-year-old FOP patient: (**a**) previous CT image, (**b**) current CT image, and (**c**) TS (subtraction) image. The emerging lesion adjacent to the thoracic spine (arrow) is difficult to detect on the current CT image, but is clearly visible in the TS image.

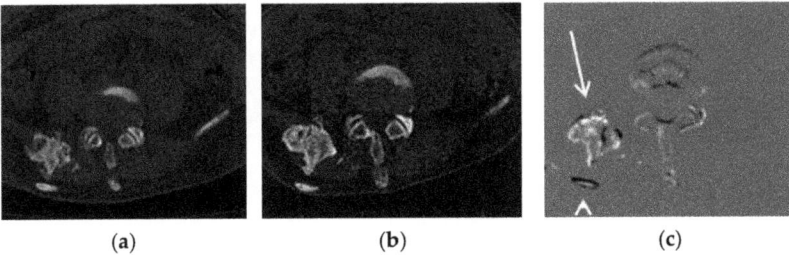

Figure 2. Example of a growing lesion. CT images of a 16-year-old FOP patient: (**a**) previous CT image, (**b**) current CT image, and (**c**) TS (subtraction) image. The growing lesion near the ilium (arrow) is difficult to detect in the current CT image, but is clearly visible in the TS image. The dorsal rib of this lesion (arrowhead) is shown due to misregistration.

4. Discussion

This study investigated the utility of TS imaging by evaluating observers' performance in detecting emerging or growing ectopic bone lesions in FOP patients. The accurate detection of new ectopic bone lesions during the follow-up of FOP patients is considered important in routine diagnostic imaging, which requires professional and substantial efforts by radiologists during routine CT scans, and would be challenging for orthopedists or pediatricians who consult with FOP patients in clinical practice.

Sensitivity when using CT images with TS in detecting emerging or growing ectopic bone lesions was found to be higher than when using CT images without TS, which was in agreement with the previous study investigating the TS detectability of bone metastases [15]. These results indicate the usefulness of TS in the detection of emerging or growing ectopic bone lesions, which is sometimes challenging with conventional CT images, as these lesions can develop in any part of the skeleton [16] and are uncommon for radiologists as well as residents. In addition, there is no additional acquisition time or radiation exposure necessary for generating TS images, as TS images are calculated from CT images acquired in routine clinical practice. The processing time was comparable to that reported in a previous study [14,15], and drastically shortened compared to the initial investigation [12] due to the improvements in the TS processing software. We expect that, with a shorter processing time, TS can be made more readily available in clinical settings.

Sensitivity when using TS to detect new ectopic lesions was 30.2–51.2%, which was inferior to the results reported for a previous investigation (54%) that evaluated the diagnostic performance value of TS in detecting bone metastases. Sensitivity was also variable, perhaps due to the rarity of FOP patients and thus the lack of experience in reading such images. However, a slightly inferior sensitivity in the detection of bone lesions in FOP patients compared to bone metastasis in cancer patients would still be of value for both patients and radiologists, providing more effective and efficient detection of issues that are challenging to detect due to the nonspecific location of potential lesions and the rarity of the disease.

In addition to the improvement in sensitivity, the number of false positives per case when using TS tended to be higher than when not using TS for three out of the four interpreters. This was partially due to the misregistrations of TS in some cases (Figure 2 and [12]). It is well known that the image quality of TS images significantly affect diagnostic performance [17], and a further improvement in the image registration algorithm would be desirable for more accurate diagnosis.

All the interpreters found the TS images useful for detecting new bone lesions (3–4 scores); however, the visibility of FOP lesions showed no significant difference, whether using TS or not. Once the interpreters had detected the new bone lesions, there seems to have been little value added by TS in their visibility, as they were calcified lesions with high contrast in CT images.

The level of confidence in their interpretation of each scan was variable among interpreters, except for the significantly higher confidence level of radiologist A when using TS compared to when not using TS. Ectopic bone lesions, unlike bone metastases, often occur adjacent to normal bones [3,18], such as continuous sclerosis protruding from the bone or isolated periosteal sclerosis, as opposed to a lesion within the normal bone. As the error signals arising from misregistration in TS appear at the edge of bones [12], three interpreters might have had difficulty in distinguishing true ectopic bone lesions from misregistration errors when reading TS.

The reading time was significantly shortened when using TS for each interpreter except for resident A, which indicates the ability of TS to provide an efficient diagnostic enhancement in the detection of new bone lesions. The significantly longer TS image reading time for one resident might have been due to the complexity of the evaluation task.

Our study suggests that bone TS images have the potential to be applied in other areas, including the detection of systemic bone diseases, such as osteomalacia, ankylosing spondylitis, or diffuse idiopathic skeletal hyperostosis. As comparison of images at two time points is fundamental to evaluating lesion progression, the TS technique is expected to be used in a wide range of diseases.

There are several limitations in this study. First, this was a retrospective single-center study with a small number of patients, because FOP is a rare disease.

A study with a larger population and longer duration will need to be conducted in the near future to validate these results. Moreover, the prediction of ectopic bone emergence could be investigated, as CT analysis has been found to be useful for the prediction of bone lesions' emergence, such as metastasis. Changes in bone mineral density obtained from CT images might also be potentially sensitive to fracture-related bone changes [11].

Second, there was a small number of interpreters, as this was a preliminary study to investigate whether TS images can be applied to follow-up evaluation of FOP lesions. Third, only pairs of thin-slice (1 mm) CT images were evaluated, whereas pairs of thin-slice CT images are not always available in clinical settings. Fourth, the generation of TS images requires both current and previous images. This method might not be useful for the initial evaluation, however, it is worth considering in the follow-up of lesions in the long term.

In conclusion, this evaluation of the use of TS in detecting emerging or growing ectopic bone lesions in FOP patients showed a higher sensitivity among residents and radiologists. However, there were more false-positive scans in datasets evaluated using TS compared to those without TS. TS might provide better diagnostic performance in follow-ups of FOP patients.

Author Contributions: Conceptualization, M.I., R.S. and J.T.; methodology, M.I. and R.S.; software, R.S.; formal analysis, M.I. and R.S.; investigation, M.I., R.S., T.K. and J.T.; resources, M.I., R.S., A.Y., B.O., Y.N., J.T. and S.M.; data curation, M.I., R.S., T.K., A.Y., B.O., Y.N. and S.M.; writing—original draft preparation, M.I. and R.S.; writing—review and editing, M.I., R.S., T.K., A.Y., B.O., Y.N., J.T. and S.M.; validation, M.I., R.S., T.K. and J.T.; visualization, M.I., R.S. and T.K.; supervision, Y.N., J.T. and S.M.; project administration, J.T. and S.M.; funding acquisition, J.T. and S.M. All authors have read and agreed to the published version of the manuscript.

Funding: This study was partially supported by Nobelpharma Co., Ltd.

Institutional Review Board Statement: The study was conducted in accordance with the Declaration of Helsinki, and approved by the Institutional Review Board of Kyoto University Hospital (protocol code R0610, approved on 19 August 2016).

Informed Consent Statement: Patient consent was waived due to the retrospective design.

Data Availability Statement: Not applicable.

Acknowledgments: The authors would like to thank Morimi Kusakabe and Eriko Nakaishi for participating in the image interpretation experiment. The authors would also like to thank RT Ryu Mabuchi and RT Satoshi Kozawa for generating the TS images, and Yasuyo Kusunoki for coordinating the study.

Conflicts of Interest: The authors declare no conflict of interest.

References

1. Pignolo, R.J.; Baujat, G.; Brown, M.A.; De Cunto, C.; Di Rocco, M.; Hsiao, E.C.; Keen, R.; Mukaddam, M.A.; Sang, K.-H.L.Q.; Wilson, A.; et al. Natural history of fibrodysplasia ossificans progressiva: Cross-sectional analysis of annotated baseline phenotypes. *Orphanet J. Rare Dis.* **2019**, *14*, 98. [CrossRef] [PubMed]
2. Kaplan, F.S.; Zasloff, M.A.; Kitterman, J.A.; Shore, E.M.; Hong, C.C.; Rocke, D.M. Early mortality and cardiorespiratory failure in patients with fibrodysplasia ossificans progressiva. *J. Bone Jt. Surg. Am. Vol.* **2010**, *92*, 686. [CrossRef] [PubMed]
3. Smilde, B.J.; Botman, E.; de Ruiter, R.D.; Smit, J.M.; Teunissen, B.P.; Lubbers, W.D.; Schwarte, L.A.; Schober, P.; Eekhoff, E.M.W. Monitoring and Management of Fibrodysplasia Ossificans Progressiva: Current Perspectives. *Orthop. Res. Rev.* **2022**, *14*, 113. [CrossRef] [PubMed]
4. Al Mukaddam, M.; Rajapakse, C.S.; Pignolo, R.J.; Kaplan, F.S.; Smith, S.E. Imaging assessment of fibrodysplasia ossificans progressiva: Qualitative, quantitative and questionable. *Bone* **2018**, *109*, 147–152. [CrossRef] [PubMed]
5. Rajapakse, C.S.; Lindborg, C.; Wang, H.; Newman, B.T.; Kobe, E.A.; Chang, G.; Shore, E.M.; Kaplan, F.S.; Pignolo, R.J. Analog method for radiographic assessment of heterotopic bone in fibrodysplasia ossificans progressiva. *Acad. Radiol.* **2017**, *24*, 321–327. [CrossRef] [PubMed]
6. Warner, S.E.; Kaplan, F.S.; Pignolo, R.J.; Smith, S.E.; Hsiao, E.C.; De Cunto, C.; Rocco, M.D.; Harnett, K.; Grogan, D.; Genant, H.K. Whole-body Computed Tomography Versus Dual Energy X-ray Absorptiometry for Assessing Heterotopic Ossification in Fibrodysplasia Ossificans Progressiva. *Calcif. Tissue Int.* **2021**, *109*, 615–625. [CrossRef] [PubMed]
7. Ishida, T.; Ashizawa, K.; Engelmann, R.; Katsuragawa, S.; MacMahon, H.; Doi, K. Application of temporal subtraction for detection of interval changes on chest radiographs: Improvement of subtraction images using automated initial image matching. *J. Digit. Imaging* **1999**, *12*, 77. [CrossRef] [PubMed]
8. Abe, H.; Ishida, T.; Shiraishi, J.; Li, F.; Katsuragawa, S.; Sone, S.; MacMahon, H.; Doi, K. Effect of temporal subtraction images on radiologists' detection of lung cancer on CT: Results of the observer performance study with use of film computed tomography images1. *Acad. Radiol.* **2004**, *11*, 1337–1343. [CrossRef] [PubMed]
9. Sakamoto, R.; Mori, S.; Miller, M.I.; Okada, T.; Togashi, K. Detection of time-varying structures by large deformation diffeomorphic metric mapping to aid reading of high-resolution CT images of the lung. *PLoS ONE* **2014**, *9*, e85580. [CrossRef] [PubMed]
10. Aoki, T.; Murakami, S.; Kim, H.; Fujii, M.; Takahashi, H.; Oki, H.; Hayashida, Y.; Katsuragawa, S.; Shiraishi, J.; Korogi, Y. Temporal subtraction method for lung nodule detection on successive thoracic CT soft-copy images. *Radiology* **2014**, *271*, 255–261. [CrossRef] [PubMed]
11. Hoff, B.A.; Toole, M.; Yablon, C.; Ross, B.D.; Luker, G.D.; Van Poznak, C.; Galbán, C.J. Potential for Early Fracture Risk Assessment in Patients with Metastatic Bone Disease Using Parametric Response Mapping of CT Images. *Tomography* **2015**, *1*, 98–104. [CrossRef] [PubMed]
12. Sakamoto, R.; Yakami, M.; Fujimoto, K.; Nakagomi, K.; Kubo, T.; Emoto, Y.; Akasaka, T.; Aoyama, G.; Yamamoto, H.; Miller, M.I.; et al. Temporal subtraction of serial CT images with large deformation diffeomorphic metric mapping in the identification of bone metastases. *Radiology* **2017**, *285*, 629–639. [CrossRef] [PubMed]
13. Akasaka, T.; Yakami, M.; Nishio, M.; Onoue, K.; Aoyama, G.; Nakagomi, K.; Iizuka, Y.; Kubo, T.; Emoto, Y.; Satoh, K.; et al. Detection of suspected brain infarctions on CT can be significantly improved with temporal subtraction images. *Eur. Radiol.* **2019**, *29*, 759–769. [CrossRef] [PubMed]

14. Onoue, K.; Nishio, M.; Yakami, M.; Aoyama, G.; Nakagomi, K.; Iizuka, Y.; Kubo, T.; Emoto, Y.; Akasaka, T.; Satoh, K.; et al. CT temporal subtraction improves early detection of bone metastases compared to SPECT. *Eur. Radiol.* **2019**, *29*, 5673–5681. [CrossRef] [PubMed]
15. Onoue, K.; Yakami, M.; Nishio, M.; Sakamoto, R.; Aoyama, G.; Nakagomi, K.; Iizuka, Y.; Kubo, T.; Emoto, Y.; Akasaka, T.; et al. Temporal subtraction CT with nonrigid image registration improves detection of bone metastases by radiologists: Results of a large-scale observer study. *Sci. Rep.* **2021**, *11*, 18522. [CrossRef]
16. Pignolo, R.J.; Shore, E.M.; Kaplan, F.S. Fibrodysplasia ossificans progressiva: Diagnosis, management, and therapeutic horizons. *Pediatr. Endocrinol. Rev.* **2013**, *10* (Suppl. S2), 437–448. [PubMed]
17. Aoki, T.; Kamiya, T.; Lu, H.; Terasawa, T.; Ueno, M.; Hayashida, Y.; Murakami, S.; Korogi, Y. CT temporal subtraction: Techniques and clinical applications. *Quant. Imaging Med. Surg.* **2021**, *11*, 2214. [CrossRef] [PubMed]
18. Carlier, R.Y.; Safa, D.M.L.; Parva, P.; Mompoint, D.; Judet, T.; Denormandie, P.; Vallée, C.A. Ankylosing neurogenic myositis ossificans of the hip: An enhanced volumetric CT study. *J. Bone Jt. Surg. Br. Vol.* **2005**, *87*, 301–305. [CrossRef] [PubMed]

Disclaimer/Publisher's Note: The statements, opinions and data contained in all publications are solely those of the individual author(s) and contributor(s) and not of MDPI and/or the editor(s). MDPI and/or the editor(s) disclaim responsibility for any injury to people or property resulting from any ideas, methods, instructions or products referred to in the content.

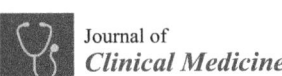

Article

Texture Analysis for the Bone Age Assessment from MRI Images of Adolescent Wrists in Boys

Rafal Obuchowicz [1], Karolina Nurzynska [2,*], Monika Pierzchala [3], Adam Piorkowski [4] and Michal Strzelecki [5]

[1] Department of Diagnostic Imaging, Jagiellonian University Medical College, 31-008 Krakow, Poland; rafalobuchowicz@su.krakow.pl
[2] Department of Algorithmics and Software, Silesian University of Technology, 44-100 Gliwice, Poland
[3] Selvita S.A., 30-348 Krakow, Poland; monika.pierzchala@selvita.com
[4] Department of Biocybernetics and Biomedical Engineering, AGH University of Science and Technology, 30-059 Krakow, Poland; pioro@agh.edu.pl
[5] Institute of Electronics, Lodz University of Technology, 93-590 Lodz, Poland; michal.strzelecki@p.lodz.pl
* Correspondence: karolina.nurzynska@polsl.pl

Abstract: Currently, bone age is assessed by X-rays. It enables the evaluation of the child's development and is an important diagnostic factor. However, it is not sufficient to diagnose a specific disease because the diagnoses and prognoses may arise depending on how much the given case differs from the norms of bone age. Background: The use of magnetic resonance images (MRI) to assess the age of the patient would extend diagnostic possibilities. The bone age test could then become a routine screening test. Changing the method of determining the bone age would also prevent the patient from taking a dose of ionizing radiation, making the test less invasive. Methods: The regions of interest containing the wrist area and the epiphyses of the radius are marked on the magnetic resonance imaging of the non-dominant hand of boys aged 9 to 17 years. Textural features are computed for these regions, as it is assumed that the texture of the wrist image contains information about bone age. Results: The regression analysis revealed that there is a high correlation between the bone age of a patient and the MRI-derived textural features derived from MRI. For DICOM T1-weighted data, the best scores reached 0.94 R2, 0.46 RMSE, 0.21 MSE, and 0.33 MAE. Conclusions: The experiments performed have shown that using the MRI images gives reliable results in the assessment of bone age while not exposing the patient to ionizing radiation.

Keywords: bone age; image texture; bone MRI; pediatric radiology; regression analysis

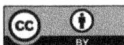

1. Introduction

Age is an imprinted parameter both from a medical and legal point of view [1,2]. There are many surgical and non-surgical procedures where precise estimation is very important [3]. In addition to medical issues, there are a wide range of non-medical subjects, e.g., legal problems and qualifications in competitive sports, where a precise age estimation is mandatory [4,5]. Legal issues become more important due to migration, especially in countries where birth records can be lost [6,7].

In the past century, it has emerged that the most accurate biological indicator of bone age is skeletal maturity. Bone age reflects the biological age of the patient, including hormonal and socioeconomic factors that are modulators of the growth and maturation of the child [8–10]. Therefore, this may be different from chronological age, especially in cases where factors that affect development are pushed to extremes, such as stress, malnutrition, or endocrine disorders [11]. With the development of radiological techniques, it has emerged that methods used for bone scanning could also be used for age determination. Therefore, X-ray-based techniques have emerged, exclusively in upper- and middle-class Caucasian populations [12,13], which nowadays gain criticism for their applicability due to racial and social differences [14–18]. With the advent of modern diagnostic techniques, there are attempts to use them in scanning for the estimation of the age of patients. Additionally, as a consequence, ultrasound, magnetic resonance (MR), and even computed tomography (CT) were employed [19–23]. The MR approach is of great interest because it is radiation-free and provides a detailed representation of tissues, including growth plates and nuclei [24–26]. The texture of such an image reflects the bone structure that is visualized in MR images. Textures represent complex patterns that are coded in the data and are built from points of different brightness and distribution. The distribution of the pixels and their characteristics can be analyzed by many textural features [27,28], such as phase frequency, coarseness, and regularity of randomness direction, to name a few [1]. Careful analysis of the initial textural pattern provides standardized feature extraction, which goes beyond the recognizable abilities of the human eye [29–31], allowing quantitative analysis of various medical images [32,33]. Changes in the growth zone and bone marrow composition reflect the maturation of the long bone as the site of dynamic morphological changes [34–38].

Since a bone age assessment is of great importance, this topic has been addressed in order to support physicians with an automated analysis of the data, making this task less labor intensive. In the literature, there are many approaches to address this problem, when analyzing X-ray images of hands [39–45], the chest [40,46], or whole-body images [47,48]. In the case of a fully automated deep learning approach, first the hand region was determined in the image using the U-Net network for semantic segmentation of the hand region, then the image registration was applied to allow for an easy determination of hand regions corresponding to each other between various images. Here, a deep learning approach for key point selection was also adopted. Finally, another network was used to solve the regression task and predict age. A similar pipeline was introduced in previous studies [40,44,45], yet the authors underlined the importance of transfer learning when preparing regression models. There were also approaches that used one network for the evaluation of bone age, as presented in the research in which whole-body scans were analyzed using well-known deep architectures, such as VGGNet, GoogLeNet, and ResNet, to find the best solution [47], or the hand X-ray image was analyzed with the attention-Xception network [43]. In [46] not only was the age determined from the chest radiograph images, but also, they analyzed the activation maps to find the most characteristic regions that influence the patient's age. Instead of using regression models, generative adversarial networks (GANs) were exploited to decide bone age [42]. It was also possible to estimate the age from the bone mineral density at Ward's triangle and the trabecular volume measured in the iliac crest [49,50]. We should not resign from more traditional approaches based on histogram thresholding, which allowed a precise determination of the chondrous part of the growth plate [51–53].

Most bone age assessment techniques implement X-ray-based imaging modalities that are invasive to some extent for patients. In this work, we would like to test whether other, non-invasive imaging techniques enable an accurate age estimation from acquired images that contain bone tissue. The aim of the present study was to explore whether the long bone textural analysis of the growth region on MRI images reflects changes in the age of the child and can possibly be applied for the determination of the bone age. To perform that examination, a dedicated database of MRI scans of adolescent hands was prepared. The descriptive region in the scan was marked manually, and then the textural features were extracted and the regression analysis was applied.

2. Materials and Methods

To verify whether it is possible to determine bone age from MRI images, a suitable dataset had to be prepared. The data acquisition is described in detail. The dataset gathered is briefly described. Next, the proposed textural features are presented, and details concerning the experiment quality measurements are given, followed by a description of experiment methodology.

2.1. Data Acquisition

This study was carried out according to the guidelines of good medical practice. The images were taken from a group of male volunteers, and the acquisition was approved by the Ethics Committee of Jagiellonian University (permission no. 1072.6120.16.2017) and complied with the Declaration of Helsinki. Written informed consent for participants was obtained from their legal guardians. The left hand of 30 healthy boys was examined by a 1.5 T system (GE Optima 360, Chicago, IL, USA) with a dedicated four-channel wrist coil. The acquisition was performed in a prone 'superman', e.g., with a hand erected in the overhead position.

Table 1 presents the parameters used to create T1-weighted and T2-weighted images. During the acquisition, 286 × 286 matrix size was used for the study. The scanning time of one sequence was in the range of 87–124 s. Radius growth plates were analyzed in coronal scans. Images were archived using the SIEMENS PACS (SYNGO, Siemens Healthineers, Erlangen, Germany). Anonymized studies were subsequently retrieved for image post-processing. The qMaZda software [54] was used for the computation of texture feature maps. Images with non-correctable motion artifacts were rejected. Small corrections of movement artifacts were performed with the use of pixel-by-pixel positioning of the overlaid images, and masks were developed that could compensate for the horizontal and vertical movements by a given number of pixels in case of minor movements.

Table 1. Parameters used for acquisition of T1- and T2-weighted images.

Parameter	T1-Weighted	T2-Weighted
Slice thickness	3 mm	3 mm
Repetition Time	435 ms	2749 ms
Echo Time	16 ms	106 ms
Number of averages	2	2
Spacing	3.5 mm	3.5 mm
Echo train length	23	23
Bandwidth	81 MHz	97 MHz

2.2. Dataset Description

The dataset consists of images that show the bone structure of the non-dominant hand (left in all cases analyzed). The subject's ages ranged from 9 to 17, with an average age of 12.43 and a median age of 12. The detailed distribution of age within the dataset is presented in Figure 1. There were accessible original DICOM (Digital Imaging and Communications in Medicine) images, and the visual information was stored in 12 bits. Furthermore, these images were normalized to the 0–255 range and stored as an 8-bit PNG image. In both cases, the image resolution is 512 × 512 pixels. Figure 2 presents an example of such a scan. In total, there are 55 images recorded with T1-weighted MRI and the same number of scans are collected with T2-weighted MRI. In image acquisition, we used a coronal plane of 3 mm thick, where a maximum of 10 layers were used in the plane with radius. From these data, up to three images per patient were considered usable considering their quality and visibility of the region of interest. In the case of the bone analysis, we used all 55 images; however, for radius growth region, only 30 images were used. The pixel spacing of the recorded data varies from 0.2539 to 0.3516 pixels, where the largest group of images was obtained for a 0.293 pixel spacing.

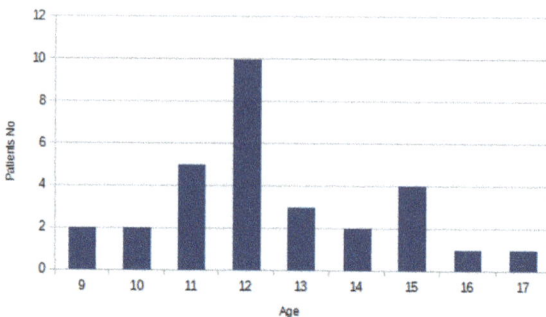

Figure 1. Distribution of the age of the patient within the dataset.

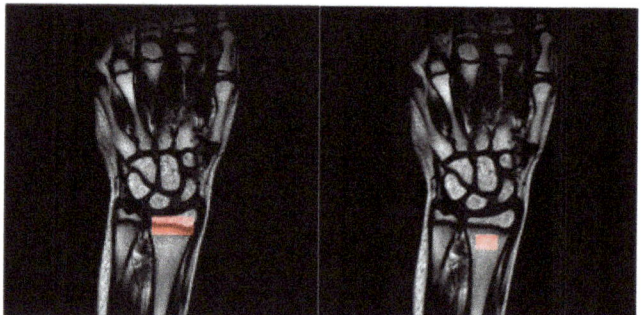

Figure 2. Exemplary magnetic resonance imaging. The red rectangle shows the growth region in the image on the right and bone region on the left scan.

2.3. Data Analysis Methods and Methodology

The starting point of the data analysis was to select a descriptive region of interest (ROI), which well characterizes bone structure and allows for calculating the textural features, which become the mathematical description of the data. Since the pixel spacing of the data differs, we have decided to test two approaches. Firstly, a constant ROI size was selected in the MRI of the forearm. Second, the ROI size differed assuring the same metric units. These regions were applied to the DICOM and PNG versions of the data. Moreover, two regions with different medical meanings were considered: the bone and the growth region; please refer to Figure 2 for visualization.

For each region, the textural features were calculated using the qMaZda software. The software supports rich functionality, from which we have chosen several options. At the beginning, $\pm 3\sigma$ normalization of the input region $I(x,y)$ was applied. It is beneficial when the image histogram is close to the Gaussian, and it was also proved that better results are obtained for MR data. For an image, the mean μ and standard deviation σ of illuminance were calculated. Then, the image was scaled by recalculating $\min_{norm} = \mu - 3\sigma$ and $\max_{norm} = \mu + 3\sigma$, and finally, thresholded, according to Equations (1) and (2):

$$N(x,y) = \frac{I(x,y) - \min_{norm}}{\max_{norm} - \min_{norm}}, \quad (1)$$

$$I_{norm}(x,y) = \begin{cases} 255 & N(x,y) > 255 \\ N(x,y) & 0 \leq N(x,y) \leq 255 \\ 0 & N(x,y) < 0 \end{cases} \quad (2)$$

Then, for the region, the textural features were calculated. Starting from the first-order features that describe illumination distribution within the histogram, by 9 parameters: mean, variance, skewness, kurtosis, and percentiles 1, 10, 50, 90, and 99. The spatial relations between pixels were also exploited to derive features from the gray-level co-occurrence matrix (GLCM) [27], run-length matrix (RLM) [55], gradient matrix [27], first-order autoregressive model (AR) [56], Haar wavelet transform (HW) [57], Gabor transforms, and histogram of oriented gradients (HOG) [58]. There are 11 parameters calculated from the GLCM matrix in four spatial directions: horizontal, vertical, and two diagonals. This method is additionally parametrized with a distance between pixels treated as neighbors. In our research, this distance was set in a range from 1 to 5 pixels. Taking into account all those combinations ($11 \times 4 \times 5$), 220 features were obtained. From the RLM method, 20 additional parameters were calculated. This method gives five features, and they were calculated using the same four directions as in the GLCM method. There were five gradient matrices built with a high-pass filter using a 3×3 pixel mask. There were five features derived from the AR method. Their idea is based on the finding that brightness depends on the weighted sum of the neighboring pixels. The HW transform brings 16 parameters, which result from four down-sampled sub-images representing the energy of the data after conversion to the wavelet transform. In the case of the Gabor filter, the transformation was calculated in four directions (as for GLCM) using six Gaussian envelopes of the following sizes: 4, 6, 8, 12, 16, and 24. That gives 24 parameters. Finally, an eight-bin histogram of occurrences of gradient orientation in the image was calculated as a feature of the HOG method. After all, those transformations' 307 features were obtained. The details on how to calculate each of these features are given in Appendix A.

Since the number of calculated features was large compared to the number of training samples, the reduction in feature space was necessary to remove redundancies and highly correlated data and improve the model's possibility to derive patterns from the data. This was achieved by using principal component analysis (PCA). Finally, the bilayered perceptron neural network implemented in the Matlab Regression Learner toolbox was applied to perform the analysis. Since the datasets are small, the leave-one-out (LOO) cross-validation schema was used to validate the neural network. This means that the network was trained for all data samples except one. The remaining sample was used for validation. This process was repeated for all samples in the dataset, so that each sample was validated separately. In the LOO approach, the bias associated with the random selection of data for folds (as in the case of cross-validation) or with the selection of the test set (as in the case of train-test split) is reduced. Furthermore, the performance of the model can be assessed for each sample. The LOO method is recommended and is quite commonly used in the case of small datasets (from a dozen to several dozen samples) [59–63].

The quality regression model was evaluated by mean square error (MSE), root mean square error (RMSE), mean absolute error (MAE), and coefficient of determination (R2).

2.4. Experiment Setup

In the experiments performed, images of bone and growth regions have been analyzed. In the case of bones, all 55 images were used. However, for the growth region analysis, each patient was represented by only one image, which reduced the number of samples to 30. In this research, we have focused on the metric version of the annotation. Since the textural features depend strongly on the pixel relations, varying sizes of pixels might influence the outcomes, whereas when we had each time data with similar pixel spacing, this problem and its influence on results could be neglected. We performed a regression analysis regarding the patient's full age. However, we noticed that the correlation improved when comparing texture features with the age given in months. Although that was an interesting finding, because of the small number of samples, it was abandoned for further investigation. The image preprocessing with the qMaZda software generated many texture features (307) to describe each sample. Using so many features can decrease regressor capabilities when most of them may not be correlated with the patient's age. Therefore, a Spearman correlation between textural features and outcomes was calculated, which helped us choose 15 highly correlated, representative features. This procedure was applied to the training data separately for each model. Furthermore, as proven by previous research, these indicated the best textural features [64]. For this set of data, PCA was applied to derive the most discriminative parameters and remove any existing correlation between them. For bone and growth region analysis, the first 3 PCA eigenvectors were selected. The assumed number of PCA features used in regression analysis reflected the number of samples analyzed (55 in the case of bone image experiments and 30 when the growth region was evaluated). Experiments were performed for all four datasets: DICOM T1-weighted, DICOM T2-weighted, PNG T1-weighted, and PNG T2-weighted images. Furthermore, two tasks were evaluated: (1) finding the relation between the textural features of the bone region and the age of the patient; and (2) evaluating the dependence of the textural features in the growth region on the age of the patient.

3. Results

Tables 2 and 3 collect the best results obtained after applying a two-layer neural network from the Matlab Regression Learner toolbox. The visualization of the results is depicted in Figures 3 and 4. The results presented in Tables 2 and 3 are the average values of the regression errors obtained for each of the samples. The plots summarize the results of all the LOO trials. From the results presented, we can see that the regression analysis in all cases allowed the prediction of the age of a patient based on the textural features analysis of the MRI data. The gathered results suggest that, considering the bone region, we achieved more stable results with fewer errors. However, due to the limited amount of data, these discrepancies between the analyzed regions could be due to decreasing the number of samples from 55 (for the bone) to 30 (for the growth region). The dispersion coefficient is very high, yet significantly better results were obtained when a T1-weighted image using the original 12-bit DICOM data was considered. We achieved the best score, which was R2 equal to 0.94 for the original 12-bit representation (DICOM) when the bone region was evaluated. In this scenario, second place was taken by the T2-weighted image with a reduced number of bits to eight (R2 equals 0.87). When analyzing the results obtained for the growth region (see Table 3), again, the T1-weighted image in 12-bit format returns the best outcomes, yet other results deteriorate significantly. This finding was also reflected in the other error metrics showing the smallest error in the case of DICOM T1-weighted datasets (see bold font in Tables 2 and 3). The slight difference in the quality of age prediction by the chosen regressors was also noticeable in the plots presented in Figures 3 and 4. Here, the predictions go through all observations in the case of analyzing textural features from bone DICOM T1-weighted images (see Figure 3a) and are very close to this line when the growth region DICOM T1-weighted images are considered (see Figure 4a). Since the true age was rounded to an integer value, the small discrepancies should not be surprising, as in reality, patients had a different number of months. As we noticed previously, the data reflected better when a shorter period was considered.

Table 2. Quantitative regression parameters for different types of data and bone images (metric). Results for 3 features derived from 15 by applying principal component analysis.

Data	R^2	RMSE	MSE	MAE
DICOM T1-weighted	0.9383	0.4584	0.2101	0.3300
DICOM T2-weighted	0.7510	0.8365	0.6997	0.6229
PNG T1-weighted	0.7283	0.9344	0.8732	0.6922
PNG T2-weighted	0.8711	0.5731	0.3284	0.4429

Table 3. Quantitative regression parameters for different types of data and growth region images (metric). Results for 3 features derived from 15 by applying principal component analysis.

Data	R^2	RMSE	MSE	MAE
DICOM T1-weighted	0.8041	0.8194	0.6714	0.6142
DICOM T2-weighted	0.6621	1.4104	1.9892	1.0969
PNG T1-weighted	0.6743	1.0550	1.1130	0.8740
PNG T2-weighted	0.5216	1.1058	1.2228	0.9228

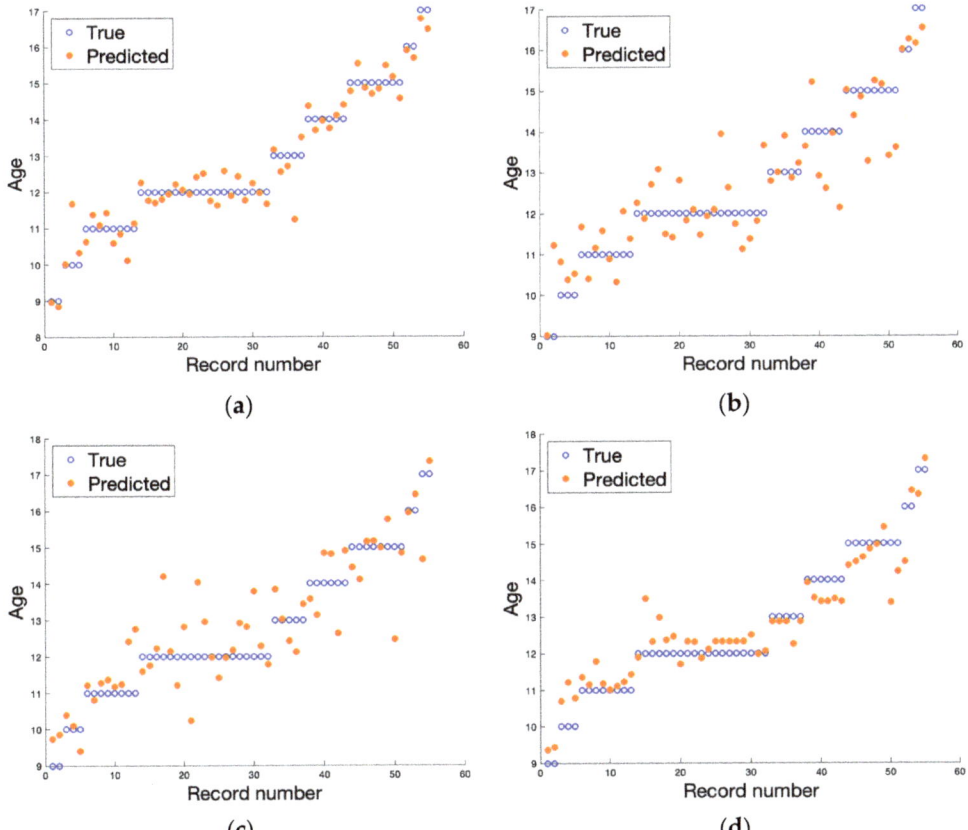

Figure 3. The result of regression algorithms for all cases examined for data describing bone images (metric). The real age is presented by blue circles and estimated age with a regression algorithm is depicted by orange dots. The samples are ordered on the y axis with increasing age. (**a**) DICOM T1-weighted, (**b**) DICOM T2-weighted, (**c**) PNG T1-weighted, and (**d**) PNG T2-weighted.

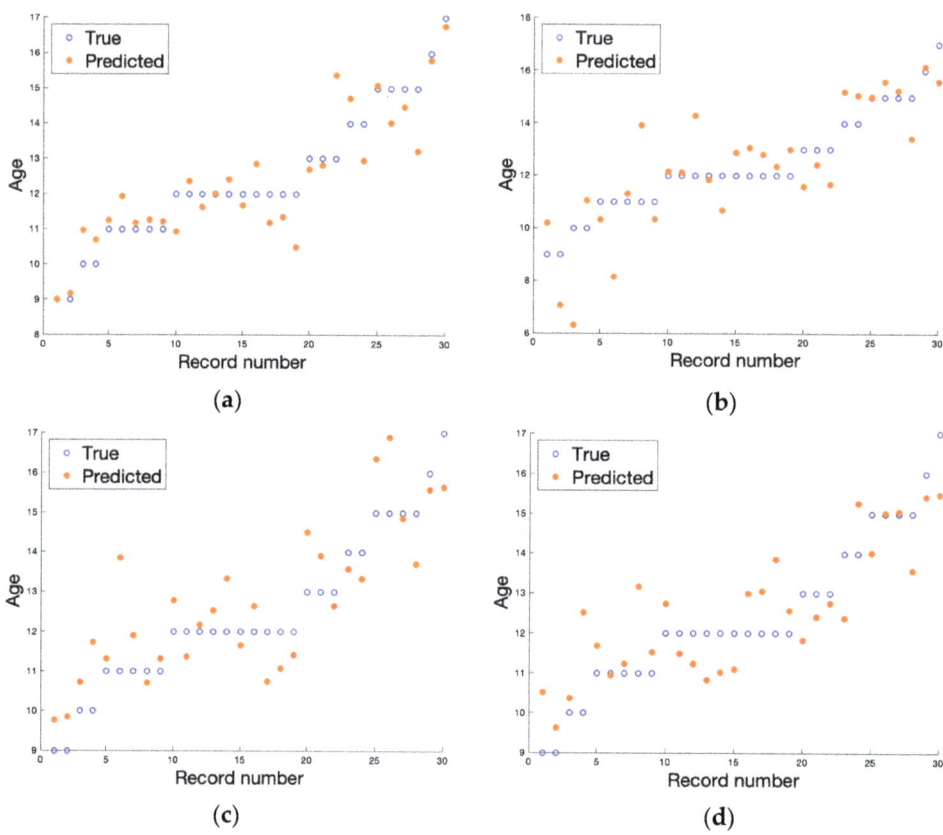

Figure 4. The result of regression algorithms for all examined cases for data describing growth region images (metric). The real age is given as a blue circle and age estimated with a regression algorithm is depicted as orange dot. The samples are ordered on the y axis with increasing age. (**a**) DICOM T1-weighted, (**b**) DICOM T2-weighted, (**c**) PNG T1-weighted, and (**d**) PNG T2-weighted.

4. Discussion

Radiographic techniques are well-established methods that are used for the determination of bone age [12,13]. There are techniques that are based not only on the wrist estimation but also on other parts of the skeleton, including the clavicle [65], elbow [66], pelvis [67,68], humerus [69], or calcaneus [70,71]. Dental studies become a focus as body parts are used for age estimation [72–74].

Moreover, with the development of computer hardware, different techniques were proposed to obtain information from the image, allowing for the creation of efficient age evaluation systems, for example, Shorthand and BoneXpert to name a few [75,76]. There are many modern techniques that are based on shape extraction algorithms with comparative techniques, including those based on artificial intelligence [77–80]. However, many of these methods are still based on an X-ray analysis, where X-ray dose issues cannot be omitted.

Age determination based on a single radiograph is associated with low doses [81]. However, a cumulative dose in cases where multiple X-rays must be performed might not be acceptable. Ultrasonography, however, which is free from radiation and easy to use, is known as an operator-dependent method, which is a serious drawback of this otherwise useful technique [82].

MR was proposed as a method free of radiation exposure, but it is also repetitive, and in this regard, according to the results, it is stable. Table 4 provided a comparison of the MAE metric for our solution and other approaches working on X-ray data. As we can see, it outperformed other methods markedly. A certain drawback of MRIs is the time needed for the exam, which forces cooperation with young patients. Regarding the success of the MR examination, parental assistance is very important [24]. Child safety and comfort was assured in this study. That was very important as unintentional movement caused by inconvenient body alignment disturbs image creation. This is especially important in a proposed method where a small region of interest in the growth plate is used; therefore, a perfect image is key to the success of the proposed solution. Child cooperation is mandatory. However as described by Terada et al. [23] and Dvorak et al [22], short exam time was sufficient condition to ensure the creation of proper images. In our study, in contradiction to the protocol proposed by Dvorak et al. [22], Hojreh et al. [26], Stern et al. [83], and Quasim et al. [84], in addition to the T1-weighted spin echo and the gradient echo sequence (as applied in [23,24]), a T2-weighted spin echo was used. The choice of a T2-weighted sequence was dictated by the need to discriminate the number of watery progenitor cells because the amount of signals from these watery compounds was used as an indicator of the immaturity of the growth zone. The dependence of the growth zone composition on age with possible detection with the MR technique was described in experimental and clinical studies by Ecklund et al. [85], who described the dependence of the signal of the growth region composition. This agrees with histological studies proposed by Ballock et al. [86] and Breur et al. [87], who precisely described the basis of the known fact that the pattern of ongoing calcification of the growth region reflects maturation with age, which is at the core of the signal changes that are analyzed in our study as one of the discriminators of long bone maturation. In a study by Yun et al. [88], the dependence between the MR growth plate signal assessed in MR and skeletal maturation was not presented; however, the authors performed a study in the younger children group. One must remember that the proposed analysis of the growth plate is based on the narrow tissue element of progenitor cells, which is less than 3 mm and is a niche compared to the surrounding bone [89,90].

Table 4. Results of performance of the presented method and other solutions for the estimation of bone age based on hand.

References	MAE (Months)
Liu et al. [42]	6.01
Iglovikov et al. [39]	6.10
Salim and Hamza [40]	6.38
Zulkifley et al. [43]	7.70
	MAE (years)
Nguyen et al. [47]	4.856
Our method	0.330 (T1 DICOM), 0.692 (T1 PNG)

Despite the relatively low volume of the growth region in the composition of highly watery cells, it is highly detectable by high MR sequences, which in the image analysis, were reflected by a high correlation with histogram parameters (a sensitive indicator of brightness distribution but not necessarily structure) and supported by the presented regression analysis. This is logical because, in the zone of highly watery progenitor cells, the defined structure is very sparse, but the signal is strong. It can be observed that the younger the patient (with a wider growth region and more fluid), the brighter the signal. In older children, the amount of watery progenitor cells was reduced at the expense of the calcified bone rim, with a subsequent reduction in the influence of the bright area.

In a comparison of the T1-weighted and T2-weighted sequences, regression occurred more accurately for T1-weighted images than for T2-weighted signals, which is at least in part due to a high tissue contrast created between less hydrated trabeculae due to hydroxyapatite and therefore, low signal bone elements and high signal bone marrow [37,38]. The discriminative effect of the T2-weighted image due to the good differentiation between the unconverted bone marrow and the trabeculae can be partially spoiled by shift artifacts due to chemical composition, but also by the thickness of the trabeculae [91,92].

A slight influence on the results was observed regarding the type of encoding, the DICOM format was better with the T1-weighted sequence, which might be due to the overall contrast in the image where the T1-weighted sequence sensitive to water produces high signal differentiation in the image that is associated with a significant amount of blood morphotic elements in the immature marrow. This observation is consistent with clinical observations where sequences with a high TR time are used to differentiate lesions due to high visual contrast [93]. It is also worth mentioning that comparing different MRI sequences is problematic; however, there are works showing that the registration of two series of MRI data is possible to some extent [94].

Recently, new algorithms for automated bone marrow segmentation from MRI data have been developed [95,96]. We are going to implement such algorithms in our future research, especially when a large image database will be collected. The challenge will be to modify these algorithms in such a way as to select a specific ROI from the segmented, whole bone marrow. We know that radiomic features are prone to many problems. One of them is the low repeatability of texture features when multicenter studies are performed. On the other hand, such studies are essential to ensure the reliable validation of the developed machine learning models. It was shown in [97] that normalization applied to muscle tissue images acquired by different MR scanners improved the reproducibility of the calculated selected texture features. We will further investigate the influence of various ROI normalization schemes' texture feature repeatability and reproducibility. Another factor that affects the calculation of bone marrow radiomic features is the variation of signal intensity between different scanners [98] as well as its dependence on signal blur phenomena. It is mostly caused by a chemical shift and magnetic susceptibility artifact, which belong to a class of tissue-specific artifacts. Other, less important might be also geometric artifacts that come from tissue tilt. Bone marrow analysis is always challenging and requires optimal image acquisition and compensation of acquisition artifacts.

There are some limitations to this study. First, the image acquisition was relatively long. However, the scanning time was successfully overcome by the cooperative and motivated children. Since it was a pilot study and we only wanted to verify the hypothesis that it is possible to determine the bone age with high accuracy from the MRI images, a small group of patients was examined. For further studies, it should be extended. Finally, the error in the segmentation of the growth plate must be considered, given the small area of interest and the averaging effect due to the influence of the surrounding tissues.

5. Conclusions

This preliminary study presented the feasibility of implementing MRI bone scans in the bone age estimation protocols as a novel approach based on an analysis of the internal bone structure based on tissue texture. This is a different approach in comparison to shape and volume analyses based on X-ray techniques that are used today. To verify the hypothesis that it is possible to estimate the patient's age based on an MRI hand scan, a database of non-dominant hands of 30 children was acquired. On those scans, the regions of interest were manually selected, distinguishing the bone and growth regions, both annotated with a constant pixel spacing. For these regions, textural features were calculated using the qMaZda software. To select the most representative data, a correlation analysis was performed followed by the PCA transform. Then, regression analysis was applied, which revealed a high correlation between the DICOM T1 images and the age of the patients (for the remaining types of analyzed data, the correlation was moderate). This is a significant finding, as it supports the claim that the use of the radiation-free technique can replace the current protocol based on X-ray scans. Moreover, we see that the magnetic resonance images convey complete information about bone structure and can be used interchangeably with X-ray images. The presented approach that implements machine learning on textures visualized in MRI scans is a novel solution toward the most complete analysis of bone age information, allowing for an accurate assessment of the biological age of the patient.

Author Contributions: Conceptualization, R.O. and A.P.; methodology, R.O., A.P., K.N. and M.S.; software, R.O., M.P., A.P. and M.S.; validation, R.O. and K.N.; formal analysis, R.O., M.P. and M.S.; investigation, R.O., K.N., M.P. and A.P.; resources, R.O., A.P. and M.S.; data curation, R.O., M.P., A.P. and M.S.; writing—original draft preparation, R.O., K.N. and M.S.; writing—review and editing, R.O., K.N., A.P. and M.S.; visualization, R.O., K.N., M.P. and A.P.; supervision, R.O., A.P. and M.S.; project administration, R.O., A.P. and M.S. All authors have read and agreed to the published version of the manuscript.

Funding: This research received no external funding.

Institutional Review Board Statement: The study was carried out in accordance with the Declaration of Helsinki and approved by the Institutional Review Board (or Ethics Committee) of Jagiellonian University (protocol code: 1072.6120.16.2017 and date of approval: 21 December 2017).

Informed Consent Statement: Patient consent was waived due to the retrospective nature of the research and access to the anonymized data.

Data Availability Statement: Data is unavailable due to privacy.

Acknowledgments: We thank Wiesław Guz for his assistance during the completion of the MR images.

Conflicts of Interest: The authors declare no conflict of interest.

Appendix A

Here, the following points provide detailed information about the definition of the texture feature parameters that were used in presented research.

1. First-order features

First-order features are calculated for a gray-scale image using formulae presented in Table A1. Here, h stands for the normalized histogram function of occurrences at the G pixel level for image of width W and height H.

Table A1. Formulae to calculate first order features from the gray-scale image.

Feature Name	Formulae	
Mean	$\mu = \frac{1}{W \cdot H} \sum_{x=0}^{W-1} \sum_{y=0}^{H-1} I(x,y) = \sum_{i=0}^{G-1} i \cdot h(i)$	(A1)
Variance	$\sigma^2 = \frac{1}{W \cdot H} \sum_{x=0}^{W-1} \sum_{y=0}^{H-1} (I(x,y) - \mu)^2 = \sum_{i=0}^{G-1} (i - \mu)^2 \cdot h(i)$	(A2)
Skewness	$\sigma^{-3} \sum_{i=0}^{G-1} (i - \mu)^3 \cdot h(i)$	(A3)
Kurtosis	$\sigma^{-4} \sum_{i=0}^{G-1} (i - \mu)^4 \cdot h(i) - 3$	(A4)
Percentile	$\sum_{i=0}^{G-1} h(i) \geq percentile$	(A5)

2. Gray-level co-occurrence matrix [27]

Table A2 presents the features derived from the gray-level co-occurrence matrix p. This matrix saves the information of the number of existing co-occurrence of pixels of intensities indexing this cells within an image in cells. It is calculated separately in four directions (horizontal, vertical, and two diagonals). It is also possible to parametrize the distance d between pixels considered as adjoining in our research $d = 1 \ldots 5$. The G stands for the pixel gray-level values.

Table A2. Formulae to calculate gray level co-occurrence matrix from the gray-scale image.

Feature Name	Formulae	
Contrast	$\sum_{i=0}^{G-1}\sum_{j=0}^{G-1}(i-j)^2 p(i,j)$	(A6)
Correlation	$\sum_{i=0}^{G-1}\sum_{j=0}^{G-1}\frac{ijp(i,j)-\mu_i\mu_j}{\delta_i\delta_j}$ where μ_i is average and δ_i is standard deviation for p_i	(A7)
Homogeneity	$\sum_{i=0}^{G-1}\sum_{j=0}^{G-1}\frac{p(i,j)}{1+(i-j)^2}$	(A8)
Entropy	$-\sum_{i=0}^{G-1}\sum_{j=0}^{G-1}p(i,j)\log_2(p(i,j))$	(A9)
Angular second moment	$\sum_{i=0}^{G-1}\sum_{j=0}^{G-1}p^2(i,j)$	(A10)
Sum average	$\sum_{m=1}^{G}mp_{sum}(m)$	(A11)
Sum variance	$\sum_{m=1}^{G}(m-sum-avg)^2 p_{sum}(m)$	(A12)
Difference variance	$\sum_{m=1}^{G}(i-\mu_{dif})^2 p_{dif}(m)$	(A13)
Difference entropy	$-\sum_{m=1}^{G}p_{dif}(m)\log(p_{sum}(m))$	(A14)
Sum entropy	$-\sum_{m=1}^{G}p_{sum}(m)\log(p_{sum}(m))$	(A15)
Sum of squares	$\sum_{i=0}^{G-1}\sum_{j=0}^{G-1}(i-\mu)^2 p(i,j)$	(A16)

3. Run-length matrix [55]

The run-length matrix p stores information about the length of pixel runs having the same pixel value. Thus, here, each matrix cell is indexed by the pixel gray-level value G, and the length L. The total number of recorded runs is denoted by n_r. Features derived from the run-length matrix are given in Table A3.

Table A3. Formulae to calculate run-length matrix features from the gray-scale image.

Feature Name	Formulae	
Short run emphasis	$\frac{1}{n_r}\sum_{i=0}^{G-1}\sum_{j=1}^{L}\frac{p(i,j)}{j^2}$	(A17)
Long run emphasis	$\frac{1}{n_r}\sum_{i=0}^{G-1}\sum_{j=1}^{L}p(i,j)\cdot j^2$	(A18)
Gray-level non-uniformity	$\frac{1}{n_r}\sum_{i=0}^{G-1}\left(\sum_{j=1}^{L}p(i,j)\right)$	(A19)
Run-length non-uniformity	$\frac{1}{n_r}\sum_{j=1}^{L}\left(\sum_{i=0}^{G-1}p(i,j)\right)$	(A20)
Run percent	$\frac{n_r}{W\cdot H}$	(A21)

4. Gradient matrix [27]

The gradient magnitude for image region of interest I is calculated as follows:

$$|\mathcal{D}| = \sqrt{(I(x,y+1)-I(x,y-1))^2 + (I(x+1,y)-I(x-1,y))^2} \quad (A22)$$

and within this region the mean, variance, skewness, and kurtosis are calculated (see formulas already presented for first-order features in Table A1) and additionally, the non-zeros parameter is computed as a ratio of $|T| > 0$ to all pixels in region of interest.

5. First order autoregressive model [56]

The autoregressive model with four θ parameters is given with formulae:

$$I(x,y) = \theta_1(I(x-1,y)-\mu) + \theta_2(I(x,y-1)-\mu) + \theta_3(I(x-1,y-1)-\mu) + \theta_4(I(x+1,y-1)-\mu) + \mu + e(x,y) \quad (A23)$$

where

$$\mu = \frac{\sum_{x,y\in ROI}I(x,y)}{\sum_{x,y\in ROI}1} \quad (A24)$$

and e stands for error.

6. Haar wavelet transform [57]

A Haar discrete wavelet transform with its energies and frequencies is applied to four sub-band images returning the energy and three low-pass (L) and high-pass (H) filters in horizontal and vertical directions: HH, LH, and HL.

7. Gabor transform

The Gabor transform locally decomposes the image and is calculated separately in four directions (horizontal, vertical, and both diagonals). The frequency components are computed by convolution with a kernel:

$$k(x,y) = e^{\frac{-(x^2+y^2)}{2\delta^2}} (cos(\beta) + jsin(\beta)) \text{ where } \beta = \omega(x\cos\alpha + y\sin\alpha) \quad (A25)$$

where the parameters define the frequency ω, orientation α, and standard deviation of the Gaussian envelope δ. The average magnitude is calculated as follows:

$$Mag = \frac{\sum_{x,y \in ROI'} k(x,y)}{\sum_{x,y \in ROI'} 1} \quad (A26)$$

and the ROI' is morphologically eroded.

8. Histogram of oriented gradients [58]

Histogram of oriented gradients divides the image into 8×8 pixels cells, where the gradient's magnitudes and directions are calculated. This information is coded into an 8-bin histogram, where the bins reflect the quantized gradient directions.

References

1. Schmitt, A. *Forensic Anthropology and Medicine: Complementary Sciences from Recovery to Cause of Death*; Humana: Paramus, NJ, USA, 2006; pp. 212–219.
2. Abdelbary, M.H.; Abdelkawi, M.M.; Nasr, M.A. Age determination by MR imaging of the wrist in Egyptian male foot ballplayers How far is it reliable? *Egypt. J. Radiol. Nucl. Med.* **2018**, *49*, 146–151. [CrossRef]
3. Dekhne, M.S.; Kocher, I.D.; Hussain, Z.B.; Feroe, A.G.; Sankarankutty, S.; Williams, K.A.; Heyworth, B.E.; Milewski, M.D.; Kocher, M.S. Tibial tubercle apophyseal stage to determine skeletal age in pediatric patients undergoing ACL Reconstruction: A validation and reliability study. *Orthop. J. Sports Med.* **2021**, *9*, 23259671211036897. [CrossRef] [PubMed]
4. Schmidt, S.; Koch, B.; Schulz, R.; Reisinger, W.; Schmeling, A. Studiesin use of the Greulich–Pyle skeletal age method to assess criminal liability. *Legal Med.* **2008**, *10*, 190–195. [CrossRef]
5. Malina, R.M. Skeletal age and age verification in youth sport. *Sports Med.* **2011**, *41*, 925–947. [CrossRef] [PubMed]
6. Schmeling, A.; Reisinger, W.; Geserick, G.; Olze, A. Age estimation of unaccompanied minors: Part I. General considerations. *Forensic Sci. Int.* **2006**, *159*, S61–S64. [CrossRef] [PubMed]
7. Menjívar, C.; Perreira, K.M. Undocumented and unaccompanied: Children of migration in the European Union and the United States. *J. Ethn. Migr. Stud.* **2019**, *45*, 197–217. [CrossRef] [PubMed]
8. Reinehr, T.; de Sousa, G.; Wabitsch, M. Relationships of IGF-I and androgens to skeletal maturation in obese children and adolescents. *J. Pediatr. Endocrinol. Metab.* **2006**, *19*, 1133–1140. [CrossRef] [PubMed]
9. Phillip, M.; Moran, O.; Lazar, L. Growth without growth hormone. *J. Pediatr. Endocrinol. Metab.* **2002**, *15*, 1267–1272. [PubMed]
10. Cox, L.A. The biology of bone maturation and ageing. *Acta Paediatr. Suppl.* **1997**, *423*, 107–108. [CrossRef]
11. Kaplowitz, P.; Srinivasan, S.; He, J.; McCarter, R.; Hayeri, M.R.; Sze, R. Comparison of bone age readings by pediatric endocrinologists and pediatric radiologists using two bone age atlases. *Pediatr. Radiol.* **2010**, *41*, 690–693. [CrossRef]
12. Greulich, W.W.; Pyle, S.I. *Radiographic Atlas of Skeletal Development of the Hand and Wrist*, 2nd ed.; Stanford University Press: Stanford, CA, USA, 1959.
13. Tanner, J.M.; Whitehouse, R.H.; Healy, M. *A New System for Estimating Skeletal Maturity from the Hand and Wrist with Standards Derived from a Study of 2600 Healthy British Children*; Centre International de L'enfance: Paris, France, 1962.
14. Alshamrani, K.; Messina, F.; Offiah, A.C. Is the Greulich and Pyle atlas applicable to all ethnicities? A systematic review and meta-analysis. *Eur. Radiol.* **2019**, *29*, 2910–2923. [PubMed]
15. Alshamrani, K.; Offiah, A.C. Applicability of two commonly used bone age assessment methods to twenty-first century UK children. *Diag. Interv. Radiol.* **2020**, *30*, 504–513. [CrossRef]
16. van Rijn, R.R.; Lequin, M.H.; Robben, S.G.; Hop, W.C.; van Kuijk, C. Is the Greulich and Pyle atlas still valid for Dutch Caucasian children today. *Pediatr. Radiol.* **2021**, *31*, 748–752. [CrossRef]

17. Cantekin, K.; Celikoglu, M.; Miloglu, O.; Dane, A.; Erdem, A. Bone age assessment: The applicability of the Greulich-Pyle method in eastern Turkish children. *J. Forensic Sci.* **2012**, *57*, 679–682. [CrossRef] [PubMed]
18. Dembetembe, K.A.; Morris, A.G. Is Greulich-Pyle age estimation applicable for determining maturation in male Africans. *South Afr. Sci. Suid-Afrik. Wet.* **2012**, *108*, 1–6. [CrossRef]
19. Mentzel, H.-J.; Vilser, C.; Eulenstein, M.; Schwartz, T.; Vogt, S.; Böttcher, J.; Yaniv, I.; Tsoref, L.; Kauf, E.; Kaiser, W.A. Assessment of skeletal age at the wrist in children with a new ultrasound device. *Pediatr. Radiol.* **2005**, *35*, 429–433. [CrossRef] [PubMed]
20. Khan, K.M.; Miller, B.S.; Hoggard, E.; Somani, A.; Sarafoglou, K. Application of ultrasound for bone age estimation in clinical practice. *J. Pediatr.* **2009**, *154*, 243–247. [CrossRef]
21. Bilgili, Y.; Hizel, S.; Kara, S.A.; Sanli, C.; Erdal, H.H.; Altinok, D. Accuracy of skeletal age assessment in children from birth to 6 years of age with the ultrasonographic version of the Greulich-Pyle atlas. *J. Ultrasound Med.* **2003**, *22*, 683–690. [CrossRef]
22. Dvorak, J.; George, J.; Junge, A.; Hodler, J. Age determination by magnetic resonance imaging of the wrist in adolescent male football players. *Br. J. Sports Med.* **2007**, *41*, 45–52. [CrossRef]
23. Terada, Y.; Kono, S.; Tamada, D.; Uchiumi, T.; Kose, K.; Miyagi, R.; Yamabe, E.; Yoshioka, H. Skeletal age assessment in children using an open compact MRI system. *Magn. Reson. Med.* **2013**, *69*, 1697–1702. [CrossRef]
24. Terada, Y.; Kono, S.; Uchiumi, T.; Kose, K.; Miyagi, R.; Yamabe, E.; Fujinaga, Y.; Yoshioka, H. Improved reliability in skeletal age assessment using a pediatric hand MR scanner with a 0. 3T permanent magnet. *Magn. Reson. Med. Sci.* **2014**, *13*, 215–219. [CrossRef] [PubMed]
25. Tomei, E.; Sartori, A.; Nissman, D.; Al Ansari, N.; Battisti, S.; Rubini, A.; Stagnitti, A.; Martino, M.; Marini, M.; Barbato, E.; et al. Value of MRI of the hand and the wrist in evaluation of bone age: Preliminary results. *J. Magn. Reson. Imaging* **2014**, *39*, 1198–1205. [CrossRef] [PubMed]
26. Hojreh, A.; Gamper, J.; Schmook, M.T.; Weber, M.; Prayer, D.; Herold, C.J.; Noebauer-Huhmann, I.M. Hand MRI and the Greulich-Pyle atlas in skeletal age estimation in adolescents. *Skelet. Radiol.* **2018**, *47*, 963–971. [CrossRef] [PubMed]
27. Haralick, R.M. Statistical and structural approaches to texture. *Proc. IEEE* **1979**, *67*, 786–804. [CrossRef]
28. Haralick, R.M.; Shanmugam, K.; Dinstein, I. Textural Features for Image Classification. *IEEE Trans. Syst. Man. Cybern.* **1973**, *3*, 610–621. [CrossRef]
29. Kociołek, M.; Strzelecki, M.; Klepaczko, A. *Functional kidney analysis based on textured DCE-MRI images, In Advances in Intelligent Systems and Computing*; Piętka, E., Badura, P., Kawa, J., Wieclawek, W., Eds.; Springer Verlag: Berlin/Heidelberg, Germany, 2019; pp. 38–49.
30. Szczypiński, P.M.; Strzelecki, M.; Materka, A.; Klepaczko, A. MaZda—The software package for textural analysis of biomedical images. *Adv. Intell. Soft Comput.* **2009**, *65*, 73–84.
31. Materka, A. Texture analysis methodologies for magnetic resonance imaging. *Dialogues Clin. Neurosci.* **2022**, *6*, 243–250. [CrossRef]
32. Chrzanowski, L.; Drozdz, J.; Strzelecki, M.; Krzeminska-Pakula, M.; Jedrzejewski, K.; Kasprzak, J. Application of neural networks for the analysis of histological and ultrasonic aortic wall appearance—An in-vitro tissue characterization study. *Ultrasound Med. Biol.* **2008**, *34*, 103–113. [CrossRef]
33. Obuchowicz, R.; Kruszyńska, J.; Strzelecki, M. Classifying median nerves in carpal tunnel syndrome: Ultrasound image analysis. *Biocybern. Biomed. Eng.* **2021**, *41*, 335–351. [CrossRef]
34. Hochberg, Z. Clinical physiology and pathology of the growth plate. *Best Pract. Res. Clin. Endocrinol. Metab.* **2002**, *16*, 399–419. [CrossRef]
35. Jaramillo, D.; Laor, T.; Zaleske, D.J. Indirect trauma to the growth plate: Results of MR imaging after epiphyseal and metaphyseal injury in rabbits. *Radiology* **1993**, *187*, 171–178. [CrossRef] [PubMed]
36. Wilsman, N.J.; Farnum, C.E.; Green, E.M.; Lieferman, E.M.; Clayton, M.K. Cell cycle analysis of proliferative zone chondrocytes in growth plates elongating at different rates. *J. Orthop. Res.* **1996**, *14*, 562–572. [CrossRef] [PubMed]
37. Burdiles, A.; Babyn, P.S. Pediatric bone marrow MR imaging. *Magn. Reson. Imaging Clin. N Am.* **2009**, *17*, 391–409. [CrossRef]
38. Chan, B.Y.; Gill, K.G.; Rebsamen, S.L.; Nguyen, J.C. MR Imaging of Pediatric Bone Marrow. *Radiographics* **2016**, *36*, 1911–1930. [CrossRef] [PubMed]
39. Iglovikov, V.I.; Rakhlin, A.; Kalinin, A.A.; Shvets, A.A. Pediatric bone age assessment using deep convolutional neural networks. In *Deep Learning in Medical Image Analysis and Multimodal Learning for Clinical Decision Support*; Springer: Cham, Switzerland, 2018; pp. 300–308.
40. Salim, I.; Hamza, A.B. Ridge regression neural network for pediatric bone age assessment. *Multimed. Tools Appl.* **2021**, *80*, 30461–30478. [CrossRef]
41. Marouf, M.; Siddiqi, R.; Bashir, F.; Vohra, B. Automated hand X-ray based gender classification and bone age assessment using convolutional neural network. In Proceedings of the 2020 3rd International Conference on Computing, Mathematics and Engineering Technologies (iCoMET), Sukkur, Pakistan, 29–30 January 2020; pp. 1–5.
42. Liu, B.; Zhang, Y.; Chu, M.; Bai, X.; Zhou, F. Bone age assessment based on rank-monotonicity enhanced ranking CNN. *IEEE Access* **2019**, *7*, 120976–120983. [CrossRef]
43. Zulkifley, M.A.; Mohamed, N.A.; Abdani, S.R.; Kamari, N.A.M.; Moubark, A.M.; Ibrahim, A.A. Intelligent bone age assessment: An automated system to detect a bone growth problem using convolutional neural networks with attention mechanism. *Diagnostics* **2021**, *11*, 765. [CrossRef] [PubMed]

44. Lee, H.; Tajmir, S.; Lee, J.; Zissen, M.; Yeshiwas, B.A.; Alkasab, T.K.; Choy, G.; Do, S. Fully automated deep learning system for bone age assessment. *J. Digit. Imaging* **2017**, *30*, 427–441. [CrossRef]
45. Castillo, J.; Tong, Y.; Zhao, J.; Zhu, F. RSNA Bone-Age Detection Using Transfer Learning and Attention Mapping. In *ECE228 and SIO209 Machine Learning for Physical Applications*; 2018; pp. 1–5. Available online: http://noiselab.ucsd.edu/ECE228_2018/Reports/Report6.pdf (accessed on 1 February 2020).
46. Karargyris, A.; Kashyap, S.; Wu, J.T.; Sharma, A.; Moradi, M.; Syeda-Mahmood, T. Age prediction using a large chest X-ray dataset. In Proceedings of the Medical Imaging 2019: Computer-Aided Diagnosis, San Diego, CA, USA, 16–21 February 2019; p. 10950.
47. Nguyen, H.; Soohyung, K. Automatic whole-body bone age assessment using deep hierarchical features. *arXiv* **2019**, arXiv:1901.10237.
48. Janczyk, K.; Rumiński, J.; Neumann, T.; Głowacka, N.; Wiśniewski, P. Age prediction from low resolution, dual-energy X-ray images using convolutional neural networks. *Appl. Sci.* **2022**, *12*, 6608. [CrossRef]
49. Castillo, R.F.; Ruiz, M.D.C.L. Assessment of age and sex by means of DXA bone densitometry: Application in forensic anthropology. *Forensic Sci. Int.* **2011**, *209*, 53–58. [CrossRef] [PubMed]
50. Navega, D.; Coelho, J.D.O.; Cunha, E.; Curate, F. DXAGE: A new method for age at death estimation based on femoral bone mineral density and artificial neural networks. *J. Forensic Sci.* **2017**, *63*, 497–503. [CrossRef] [PubMed]
51. Pietka, B.E.; Pośpiech, S.; Gertych, A.; Cao, F.; Huang, H.K.; Gilsanz, V. Computer automated approach to the extraction of epiphyseal regions in hand radiographs. *J Digit Imaging.* **2001**, *14*, 165–172.
52. Pietka, E.; Gertych, A.; Pospiech-Kurkowska, S.; Cao, F.; Huang, H.K.; Gilsanz, V. Computer assisted bone age assessment: Graphical user interface for image processing and comparison. *J. Digit. Imaging* **2004**, *17*, 175–188. [CrossRef] [PubMed]
53. Gertych, A.; Piętka, E.; Liu, B.J. Segmentation of regions of interest and post-segmentation edge location improvement in computer-aided bone age assessment. *Pattern Anal. Appl.* **2007**, *10*, 115. [CrossRef]
54. Szczypinski, P.M.; Klepaczko, A.; Kociolek, M. QMaZda—Software tools for image analysis and pattern recognition. In Proceedings of the 2017 Signal Processing: Algorithms, Architectures, Arrangements, and Applications (SPA), Poznan, Poland, 20–22 September 2017; pp. 217–221.
55. Galloway, M.M. Texture analysis using grey level run lengths. *Comput. Graph. Image Process.* **1975**, *4*, 172–179. [CrossRef]
56. Kashyap, R.; Chellappa, R. Estimation and choice of neighbors in spatial-interaction models of images. *IEEE Trans. Inf. Theory* **1983**, *29*, 60–72. [CrossRef]
57. Porter, R.; Canagarajah, N. Rotation invariant texture classification schemes using GMRFs and wavelets. In Proceedings of the Proceedings IWISP'96, Manchester, UK, 4–7 November 1996; pp. 183–186.
58. Pierzchała, M.; Obuchowicz, R.; Guz, W.; Piórkowski, A. Correlation of the results of textural analysis of wrist MRI images with age in boys aged 9–17. *Bio-Algorithms Med-Syst.* **2021**, *17*, eA18–eA19.
59. Hu, J.; Wang, Y.; Guo, D.; Qu, Z.; Sui, C.h.; He, G.; Wang, S.; Chen, X.; Wang, C.h.; Liu, X. Diagnostic performance of magnetic resonance imaging–based machine learning in Alzheimer's disease detection: A meta-analysis. *Neuroradiology* **2023**, *65*, 513–527. [CrossRef]
60. Snider, E.J.; Hernandez-Torres, S.I.; Hennessey, R. Using ultrasound image augmentation and ensemble predictions to prevent machine-learning model overfitting. *Diagnostics* **2023**, *13*, 417. [CrossRef]
61. Shao, Y.; Hashemi, H.S.; Gordon, P.; Warren, L.; Wang, J.; Rohling, R.; Salcudean, S. Breast cancer detection using multimodal time series features from ultrasound shear wave absolute vibro-elastography. *IEEE J. Biomed. Health Inform.* **2022**, *26*, 704–714. [CrossRef] [PubMed]
62. d'Este, S.H.; Nielsen, M.B.; Hansen, A.E. Visualizing glioma infiltration by the combination of multimodality imaging and artificial Intelligence, a systematic review of the literature. *Diagnostics* **2021**, *11*, 592. [CrossRef] [PubMed]
63. Hoar, D.; Lee, P.Q.; Guida, A.; Patterson, S.; Bowen, C.V.; Merrimen, J.; Wang, C.; Rendon, R.; Beyea, S.D.; Clarke, S.E. Combined transfer learning and test-time augmentation improves convolutional neural network-based semantic segmentation of prostate cancer from multi-parametric MR images. *Comput. Methods Programs Biomed.* **2021**, *210*, 106375. [CrossRef] [PubMed]
64. Dalal, N.; Triggs, B. Histograms of oriented gradients for human detection. In Proceedings of the 2005 IEEE Computer Society Conference on Computer Vision and Pattern Recognition (CVPR'05), San Diego, CA, USA, 20–26 June 2005; Volume 1, pp. 886–893. [CrossRef]
65. Kreitner, K.F.; Schweden, F.J.; Riepert, T.; Nafe, B.; Thelen, M. Bone age determination based on the study of the medial extremity of the clavicle. *Eur. Radiol.* **1998**, *8*, 1116–1122. [CrossRef]
66. Charles, Y.P.; Dimeglio, A.; Canavese, F.; Daures, J.-P. Skeletal age assessment from the olecranon for idiopathic scoliosis at Risser grade 0. *J. Bone Joint Surg. Am.* **2007**, *89*, 2737–2744. [CrossRef] [PubMed]
67. Risser, J.C. The Iliac apophysis; an invaluable sign in the management of scoliosis. *Clin. Orthop.* **1958**, *11*, 111–119. [CrossRef]
68. Little, D.G.; Sussman, M.D. The Risser sign: A critical analysis. *J. Pediatr. Orthop.* **1994**, *14*, 569–575. [CrossRef]
69. Li, D.T.; Cui, J.J.; DeVries, S.; Nicholson, A.D.; Li, E.; Petit, L.; Kahan, J.B.; Sanders, J.O.; Liu, R.W.; Cooperman, D.R.; et al. Humeral head ossification predicts peak height velocity timing and percentage of growth remaining in children. *J. Pediatr. Orthop.* **2018**, *38*, E546–E550. [CrossRef] [PubMed]
70. Nicholson, A.D.; Liu, R.W.; Sanders, J.O.; Cooperman, D.R. Relationship of calcaneal and iliac apophyseal ossification to peak height velocity timing in children. *J. Bone Joint Surg. Am.* **2015**, *97*, 147–154. [CrossRef]

71. Li, S.Q.; Nicholson, A.D.; Cooperman, D.R.; Liu, R.W. Applicability of the calcaneal apophysis ossification staging system to the modern pediatric population. *J. Pediatr. Orthop.* **2019**, *39*, 46–50. [CrossRef]
72. Demirjian, A.; Goldstein, H.; Tanner, J.M. A new system of dental age assessment. *Hum. Biol.* **1973**, *45*, 211–227. [PubMed]
73. Sehrawat, J.S.; Singh, M. Willems method of dental age estimation in children: A systematic review and meta-analysis. *J. Forensic Leg. Med.* **2017**, *52*, 122–129. [CrossRef] [PubMed]
74. Malik, P.; Saha, R.; Agarwal, A. Applicability of Demirjian's method of age assessment in a North Indian female population. *Eur. J. Paediatr. Dent.* **2012**, *13*, 133–135.
75. Heyworth, B.E.; Osei, D.A.; Fabricant, P.D.; Schneider, R.; Doyle, S.h.M.; Green, D.W.; Widmann, R.F.; Lyman, S.; Burke, S.W.; Scher, D.M. The shorthand bone age assessment: A simpler alternative to current methods. *J. Pediatr. Orthop.* **2013**, *33*, 569–574. [CrossRef]
76. Thodberg, H.H.; Kreiborg, S.; Juul, A.; Pedersen, K.D. The BoneXpert method for automated determination of skeletal maturity. *IEEE Trans. Med. Imaging* **2009**, *28*, 52–66. [CrossRef] [PubMed]
77. Wang, F.; Gu, X.; Chen, S.; Liu, Y.; Shen, Q.; Pan, H.; Shi, L.; Jin, Z. Artificial intelligence system can achieve comparable results to experts for bone age assessment of Chinese children with abnormal growth and development. *PeerJ* **2020**, *8*, e8854. [CrossRef]
78. Liu, Y.; Zhang, C.; Cheng, J.; Chen, X.; Wang, Z.J. A multi-scale data fusion framework for bone age assessment with convolutional neural networks. *Comput. Biol. Med.* **2019**, *108*, 161–173. [CrossRef] [PubMed]
79. Ren, X.; Li, T.; Yang, X.; Wang, S.; Ahmad, S.; Xiang, L.; Stone, S.R.; Li, L.; Zhan, Y.; Shen, D.; et al. Regression convolutional neural network for automated pediatric bone age assessment from hand radiograph. *IEEE J. Biomed. Health Inform.* **2019**, *23*, 2030–2038. [CrossRef]
80. Tong, C.; Liang, B.; Li, J.; Zheng, Z. A Deep Automated Skeletal Bone Age Assessment Model with Heterogeneous Features Learning. *J. Med. Syst.* **2018**, *42*, 249. [CrossRef]
81. Mettler, F.A.; Huda, W.; Yoshizumi, T.T.; Mahesh, M. Effective doses in radiology and diagnostic nuclear medicine: A catalog 1. *Radiology* **2008**, *248*, 254–263. [CrossRef]
82. Xu, H.; Shao, H.; Wang, L.; Jin, J.; Wang, J. A Methodological comparison between ultrasound and X-ray evaluations of bone age. *J. Sports Sci.* **2008**, *6*, 27.
83. Stern, D.; Ebner, T.; Bischof, H.; Grassegger, S.; Ehammer, T.; Urschler, M. Fully automatic bone age estimation from left hand MR images. In *Medical Image Computing and Computer-Assisted Intervention—MICCAI 2014*; Golland, P., Hata, N., Barillot, C., Hornegger, J., Howe, R., Eds.; Lecture Notes in Computer Science; Springer: Berlin/Heidelberg, Germany, 2014; Volume 8674.
84. Qasim, M.S.h.; Abdullateef, A.; Mohammed, A.l.-H.; Najah, R.R. Magnetic resonance imaging of the left wrist: Assessment of the bone age in a sample of healthy Iraqi adolescent males. *J. Fac. Med.* **2015**, *57*, 22–26.
85. Ecklund, K.; Jaramillo, D. Patterns of premature physeal arrest: MR imaging of 111 children. *AJR Am. J. Roentgenol.* **2002**, *178*, 967–972. [CrossRef] [PubMed]
86. Ballock, R.T.; O'Keefe, R.J. The biology of the growth plate. *J. Bone Joint Surg. Am.* **2003**, *85*, 715–726. [CrossRef]
87. Breur, G.J.; van Enkevort, B.A.; Farnum, C.E.; Wilsman, N.J. Linear relationship between the volume of hypertrophic chondrocytes and the rate of longitudinal bone growth in growth plates. *J. Orthop. Res.* **1991**, *9*, 348–359. [CrossRef]
88. Yun, H.H.; Kim, H.J.; Jeong, M.S.; Choi, Y.S.; Seo, J.Y. Changes of the growth plate in children: 3-dimensional magnetic resonance imaging analysis. *Korean. J. Pediatr.* **2018**, *61*, 226–230. [CrossRef]
89. Craig, J.G.; Cody, D.D.; van Holsbeeck, M. The distal femoral and proximal tibial growth plates: MR imaging, three-dimensional modeling and estimation of area and volume. *Skelet. Radiol.* **2004**, *33*, 337–344. [CrossRef] [PubMed]
90. Stokes, I.A. Growth plate mechanics and mechanobiology. *A survey of present understanding. J. Biomech.* **2009**, *42*, 1793–1803.
91. Mitchell, D.G.; Kim, I.; Chang, T.S.; Vinitski, S.; Consigny, P.M.; Saporano, S.A.; Ehrlich, S.M.; Rifkin, M.D.; Rubin, R. Fatty liver: Chemical shift phase-difference and suppression magnetic resonance imaging techniques in animals, phantoms, and humans. *Invest. Radiol.* **1991**, *26*, 1041–1052. [CrossRef]
92. Bley, T.A.; Wieben, O.; François, C.J.; Brittain, J.H.; Reeder, S.B. Fat and water magnetic resonance imaging. *J. Magn. Reson. Imaging* **2010**, *31*, 4–18. [CrossRef]
93. Moon, W.J.; Lee, M.H.; Chung, E.C. Diffusion-weighted imaging with sensitivity encoding (SENSE) for detecting cranial bone marrow metastases: Comparison with T1-weighted images. *Korean J. Radiol.* **2007**, *8*, 185–191. [CrossRef]
94. Bzowski, P.; Borys, D.; Guz, W.; Obuchowicz, R.; Piórkowski, A. Evaluation of the MRI Images Matching Using Normalized Mutual Information Method and Preprocessing Techniques. *Adv. Intell. Syst. Comput.* **2020**, *1062*, 92–100. [CrossRef]
95. Wennmann, M.; Klein, A.; Bauer, F.; Chmelik, J.; Grözinger, M.; Uhlenbrock, C.; Lochner, J.; Nonnenmacher, T.; Rotkopf, L.T.; Sauer, S.; et al. Combining deep learning and radiomics for automated, objective, comprehensive bone marrow characterization from whole-body MRI. *A multicentric feasibility study. Invest. Radiol.* **2022**, *57*, 752–763. [CrossRef] [PubMed]
96. Wennmann, M.; Neher, P.; Stanczyk, N.; Kahl, K.C.; Kächele, J.; Weru, V.; Hielscher, T.; Grözinger, M.; Chmelik, J.; Zhang, K.S.; et al. Deep learning for automatic bone marrow apparent diffusion coefficient measurements from whole-body magnetic resonance imaging in patients with multiple myeloma: A retrospective multicenter study. *Invest. Radiol.* **2023**, *58*, 273–282. [CrossRef] [PubMed]

97. Wennmann, M.; Bauer, F.; Klein, A.; Chmelik, J.; Grözinger, M.; Rotkopf, L.T.; Neher, P.; Gnirs, R.; Kurz, F.T.; Nonnenmacher, T.; et al. In vivo repeatability and multiscanner reproducibility of MRI radiomics features in patients with monoclonal plasma cell disorders: A prospective bi-institutional study. *Invest Radiol.* **2023**, *58*, 253–264. [CrossRef] [PubMed]
98. Wennmann, M.; Thierjung, H.; Bauer, F.; Weru, V.; Hielscher, T.; Grözinger, M.; Gnirs, R.; Sauer, S.; Goldschmidt, H.; Weinhold, N.; et al. Repeatability and Reproducibility of ADC Measurements and MRI Signal Intensity Measurements of Bone Marrow in Monoclonal Plasma Cell Disorders: A Prospective Bi-institutional Multiscanner.; Multiprotocol Study. *Invest. Radiol.* **2022**, *57*, 272–281. [CrossRef]

Disclaimer/Publisher's Note: The statements, opinions and data contained in all publications are solely those of the individual author(s) and contributor(s) and not of MDPI and/or the editor(s). MDPI and/or the editor(s) disclaim responsibility for any injury to people or property resulting from any ideas, methods, instructions or products referred to in the content.

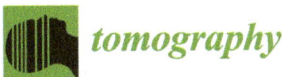

Article

Strain and Strain Rate Tensor Mapping of Medial Gastrocnemius at Submaximal Isometric Contraction and Three Ankle Angles

Ryan Hernandez [1,†], Usha Sinha [1,†], Vadim Malis [2], Brandon Cunnane [1], Edward Smitaman [3] and Shantanu Sinha [2,*]

1 Department of Physics, San Diego State University, San Diego, CA 92182, USA
2 Muscle Imaging and Modeling Lab., Department of Radiology, University of California San Diego, San Diego, CA 92037, USA
3 Department of Radiology, University of California San Diego, San Diego, CA 92182, USA
* Correspondence: shsinha@ucsd.edu; Tel.: +1-310-435-3994
† These authors contributed equally to this work.

Abstract: Introduction: The aim of this study is to analyze the muscle kinematics of the medial gastrocnemius (MG) during submaximal isometric contractions and to explore the relationship between deformation and force generated at plantarflexed (PF), neutral (N) and dorsiflexed (DF) ankle angles. Method: Strain and Strain Rate (SR) tensors were calculated from velocity-encoded magnetic resonance phase-contrast images in six young men acquired during 25% and 50% Maximum Voluntary Contraction (MVC). Strain and SR indices as well as force normalized values were statistically analyzed using two-way repeated measures ANOVA for differences with force level and ankle angle. An exploratory analysis of differences between absolute values of longitudinal compressive strain ($E_{\lambda 1}$) and radial expansion strains ($E_{\lambda 2}$) and maximum shear strain (E_{max}) based on paired t-test was also performed for each ankle angle. Results: Compressive strains/SRs were significantly lower at 25%MVC. Normalized strains/SR were significantly different between %MVC and ankle angles with lowest values for DF. Absolute values of $E_{\lambda 2}$ and E_{max} were significantly higher than $E_{\lambda 1}$ for DF suggesting higher deformation asymmetry and higher shear strain, respectively. Conclusions: In addition to the known optimum muscle fiber length, the study identified two potential new causes of increased force generation at dorsiflexion ankle angle, higher fiber cross-section deformation asymmetry and higher shear strains.

Keywords: muscle strain mapping; velocity-encoded MRI; fiber deformation asymmetry; shear strain

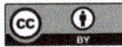

1. Introduction

Dynamic MRI studies using velocity-encoded phase-contrast imaging have enabled the extraction of 2D and 3D strain and strain rate tensors which provide information beyond one-dimensional strain measurements along the fiber [1–4]. The ability to measure both the compressive and radial expansion strains as well as shear strains enables a more detailed look at muscle and muscle fiber shape change during different types of contraction [5,6]. Further, principal strains can be extracted without the requirement for identifying the muscle fiber; this provides a lot of flexibility when muscle fibers are not visualized readily. Earlier studies on strain and strain rate tensor mapping have identified several features including, the anisotropy of deformation in the cross-section of the muscle fiber and deviation of the principal strain direction from the muscle fiber orientation [1,2,7]. There are several hypotheses and predictions from computational models that are related to some of these experimentally observed features [8]. For example, computational models have shown that the force output is increased when constraints to deformation are introduced in the fiber cross-section, i.e., a larger anisotropy of deformation in the fiber cross-section leads to larger forces being generated [8]. Computational models exploring force transmission from non-spanning fibers have identified that the shear in the endomysium can effectively transmit the force to the tendon [9]. Regarding anisotropy of deformation and muscle shape changes, Eng et al. used a physical model based on an array of actuators to show that when the actuators contract against a load the actuators radially expand in the width direction but are prevented from expanding in the height direction. These constraints determine the final shape change of the muscle on contraction [5]. Most studies on shape changes monitor at the entire muscle level while the shape changes also occur at the muscle fiber level [6]. In contrast to ultrasound, VE-PC MRI and strain/SR tensor mapping also provides a convenient way to monitor shape changes in muscle fiber bundles (at the level of the voxel).

Muscle sarcomere force-length (FL) relationship is well established and describes the dependence of the steady-state isometric force of a muscle (or fiber, or sarcomere) as a function of muscle (fiber, sarcomere) length [10,11]. Muscle fiber architecture (fiber length and pennation angle) will clearly influence force production. Several researchers have examined the force produced by the Medial Gastrocnemius (MG) during isometric, concentric, and eccentric plantarflexion contraction for combinations of knee flexion and ankle positions [12–15]. The initial muscle fiber length and pennation angle of the MG changes with knee flexion and ankle angle. Earlier studies have used electromyography (EMG) and ultrasound (US) to study muscle isometric plantarflexion force, activation, and muscle architecture changes in the MG for combinations of knee flexion and ankle angles [13–15]. These studies are in general agreement that there is a decrease in force accompanied by a decrease in the activation of the MG at pronounced knee flexion positions, i.e., short muscle lengths.

Phase-contrast MR imaging has been successfully implemented to study muscle kinematics under different contraction paradigms as well as under different muscle conditions [1,3,4]. Strain describes how the tissue is deformed with respect to a reference state and requires tissue tracking. SR describes the rate of regional deformation and does not require 3D tracking or a reference state. A positive Strain or SR indicates a local expansion while a negative strain or SR indicates a local contraction. Strain and strain rate in the direction closest to the fiber provides information on the fiber contractility, while in the orthogonal directions it provides information about the deformation in the fiber cross-section allowing one to explore radial deformation and asymmetry of radial deformation. Another relevant index derived from the tensors is the shear strain and shear strain rate; these two indices may potentially reflect extent of lateral transmission of force [1,9]. The current paper focuses on analyzing the 2D strain and SR tensor during submaximal isometric contraction at two force levels and three ankle positions (dorsiflexed, neutral and plantarflexed) in order to extract principal (longitudinal compression and radial expansion) strains and shear strains. The hypothesis of the paper is that the dorsiflexed ankle position (i) will be the most efficient for force production, i.e., yield the smallest normalized compressive strain (normalized to force), (ii) have the highest anisotropy of deformation in the fiber cross-section, and (iii) largest shear strain compared to the longitudinal compressive strains. These three factors will together lead to a higher force generated at the dorsiflexed ankle angle compared to the neutral and plantarflexed angle.

2. Materials and Methods

A total of six male subjects (33.2 ± 16.3 yrs, height: 172.5 ± 7.0 cm, mass: 73.3 ± 6.5 kg) were included in this study; the criterion for inclusion was that subjects should be moderately active (defined as 150 to 300 min per week of moderate intensity activity such as brisk walking). The cohort included five young subjects (mean age: 26 years) and one old subject (66 years) so the current study lacked statistical power to look at age related differences; however, this will be the subject for future studies. Subjects participating in competitive sports or those with any surgical procedures on the lower leg were excluded. In addition, subjects were asked not to perform strenuous exercise during the preceding 24 h before the imaging session. The study was approved by the Medical Research Ethics Board of University of California San Diego and conformed to all standards for the use of human subjects in research as outlined in the Declaration of Helsinki on the use of human subjects in research. Dynamic MR images were obtained of the subjects' lower dominant leg with a 1.5 T Signa HD16 MR scanner (General Electric Medical Systems, Milwaukee, WI, USA). The subjects were placed feet first in the supine position in the scanner and Figure 1 is a schematic that shows the positioning, visual feedback, force measurement and scan trigger setup. The dominant leg was placed into the foot pedal with the cardiac flex coil wrapped around the lower leg (the cardiac rather than a smaller coil was used in order to accommodate the foot pedal). The foot pedal device allowed for positioning and anchoring the foot at different ankle angles. In this study, the foot was positioned at three nominal angles—dorsiflexion (DF) 5°, neutral (N) $-25°$, and plantarflexion (PF) $-40°$. A large FOV image that included the ankle was collected at each foot position using the body coil to verify/estimate the ankle angle.

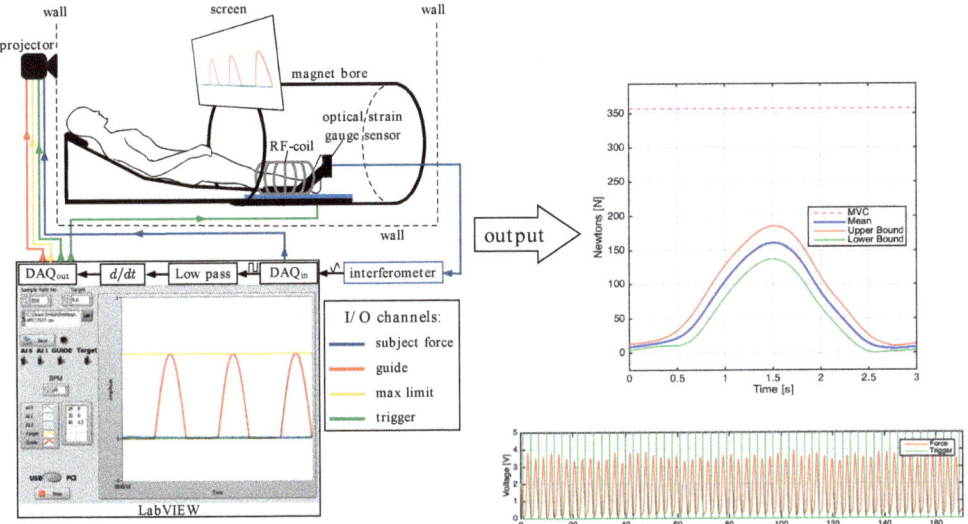

Figure 1. Left top panel: Subject setup with dominant leg in the foot pedal device, centered in a cardiac flex coil (labeled RF coil), with visual feedback projected onto the screen for the subject to follow. Pressure against the carbon-fiber plate in the foot pedal was detected by the transducer and converted into voltage and then converted into measurements of force. **Left bottom** panel: The foot pedal output was processed to generate a trigger to synchronize with the MR acquisition and also displayed to the subject on a screen. **Right top** panel: The force curve averaged over ~53 contractions (required to acquire the MR images) is shown along with upper and lower boundaries of the force curve. **Right lower** panel: Plot of the force curves for one VE-PC acquisition and the green vertical lines are the triggers. The foot positioning for neutral (N) ankle angle is shown here, dorsiflexed (DF) and plantarflexed (PF) positions were obtained by adjusting the ankle angle of the foot.

The ball of the foot rested on a carbon-fiber plate onto which an optical pressure transducer (Luna Innovations, Roanoke, VA, USA) was embedded (Figure 1). Pressure against the plate was detected by the transducer which was subsequently converted to a voltage and used to trigger the MR image acquisition. In addition to serving as a trigger for the MR acquisition, the pressure transducer voltage output was recorded at a sampling rate of 200 Hz (averaged during analysis to produce curves of mean force) and later converted into units of force (N) based on a calibration of the system using disc weights. The Maximum Voluntary Contraction (MVC) was determined for each subject as the best of three trials recorded prior to MR imaging. MVC was measured for each ankle position and sub-maximal contraction levels were set based on the MVC at that ankle position.

Images were acquired under different experimental conditions: during two submaximal, isometric contraction of the plantarflexor muscles (at 25% and 50% of the subject's MVC) with the foot at three ankle positions: dorsiflexed (DF), neutral (N), plantarflexed (PF). MR image acquisition required ~53 repeated contractions; thus, it was important to ensure consistency of motion. The subject was provided with the feedback of the actual force generated by the subject superposed on the desired force curve to facilitate consistent contractions.

Imaging Protocol: A large FOV sagittal scout was acquired using the body coil in order to measure the ankle angle from the images. A set of high-resolution water-saturated oblique sagittal fast spin echo (FSE) images of the MG (TE: 12.9 ms, TR: 925 ms, NEX: 4, slice thickness: 3 mm, interslice gap: 0 mm, FOV: 30 cm × 22.5 cm, 512 × 384 matrix) was initially acquired. This sequence provides high-tissue contrast from the high signal from fat in fascicles in the background of suppressed muscle water signal and was used to visualize fascicles. The slice that best depicted the fascicles was selected for the Velocity-Encoded Phase-Contrast (VE-PC) scan. The VE-PC sequence had three-directional velocity encoding and a single oblique sagittal slice was acquired (TE: 7.7 ms, TR: 16.4 ms, NEX: 2, FA: 20°, slice thickness: 5 mm, FOV: 30 cm × 22.5 cm, partial-phase FOV = 0.55, 256 × 192 matrix, 4 views/segment, 1 slice, 22 phases, 10 cm·s^{-1} 3 direction velocity encoding). This resulted in 53 repetitions [([192 (phase encode lines) × 0.55 (partial FOV) × 2 (NEX)/4 (views per segment) = 53])] for the image acquisition. In total, twenty-two phases (using view-sharing) were collected within each contraction–relaxation cycle of ~3 s (isometric contraction). At each ankle position, diffusion tensor images (DTI) using 30 diffusion directions at b = 400 s/mm^2 with geometric parameters matched to the VE-PC images were acquired. The study protocol included at each ankle angle: large FOV image, VE-PC at 50%, followed by the 5-min DTI acquisition and then 25%MVC. The foot was then repositioned before repeating the imaging protocol. It should be noted that this order of imaging was implemented to minimize fatigue between the different dynamic acquisitions. The DTI data are not used in the current study but in a separate analysis to identify fascicles to derive fiber strains.

Image Analysis: The phase images of the VE-PC data directly quantify velocity in the direction of the velocity-encoding gradient. Prior to extracting the velocity data, the phase images were corrected for phase artifacts arising from sources such as B$_0$ inhomogeneities and chemical shift and not from the velocity-encoding gradient. Velocity images extracted from the phase-corrected data are inherently noisy. As the calculation of the strain or SR tensor involves estimation of the spatial gradients of the displacement/velocity images that introduces additional noise into the image, the velocity images were first denoised using a 2D anisotropic diffusion filter [16]. The anisotropic diffusion filter reduces noise in homogenous regions while preserving edges, maintaining the effective resolution of the original velocity image. The filter was applied iteratively to reduce noise in homogenous regions, and was defined by the equation:

$$c(||\nabla I||) = \exp\left(-\left(\frac{||\nabla I||}{K}\right)^2\right) \tag{1}$$

where c is the diffusion coefficient, I is the image to be denoised, and ∇I is the image gradient. The extent of denoising is controlled by the value of K and the number of iterations. K was held at a low value of 2 since there are no strong edges in the phase images. The level of denoising was explored at two values of the number of iterations, N: 10 and 15. The number of iterations at 10 was chosen as an optimum, a trade-off between noise reduction in the strain indices and excessive blurring. Figure S1 shows the phase images acquired from velocity encoded in the x-, y- and z-directions, respectively, along with corresponding noise-filtered images at two values of N (10 and 15). The reduction in noise is readily visualized at both iterations while an increase in blurring is seen at N = 15 iteration.

Strain and SR tensor: Voxels in the entire volume were tracked to obtain (in-plane) displacements using the velocity information in the phase images. The displacement maps (in x- and y-directions) as well as the velocity maps were processed as outlined below to obtain 2D strain and strain rate tensors in the principal frame of reference. For each voxel in the displacement and velocity maps, the 2D spatial gradient maps, L, of the displacement and velocity vector were calculated as detailed in [1]:

$$L = \begin{bmatrix} \frac{\partial u}{\partial x} & \frac{\partial v}{\partial x} \\ \frac{\partial u}{\partial y} & \frac{\partial v}{\partial y} \end{bmatrix} \qquad (2)$$

where u and v are the x and y components of either the displacement or the velocity vector. The symmetric form of the spatial gradient of displacement or velocity is generated from:

$$D = 0.5\left(L + L^T\right) \qquad (3)$$

The symmetric tensor D was diagonalized to yield the 2×2 strain (E, Eulerian strain) and SR tensor in the principal frame of reference. The principal components of the strain or strain rate tensor (eigenvalues arranged in ascending order) were labeled as follows: $E_{\lambda 1}$ and $E_{\lambda 2}$ are the normal principal strains while $SR_{\lambda 1}$ and $SR_{\lambda 2}$, the normal principal strain rates (defined as perpendicular to the face of an element and represented by the diagonal terms of the E or SR tensor). It should be noted that during the compression part of the cycle, the eigenvector corresponding to $E_{\lambda 1}$ and $SR_{\lambda 1}$ is in a direction close to the muscle fiber direction while in the relaxation phase the eigenvectors are in a direction approximately orthogonal to the fiber direction. The reverse is true for $E_{\lambda 2}$ and $SR_{\lambda 2}$. Two other strain and SR indices are calculated from the tensors: the out-of-plane strain denoted by $E_{\text{out-plane}}$ and $SR_{\text{out-plane}}$ and the maximum shear strain or shear strain rate denoted by $E_{\max}$ and $SR_{\max}$, respectively. The out-of-plane strain and strain rate, which is in the fiber cross-section perpendicular to the imaging plane, was calculated from the sum of the principal eigenvalues at each voxel based on the assumption that muscle tissue is incompressible. A local contraction along the muscle will be accompanied by a local expansion in the plane perpendicular to the fiber. If considered in 3D, the sum of the three strain rates for an incompressible volume should be zero. However, only the 2D tensor is calculated here due to the constraints of single slice imaging, so the negative of the sum of the two eigenvalues (E or SR) yields the magnitude of the third eigenvalue.

$$E_{\text{out-plane}} = -\left(E_{\lambda_1} + E_{\lambda_2}\right) \qquad (4a)$$

$$SR_{\text{out-plane}} = -\left(SR_{\lambda_1} + SR_{\lambda_2}\right) \qquad (4b)$$

Shear strain and strain rate (represented by the off-diagonal terms of the E and SR tensors) are dependent on the frame of reference; it is zero in the principal frame and is a maximum when the 2D tensor is rotated from the principal frame by 45°. In this frame, the diagonal terms are zero and one can obtain the maximum shear strain or strain rate. Mathematically, the maximum shear strain or strain rate is also found from:

$$E_{\max} = 0.5\left(E_{\lambda_1} - E_{\lambda_2}\right) \qquad (5a)$$

$$SR_{\max} = 0.5\left(SR_{\lambda_1} - SR_{\lambda_2}\right) \qquad (5b)$$

Shear strains or strain rates are defined as parallel to the face of an element and represented by off-diagonal terms in the E or SR tensor).

Strain and SR indices in ROIs positioned at the proximal, middle and distal regions of the MG muscle (corresponding to a location at approximately 75%, 50% and 25% of the total length of the MG) were extracted. The ROIs were positioned in the first frame of the dynamic data and the pixels in the ROI were tracked using the velocity data to ensure that the measurement is performed on the same pixels even if they have moved to different locations. The tracked ROIs were also checked manually in a cine loop to confirm that the entire ROI stayed in the MG. Statistical analysis was performed on the average of values extracted from the proximal and middle ROIs; the distal ROI was not used as the values were noisy. An analysis of the spatial variation of the strain and strain rate between the proximal and middle regions would be interesting. However, the current study lacks the statistical power to introduce another factor in the analysis; this will be the subject of a future study. Values of all strain and strain rate indices values were extracted from the temporal frame corresponding to the peak in $SR_{\lambda1}$ for all strain rate indices and at the peak of $E_{\lambda1}$ for the strain indices.

Strain Deformation in the Fiber Cross-Section: In the following discussion, all strain values refer to absolute values.

Case 1: Symmetric deformation in fiber cross-section: In this case, the deformation in the fiber cross-section is symmetric, i.e., the deformation is the same in both directions. This leads to $E_{\lambda2} \sim E_{\text{out-plane}}$ and by the incompressibility of muscle tissue, these two strains will be equal to the half of $E_{\lambda1}$. The maximum shear strain will be $\sim 0.75 |E_{\lambda1}|$. This is illustrated in Figure 2a.

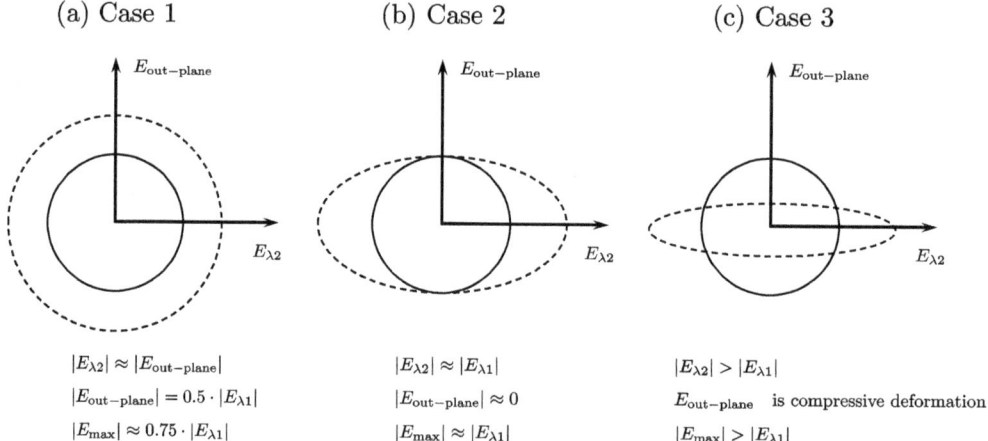

Figure 2. Schematic of different deformation patterns in the fiber cross-section, the non-deformed state is shown as a solid line and the deformed state with a dashed line. (**a**): Symmetric deformation in fiber cross-section leads to $|E_{\lambda2}| \sim |E_{\text{out-plane}}| \sim 0.5 |E_{\lambda1}|$ and $|E_{\max}| \sim 0.75 |E_{\lambda1}|$. (**b**): Asymmetric deformation in fiber cross-section with little to no deformation in the out-plane direction leads to $|E_{\lambda2}| \sim |E_{\lambda1}|$, $E_{\text{out-plane}} \sim 0$ and $|E_{\max}| \sim |E_{\lambda1}|$. (**c**): Highly asymmetric deformation in fiber cross-section with $|E_{\lambda2}| > |E_{\lambda1}|$ will lead to $E_{\text{out-plane}}$ being negative (compressive strain in the fiber cross-section) and $|E_{\max}| > |E_{\lambda1}|$.

Case 2: Asymmetric deformation in fiber cross-section: In this case, the deformation in the fiber cross-section is along one direction, say along $E_{\lambda2}$. Then, deriving from the incompressibility of muscle tissue, $E_{\text{out-plane}}$ will be close to zero or very low values and $E_{\lambda2}$ will be equal to $E_{\lambda1}$. The maximum shear strain will be $\sim E_{\lambda1}$. This is illustrated in Figure 2b.

Case 3: Highly asymmetric deformation in the fiber cross-section with $E_{\lambda2}$ greater than $E_{\lambda1}$. In this case, the deformation in the fiber cross-section is such that the radial expansion in the in-plane direction exceeds that of the compressive strain in the fiber direction. From the incompressibility of the muscle tissue, this will lead to a compressive deformation in the out-plane direction. The maximum shear strain will be greater than $E_{\lambda 1}$. This is illustrated in Figure 2c.

Statistical analysis: The outcome variables of the analysis are the eigenvalues of the strain tensor ($E_{\lambda 1}$, $E_{\lambda 2}$, $E_{\text{out-plane}}$, $E_{\max}$) and the strain rate tensor ($SR_{\lambda 1}$, $SR_{\lambda 2}$, $SR_{\text{out-plane}}$, $SR_{\max}$). Strain is unitless and the SR eigenvalues are in units of s^{-1}. Normality of data was tested by using both, the Shapiro–Wilke test and visual inspection of Q-Q plots. Principal strains and strains rates as well the normalized strains and strain rates were normally distributed. Thus, changes between ankle angles, %MVC as well as potential interaction effects (ankle angle × %MVC), were assessed using two-way repeated measures ANOVAs and in case of significant ANOVA results for the factor 'ankle angles', Bonferroni-adjusted post hoc analyses were performed. Data are reported as mean ± SD for the variables since they were normally distributed. For all tests, the level of significance was set at $\alpha = 0.05$. In addition to the above statistical tests, exploratory analysis using paired t-test was performed at each ankle angle between (i) absolute values of $E_{\lambda 1}$ and $E_{\lambda 2}$ using data from both force levels and (ii) absolute values of $E_{\lambda 1}$ and $E_{\max}$ using data from both force levels. The statistical analyses were carried out using SPSS for Mac OSX (SPSS 28.0.1.1, SPSS Inc., Chicago, IL, USA).

3. Results

3.1. MVC at Different Ankle Angles

Maximum Voluntary Contraction (MVC) was measured for each subject at each ankle angle as the best of three trials recorded prior to imaging: $MVC_{DF} = 289 \pm 9$ N, $MVC_N = 143 \pm 14$ N, $MVC_{PF} = 65 \pm 10$ N (average over all 6 subjects). The MVCs were significantly different between the three ankle angles: MVC_{DF-N} ($p = 0.0012$), MVC_{N-PF} ($p = 0.0003$), and MVC_{DF-PF} ($p = 0.0012$), where the subscripts are the two ankle angles compared in paired t-tests.

3.2. Strain and Strain Rate Maps and Temporal Plots of Deformation Indices

Figure 3 shows for one subject, the compressive strain ($E_{\lambda 1}$) and strain rate ($SR_{\lambda 1}$) maps through select frames of the dynamic cycle of 22 temporal frames for the three ankle angles at 50%MVC. The values of $E_{\lambda 1}$ and $SR_{\lambda 1}$ are superposed on the magnitude images of the VE-PC dataset using a colormap. Negative values of strain or strain rate (blue hue) are seen in the medial gastrocnemius and in the soleus (plantar flexor muscles) around frame 11 for the strain and around frames 8 and 16 for the strain rate maps. The temporal variation of strain and strain rate are shown in Figure 4a,b for one subject for a ROI placed in middle of the MG muscle for the three ankle angles and two %MVCs. Figure S2 shows for one subject, $E_{\lambda 2}$ and $SR_{\lambda 2}$ maps through select frames of the dynamic cycle of 22 temporal frames for the three ankle angles at 50%MVC. The values of $E_{\lambda 2}$ and $SR_{\lambda 2}$ are superposed on the magnitude images of the VE-PC dataset using a colormap. Positive values of strain or strain rate (red hue) are seen in the medial gastrocnemius and in the soleus (plantar flexor muscles) around frame 11 for the strain and around frames 8 and 16 for the strain rate maps.

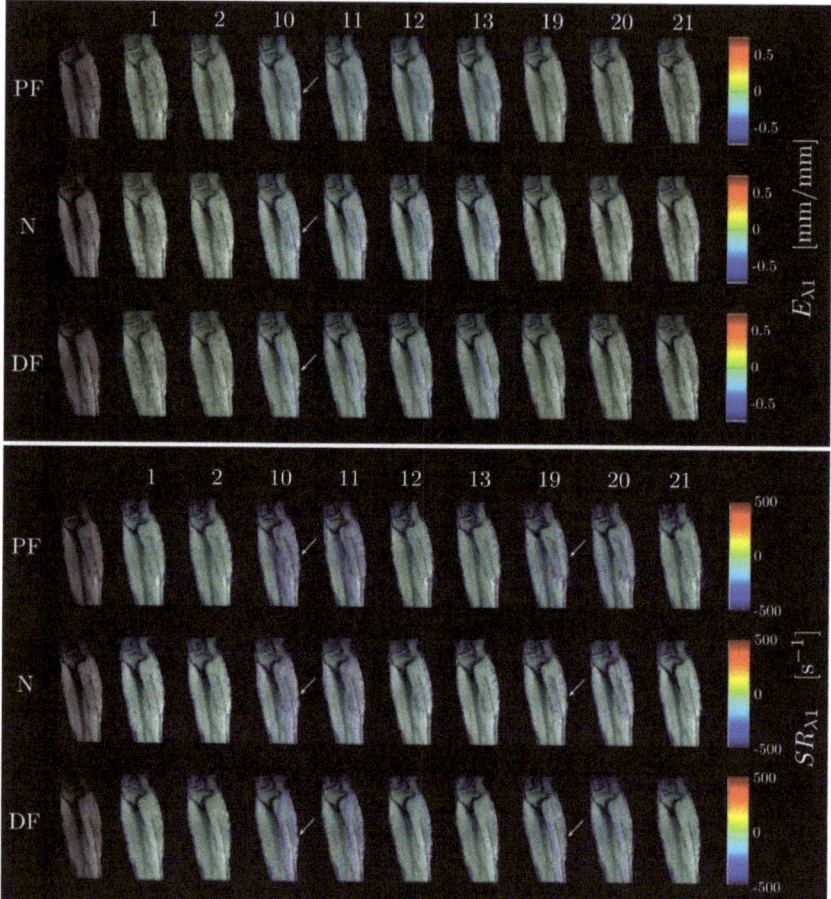

Figure 3. Maps of the negative strain ($E_{\lambda 1}$) (**top** panel) and negative strain rate ($SR_{\lambda 1}$) (**bottom** panel) projected on magnitude images at the corresponding temporal frame. Images shown here were acquired at 50%MVC, at each foot position PF, N, DF (order of rows **top** to **bottom**). Overlay allows for better identification of the underlying muscle, aponeuroses, and fascicles. The color maps are color-coded according to the legend with the figures. Select frames (from the acquired 22 dynamic frames) where peak strains and strain rates occur are shown here, the frame number is indicated on the top row. The peak of the strain occurs around frame 10–11 (arrow points to MG) where the blue shade corresponding to compressive strains in the MG and in the soleus can be seen. The peak of the strain rate occurs in the contraction (~frame 7–8, arrow to MG) and relaxation (~frame 16) phases and this is visualized as blue shades in the MG and in the soleus around these frames. The regions of interest in the MG (seen as red boxes in the first frame of each row) used to extract the deformation indices are shown in the first frame.

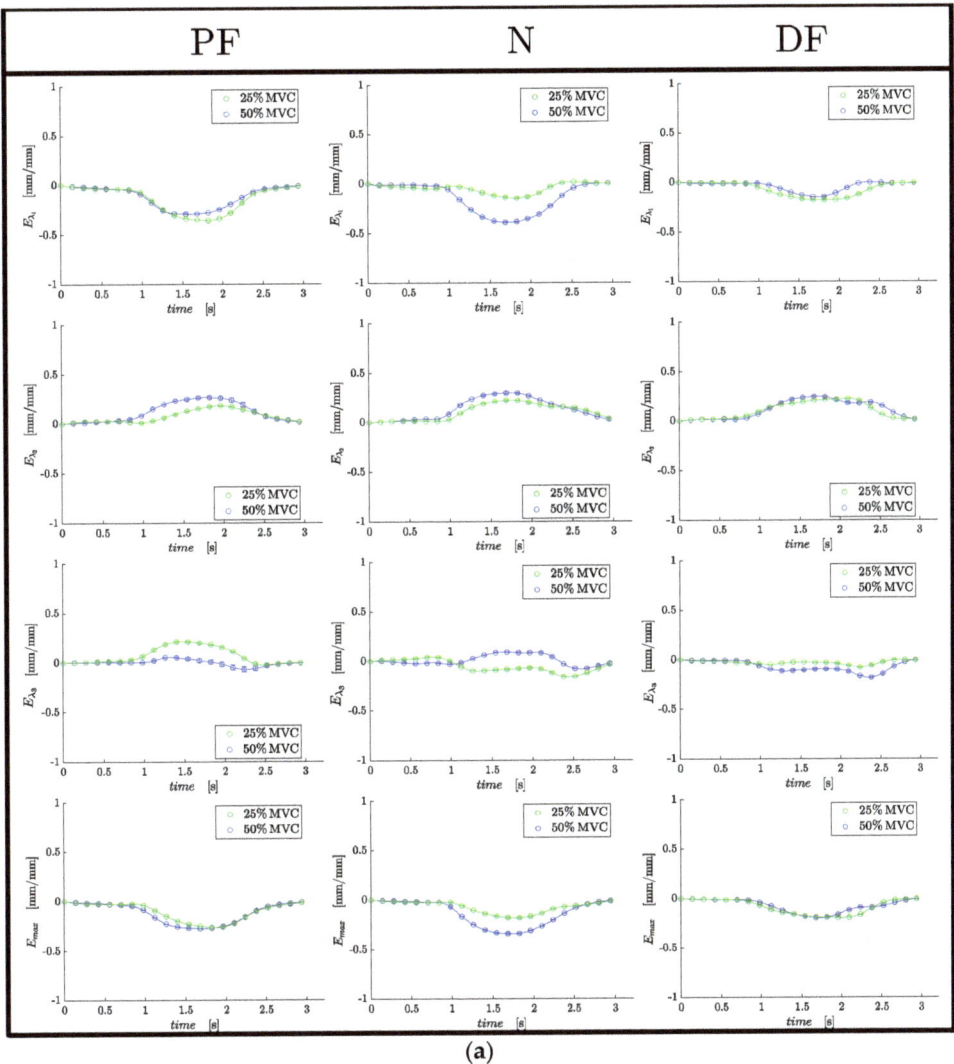

Figure 4. *Cont.*

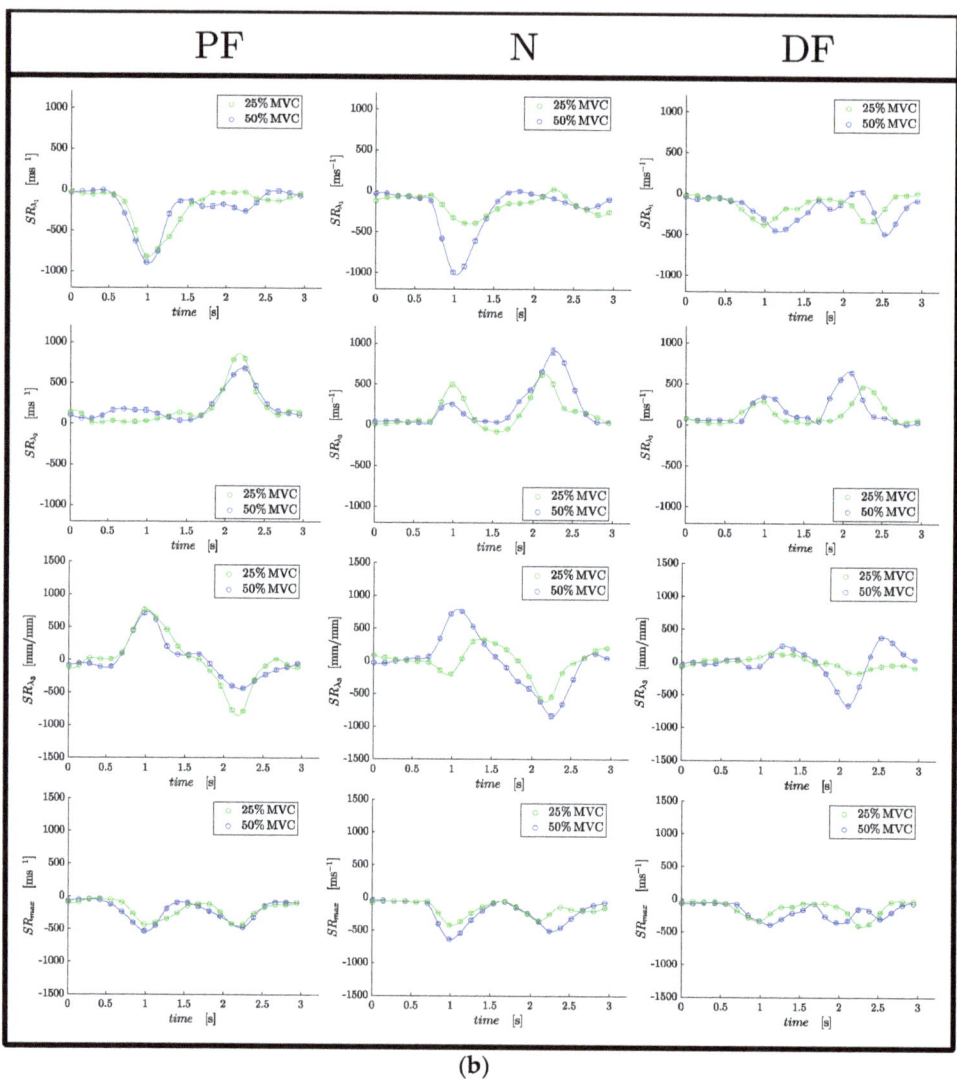

Figure 4. (a) Temporal plots for strain indices for one subject for an ROI placed in the middle of the MG muscle for the three ankle angles (PF, N, DF). Organized in column by foot angle position, and in row order of: $E_{\lambda 1}$, $E_{\lambda 2}$, $E_{\lambda 3 \text{ (or out-plane)}}$, and $E_{\max}$. (b) Temporal plots for strain rate indices for one subject for an ROI placed in the middle of the MG muscle for the three ankle angles (PF, N, DF). Organized in column by foot angle position, and in row order of: $SR_{\lambda 1}$, $SR_{\lambda 2}$, $SR_{\lambda 3 \text{ (or out-plane)}}$, and $SR_{\max}$.

3.3. Region of Interest Values of Deformation Indices at Peak Contraction

Table 1 and Table S1 list the peak strain and strain rate indices, respectively, averaged over all subjects for the three ankle angles and %MVC (data shown is the average for proximal and middle ROIs). Compressive strain and strain rate values ($E_{\lambda 1}$ and $SR_{\lambda 1}$) showed significantly lower absolute values at 25%MVC compared to 50%MVC while showing no significant changes between ankle angles. Radial strains and strain rates ($E_{\lambda 2}$, $SR_{\lambda 2}$, $E_{\text{out-plane}}$, $SR_{\text{out-plane}}$) in the fiber cross-section showed no significant changes with

%MVC or with ankle angle though $E_{\lambda2}$ was consistently higher at 50%MVC. The absolute values of $E_{\text{out-plane}}$ and $SR_{\text{out-plane}}$ are much smaller than the strains and strain rates in the other two directions, indicating that deformation is the smallest in this direction. Further, while $E_{\lambda2}$ and $SR_{\lambda2}$ are clearly radial expansion strain and strain rates, respectively, in the fiber cross-section, $E_{\text{out-plane}}$ and $SR_{\text{out-plane}}$ are smaller in magnitude and exhibit negative signs indicating that these are small radial compressive strain and strain rates, respectively, in the out-of-plane direction. This indicates that the deformation is close to that shown in Figure 2, between Case 2 and Case 3. It should be noted that the largest absolute values of $E_{\text{out-plane}}$ and $SR_{\text{out-plane}}$ occur for the dorsiflexed ankle position. The maximum shear strain showed no significant changes with either %MVC (though larger absolute values at 50%MVC) or ankle angle. Maximum shear strain rate showed significant changes with %MVC (higher absolute values at 50%MVC) but no significant change with ankle angle.

Table 1. Strain indices for different ankle angles and %MVC.

Ankle Position	%MVC	Peak Force (N)	$E_{\lambda1}$ *	$E_{\lambda2}$	$E_{\text{out-plane}}$	$E_{\max}$
Plantarflexion	50	32 ± 6.959	−0.141 ± 0.009	0.168 ± 0.03	−0.036 ± 0.031	−0.151 ± 0.019
	25	16.72 ± 3.694	−0.102 ± 0.022	0.137 ± 0.031	−0.046 ± 0.019	−0.117 ± 0.026
Neutral	50	74.24 ± 9.655	−0.185 ± 0.015	0.208 ± 0.025	−0.013 ± 0.033	−0.19 ± 0.014
	25	37.68 ± 4.883	−0.134 ± 0.024	0.202 ± 0.037	−0.068 ± 0.052	−0.165 ± 0.022
Dorsiflexion	50	141.2 ± 9.246	−0.143 ± 0.019	0.209 ± 0.008	−0.083 ± 0.023	−0.173 ± 0.006
	25	73.82 ± 4.26	−0.095 ± 0.027	0.169 ± 0.018	−0.092 ± 0.025	−0.129 ± 0.019

* Significant difference between 25% and 50%MVC.

Table 2 and Table S2 list the peak strain indices normalized to force and peak strain rate indices normalized to force, respectively, averaged over all subjects for the three ankle angles and %MVC (data shown are the average for proximal and middle ROIs). Comparing the absolute values across all %MVC and ankle angles, the lowest normalized strains were at 50%MVC and the dorsiflexed ankle angle while the highest values were at the 25%MVC and the plantarflexed ankle angle. $E_{\lambda1}$ normalized to force significantly changed with ankle angle, pairwise comparison revealed changes between (PF and DF), (PF and N), (N and DF) but showed no significant change with %MVC. $SR_{\lambda1}$ normalized to force significantly changed with %MVC and also with ankle angle, pairwise comparison revealed changes between PF and N. $E_{\lambda2}$ normalized to force showed significant change with %MVC as well as with ankle angles, pairwise comparison revealed changes between (PF and DF) and (N and DF). $SR_{\lambda2}$ normalized to force showed significant change with %MVC as well as with ankle angles, pairwise comparison revealed changes between (PF and N) and (PF and DF). Normalized $E_{\text{out-plane}}$ and $SR_{\text{out-plane}}$ showed no significant changes with either %MVC or with ankle angle. $E_{\max}$ and $SR_{\max}$ normalized to force significantly changed with %MVC and also with ankle angle, pairwise comparison revealed changes between (PF and DF), (N and DF).

Table 3 lists the absolute value of $E_{\lambda1}$, $E_{\lambda2}$ and $E_{\max}$ for each ankle angle averaged over all subjects and both force levels. The mean of $E_{\lambda2}$ was greater than $E_{\lambda1}$ for all three ankle angles and paired t-tests comparing the absolute values of $E_{\lambda1}$ and $E_{\lambda2}$ yielded the following results: for PF ankle angle, the absolute values of $E_{\lambda1}$ and $E_{\lambda2}$ were significantly different ($p = 0.04$), for neutral ankle angle the difference was not significant while for the dorsiflexed ankle the difference was highly significant ($p = 0.002$) and the largest difference in means of the absolute values of $E_{\lambda1}$ and $E_{\lambda2}$ was seen in the DF ankle angle (~59% compared to ~26% for the other two ankle angles). The mean of $E_{\max}$ was greater than $E_{\lambda1}$ for all three ankle angles and paired t-tests comparing the absolute values of $E_{\lambda1}$ and $E_{\max}$ showed significant differences between the two values only for the dorsiflexed ankle angle ($p = 0.004$) and the size effect was also largest at the DF ankle angle (~27% compared to ~10%).

Table 2. Strain indices normalized to force for different ankle angles and %MVC.

Ankle Position	%MVC	Peak Force (N)	$E_{\lambda 1}$ o,l,δ	$E_{\lambda 2}$ o,l,*	$E_{\text{out-plane}}$	$E_{\max}$ o,l,*
PF	50	32 ± 6.96	−0.0053 ± 0.001	0.0061 ± 0.0012	−0.001 ± 0.0016	−0.0056 ± 0.001
	25	16.72 ± 3.69	−0.0069 ± 0.0007	0.01 ± 0.0012	−0.0041 ± 0.0009	−0.0083 ± 0.0009
N	50	74.24 ± 9.65	−0.0027 ± 0.0004	0.0032 ± 0.0004	−0.0003 ± 0.0004	−0.0028 ± 0.0003
	25	37.68 ± 4.88	−0.0043 ± 0.0011	0.0058 ± 0.0007	−0.0012 ± 0.0018	−0.005 ± 0.0006
DF	50	141.2 ± 9.25	−0.001 ± 0.0002	0.0015 ± 0.0001	−0.0006 ± 0.0002	−0.0012 ± 0.0001
	25	73.82 ± 4.26	−0.0015 ± 0.0005	0.0025 ± 0.0003	−0.0013 ± 0.0004	−0.0019 ± 0.0003

* Significant difference between 25% and 50%MVC; l Significant difference between PF and DF; δ Significant difference between PF and N; o Significant difference between N and DF.

Table 3. Comparison of absolute values (std dev) of $E_{\lambda 1}$ to $E_{\lambda 2}$ and $E_{\lambda 1}$ to $E_{\max}$ for PF, N, DF.

Ankle Position	Abs ($E_{\lambda 1}$)	$E_{\lambda 2}$	Abs ($E_{\max}$)	%Diff ($E_{\lambda 1}, E_{\lambda 2}$)	%Diff ($E_{\lambda 1}, E_{\max}$)
Plantarflexion *	0.121(0.044)	0.152(0.073)	0.134(0.056)	25.50%	10.10%
Neutral	0.160(0.054)	0.205(0.073)	0.178(0.044)	28.60%	11.40%
Dorsiflexion *,**	0.119(0.060)	0.189(0.039)	0.151(0.040)	59.40%	27.30%

* Significant difference between absolute values of $E_{\lambda 1}$ and $E_{\lambda 2}$; ** Significant difference between $E_{\lambda 1}$ and $E_{\max}$.

4. Discussion

The force attained at Maximum Voluntary Contraction (MVC) at the three ankle angles were significantly different ($p < 0.001$) with the maximum MVC at the dorsiflexed ankle position and the minimum MVC at the plantarflexed position. This clearly shows that the most efficient ankle position for force generation is the dorsiflexed position. This has also been observed in previous studies [13–15]. Moreover, this finding highlights the importance of maintaining the ankle angle in the same position for longitudinal or cross-sectional dynamic cohort studies (e.g., young vs. old subjects).

Strain and strain rate are deformation indices; strain requires a frame of reference while strain rate is an instantaneous measurement. Strain rate is equal to differential velocities of the tissue, while strain is equal to differential displacement. Thus, strain rate maps reported herein are derived from the acquired velocity images, while the strain maps are computed from displacement maps tracked from the acquired velocity images. While strain and strain rate are related, SR can be different for tissue regions having the same strain. This is the first study of principal strains and strain rates during isometric contraction at different ankle positions. It has the advantage that compared to fiber strains, there is no need to identify the direction of the muscle fibers. In ultrasound and prior dynamic MR studies, muscle fibers were identified via fascicle locations [1,13]. This latter process is prone to error (since fascicles may not entirely run in the plane of the image) and suffers from low contrast (e.g., the lack of fat tissue in young subjects close to the fascicles prevents visualization of the fascicles in MRI). Further, the 2D strain/SR tensor analysis used in the current paper provides measurements of the deformation in the fiber cross-section as well as the shear strain in addition to the contractile strain. In contrast, 1D strain analysis (either US or MRI) can only provide information about muscle contractility [13]. In-plane deformation and shear strain/SR are influenced by the material properties of the extracellular matrix (ECM) and thus, measurement of the in-plane deformation and shear strain/shear strain rate with ankle angle could potentially provide information on the effect of the ECM on force production. Further, the ability to measure or deduce deformations in the fiber cross-section affords an opportunity to monitor fiber shape changes during isometric contraction at the different ankle angle positions.

At each ankle position, absolute values of the strain indices increased with submaximal %MVC, although it was significant only for $E_{\lambda 1}$, $SR_{\lambda 1}$ and $SR_{\max}$ (Table 1). Significant differences in $E_{\lambda 1}$ and $SR_{\lambda 1}$ with %MVC are anticipated as the higher force at the higher %MVC requires a larger contraction (strain). Surprisingly, there were no significant differences in the strain or SR indices between the different ankle angles despite a highly significant difference in force between the different ankle angles. This implies that similar strains (amount of contraction) at the different ankle angles were capable of producing significantly different forces. The deduced absolute values of $E_{\text{out-plane}}$ and $SR_{\text{out-plane}}$ are much smaller than the strains and strain rates in the orthogonal direction of the fiber cross-section indicating a strong anisotropy of deformation; this is true for all ankle angles. Anisotropy of fiber cross-section deformation has been reported in earlier studies for the neutral ankle angle [1–4,17]. The results from this study also show that anisotropy holds at plantarflexed and dorsiflexed ankle angles.

The normalized strain indices (normalized to the force for the ankle position/%MVC) showed significant differences for both force levels and ankle positions (Table 2). The absolute value of the normalized strain/SR indices was higher for the lower %MVC than for the higher %MVC: this implies a lack of linearity between strain and %MVC and that larger contraction/force (strains) is needed to achieve lower %MVCs. This may also arise from the MG contributing more to force production at lower %MVCs and the soleus contributing more at the higher %MVCs. All the normalized strain and strain rate indices were lower in the dorsiflexed position than in the plantarflexed or neutral ankle positions and most of these changes were significant (Table 2). The changes in the normalized principal compressive strain can be understood in terms of the muscle force–length (FL) curve. The FL relationship describes the dependence of the steady-state isometric force of a muscle fiber or sarcomere on muscle fiber or sarcomere length and the 'sliding filament' theory has been used to explain the FL curve [10,11]. In this theory, the maximal isometric force of a sarcomere is determined by the amount of overlap between the contractile filaments, actin, and myosin [10]. Starting from short muscle lengths, force increases as sarcomere length increases (ascending slope), reaches a plateau at intermediate lengths (optimal length for maximum force production), followed by a decrease in force as sarcomere length increases (descending slope) at long muscle lengths. Lower normalized strain at the DF ankle position implies that small contractions at this ankle angle are capable of producing large forces from which it can be deduced that the muscle fiber length in the dorsiflexed position is close to the optimal length of the force–length curve. Compared to the dorsiflexed position, the plantarflexed position is inefficient for force production—essentially implying that it is far from the optimal length for isometric force production. Normalized strains in the neutral ankle position were intermediate between the plantar and dorsiflexion states. Prior studies have identified that, in vivo, the plantar flexors work on the ascending limb of the force–length relationship due to the anatomical constraints of the ankle- and knee-joints [11–13]. The lower force of the plantarflexed angle can thus be attributed to the shorter length of the muscle fiber at this ankle angle which places it lower on the ascending limb of the FL curve and consequently, lower force production.

Arampatzis et al. studied MG fiber lengths and electrical activity using US and EMG, respectively [13]. They reported that active fiber lengths at MVC were not significantly different between knee flexion/ankle angle positions even though resting fiber lengths were significantly different between knee flexion/ankle angle positions [13]. Furthermore, EMG was significantly reduced in the most plantarflexed position despite active fiber lengths being the same in all the knee flexion/ankle angle positions. Arampatzis et al. identified that the main mechanism for the decrease in EMG activity is a neural inhibition mechanism [13]. This neural inhibition occurs because the muscle reaches a critical shortened length and since it is further down in the ascending limb of the force–length relationship, the torque output cannot be increased even if the muscle is fully activated [18]. Compared to Arampatzis' study that reported a reduction in EMG at the plantarflexed position, the current study did not see a reduction in strain (no significant difference in strain or SR between the ankle angles) at PF [13]. One source of discrepancy could be that the maximum force level was at 50%MVC in the current study compared to 100%MVC for the US/EMG studies. However, it should be noted that the current study, similar to previous studies, also identified the plantarflexed position as the least efficient in force production.

The above analysis of the contractile strain/SR attributes the lower force generation at the plantarflexed ankle angle (compared to the neutral/dorsiflexed ankle angle) entirely to the critical shortened length and the relative position on the force length curve for the three ankle angles. While this is likely the biggest contributor to the reduced force and to the increase in normalized strains at PF (larger strains/force compared to the DF ankle angle), the current analysis shows there may potentially be other contributors to the loss of force. Azizi et al. advanced the hypothesis that constraints to radial expansion in the fiber cross-section could limit the extent of contraction, limiting force generation and verified this in a physical model and in vivo; the latter by applying external constraints in the muscle cross-section [19]. An analysis of the absolute values of $E_{\lambda 1}$ and $E_{\lambda 2}$ for the three ankles showed that the dorsiflexed ankle position had the largest and most significant difference ($|E_{\lambda 2}| > |E_{\lambda 1}|$); the deformation is similar to that shown in Figure 2c. On the other hand, while $|E_{\lambda 2}| > |E_{\lambda 1}|$ for both plantarflexor and neutral ankle angles, the differences were smaller and tentatively, the deformation patterns in these two ankle angles may be between the schematics shown in Figure 2b,c. One explanation for the PF and N to have smaller in-plane deformations (smaller $E_{\lambda 2}$) compared to the dorsiflexed position may be related to the initial (at rest) fiber radial size. The plantarflexed position has the largest fiber cross-section of the three ankle angles and the larger initial radial size may provide a constraint to further radial expansion. Azizi et. al. showed with a physical model that constraints to radial expansion limits the contractility and thus, the force generated [19]. Thus, the constraints to radial expansion in the PF (arising from the larger radius) may also be a contributor to force reduction in this ankle angle position. Further, computational modeling studies have predicted that when there is a strongly anisotropic constraint the force output may increase by a factor of two [8]. This latter computational model showed that maximum force output was obtained by introducing anisotropy of passive material stiffness along the fiber cross-sectional axes such that there was very little deformation along one axis (the through-plane axis) during a muscle length change. In this anisotropic model, the stiffness in one direction was reinforced such that it was stiffer by a factor of 4 compared to the orthogonal direction that resulted in a near doubling in force compared to an isotropically stiff material. The authors postulated that the structural muscle proteins called costameres were a potential candidate for introducing such an anisotropy in the passive material properties [8]. Highly asymmetric deformation in the fiber cross-section seen in DF may be facilitated since in this ankle position, the fiber is longest and consequently, the fiber cross-section area is the smallest allowing larger radial expansions. A strongly anisotropic constraint, as is seen in DF, provides another potential mechanism of higher force in DF from the highly asymmetric deformation at this ankle angle. It should be noted that the strain in the fiber cross-section ($E_{\lambda 2}$) is also highly likely to be determined by the extracellular matrix (e.g., a stiffer ECM will offer a greater constraint to deformation).

An analysis of the difference in absolute values of $E_{\lambda 1}$ and E_{max} at each ankle angle also showed that E_{max} was greater than $E_{\lambda 1}$ in all three ankle angles but was significantly so only for the dorsiflexed ankle angle. In terms of the deformation pattern, this also indicates that while PF and N ankle angles are potentially between the schematics shown for asymmetric to highly asymmetric (Figure 2b,c), the dorsiflexion case may potentially correspond to highly asymmetric. Prior MR studies found a significant positive correlation of force in a cohort of young and old subjects or force loss due to unloading to the absolute value of the max shear strain (E_{max}) [7,20]. Thus, another potential reason for the higher force generated may arise for higher absolute values of E_{max} in the dorsiflexed position.

A recent study measured intramuscular pressure (IMP) and EMG during isometric dorsiflexion (DF) MVC and isometric DF ramp contractions at DF, N, and plantarflexion (PF) ankle positions [21]. IMP was significantly correlated to the ankle torque during ramp contractions at each ankle position tested. However, the IMP did not reflect the change in the ankle torque which changed significantly at different ankle positions. Similar to the IMP study, the current study also showed that compressive strains at each ankle angle did not reflect the change in MVC at different ankle angles. However, normalized strains

(strains normalized to force) were significantly different between the ankle angles with an inverse correlation (higher force at DF was associated with the lowest normalized strain). An application of studying skeletal muscle under different ankle angle positions is in the examination of the EMG-torque slope in chronic stroke survivors [22]. The findings of the latter study suggest that muscular contraction efficiency is affected by hemispheric stroke, but in an angle-dependent and non-uniform manner. A future extension of the current work could be to study MRI-derived strain–force or strain–torque relationships in chronic stroke survivors to explore whether the patterns are similar to normal subjects or affected like the EMG-torque relationship [22]. It should also be noted that with the development of fast diffusion tensor imaging techniques such as the B-matrix spatial distribution method (BSD-DTI), it becomes more feasible to integrate dynamic strain mapping with diffusion tensor imaging [23].

There are some limitations to this study: (i) A single slice is acquired, limiting the strain analysis to a 2D tensor. In reality, the strain is a 3D tensor and volume imaging is required to capture the full trajectory of 3D tissue motion. However, it has been shown in earlier studies as well as in this study that the deformation is predominantly planar. It is demonstrated in this paper by the relatively small values of $E_{out\text{-}plane}$ or $SR_{out\text{-}plane}$. Further, care was taken to ensure that the acquired oblique sagittal slice captured the MG fibers in the imaging plane. (ii) The cohort size is small but the repeated measures design provides higher statistical power and statistically significant differences were seen between the normalized strain and strain rate values between the different ankle angles. This is a proof-of-concept paper where a new technique is established (2D strain tensor analysis to track changes of compressive, radial expansive and shear strains for different fiber architecture). The technique will be expanded in a future study to include a larger number of subjects and applied to studying differences with age and in disease conditions such as muscular dystrophy. The proposed MRI-based strain technique can also be adapted for elastography and compared to other techniques such as elastosonography [24].

5. Conclusions

In summary, 2D strain and strain rate tensor mapping of muscle deformation at three ankle angles provided insight on the effect of resting fiber length on the force generated. The decrease in MVC at the plantarflexed ankle angle position could tentatively be attributed to the shortened rest length which places it lower on the ascending arm of the FL curve. In addition to changes in contractile strain, this study revealed a strong asymmetry in deformation in the fiber cross-section with the highest asymmetry at the dorsiflexed ankle angle. The highest values of shear strain (relative to the contractile strain) were also seen at the dorsiflexed ankle angle. This study points to the potential contribution of factors besides the known contribution from the resting length of the muscle being close to optimum for force production in the dorsiflexed position. These additional factors are the increased deformation asymmetry and increased relative shear strain, representing two parameters that may also increase force production at the dorsiflexed position.

Supplementary Materials: The following supporting information can be downloaded at: https://www.mdpi.com/article/10.3390/tomography9020068/s1, Figure S1: Maps of the acquired velocity (phase) images and after denoising with 10 and 15 iterations respectively of the anisotropic diffusion filter. Figure S2: Maps of the positive strain ($E_{\lambda 2}$) and positive strain rate ($SR_{\lambda 2}$). Table S1: Strain rate indices for different ankle angles and %MVC. Table S2: Strain rate indices normalized to force for different ankle angles and %MVC.

Author Contributions: Conceptualization, U.S.; Formal analysis, R.H. and U.S.; Funding acquisition, S.S.; Methodology, V.M., B.C. and S.S.; Software, R.H. and V.M.; Supervision, U.S. and V.M.; Writing—original draft, U.S.; Writing—review and editing, R.H., U.S., V.M., B.C., E.S. and S.S. All authors have read and agreed to the published version of the manuscript.

Funding: This research was funded by National Institute on Aging (National Institute of Health, USA), grant number R01AG056999.

Institutional Review Board Statement: The study was conducted in accordance with the Declaration of Helsinki, and approved by the Institutional Review Board (or Ethics Committee) of University of California at San Diego (UCSD IRB# 171489, 6 July 2021) for studies involving humans.

Informed Consent Statement: Informed consent was obtained from all subjects involved in the study.

Data Availability Statement: The data presented in this study are available on request from the corresponding author.

Conflicts of Interest: The authors declare no conflict of interest. The funders had no role in the design of the study; in the collection, analyses, or interpretation of data; in the writing of the manuscript; or in the decision to publish the results.

References

1. Sinha, U.; Malis, V.; Csapo, R.; Moghadasi, A.; Kinugasa, R.; Sinha, S. Age-related differences in strain rate tensor of the medial gastrocnemius muscle during passive plantarflexion and active isometric contraction using velocity encoded MR imaging: Potential index of lateral force transmission. *Magn. Reson. Med.* **2014**, *73*, 1852–1863. [CrossRef]
2. Englund, E.K.; Elder, C.P.; Xu, Q.; Ding, Z.; Damon, B.M. Combined diffusion and strain tensor MRI reveals a heterogeneous, planar pattern of strain development during isometric muscle contraction. *Am. J. Physiol. Regul. Integr. Comp. Physiol.* **2011**, *300*, R1079–R1090. [CrossRef]
3. Malis, V.; Sinha, U.; Sinha, S. 3D muscle deformation mapping at submaximal isometric contractions: Applications to aging muscle. *Front. Physiol.* **2020**, *11*, 600590. [CrossRef]
4. Mazzoli, V.; Gottwald, L.M.; Peper, E.S.; Froeling, M.; Coolen, B.F.; Verdonschot, N.; Sprengers, A.M.; van Ooij, P.; Strijkers, G.J.; Nederveen, A.J. Accelerated 4D phase contrast MRI in skeletal muscle contraction. *Magn. Reason. Med.* **2018**, *80*, 1799–1811. [CrossRef]
5. Eng, C.M.; Azizi, E.; Roberts, T.J. Structural determinants of muscle gearing during dynamic contractions. *Integr. Comp. Biol.* **2018**, *58*, 207–218. [CrossRef]
6. Raiteri, B.J.; Cresswell, A.G.; Lichtwark, G.A. Three-dimensional geometrical changes of the human tibialis anterior muscle and its central aponeurosis measured with three-dimensional ultrasound during isometric contractions. *PeerJ* **2016**, *4*, e2260. [CrossRef]
7. Sinha, U.; Malis, V.; Csapo, R.; Narici, M.; Sinha, S. Shear strain rate from phase contrast velocity encoded MRI: Application to study effects of aging in the medial gastrocnemius muscle. *J. Magn. Reson. Imaging.* **2018**, *48*, 1351–1357. [CrossRef] [PubMed]
8. Hodgson, J.A.; Chi, S.W.; Yang, J.P.; Chen, J.S.; Edgerton, V.R.; Sinha, S. Finite element modeling of passive material influence on the deformation and force output of skeletal muscle. *J. Mech. Behav. Biomed. Mater.* **2012**, *9*, 163–183. [CrossRef] [PubMed]
9. Sharafi, B.; Blemker, S.S. A mathematical model of force transmission from intrafascicularly terminating muscle fibers. *J. Biomech.* **2011**, *44*, 2031–2039. [CrossRef] [PubMed]
10. Moo, E.K.; Leonard, T.R.; Herzog, W. The sarcomere force-length relationship in an intact muscle-tendon unit. *J. Exp. Biol.* **2020**, *223*, jeb215020. [CrossRef]
11. Maganaris, C.N. Force-length characteristics of in vivo human skeletal muscle. *Acta Physiol. Scand.* **2001**, *172*, 279–285. [CrossRef]
12. Maganaris, C.N. Force-length characteristics of the in vivo human gastrocnemius muscle. *Clin. Anat.* **2003**, *16*, 215–223. [CrossRef] [PubMed]
13. Arampatzis, A.; Karamanidis, K.; Stafilidis, S.; Morey-Klapsing, G.; DeMonte, G.; Brüggemann, G.P. Effect of different ankle- and knee-joint positions on gastrocnemius medialis fascicle length and EMG activity during isometric plantar flexion. *J. Biomech.* **2006**, *39*, 1891–1902. [CrossRef]
14. Wakahara, T.; Kanehisa, H.; Kawakami, Y.; Fukunaga, T. Fascicle behavior of medial gastrocnemius muscle in extended and flexed knee positions. *J. Biomech.* **2007**, *40*, 2291–2298. [CrossRef]
15. Wakahara, T.; Kanehisa, H.; Kawakami, Y.; Fukunaga, T. Effects of knee joint angle on the fascicle behavior of the gastrocnemius muscle during eccentric plantar flexions. *J. Electromyogr. Kinesiol.* **2009**, *19*, 980–987. [CrossRef] [PubMed]
16. Maesli, B. Nonlinear anisotropic diffusion methods for image denoising problems: Challenges and future research opportunities. *Array* **2023**, *17*, 100265. [CrossRef]
17. Kinugasa, R.; Hodgson, J.A.; Edgerton, V.R.; Sinha, S. Asymmetric deformation of contracting human gastrocnemius muscle. *J. Appl. Physiol.* **2012**, *112*, 463–470. [CrossRef]
18. Kennedy, P.M.; Cresswell, A.G. The effect of muscle length on motor-unit recruitment during isometric plantar flexion in humans. *Exp. Brain Res.* **2001**, *137*, 58–64. [CrossRef] [PubMed]
19. Azizi, E.; Deslauriers, A.R.; Holt, N.C.; Eaton, C.E. Resistance to radial expansion limits muscle strain and work. *Biomech. Model. Mechanobiol.* **2017**, *16*, 1633–1643. [CrossRef]
20. Malis, V.; Sinha, U.; Csapo, R.; Narici, M.; Sinha, S. Relationship of changes in strain rate indices estimated from velocity-encoded MR imaging to loss of muscle force following disuse atrophy. *Magn. Reson. Med.* **2018**, *79*, 912–922. [CrossRef]
21. Ateş, F.; Davies, B.L.; Chopra, S.; Coleman-Wood, K.; Litchy, W.J.; Kaufman, K.R. intramuscular pressure of tibialis anterior reflects ankle torque but does not follow joint angle-torque relationship. *Front. Physiol.* **2018**, *9*, 22. [CrossRef] [PubMed]

22. Son, J.; Rymer, W.Z. Effects of changes in ankle joint angle on the relation between plantarflexion torque and EMG magnitude in major plantar flexors of male chronic stroke survivors. *Front. Neurol.* **2020**, *11*, 224. [CrossRef] [PubMed]
23. Mazur, W.; Urbańczyk-Zawadzka, M.; Banyś, R.; Obuchowicz, R.; Trystuła, M.; Krzyżak, A.T. diffusion as a natural contrast in MR imaging of peripheral artery disease (PAD) tissue changes. A case study of the clinical application of DTI for a patient with chronic calf muscles ischemia. *Diagnostics* **2021**, *11*, 92. [CrossRef] [PubMed]
24. Pichiecchio, A.; Alessandrino, F.; Bortolotto, C.; Cerica, A.; Rosti, C.; Raciti, M.V.; Rossi, M.; Berardinelli, A.; Baranello, G.; Bastianello, S.; et al. Muscle ultrasound elastography and MRI in preschool children with Duchenne muscular dystrophy. *Neuromuscul. Disord.* **2018**, *28*, 476–483. [CrossRef]

Disclaimer/Publisher's Note: The statements, opinions and data contained in all publications are solely those of the individual author(s) and contributor(s) and not of MDPI and/or the editor(s). MDPI and/or the editor(s) disclaim responsibility for any injury to people or property resulting from any ideas, methods, instructions or products referred to in the content.

Article

Effect of Anthropometric Parameters on Achilles Tendon Stiffness of Professional Athletes Measured by Shear Wave Elastography

Claudia Römer [1,*], Enrico Zessin [1], Julia Czupajllo [1], Thomas Fischer [2], Bernd Wolfarth [1] and Markus Herbert Lerchbaumer [2]

1. Department of Sports Medicine, Charité Universitätsmedizin Berlin, 10115 Berlin, Germany
2. Department of Radiology, Charité–Universitätsmedizin Berlin, Charitéplatz 1, 10117 Berlin, Germany
* Correspondence: claudia.roemer@charite.de

Abstract: Background: Shear wave elastography (SWE) is currently used to detect tissue pathologies and, in the setting of preventive medicine, may have the potential to reveal structural changes before they lead to functional impairment. Hence, it would be desirable to determine the sensitivity of SWE and to investigate how Achilles tendon stiffness is affected by anthropometric variables and sport-specific locomotion. Methods: To investigate the influence of anthropometric parameters on Achilles tendon stiffness using SWE and examine different types of sports to develop approaches in preventive medicine for professional athletes, standardized SWE of Achilles tendon stiffness was performed in 65 healthy professional athletes (33 female, 32 male) in the longitudinal plane and relaxed tendon position. Descriptive analysis and linear regression were performed. Furthermore, subgroup analysis was performed for different sports (soccer, handball, sprint, volleyball, hammer throw). Results: In the total study population (n = 65), Achilles tendon stiffness was significantly higher in male professional athletes ($p < 0.001$) than in female professional athletes (10.98 m/s (10.15–11.65) vs. 12.19 m/s (11.25–14.74)). Multiple linear regression for AT stiffness did not reveal a significant impact of age or body mass index (BMI) ($p > 0.05$). Subgroup analysis for type of sport showed the highest AT stiffness values in sprinters (14.02 m/s (13.50–14.63)). Conclusion: There are significant gender differences in AT stiffness across different types of professional athletes. The highest AT stiffness values were found in sprinters, which needs to be considered when diagnosing tendon pathologies. Future studies are needed to investigate the benefit of pre- and post-season musculoskeletal SWE examinations of professional athletes and a possible benefit of rehabilitation or preventive medicine.

Keywords: elastography; shear wave elastography; SWE; tendon; ultrasound; professional athlete

1. Introduction

The Achilles tendon (AT) is the largest tendon in the body, making it very easily accessible and suitable for ultrasound (US) examinations. Achilles tendinopathy is very common in both active individuals and in the general population and causes pain and severe limitations in mobility. Acute and chronic Achilles tendinopathy is one of the most common overuse injuries in professional athletes such as runners, jumpers and triathletes [1]. Runners have a lifetime prevalence of developing Achilles tendinopathy of 52% [2,3]. Furthermore, AT rupture is one of the most severe injuries of the lower limb, in terms of loss of training days in triathletes [4].

Tendon disorders cause pain and severe limitations in mobility. Since the pathogenesis of tendinopathy is considered a multifactorial process with inflammation and degeneration [1,5,6], established ultrasound techniques and MRI are limited tools in assessing morphological changes, which are required for clinical diagnosis of tendinopathies [7,8]. As it is reported that there are discrete areas of pathology in disordered tendons, it is even more relevant that SWE can provide direct measurements of specific areas within the tendon [2].

Shear wave elastography (SWE) has been reported to be a suitable technique to assess tissue stiffness and to allow the identification of injuries in professional athletes [9,10]. SWE has shown its potential and is already established in breast, liver, thyroid and prostate imaging [7]. Dirrichs et al. showed that SWE had higher sensitivity than B-mode and power Doppler US, which were established for the examination of tendinopathy [10]. In contrast to strain elastography (also known as compression elastography), in which the tissue is subjected to strain stress with uniform repetitive pressure and the resulting compression/deformation can be recorded, SWE uses a different basic physical principle. In addition to the ultrasound wave, another low-frequency shear wave is applied; the modulus of elasticity can be calculated from the propagation speed of this transverse wave [11]. Formed by ultrasonic pulses radiated perpendicular to the surface, the propagation of the shear wave front can be recorded and its propagation velocity calculated, which correlates with the modulus of elasticity. The technical advantage of the method is the independence of the externally applied pressure and thus an improved standardization with less susceptibility to inter- and intra-observer variability.

SWE has revealed significantly lower tendon stiffness in individuals with symptomatic Achilles lesions [10]. While the effects of anthropometric parameters such as age or body mass index (BMI) on tissue stiffness assessed by SWE have been investigated in several studies [12–15], data for professional athletes are missing. Softening of tendon tissue has been attributed to very early changes in tissue elasticity in early tendinopathy [5,16]. Tendons and muscles undergo changes in composition and architecture with aging, which impacts their mechanical properties and function [12,17]. Muscle mass declines with age, which leads to a progressive reduction of muscle function and strength. These changes impair daily life in the elderly. On the other hand, it has been shown that tendons maintain their dimensions and mechanical properties with aging [15,18]. Mechanical stress such as regular exercising can modulate age-related alterations and counteract a loss of function of the muscle–tendon unit [12]. In another study, participants with Achilles tendinopathy were older and had significantly higher BMIs compared to a control group [2]. The body fat percentage seemed to be more relevant for tendon stiffness than BMI, which could be explained by metabolic pro-inflammatory effects due to larger amounts of adipose tissue.

Shear wave elastography holds great potential for detecting early changes in tendon structure, even before functional impairment becomes apparent [9].

Due to the increasing availability of SWE in commercial US systems, the number of publications on the topic of elastography increased in recent years. Despite this, musculoskeletal imaging (MSK) has seen only a limited increase in the level of evidence in a small number of musculoskeletal questions [19]. However, with the increasing use of elastography in musculoskeletal US, the growing number of studies may have the potential to establish this application in routine clinical practice for diagnosis and prevention.

Before SWE can be used to diagnose soft tissue injuries such as tendinopathy, we need to develop valid diagnostic criteria to differentiate between healthy and abnormal tendons and to identify preclinical changes. To establish such criteria, we need to know how anthropometric parameters alter tissue stiffness in professional athletes and in different types of sports.

Objective

The objective of this study is to investigate the influence of anthropometric parameters on the tendon and muscle stiffness of the lower limb using SWE and to determine the reference. Standarized SWE examinations of Achilles tendons in the longitudinal plane and relaxed tendon position were performed in 65 healthy professional athletes.

2. Methods

2.1. Study Population

The prospective study included 65 healthy professional athletes, who were examined at Charité–Universitätsmedizin Berlin. Inclusion criteria were: (I) healthy professional athletes, (II) without any acute (>6 months) musculoskeletal, rheumatic or vascular comorbidities and no previous injuries of the Achilles tendon and (III) written informed consent to participate in the study. Exclusion criteria were: tendon neovascularization, hypoechogenity and tendon thickening. The study was conducted in accordance with the Declaration of Helsinki and was approved by the local ethics committee of Charité University Medicine Berlin (ethical vote number EA2/162/19).

Baseline participant characteristics were obtained by a questionnaire at the time of examination. On the day of the examination, no training was performed. Professional athletes (handball, soccer, volleyball, sprint, hammer throw) with more than 10 h training per week were included. All measurements were jointly performed by a trained sonographer and a highly experienced radiologist who were blinded to the type of sport.

2.2. Shear Wave Elastography Examination

All US-SWE examinations were performed using a standardized protocol. For assessment of the Achilles tendon (mid portion), participants were examined in the prone position with both feet hanging over the edge of the examination couch in a relaxed position. Prior to US-SWE, gray-scale B-mode US was performed in the transverse and longitudinal planes for the adequate assessment of the Achilles tendon and probe position. All examinations were performed using a high-end US system with a 4–10 MHz multifrequency linear array transducer and a center frequency of 7 MHz (Acuson Sequoia, Siemens Healthineers, Erlangen, Germany). The US-SWE software (Virtual Touch™) allows real-time measurement using Acoustic Radiation Force Impulse (ARFI) imaging technology for the quantitative evaluation of shear wave speed.

US-SWE examinations were performed in the longitudinal plane to depict each tendon and the area of interest in one single image (Figure 1). Using the respective 2D SWE approach, the examiner acquired four US images of the AT of the right leg of each professional athlete, with a total of 650 consecutive SWE measurements using a 3-mm circular region of interest (ROI) placed in the center of each target tendon, avoiding areas of visible artifacts. Thus, representative tendon stiffness is given as the median of 10 measurements and the corresponding interquartile range (IQR). Before ROI placement, shear wave speed as a surrogate for tissue stiffness was depicted by color-coded SWE mapping. The standardized penetration depth was adapted to each participant for optimal visualization of the tendon and correct SWE measurement. Gain was not changed to avoid potential effects on US-SWE measurement.

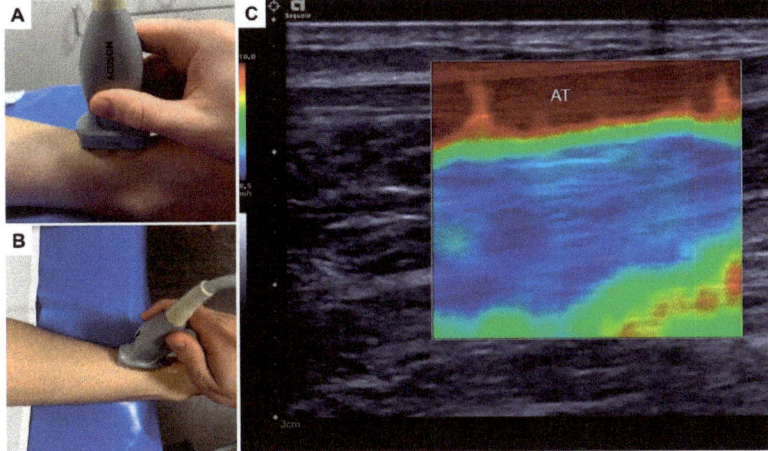

Figure 1. Example of SWE examination of a female athlete in a relaxed prone position with longitudinal probe orientation (**A**,**B**) and corresponding color-coded mapping of SWE (**C**) of the Achilles tendon (AT) in the mid-portion.

2.3. Statistical Analysis

Multiple linear regression analysis of AT stiffness was performed using anthropometric parameters such as gender, age and BMI as input parameters. Continuous variables were tested for normal distribution using the Kolmogorov–Smirnov test. Non-normally distributed variables are reported as median and IQR. A two-sided significance level of $\alpha = 0.05$ was determined as appropriate to indicate statistical significance. All statistical analyses were performed using the SPSS software (IBM Corp., released 2019. IBM SPSS Statistics for Windows, Version 26.0. Armonk, NY: IBM Corp.) and Matlab (MATLAB and Statistics Toolbox Release 2022b, The MathWorks, Inc., Natick, Massachusetts, United States).

3. Results

3.1. Athletes' Characteristics

A total of 65 professional athletes with a mean age of 20.19 years [16–29] were examined. The median BMI was 22.85 kg/m^2 (IQR 19.60–32.38 kg/m^2). The results are summarized in Table 1. One professional athlete had a history of hypothyroidism, while no other diseases such as diabetes mellitus, fatigue, hyperlipidemia, rheumatic diseases or malposition of lower limb joints were known. Overall, 14 athletes reported rupture of lower limb ligaments (ligament rupture of the ankle [n = 8], knee ligament rupture [n = 7]). None reported Achilles tendon pain, swelling, difficulty in joint movement or tendon rupture. Medications taken at the time of the examination were: hormonal contraceptives (oral [n = 9], intrauterine device [n = 2]).

Table 1. Baseline characteristics of professional athletes (n = 65).

	Male (n = 32)		Female (n = 33)	
	Mean & Range		Mean & Range	
AT	12.19	11.25–14.74	10.98	10.15–11.65
Age	19.83	18.00–21.00	20.76	18.00–24.50
BMI	23.52	22.40–24.43	23.34	21.30–24.38

3.2. Results of US-SWE in Professional Athletes

The analysis of variance (ANOVA) for AT stiffness in professional athletes is shown in Tables 2 and 3. In multiple linear regression for AT stiffness, only gender showed a significant influence ($p < 0.01$), while age, height, weight and BMI did not ($p > 0.05$). Therefore, subgroup analysis for type of sport was performed for female and male professional athletes.

Table 2. Multiple linear regression model of AT stiffness in professional athletes.

	Coefficient	Standard Error	p Value
Bias	4.24	25.48	0.8686
Gender (m = 1, f = 0)	−1.34	0.42	0.0021
Age	0.02	0.05	0.7060
Height	4.40	14.09	0.7561
Weight	−0.05	0.16	0.7545
BMI	0.16	0.53	0.7697

Shear wave speed (SWS) for male and female athletes showed normal distribution (Figure 2). Male athletes had significantly higher AT SWE values, which can be seen in the boxplot in Figure 2. There was no significant difference in age and BMI between males and females ($p > 0.05$).

Table 3. Linear regression model of AT stiffness in professional athletes only for gender.

	Coefficient	Standard Error	p Value
Bias	10.98	0.22	<0.0001
Gender (m = 1, f = 0)	1.20	0.32	0.0003
R^2 (adjusted)		0.17	
Standard error		1.29 m/s	

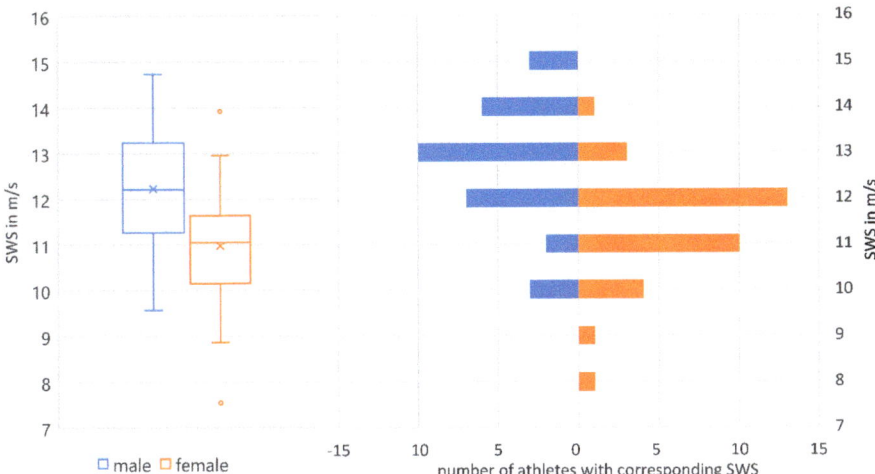

Figure 2. SWS in m/s of Achilles tendon in professional athletes (male = blue, female = orange).

For different types of sports and different load impacts on ATs, subgroup analysis was performed. In the male group, (sports: football (n = 21), handball (n = 7) and sprint (n = 4)) professional sprint athletes (14.02 m/s (13.50–14.63) showed significantly higher AT stiffness compared with handball (11.49 m/s (10.34–12.64), $p < 0.01$) and football players (12.06 m/s (11.25–12.87), $p < 0.01$), shown in Figure 3.

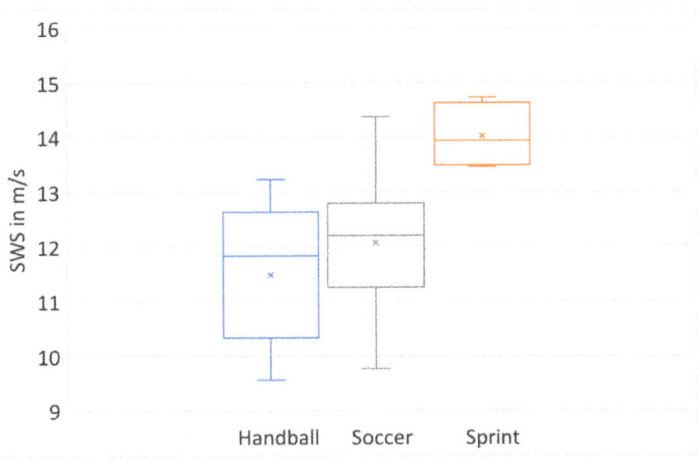

Figure 3. AT stiffness for male athletes in different sports.

In the female group (sports: handball (n = 6), volleyball (n = 14), sprint (n = 4) and hammer throw (n = 9)), professional sprint athletes (12.31 m/s (11.19–13.60)) showed significantly higher AT stiffness compared with volleyball and handball players (VB: 10.88 m/s (10.04–11.68), HB: 10.31 m/s (8.57–11.63), $p < 0.05$) and hammer throwers (11.03 m/s (10.30–11.61), $p < 0.05$), (Figures 4 and 5). No significant difference in AT stiffness was found between volleyball players and hammer throwers, volleyball and handball players and handball players and hammer throwers ($p > 0.05$).

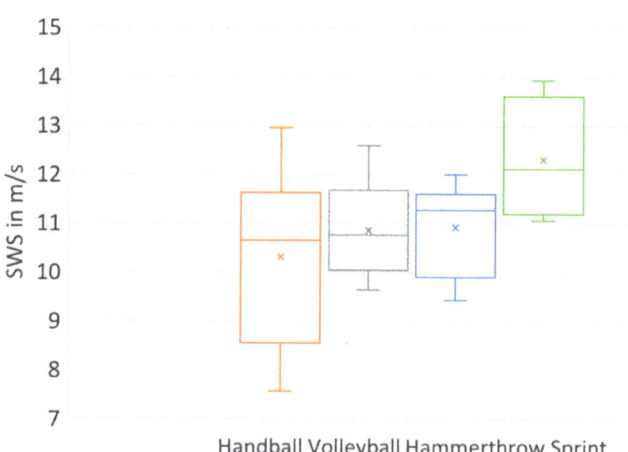

Figure 4. AT stiffness values for female athletes in different sports.

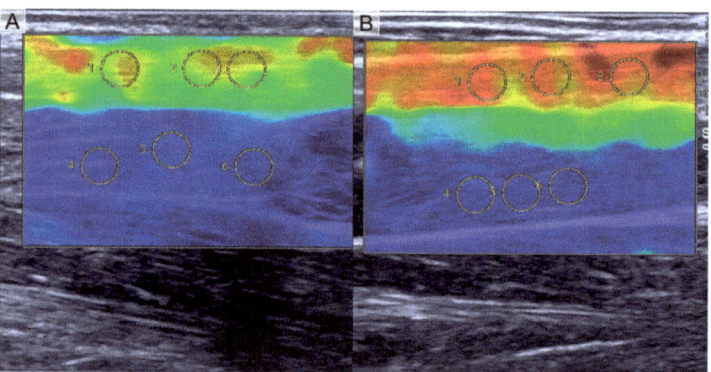

Figure 5. Color-coded mapping shows lower stiffness in SWE assessment in a female handball player (**A**, median SWS 10.31 m/s visualized as mostly green) and a female sprinter (**B**, median SWS 12.31 m/s visualized as mostly orange/red).

4. Discussion

The role of SWE imaging in musculoskeletal applications is currently under discussion. In clinical practice, it is widely used for the assessment of Achilles tendinopathy and as an additional tool to confirm findings of B-mode power Doppler US of tendons. Available data were typically obtained in smaller study populations, and there is no guideline on musculoskeletal elastography in general for a standardized clinical application. Before we can use tendon stiffness measured by SWE in rehabilitation or injury prevention, we need to establish baseline values and determine the effects of demographic characteristics such as age, sex or BMI for professional athletes.

4.1. Influence of Anthropometric Parameters on Achilles Tendon Stiffness

Our results show a significant effect of gender on AT stiffness. Stiffness values in male professional athletes were significantly higher than in female professional athletes ($p < 0.001$). This result is in line with the tendon stiffness reported for a non-athlete study population of similar size [20,21]; however, not in all degrees of dorsiflexion [20]. In another study of a non-athlete population, no significant difference in tendon stiffness was found between men and women [22]. A further study reported significant stiffness differences between professional and semi-professional athletes due to training load [23]. Training intensity is a relevant factor for Achilles tendon morphology [24], which is why caution is in order when comparing results obtained in semi-professional and professional athletes. Tendons combine elastic and viscous characteristics when undergoing deformation due to stress, so-called viscoelasticity. They transfer forces generated by muscles to bones to perform movements. The tendon structure is characterized by parallel bundles of collagen (30%) and elastin (2%), which are embedded in an extracellular matrix (68%) (water, tenocytes, mucopolysaccharide, proteoglycan gel). Mechanic loading is essential to maintaining tendon homeostasis [25]. Changes in this molecular structure have an impact on tendon stiffness and function [15].

Lower stiffness of the Achilles tendon has been reported for older individuals [12]. In our study, ANOVA did not identify age as a relevant parameter, which may be attributable to the fact that we investigated a significantly younger study population (16–29 years), which is significantly younger than other studies (20–85 years) [12–14]. In a study of 326 healthy volunteers, Fu et al. found no correlation between shear wave velocity and age [22]. Passive tissue stiffness and the correct measurement angle especially need to be considered [14] to assess further examinations in older professional athletes. Furthermore, no significant influence of BMI on tendon stiffness was found, as earlier studies also concluded [24,26,27]. Regular pre- and post-season preventive SWE examinations of the sport-specific exposed tendons in professional athletes may reduce injury risk by detecting early changes in tissue stiffness [9,28].

4.2. Achilles Tendon Stiffness in Different Sports

Tendon thickness and stiffness correlate positively with the strength of the corresponding muscle and might affect muscle function and force output, especially in the early phases of muscle contraction [25,29]. Besides gender, training load and maturation have different effects on the physical, chemical and mechanical properties of musculoskeletal tissue [24,30]. The elastic properties of tendons and muscles are influenced by activity level and show higher tissue stiffness in athletes [23,31]. Tissue stiffness might also be modulated by other factors including false locomotion patterns and sport types with high vertical forces, such as sprinting [32,33]. Athletes with greater mechanical stress and repetitive microtraumas show tendon thickening as part of structural remodeling processes and an increase in cross-sectional area [34]. Regular strength training and loading of muscles and tendons is known to lead to increased tendon size [18]. This increase is considered a compensatory mechanism to reduce mechanical loads on tendons and deformation resulting from increased body mass or muscle strength [29,35]. Therefore, we performed subgroup analysis for sports type to investigate AT stiffness in relation to different locomotion patterns, as all athletes included had training loads of >10 h per week in our study. AT stiffness values of professional female sprinters were significantly higher than in other sports such as handball, volleyball and hammer throw. The significant difference we found between professional sprinters and professional male soccer players is remarkable, as training patterns and running workload are comparable in these sports [36]. However, the running surface seems to have an important impact on AT maturation, stiffness and injury [33,37] and variable sprinting patterns from different angles, especially in a soccer game, needed to be considered and may influence tendon load and stiffness [36]. Soccer involves more stop-and-go movement, which may be a higher risk for injury [38] and could explain the lower AT stiffness values. Achilles tendon rupture is a critical injury for athletes, with return-to-sport rates of around 70% [39]. Return-to-sport is not exactly defined considering return-to-play in the same sports and at the same intensity as before [38]. In this context, AT tendinopathy and rupture can end an athlete's career [39]. Two studies reported the strength of the lower limb with AT rupture to be significantly lower in comparison to the other limb after conservative or surgical therapy [38,40]. Sport-specific return-to-play guidelines are necessary to ensure optimal rehabilitation for injured athletes [39], and objective criteria are needed [41,42]. With both surgical and conservative treatment, AT rehabilitation is a complex and long process [43–45]. SWE can be a useful tool to regularly monitor tendon stiffness changes during rehabilitation, as stiffness might be the best parameter to assess the multifactorial risk factors for AT injuries [33]. Further studies are necessary to investigate the potential of SWE in rehabilitation after acute or chronic tendinopathy and in the rehabilitation process after AT rupture in professional athletes.

Not only do stiffness differences between professional and semiprofessional athletes need to be considered when SWE is used to detect abnormalities [10], but also differences in stiffness between different sports. Overall, SWE is an easy-to-use US technique to assess tissue stiffness in rehabilitation and preventive medicine. It is characterized by high intra- and inter-operator reliability [46], allowing faster and more cost-efficient diagnosis than MRI.

4.3. Role of SWE in Assessment of Achilles Tendon

US has been considered the primary imaging modality of choice, with improved diagnostic performance in the evaluation of tendinopathic changes. Furthermore, the dynamic assessment established US as part of the functional investigation in acute ruptures linked to clinical examination as a point-of-care US tool. Compared to other anatomical regions such as the patellar tendon or quadriceps tendon, there are a larger number of studies for AT, resulting in a higher experience in Achilles tendon diagnostics, especially for tendinopathies. The healthy AT usually provides a more homogeneous color map with higher stiffness values compared to the patellar tendon or quadriceps tendon, whereas the stiffness of the tendon is related to the training volume or a relevant preload and can change, especially due to intensive training [23]. Thus, in professional athletes with a high training volume, the baseline stiffness is higher than in semi-professional amateur athletes.

The use of SWE achieves high specificity in detecting tendinopathy, and the combined use of conventional US is recommended to increase the sensitivity of the diagnosis. In a meta-analysis, almost all studies described significantly reduced stiffness values in symptomatic tendons in the setting of tendinopathy, which also reflects clinical experience [47]. SWE can easily be used for diagnostic and follow-up purposes to demonstrate early changes in affected tendons and/or adaptation to the healthy contralateral side in the context of short-term follow-up.

Although acute Achilles tendon rupture is often unequivocal on B-mode imaging and dynamic examination, SWE can also be helpful in this setting. Total rupture usually shows very low SWE values due to complete retraction and loss of tendon tension. This can be used especially in partial ruptures to differentiate the ruptured and still-preserved tendon portion, with corresponding higher stiffness values. SWE can be used in patients with AT rupture to assess contralateral tendon stiffness and elasticity. Interestingly, Ivanac et al. demonstrated a lower elasticity (-23%) of contralateral ATs in patients with acute AT rupture compared to healthy individuals based on SWE findings [48]. This study's results show a potential disorder or compensation of contralateral tendons after surgery. Hence, contralateral tendons may be exposed to higher force transmission after surgery in patients who suffered from acute rupture. This may lead to a higher vulnerability for future ruptures on the contralateral side.

4.4. Future Aspects in SWE

Despite a great interest in SWE imaging, the published literature is still sparse and strongly focused on cross-sectional studies with small patient numbers. Thus, the clinically established application of SWE is mainly anchored in diagnostic questions of tendinopathy. Here, SWE is usually used additively to the established B-Mode and Doppler Imaging criteria and increases the diagnostic power. This addition of multiple newer US applications is now increasingly presented as "multiparametric ultrasound".

Currently, there is no guideline for SWE in musculoskeletal tissue. Furthermore, the metric values given by US systems from different manufacturers are not directly comparable. There is still no guideline in the field of MSK imaging that summarizes a consensus on technical principles (e.g., measurement field size, region of interest or number of measurements per area). In addition to the diagnostic approach of SWE, longitudinal studies are currently lacking, especially in the field of sports medicine, e.g., in the context of muscle injuries or prognostics (a possible preventive approach of SWE). The scientifically relevant question in the coming years will be whether the early use of SWE could prevent acute injuries in a pre-damaged tendon or an overloaded muscle. Quantitative assessment of tissue stiffness and elasticity allows metric assessment of intrinsic tissue properties, which may be of particular value in tissue healing or diagnosing early-stage disease if no pathological findings can be depicted in B-Mode US or Doppler imaging. SWE may help in the prediction of impending tendon failure, which probably helps the clinician in making decisions for the early initiation of treatment [19].

4.5. Limitations

Nine female professional athletes in our study took an oral hormonal contraceptive and this constitutes future work. Oral contraceptives have an impact on the natural fluctuation of hormones [49–51]. However, the exact effect on tendon stiffness is still a topic under debate due to less high-quality studies and contradictive results [51–53]. Other factors such as low energy availability and psychological stress, which can lead to higher cortisol levels and may also affect tissue properties, need to be considered [53,54]. We did not consider the menstrual cycle phases of female athletes, which will be considered in future studies. Further limitations of our study are the small sample sizes for the sports-specific subgroup analysis and the relatively high scatter of measured values. This results from the exclusion criteria of tendinopathy symptoms (pain, swelling) and ultrasound findings (neovascularization, hypoechogenicity and tendon thickening). Further investigations should include a larger number of athletes in different sports.

5. Conclusions

Gender and type of sports need to be considered as influencing factors when assessing AT stiffness by SWE in professional athletes. Especially for professional athletes, easy access to diagnostic tools is necessary to detect the early stages of injuries and to develop preventive treatment algorithms to avoid severe tendon and muscle injuries. Further studies are necessary to investigate larger groups of professional athletes in different sports.

Author Contributions: Conceptualization, C.R. and M.H.L.; methodology, C.R. and M.H.L.; software, C.R. and M.H.L.; validation, C.R., M.H.L. and T.F.; formal analysis, C.R. and M.H.L.; investigation, C.R., J.C., E.Z. and M.H.L.; resources, M.H.L. and T.F.; data curation, C.R., J.C., E.Z. and M.H.L.; writing—original draft preparation, C.R. and M.H.L.; writing—review and editing, C.R., J.C., E.Z., T.F., B.W. and M.H.L.; visualization, C.R. and M.H.L.; supervision, B.W. and T.F.; project administration, C.R. and M.H.L.; funding acquisition, none. All authors have read and agreed to the published version of the manuscript.

Funding: This research received no external funding.

Institutional Review Board Statement: The study was conducted in accordance with the Declaration of Helsinki and approved by the Institutional Review Board (or Ethics Committee) of Charité University Medicine (protocol code EA2/162/19, date of approval 28 October 2019).

Informed Consent Statement: Informed consent was obtained from all subjects involved in the study.

Data Availability Statement: The data presented in this study are available on request from the corresponding author. The data are not publicly available due to data privacy regulations.

Acknowledgments: The authors thank Bettina Herwig for the language editing of the manuscript.

Conflicts of Interest: The authors declare no conflict of interest regarding this publication.

Abbreviations

AT	Achilles tendon
BMI	Body mass index
MSK	Musculoskeletal
ROI	Region of interest
SWE	Shear wave elastography
SWS	Shear wave speed
US	Ultrasound

References

1. Kannus, P.; Natri, A. Etiology and pathophysiology of tendon ruptures in sports. *Scand. J. Med. Sci. Sport.* **1997**, *7*, 107–112. [CrossRef] [PubMed]
2. Coombes, B.K.; Tucker, K.; Vicenzino, B.; Vuvan, V.; Mellor, R.; Heales, L.; Nordez, A.; Hug, F. Achilles and patellar tendinopathy display opposite changes in elastic properties: A shear wave elastography study. *Scand. J. Med. Sci. Sport.* **2018**, *28*, 1201–1208. [CrossRef]
3. Zhang, L.N.; Wan, W.B.; Wang, Y.X.; Jiao, Z.Y.; Zhang, L.H.; Luo, Y.K.; Tang, P.F. Evaluation of Elastic Stiffness in Healing Achilles Tendon After Surgical Repair of a Tendon Rupture Using In Vivo Ultrasound Shear Wave Elastography. *Med. Sci. Monit.* **2016**, *22*, 1186–1191. [CrossRef] [PubMed]
4. Vleck, V.E.; Garbutt, G. Injury and training characteristics of male Elite, Development Squad, and Club triathletes. *Int. J. Sports Med.* **1998**, *19*, 38–42. [CrossRef] [PubMed]
5. Cao, W.; Sun, Y.; Liu, L.; Wang, Z.; Wu, J.Y.; Qiu, L.; Wang, Y.X.; Yuan, Y.; Shen, S.F.; Chen, Q.; et al. A Multicenter Large-Sample Shear Wave Ultrasound Elastographic Study of the Achilles Tendon in Chinese Adults. *J. Ultrasound Med.* **2019**, *38*, 1191–1200. [CrossRef]
6. Abate, M.; Silbernagel, K.G.; Siljeholm, C.; Di Iorio, A.; De Amicis, D.; Salini, V.; Werner, S.; Paganelli, R. Pathogenesis of tendinopathies: Inflammation or degeneration? *Arthritis Res. Ther.* **2009**, *11*, 235. [CrossRef]
7. Breda, S.J.; van der Vlist, A.; de Vos, R.J.; Krestin, G.P.; Oei, E.H.G. The association between patellar tendon stiffness measured with shear-wave elastography and patellar tendinopathy-a case-control study. *Eur. Radiol.* **2020**, *30*, 5942–5951. [CrossRef]
8. Ozcan, A.N.; Tan, S.; Tangal, N.G.; Ciraci, S.; Kudas, S.; Bektaser, S.B.; Arslan, H. Real-time sonoelastography of the patellar and quadriceps tendons: Pattern description in professional athletes and healthy volunteers. *Med. Ultrason.* **2016**, *18*, 299–304. [CrossRef]
9. Dirrichs, T.; Quack, V.; Gatz, M.; Tingart, M.; Kuhl, C.K.; Schrading, S. Shear Wave Elastography (SWE) for the Evaluation of Patients with Tendinopathies. *Acad Radiol.* **2016**, *23*, 1204–1213. [CrossRef]
10. Dirrichs, T.; Quack, V.; Gatz, M.; Tingart, M.; Rath, B.; Betsch, M.; Kuhl, C.K.; Schrading, S. Shear Wave Elastography (SWE) for Monitoring of Treatment of Tendinopathies: A Double-blinded, Longitudinal Clinical Study. *Acad Radiol.* **2018**, *25*, 265–272. [CrossRef]
11. Taljanovic, M.S.; Gimber, L.H.; Becker, G.W.; Latt, L.D.; Klauser, A.S.; Melville, D.M.; Gao, L.; Witte, R.S. Shear-Wave Elastography: Basic Physics and Musculoskeletal Applications. *Radiographics* **2017**, *37*, 855–870. [CrossRef] [PubMed]
12. Lindemann, I.; Coombes, B.K.; Tucker, K.; Hug, F.; Dick, T.J.M. Age-related differences in gastrocnemii muscles and Achilles tendon mechanical properties in vivo. *J. Biomech.* **2020**, *112*, 110067. [CrossRef] [PubMed]
13. Liu, X.; Yu, H.K.; Sheng, S.Y.; Liang, S.M.; Lu, H.; Chen, R.Y.; Pan, M.; Wen, Z.B. Quantitative evaluation of passive muscle stiffness by shear wave elastography in healthy individuals of different ages. *Eur. Radiol.* **2021**, *31*, 3187–3194. [CrossRef] [PubMed]
14. Pang, J.; Wu, M.; Liu, X.; Gao, K.; Liu, Y.; Zhang, Y.; Zhang, E.; Zhang, T. Age-Related Changes in Shear Wave Elastography Parameters of the Gastrocnemius Muscle in Association with Physical Performance in Healthy Adults. *Gerontology* **2021**, *67*, 306–313. [CrossRef]
15. Turan, A.; Teber, M.A.; Yakut, Z.I.; Unlu, H.A.; Hekimoglu, B. Sonoelastographic assessment of the age-related changes of the Achilles tendon. *Med. Ultrason* **2015**, *17*, 58–61. [CrossRef]
16. De Zordo, T.; Fink, C.; Feuchtner, G.M.; Smekal, V.; Reindl, M.; Klauser, A.S. Real-time sonoelastography findings in healthy Achilles tendons. *AJR Am. J. Roentgenol.* **2009**, *193*, W134–W138. [CrossRef] [PubMed]
17. Slane, L.C.; Martin, J.; DeWall, R.; Thelen, D.; Lee, K. Quantitative ultrasound mapping of regional variations in shear wave speeds of the aging Achilles tendon. *Eur. Radiol.* **2017**, *27*, 474–482. [CrossRef] [PubMed]

18. Couppe, C.; Hansen, P.; Kongsgaard, M.; Kovanen, V.; Suetta, C.; Aagaard, P.; Kjaer, M.; Magnusson, S.P. Mechanical properties and collagen cross-linking of the patellar tendon in old and young men. *J. Appl. Physiol. (1985)* **2009**, *107*, 880–886. [CrossRef] [PubMed]
19. Sconfienza, L.M.; Albano, D.; Allen, G.; Bazzocchi, A.; Bignotti, B.; Chianca, V.; Facal de Castro, F.; Drakonaki, E.E.; Gallardo, E.; Gielen, J.; et al. Clinical indications for musculoskeletal ultrasound updated in 2017 by European Society of Musculoskeletal Radiology (ESSR) consensus. *Eur. Radiol.* **2018**, *28*, 5338–5351. [CrossRef]
20. Tas, S.; Salkin, Y. An investigation of the sex-related differences in the stiffness of the Achilles tendon and gastrocnemius muscle: Inter-observer reliability and inter-day repeatability and the effect of ankle joint motion. *Foot* **2019**, *41*, 44–50. [CrossRef] [PubMed]
21. Arda, K.; Ciledag, N.; Aktas, E.; Aribas, B.K.; Kose, K. Quantitative assessment of normal soft-tissue elasticity using shear-wave ultrasound elastography. *AJR Am. J. Roentgenol.* **2011**, *197*, 532–536. [CrossRef]
22. Fu, S.; Cui, L.; He, X.; Sun, Y. Elastic Characteristics of the Normal Achilles Tendon Assessed by Virtual Touch Imaging Quantification Shear Wave Elastography. *J. Ultrasound Med.* **2016**, *35*, 1881–1887. [CrossRef] [PubMed]
23. Romer, C.; Czupajllo, J.; Zessin, E.; Fischer, T.; Wolfarth, B.; Lerchbaumer, M.H. Stiffness of Muscles and Tendons of the Lower Limb of Professional and Semiprofessional Athletes Using Shear Wave Elastography. *J. Ultrasound Med.* **2022**, *41*, 3061–3068. [CrossRef]
24. Wiesinger, H.P.; Kosters, A.; Muller, E.; Seynnes, O.R. Effects of Increased Loading on In Vivo Tendon Properties: A Systematic Review. *Med. Sci. Sport. Exerc.* **2015**, *47*, 1885–1895. [CrossRef]
25. Tas, S.; Onur, M.R.; Yilmaz, S.; Soylu, A.R.; Korkusuz, F. Shear Wave Elastography Is a Reliable and Repeatable Method for Measuring the Elastic Modulus of the Rectus Femoris Muscle and Patellar Tendon. *J. Ultrasound Med.* **2017**, *36*, 565–570. [CrossRef]
26. Al-Qahtani, M.; Al-Tayyar, S.; Mirza, E.H.; Al-Musallam, A.; Al-Suwayyid, A.; Javed, R. Body Mass Index and Segmental Mass Correlation With Elastographic Strain Ratios of the Quadriceps Tendon. *J. Ultrasound Med.* **2019**, *38*, 2005–2013. [CrossRef] [PubMed]
27. Petrescu, P.H.; Izvernariu, D.A.; Iancu, C.; Dinu, G.O.; Crisan, D.; Popescu, S.A.; Sirli, R.L.; Nistor, B.M.; RauTia, I.C.; Lazureanu, D.C.; et al. Evaluation of normal and pathological Achilles tendon by real-time shear wave elastography. *Rom. J. Morphol. Embryol.* **2016**, *57*, 785–790.
28. Romer, C.; Czupajllo, J.; Zessin, E.; Fischer, T.; Wolfarth, B.; Lerchbaumer, M.H. Muscle and Tendon Stiffness of the Lower Limb of Professional Adolescent Soccer Athletes Measured Using Shear Wave Elastography. *Diagnostics* **2022**, *12*, 2453. [CrossRef] [PubMed]
29. Abate, M.; Oliva, F.; Schiavone, C.; Salini, V. Achilles tendinopathy in amateur runners: Role of adiposity (Tendinopathies and obesity). *Muscles Ligaments Tendons J.* **2012**, *2*, 44–48.
30. Esmaeili, A.; Stewart, A.M.; Hopkins, W.G.; Elias, G.P.; Aughey, R.J. Effects of Training Load and Leg Dominance on Achilles and Patellar Tendon Structure. *Int. J. Sport. Physiol. Perform.* **2017**, *12*, S2122–S2126. [CrossRef]
31. Dirrichs, T.; Schrading, S.; Gatz, M.; Tingart, M.; Kuhl, C.K.; Quack, V. Shear Wave Elastography (SWE) of Asymptomatic Achilles Tendons: A Comparison Between Semiprofessional Athletes and the Nonathletic General Population. *Acad Radiol.* **2019**, *26*, 1345–1351. [CrossRef] [PubMed]
32. Wiesinger, H.P.; Rieder, F.; Kosters, A.; Muller, E.; Seynnes, O.R. Are Sport-Specific Profiles of Tendon Stiffness and Cross-Sectional Area Determined by Structural or Functional Integrity? *PLoS ONE* **2016**, *11*, e0158441. [CrossRef] [PubMed]
33. Lorimer, A.V.; Hume, P.A. Stiffness as a Risk Factor for Achilles Tendon Injury in Running Athletes. *Sport. Med.* **2016**, *46*, 1921–1938. [CrossRef]
34. Frankewycz, B.; Penz, A.; Weber, J.; da Silva, N.P.; Freimoser, F.; Bell, R.; Nerlich, M.; Jung, E.M.; Docheva, D.; Pfeifer, C.G. Achilles tendon elastic properties remain decreased in long term after rupture. *Knee Surg. Sport. Traumatol. Arthrosc.* **2018**, *26*, 2080–2087. [CrossRef] [PubMed]
35. Tas, S.; Yilmaz, S.; Onur, M.R.; Soylu, A.R.; Altuntas, O.; Korkusuz, F. Patellar tendon mechanical properties change with gender, body mass index and quadriceps femoris muscle strength. *Acta Orthop. Traumatol. Turc.* **2017**, *51*, 54–59. [CrossRef] [PubMed]
36. Schimpchen, J.; Skorski, S.; Nopp, S.; Meyer, T. Are "classical" tests of repeated-sprint ability in football externally valid? A new approach to determine in-game sprinting behaviour in elite football players. *J. Sport. Sci.* **2016**, *34*, 519–526. [CrossRef]
37. Lorimer, A.V.; Hume, P.A. Achilles tendon injury risk factors associated with running. *Sport. Med.* **2014**, *44*, 1459–1472. [CrossRef]
38. Kinner, B.; Seemann, M.; Roll, C.; Schlumberger, A.; Englert, C.; Nerlich, M.; Prantl, L. Sports and activities after achilles tendon injury of the recreational athlete. *Sportverletz. Sportschaden.* **2009**, *23*, 210–216. [CrossRef]
39. Caldwell, J.E.; Vosseller, J.T. Maximizing Return to Sports After Achilles Tendon Rupture in Athletes. *Foot. Ankle Clin.* **2019**, *24*, 439–445. [CrossRef]
40. Cetti, R.; Christensen, S.E.; Ejsted, R.; Jensen, N.M.; Jorgensen, U. Operative versus nonoperative treatment of Achilles tendon rupture. A prospective randomized study and review of the literature. *Am. J. Sport. Med.* **1993**, *21*, 791–799. [CrossRef]
41. Wise, P.M.; King, J.L.; Stauch, C.M.; Walley, K.C.; Aynardi, M.C.; Gallo, R.A. Outcomes of NCAA Defensive Football Players Following Achilles Tendon Repair. *Foot Ankle Int.* **2020**, *41*, 398–402. [CrossRef]
42. Mansfield, K.; Dopke, K.; Koroneos, Z.; Bonaddio, V.; Adeyemo, A.; Aynardi, M. Achilles Tendon Ruptures and Repair in Athletes-a Review of Sports-Related Achilles Injuries and Return to Play. *Curr. Rev. Musculoskelet. Med.* **2022**, *15*, 353–361. [CrossRef]

43. Knobloch, K.; Thermann, H.; Hufner, T. Achilles tendon rupture–early functional and surgical options with special emphasis on rehabilitation issues. *Sportverletz. Sportschaden.* **2007**, *21*, 34–40. [CrossRef]
44. Majewski, M.; Schaeren, S.; Kohlhaas, U.; Ochsner, P.E. Postoperative rehabilitation after percutaneous Achilles tendon repair: Early functional therapy versus cast immobilization. *Disabil. Rehabil.* **2008**, *30*, 1726–1732. [CrossRef]
45. Rettig, A.C.; Liotta, F.J.; Klootwyk, T.E.; Porter, D.A.; Mieling, P. Potential risk of rerupture in primary achilles tendon repair in athletes younger than 30 years of age. *Am. J. Sport. Med.* **2005**, *33*, 119–123. [CrossRef]
46. Payne, C.; Watt, P.; Cercignani, M.; Webborn, N. Reproducibility of shear wave elastography measuresof the Achilles tendon. *Skeletal. Radiol.* **2018**, *47*, 779–784. [CrossRef]
47. Prado-Costa, R.; Rebelo, J.; Monteiro-Barroso, J.; Preto, A.S. Ultrasound elastography: Compression elastography and shear-wave elastography in the assessment of tendon injury. *Insights Imaging* **2018**, *9*, 791–814. [CrossRef] [PubMed]
48. Ivanac, G.; Lemac, D.; Kosovic, V.; Bojanic, K.; Cengic, T.; Dumic-Cule, I.; Pecina, M.; Brkljacic, B. Importance of shear-wave elastography in prediction of Achilles tendon rupture. *Int. Orthop.* **2021**, *45*, 1043–1047. [CrossRef] [PubMed]
49. Stewart, M.; Black, K. Choosing a combined oral contraceptive pill. *Aust. Prescr.* **2015**, *38*, 6–11. [CrossRef]
50. Bennink, H.J. Reprint of Are all estrogens the same? *Maturitas* **2008**, *61*, 195–201. [CrossRef] [PubMed]
51. Romer, C.; Czupajllo, J.; Wolfarth, B.; Lerchbaumer, M.H.; Legerlotz, K. Effects of orally administered hormonal contraceptives on the musculoskeletal system of healthy premenopausal women-A systematic review. *Health Sci. Rep.* **2022**, *5*, e776. [CrossRef]
52. Arendt, E.A.; Bershadsky, B.; Agel, J. Periodicity of noncontact anterior cruciate ligament injuries during the menstrual cycle. *J. Gend Specif. Med.* **2002**, *5*, 19–26. [PubMed]
53. Legerlotz, K.; Nobis, T. Insights in the Effect of Fluctuating Female Hormones on Injury Risk-Challenge and Chance. *Front. Physiol.* **2022**, *13*, 827726. [CrossRef] [PubMed]
54. Paquette, M.R.; Napier, C.; Willy, R.W.; Stellingwerff, T. Moving Beyond Weekly "Distance": Optimizing Quantification of Training Load in Runners. *J. Orthop. Sport. Phys. Ther.* **2020**, *50*, 564–569. [CrossRef] [PubMed]

Disclaimer/Publisher's Note: The statements, opinions and data contained in all publications are solely those of the individual author(s) and contributor(s) and not of MDPI and/or the editor(s). MDPI and/or the editor(s) disclaim responsibility for any injury to people or property resulting from any ideas, methods, instructions or products referred to in the content.

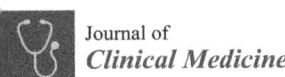

Article

3-Tesla T2 Mapping Magnetic Resonance Imaging for Evaluation of SLAP Lesions in Patients with Shoulder Pain: An Arthroscopy-Controlled Study

Patrick Stein [1,*], Felix Wuennemann [1,2], Thomas Schneider [1], Felix Zeifang [3,4], Iris Burkholder [5], Marc-André Weber [6], Hans-Ulrich Kauczor [1] and Christoph Rehnitz [1]

1. Diagnostic and Interventional Radiology, University Hospital Heidelberg, Im Neuenheimer Feld 420, 69120 Heidelberg, Germany
2. Institute of Diagnostic and Interventional Radiology & Neuroradiology, Helios Dr. Horst Schmidt Clinics Wiesbaden, Ludwig-Erhard-Straße 100, 65199 Wiesbaden, Germany
3. Center for Orthopedics, Trauma Surgery and Spinal Cord Injury, University Hospital Heidelberg, Schlierbacher Landstraße 200A, 69118 Heidelberg, Germany
4. Ethianum Clinic Heidelberg, Voßstraße 6, 69115 Heidelberg, Germany
5. Department of Nursing and Health, University of Applied Sciences of the Saarland, 66117 Saarbruecken, Germany
6. Institute of Diagnostic and Interventional Radiology, Pediatric Radiology and Neuroradiology, University Medical Center Rostock, Ernst-Heydemann-Straße 6, 18057 Rostock, Germany
* Correspondence: patrick.stein@med.uni-heidelberg.de

Abstract: This study investigated the ability of T2 mapping to assess the glenoid labrum and to differentiate between healthy labral substances and superior labral anterior posterior (SLAP) lesions using arthroscopy as the gold standard. Eighteen patients (mean age: 52.4 ± 14.72 years, 12 men) with shoulder pain were examined using 3-Tesla T2 mapping. All the patients underwent shoulder arthroscopy. Using morphological sequences for correlation, regions of interest covering the entire labral substance were placed in the corresponding T2 maps. The diagnostic cutoff values, sensitivities, and specificities, as well as the inter-reader correlation coefficients (ICCs) determined by two independent radiologists, were calculated. The mean T2 value was 20.8 ± 2.4 ms for the healthy labral substances and 37.7 ± 10.63 ms in the patients with SLAP lesions. The maximum T2 value in normal labrum (21.2 ms) was lower than the minimum T2 value in the patients with SLAP lesions (27.8 ms), leading to sensitivities, specificities, and positive and negative predictive values of 100% (95% CI 54.1–100.0) for all the cutoff values between 21.2 and 27.8 ms. The ICCs ranged from 0.91 to 0.99. In summary, the data suggest that evaluation and quantification of the labral (ultra)structural integrity using T2 mapping may allow discrimination between arthroscopically confirmed SLAP lesions and a healthy glenoid labrum. T2 mapping may therefore be helpful in diagnosing patients with suspected labral damage.

Keywords: T2 mapping; glenoid labrum; superior labral anterior posterior (SLAP) lesions; arthroscopy

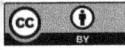

1. Introduction

Shoulder pain is a significant medical and socioeconomic problem that can lead to the inability to work and perform household or leisure activities. In a systematic review, Luime et al. reported a one-year prevalence of shoulder pain of up to 46.7% and a lifetime prevalence of up to 66.7% [1]. In addition, an age-dependent distribution has been reported, with older people being more likely to experience shoulder pain [1]. One repeatedly encountered source of shoulder pain affecting all age groups is superior labral anterior posterior (SLAP) lesions. The superior labrum plays an important role in the stability of the shoulder joint. Accordingly, SLAP lesions have been documented to cause both anterior and posterior instabilities in overhead athletes [2–4]. Microinstability, in turn, can lead to various shoulder injuries, including cartilage defects, and may progress to advanced osteoarthritis (OA) [5,6]. Despite the increasing understanding of its pathomechanisms and epidemiology, the diagnosis of superior labral lesions remains clinically and radiologically challenging.

Over the last few decades, the incidence of SLAP lesions has increased [7,8]. A study based on private insurance data from 2003 to 2013 reported a fivefold increase in the incidence of SLAP lesions [9]. In the younger population, traumatic shoulder injuries and participation in sports with overhead throwing movements are major causes of superior labral lesions, whereas chronic degeneration seems to play a major role in the development of SLAP lesions in older adults [10,11]. In 53 asymptomatic middle-aged subjects (45–60 years), non-contrast magnetic resonance imaging (MRI) revealed a prevalence of up to 72% for superior labral tears [12]. A similar study found no labral tears but observed an "abnormal labral signal" in 50% of a symptomatic subgroup in a comparatively younger cohort (25–55 years) [13]. However, in neither of these studies was the diagnosis confirmed via arthroscopy. Furthermore, histological post-mortem studies showed marked degenerative changes in the labral substance as well as the more frequent occurrence of labral tears with increasing age [14,15]. Thus, the continuous transition of age-related degenerative changes into manifest labral tears appears to be a relevant pathomechanism.

Along with the increase in incidence, there has been an increase in the number of surgically treated labral lesions [7,8,16]. While some studies have shown satisfactory postoperative outcomes [17,18], several recent studies have reported complications and the incomplete regression of symptoms, particularly in middle-aged and older patients, as well as in professional overhead athletes [8,19–21]. Therefore, timely diagnosis of early and potentially reversible damage to the collagen matrix is desirable to delay or prevent the clinical progression of manifest labral tears.

MRI, which is sometimes supplemented by MR arthrography, is the radiological gold standard for the morphological evaluation of the glenoid labrum [22,23]. The diagnostic performance of non-contrast MRI in superior labral tears has been studied several times, with variable results in terms of accuracy and sensitivity [24,25]. While some studies have reported high diagnostic accuracy for MR arthrography, others have demonstrated non-specific as well as non-sensitive results for MRI and MR arthrography in the diagnosis of SLAP lesions [26–28]. Early degenerative changes usually cannot be detected with conventional morphological MRI sequences; however, functional sequences such as delayed gadolinium-enhanced MRI of cartilage (dGEMRIC), T2* mapping, and T2 mapping allow the assessment of the biochemical composition of joint structures [29–31]. This enables the detection of damage to the ultrastructural integrity of cartilage or collagen networks. T2 mapping can detect and quantify early degenerative changes in the cartilage of numerous joints, including the wrist, ankle, metacarpophalangeal joints, and knee [29,32–34]. As high T2 values reflect disruption of the 3D collagen network and an increase in water content, T2 mapping may also be appropriate for fibrocartilaginous or collagenous structures such as the glenoid labrum and menisci, respectively. In knee OA, a correlation between high T2 values and histologically confirmed signs of meniscal degeneration was demonstrated [35]. However, the study included patients with severe OA who were scheduled for knee arthroplasty, indicating a high pre-test probability of concomitant meniscal degeneration.

To our knowledge, no studies to date have evaluated the diagnostic performance of T2 mapping for the assessment of the glenoid labrum. In addition, T2 mapping of the shoulder joint in general has hardly ever been studied, and only a few existing studies have validated this technique using arthroscopy.

Thus, the purpose of this study was to evaluate the ability of T2 mapping to assess the biochemical integrity of the superior labrum and to differentiate between individuals with and without SLAP lesions in patient cohorts with shoulder pain but not high-grade OA, using shoulder arthroscopy as the gold standard. As a secondary study aim, the interrater reliability was assessed by calculating the intraclass correlation coefficient (ICC).

2. Materials and Methods

2.1. Participants

This study included patients with shoulder pain who were to undergo arthroscopy and were referred to our department for preoperative MRI over a period of 3 months. The exclusion criteria were as follows: endoprosthetic replacement of the glenohumeral joint or osteosynthetic material involving the proximal humerus; prior tendinous or ligamentous refixation procedures; advanced OA (Kellgren–Lawrence score > 1); and age less than 18 years. Nineteen consecutive patients who met the inclusion criteria were enrolled in the study initially. As one patient, in whom only a routine MRI protocol without T2 mapping sequences was inadvertently applied, had to be excluded, 18 patients remained for inclusion.

2.2. Study Design and Reporting

After inclusion into the study, the index test (3-Tesla MRI with T2 mapping) was performed in each subject. After a maximum interval of 6 days (mean interval: 4 days) the reference test (shoulder arthroscopy) was carried out. Subsequently, the subgroups were divided into "healthy individuals" and "patients with proven SLAP lesion" depending on the arthroscopy findings. Therefore, this study can be defined as a one-stage, case–control study according to item 5 of the STARD guidelines published by the EQUATOR Network in 2015 [36].

2.3. MRI Protocol and T2 Mapping

The 3-Tesla MRI system used in this study was a Magnetom Verio (Siemens Healthineers, Erlangen, Germany) with a 70 cm gantry width and an 18-channel total imaging matrix. To ensure that the shoulder was as close as possible to the magnetic isocenter, all the patients were placed in a supine position with the head first and with the shoulder joint stabilized in external rotation. Proton density-weighted, fat-saturated MRI sequences as well as T1- and T2-weighted sequences without fat saturation were used for morphological assessment of the (fibro)cartilaginous joint structures. Oblique coronal and oblique sagittal sequences were oriented perpendicular and parallel to the glenoidal fossa, respectively. A multi-echo spin-echo sequence for inline T2 mapping provided by the manufacturer (syngo MapIT, Siemens Healthineers, Erlangen, Germany) was used as the study sequence. In this sequence, a pixel-wise, monoexponential, non-negative least squares fit analysis was used to derive the T2 relaxation times from the T2 parameters, which were then used for further analysis. A color-coded map was automatically generated from the quantitative T2 relaxation times. A detailed overview of the in-house shoulder protocol and the T2 mapping study sequence is given in Table 1.

Table 1. In-house shoulder MRI protocol and T2 mapping study sequences.

No.	Sequence	Orientation	Repetition Time (TR; ms)	Echo Time (TE; ms)	Acquisition Matrix	Flip Angle	Echo Train Length	No. of Slices	TA (Min)
1	PD fs TSE	axial	3660	24	384 × 346	176	7	27	04:32
2	PD fs TSE	oblique coronal	2490	24	384 × 307	160	7	19	03:37
3	PD fs TSE	oblique sagittal	3950	23	320 × 256	140	7	29	04:49
4	PD TSE	oblique coronal	1670	23	384 × 307	160	5	19	03:24
5	T1 SE	oblique coronal	787	10	384 × 346	90	1	19	04:51
6	T2 TSE	oblique sagittal	5640	88	384 × 307	150	15	29	02:33
7	T2 MapIt	oblique coronal	2140	13.8, 27.6, 41.4, 55.2, 69	320 × 320	180	1	16	06:50

TA = time of acquisition; PD = proton density; fs = fat-saturated, TSE = turbo spin echo.

2.4. Image Analysis and Definition of SLAP Lesions

The morphological sequences were evaluated using a picture archiving and communication system (Centricity PACS, v. 4.0; GE Healthcare IT Solutions, Barrington, IL, USA).

Two independent musculoskeletal radiologists with 19 (CR) and 6 (FW) years of experience in musculoskeletal MRI evaluated the morphological as well as the color-coded study sequences. Both readers had participated in previous training sessions on the morphological analysis of the glenoid labrum, which included cases beyond the scope of this study. In addition, both readers had experience in the evaluation of quantitative biochemical imaging techniques, particularly for cartilaginous structures. Both radiologists were blinded to the results of the arthroscopy, the clinical data of the patients, and the patients' names. There was no blinding of the study participants, who had been informed about the additional study sequences and who knew that they were scheduled for shoulder arthroscopy. In accordance with the retrospective, one-stage, case–control study design, randomization was not performed.

Both readers set parameters for slice selection, magnification, and windowing. During the reading sessions, the ambient light was reduced to a minimum.

The glenoid labrum was classified as either normal or damaged using morphological proton density-weighted, fat-saturated sequences. Following Snyder et al., irregular labral margins with increased signal intensity, stripping of the superior labrum from the glenoid, and a bucket-handle tear of the superior labrum, with or without extension into the origin of the long biceps tendon, were defined as SLAP lesions [37]. If none of these diagnostic criteria was met, the labrum was considered to be normal.

2.5. Placement of Regions of Interest

First, we used the proton density-weighted fat-saturated sequences to delineate the superior labrum and determine the optimal position for region of interest (ROI) placement. The first ROI was placed in the midsection of the glenoid fossa, where the labrum had the largest dimension and appeared triangular. To reduce the effect of artifacts or imperfect ROI placement, two additional ROIs were placed, one in the anterior slice and one in the posterior adjacent slice, leaving three sections for ROI placement (Figure 1). To provide the most accurate measurement results, the ROIs were first placed in the first echo images acquired from the multi-echo spin-echo T2-weighted sequences, which further supported the morphological delineation of the labral substance. A careful visual comparison with fat-suppressed, proton density-weighted sequences was performed to ensure that the entire labrum was captured. In the next step, the ROIs were copied into the color-coded parametric T2 map. Where necessary, the copied ROIs were adjusted to ensure that the final ROI did not include any artifacts, glenoid cartilage or cortex, joint capsule, supraspinatus muscle, or synovial fluid. The average T2 relaxation times of the three adjacent ROIs were used for further evaluation.

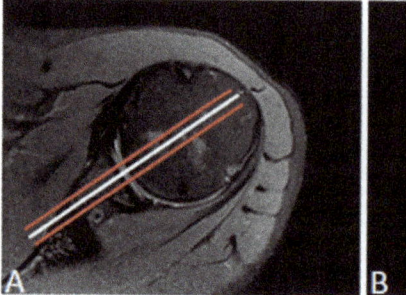 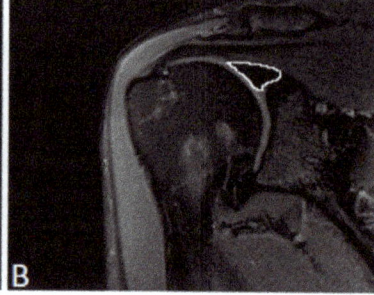

Figure 1. (**A**) Axial proton density-weighted, fat-saturated magnetic resonance image demonstrating the three oblique coronally oriented sections used for ROI placement: one midsection through the glenoid fossa (white) as well as one adjacent slice, anteriorly and posteriorly (red). (**B**) Coronal proton density-weighted, fat-saturated magnetic resonance image depicting the manually drawn ROI (white) outlining of the entirety of the glenoid labrum on a midcoronal section. The ROI was copied into the color-coded T2 mapping sequence.

The presence or absence of SLAP lesions in the morphological proton density fat-saturated (PDfs) sequences did not influence the placement of the ROIs, as the whole dimension of the labrum was always analyzed and compared with the arthroscopy. However, we also assessed the presence or absence of SLAP lesions in the morphological PDfs sequences and compared the findings with those of the arthroscopy.

2.6. Arthroscopy

Shoulder arthroscopy was performed by one of the two experienced orthopedic surgeons. According to the in-house standard, the arthroscopies were performed under general intravenous anesthesia, with all the patients placed in the beach-chair position. A posterior approach was selected for diagnostic inspection of the glenoid joint. The glenoid labrum, glenoid cartilage, and intra-articular portion of the long biceps tendon were assessed using a standardized questionnaire. The labral lesions were classified according to the method described by Snyder et al. [37]. A ventral approach was established if surgical intervention was required.

2.7. Statistical Analysis

The demographic data were analyzed descriptively. The continuous variables were summarized as mean, standard deviation, median, minimum, and maximum. For the qualitative variables, the frequency and percentage were analyzed. The patients' ages in the groups with and without lesions were compared using the exact Wilcoxon two-sample test.

The T2 imaging analysis was conducted in a descriptive manner using summary statistics and was interpreted exploratively. The Shapiro–Wilk test was used to determine whether the T2 mapping parameters were normally distributed. The groups with and without labral lesions were compared using two-sample t-tests, with the level of significance set at 5%.

The diagnostic performance of the T2 mapping for SLAP lesions was described using estimates and exact 95% confidence intervals for sensitivity (proportion of true positive patients out of all patients with SLAP lesions); specificity (proportion of true negative patients out of all patients without SLAP lesions); and positive (proportion of true positive patients out of all positive patients) and negative predictive values (proportion of true negative patients out of all negative patients).

The intraclass correlation coefficient (ICC) was used to analyze inter-reader agreement. The two readers were treated as a random sample of observers from a larger population of potential observers. According to Shrout and Fleiss (1979), for interrater reliability a two-way random effects model with subject and rater as random effects was applied for the estimation of the ICC and 95% confidence intervals [38]. All statistical analyses were performed using SAS for Windows (version 9.4; SAS Institute Inc., Cary, NC, USA) and R version 3.5.1 (www.cran.r-project.org (accessed on 10 May 2022)).

3. Results

3.1. Demographic Data

Of the 18 patients included, 12 (66.7%) were male and 6 (33.3%) were female. The mean patient age was 52.4 ± 14.72 (range, 22.0–67.0) years. Patients without SLAP lesions were only slightly younger than those with SLAP lesions (46.2 ± 18.82 [range, 22–64] years vs. 55.5 ± 11.93 [range, 29–67] years). Of the 12 patients with arthroscopically confirmed SLAP lesions, 9 (75%) were male and 3 (25%) were female. Table 2 summarizes the demographic characteristics of the patients according to the presence or absence of SLAP lesions.

3.2. Arthroscopic Evaluation of the Glenoid Labrum

Shoulder arthroscopy was performed in all patients, with a mean interval of 4 days between MRI examination and surgery (range, 0–6 days). A diagnosis of SLAP lesions was made in 12 patients (66.7%). Following Snyder et al., nine SLAP lesions were classified as type 1 (75.0%), one as type 2 (8.3%), and two as type 3 (16.7%). No SLAP lesions were diagnosed as type 4 (Table 3).

Table 2. Demographic characteristics of patients with and without SLAP lesions.

		SLAP Lesion		
		No (N = 6)	Yes (N = 12)	p-Value Wilcoxon
Gender	male	3 (50.0%)	9 (75.0%)	
	female	3 (50.0%)	3 (25.0%)	
Age (years)	n	6	12	0.2216
	Mean	46.2	55.5	
	SD	18.82	11.93	
	Median	53.5	58.5	
	Min	22.0	29.0	
	Max	64.0	67.0	

SD = standard deviation; Min = minimum; Max = maximum.

Table 3. Distribution of SLAP types according to the classification by Snyder et al.

		Total (N = 18)
SLAP lesion	no	6 (33.3%)
	yes	12 (66.7%)
SLAP Classification	SLAP 1	9 (75.0%)
	SLAP 2	1 (8.3%)
	SLAP 3	2 (16.7%)
	SLAP 4	–

Several patients with SLAP lesions were diagnosed with concomitant shoulder pathologies at arthroscopy. Focal cartilage damage was seen in 5 of the 12 patients diagnosed with SLAP lesions (41.7%), and damage to the long biceps tendon was seen in 6 of the 12 patients (50.0%). In addition, 2 out of the 12 patients (16.7%) were diagnosed with all three entities: SLAP lesion, focal cartilage damage, and lesion of the long biceps tendon.

3.3. T2 Mapping of the Glenoid Labrum

Twelve SLAP lesions were detected by MRI, which corresponded with the number of lesions detected arthroscopically. No additional lesions were observed. Table 4 shows the mean T2 mapping parameters for patients with and without SLAP lesions. The mean T2 values were 37.7 ± 10.63 ms for the patients with SLAP lesions and 20.8 ± 2.40 ms for the population without labral damage, showing a significant difference between the two groups ($p < 0.0001$). There was complete separation of the T2 mapping values between the normal and damaged glenoid labrum, as the maximum T2 value for the group without lesions (21.2 ms) was lower than the minimum T2 value for the patients with SLAP lesions (27.8 ms; Figure 2 and Table 4). Therefore, all the cutoff values between these two values yielded the same values for the sensitivity and positive predictive value of 100% with 95% CI (73.5–100.0%) and for the specificity and negative predictive value of 100% with 95% CI (54.1–100.0%). ICC analysis revealed near-perfect inter-reader agreement of 0.97 (95% CI 0.91–0.99).

Table 4. T2 mapping values (ms) for normal and damaged glenoid labrum.

		Overall	Population without Lesion	Population with Lesion
T2	n	18	6	12
	Mean	32.1	20.8	37.7
	SD	11.90	2.40	10.63
	Median	28.7	21.2	33.3
	Min	16.8	16.8	27.8
	Max	54.3	21.2	54.3

SD = standard deviation; Min = minimum; Max = maximum.

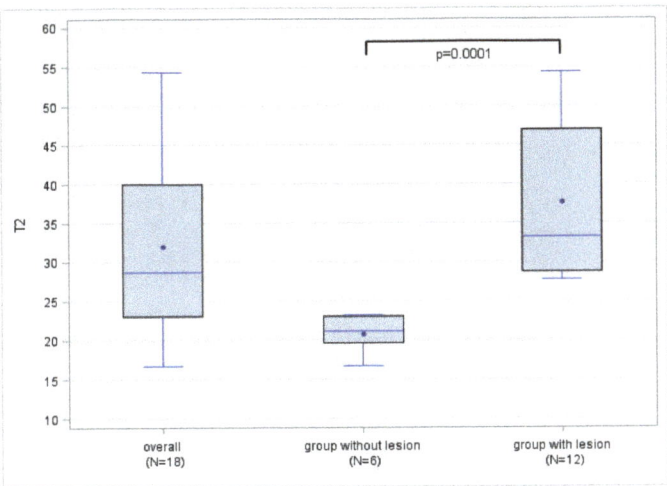

Figure 2. Boxplots of overall T2 mapping values (ms) in those with a healthy labrum and in patients with SLAP lesion. Note the complete separation of T2 values between individuals with SLAP lesion and those with a healthy labrum. The blue horizontal lines inside the box plots represent the median, the blue dots the mean T2 value.

Color-coded T2 maps depicted a visual difference between healthy and damaged labral substance (Figures 3 and 4).

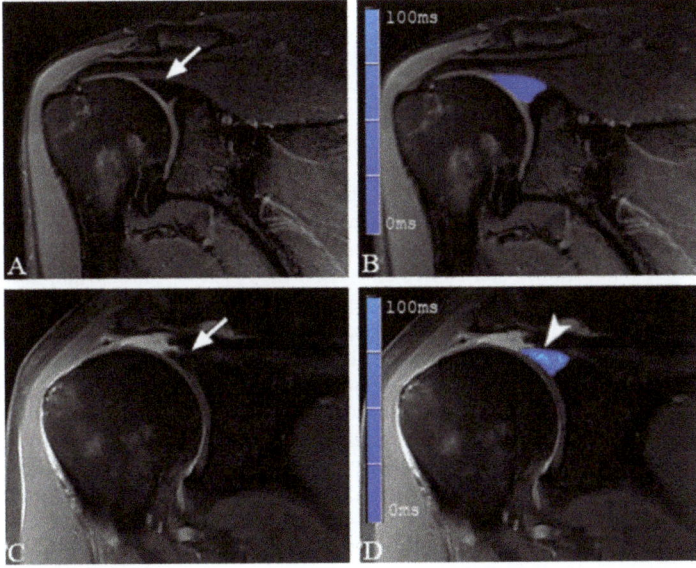

Figure 3. (**A,C**) show coronal proton density-weighted, fat-saturated magnetic resonance images of a 34-year-old woman with morphologically normal-appearing and arthroscopically proven healthy labrum (arrow in (**A**)), as well as fraying of the superior labrum in a 57-year-old man with arthroscopically proven SLAP lesion Type 1 (arrow in (**C**)). (**B,D**) show merged images of the proton density-weighted images and the corresponding color-coded T2 maps. Note the elevated average T2 mapping value of 53.9 ms in the damaged labral substance (arrowhead in (**D**)). The average T2 mapping value for the healthy labral substance was 21.3 ms (**B**).

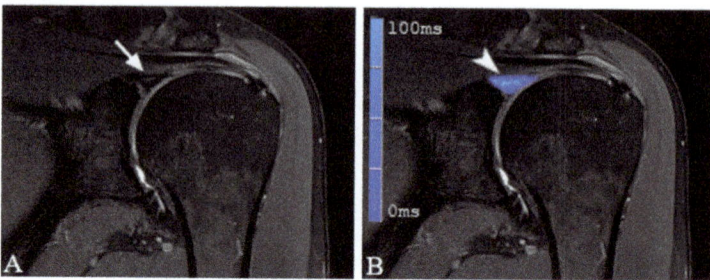

Figure 4. (**A**) shows a coronal proton density-weighted, fat-saturated magnetic resonance image of a 62-year-old man with linear hyperintensity centrally within the glenoid labrum indicating labral damage (arrow). (**B**) shows a merged image of (**A**) and the corresponding color-coded T2 map. Note the elevated average T2 mapping value of 40.5 ms (arrowhead). During arthroscopy a SLAP lesion Type 2 was present.

4. Discussion

Despite the increasing incidence over the past two decades and the improved understanding of the predisposing factors and the pathomechanism, the diagnosis of SLAP lesions remains difficult both clinically and by MRI. Early diagnosis of the pathologies of the glenoid labrum and the associated changes in biochemical composition using MRI has not yet been established, but it is desirable, for instance, to initiate therapy or modify training plans at an early stage. T2 mapping is an MRI technique that has proven to be effective in assessing the integrity of the collagen network and water content of articular cartilage in various joints [29,32–34]. However, this technique has not yet been systematically used to assess the glenoid labrum, a structure which is composed predominantly of fibrocartilaginous tissue organized in a 3D collagen network, and correlations with arthroscopy as the gold standard are lacking.

Thus, this study evaluated the ability of T2 mapping to detect and quantify labral damage containing SLAP lesions in patients with shoulder pain and to differentiate damaged labra from normal labra using shoulder arthroscopy as the gold standard. The patients with SLAP lesions had a significantly higher mean T2 value than those without (37.7 ± 10.63 ms vs. 20.8 ± 2.40 ms; $p < 0.0001$). The increase in T2 values may have been due to damage to the ultrastructural architecture of the collagen network and the associated repair mechanisms. While the exact histological composition of the glenoid labrum is still controversial, it has been shown to consist primarily of fibrocartilaginous tissue that transitions into hyaline articular cartilage towards the glenoid [39–41]. Several studies have identified loss of the collagenous matrix, with the corresponding areas of increased cellularity, vascularity, and water content, as histological correlates for degeneration in cartilaginous and fibrous tissue [42–45]. These biochemical changes are consistent not only with the increased T2 values of the labrum observed in our study but also with several other studies reporting increased T2 values in damaged articular cartilage or tendons [46–48]. While hyperintense patterns in T2-weighted images of the damaged glenoid labrum have been reported before, this is to our knowledge the first study quantifying the actual T2 relaxations times using T2 mapping [49,50]. Thus, by providing objectifiable measurements, this technique may be useful for establishing diagnostic cutoffs, or it may serve as a longitudinal biomarker for healing processes. Further studies with larger sample sizes are needed to clarify the extent to which a change in T2 relaxation times correlates with actual lesion severity.

In our study population, the highest overall T2 value in the healthy patients (21.2 ms) was lower than the lowest overall T2 value in the patients with SLAP lesions (27.8 ms). This amounts to a complete separation of the data between the two groups. Thus, all the diagnostic cutoff T2 values between 21.2 and 27.8 ms would result in the sensitivity, specificity, positive predictive value, and negative predictive value of 100% (95% CI 54.1–100.0). As this is, to our knowledge, the first study to systematically evaluate T2 relaxation times using

T2 mapping of the glenoid labrum, no appropriate data are available for direct comparison. Nevertheless, the mean T2 mapping values found in our study for healthy individuals (20.8 ± 2.4 ms), as well as for those for damaged labral substance (37.7 ± 10.63 ms), are similar to the reported T2 mapping values for the articular cartilage of the glenoid. One study described average T2 mapping values of 23.0 ± 3.0 ms for healthy glenoid cartilage and 44.8 ± 3.7 ms in patients with focal cartilage defects, thus demonstrating comparable quantitative differentiation [51]. The minor variations of the T2 mapping values may reflect the differences in histological composition, with mainly fibrocartilaginous tissue found in the labrum compared to the mainly hyaline articular cartilage.

Several studies have reported significant differences in T2 mapping values between normal and damaged cartilage [47,48,52,53]. Because the glenoid labrum is composed primarily of (fibro)cartilaginous tissue, its T2 mapping value is subject to a variety of factors known to influence the signal intensity of the articular cartilage. In particular, differences in the mechanical load, with the associated variations in water content and matrix composition, as well as the artificial signal changes such as the "magic angle" effect, have been described [31,45,54]. The latter is known to increase the T2 relaxation time in collagen fibers oriented at 55° to the magnetic field, especially when using short echo times (TE) [55–57]. In a retrospective arthroscopy-controlled study, Sasaki et al. reported increased signal intensity of the posterosuperior labrum, not only in patients with confirmed labral damage, but also in healthy individuals [58]. When a group of six asymptomatic participants was studied, the same group showed signal changes in the posterosuperior labrum, depending on the TE and positioning of the volunteers [58]. Thus, because the magic angle artifact would also cause signal alterations in healthy labral substances, complete separation of the data cannot be explained by artificial means alone. Our results could be due to the precise placement of the ROI, as well as the small study population with only six patients without SLAP lesions. Future studies with larger sample sizes may show an overlap of T2 mapping values, indicating a continuous progression of degenerative labral changes manifesting as SLAP lesions.

The T2 mapping values for the normal and damaged cartilage showed near-perfect interrater agreement, with respective ICCs of 0.97 (95% CI 0.91–0.99), which may be interpreted as a promising sign for the reliable application of this technique in clinical practice. These findings are consistent with the previously published studies of T2 mapping of the glenoid joint in healthy subjects, reporting good to excellent interrater agreement [59,60]. However, considering the small sample size and the associated small number of patients with SLAP lesions ($n = 12$), our results should be interpreted with caution and could be at least partially explained artificially.

While this study focused on differentiating labra containing SLAP lesions from the normal glenoid labrum, T2 mapping may also detect early degenerative changes that are not readily apparent in morphological sequences. In a post-mortem study, Pfahler et al. investigated histological changes in the labral substance in different age groups and reported a significant increase in the number and severity of micro- and macrolesions in the labrum with increasing age [14]. Additionally, Schwartzberg et al. reported a prevalence of up to 72% for superior labral tears in asymptomatic middle-aged individuals [12]. This finding is comparable with the 66.7% prevalence of SLAP lesions observed in our symptomatic study population. The continuous transformation of early degenerative changes into manifest labral lesions with increasing age may be accentuated by individual (micro)traumas, which could be a possible pathomechanism for the development of SLAP lesions. The detection of early degenerative changes could allow the timely initiation of protective conservative measures, such as physical therapy, to delay or prevent further disease progression. Future studies should investigate the extent to which differing T2 mapping values in morphologically normal-appearing labrums can be interpreted as an indicator of early degenerative changes. T2 mapping could then be used to assess the effect of early conservative interventions, such as physiotherapy. Additionally, several studies have shown that T2 mapping is effective in monitoring biochemical changes after cartilage repair procedures [61,62]. Xie et al. reported a correlation between a decrease in T2 mapping values and an improvement in clinical outcomes in the first year after arthroscopic rotator cuff repair, further highlighting the potential clinical utility of this technique [46].

Our study has some limitations. The small sample size may have contributed to the complete separation of T2 mapping values between the normal and damaged labral substances, resulting in a statistically perfect discrimination. In particular, the wide confidence interval (CI) of 54.1 to 100%, which is at least partly due to the small sample size, has several statistical implications. First, the small sample size affects the calculation of the confidence interval (CI) by overweighting extreme values, thus resulting in a wider CI range. Second, the sample size was too small to allow a statistically valid distinction between the different types of SLAP lesions. By generalizing the spectrum of lesion severity as "pathologic" versus "physiologic", the statistical calculation is susceptible to sampling biases such as spectrum bias, in which a study population has a different spectrum of lesion severity compared with the normal population. This is particularly important because the patient cohort was recruited at a tertiary referral center and was therefore highly selective, which may have affected the prevalence of SLAP lesions; this, in turn, may have had an effect on the sensitivity and specificity values. A patient population with a higher prevalence of SLAP lesions may include more patients with higher lesion grading, making the test perform better in this population. In view of these statistical limitations, as well as the above-mentioned variations in T2 values, our results may only be applicable to our patient cohort. Studies with larger sample sizes that distinguish between levels of lesion severity are needed to clarify this issue.

The large age discrepancy (22.0–67.0 years) must be considered a significant limitation, especially given the statistical implications of the small sample sizes discussed above. Although the age range was quite similar between the healthy subjects (22.0–64.0 years) and the patients with SLAP lesions (29.0–67.0 years), further studies with larger samples are required to allow better differentiation between age groups and to thereby address the process of age-related degeneration and the dehydration of cartilaginous structures beginning at 45–60 years of age.

Moreover, as this is the first study to quantify T2 relaxation times using T2 mapping in the glenoid labrum, there are no available data for a direct comparison of the labral T2 values.

Additionally, as mentioned above, the subgroup of patients with SLAP lesions was too small for statistically valid differentiation between SLAP types 1–4. The choice between surgical or conservative therapy and between the different surgical procedures depends largely on the attributed SLAP type [63,64]. Further studies with larger sample sizes may reveal significant differences in the T2 mapping values between SLAP types and might help to distinguish between conservatively treatable lesions and those requiring surgery.

We acknowledge that manual ROI placement in correlation with morphological MRI sequences is prone to human error. Although we reduced the impact of the potentially imprecise ROI placement by averaging three adjacent ROIs, high-resolution, three-dimensional T2 mapping sequences that can examine the entire labral substance are desirable for further studies as they will allow the voxel-wise evaluation of T2 mapping values. Additionally, using our method of ROI placement by averaging the T2 mapping values of midcoronal and anterior and posterior adjacent slices, lesions in a very anterior or very posterior position could have been missed. Therefore, three-dimensional T2 mapping sequences would allow for an even more precise assessment in future studies.

5. Conclusions

T2 mapping can evaluate and quantify the biochemical integrity of labral substances and differentiate between arthroscopically confirmed SLAP lesions and the healthy glenoid labrum. In addition to the mere morphological evaluation of the labrum, the quantification of T2 relaxation times using T2 mapping may provide objectifiable measures for diagnostic cutoff values and also function as a biomarker for monitoring healing processes under conservative therapy or postoperatively. By also providing information on the (ultra)structural integrity of the (fibro)cartilaginous networks, T2 mapping could prove help in therapeutic decision making, not only in labral pathologies but in several shoulder pathologies in general. The inclusion of T2 mapping sequences in the routine MRI protocol for suspected fibrocartilaginous or tendinous lesions may allow accurate diagnosis without the need for more invasive diagnostic procedures such as MR arthrography or even arthroscopy.

Author Contributions: Conceptualization, C.R., P.S. and F.W.; methodology, P.S., F.W., C.R., I.B. and T.S.; validation, C.R. and M.-A.W.; formal analysis, I.B., P.S., F.W. and C.R.; data interpretation, P.S., C.R., I.B., H.-U.K., T.S., F.Z. and M.-A.W.; writing—original draft preparation, P.S. and C.R.; writing—review and editing, P.S., C.R., F.W., I.B., H.-U.K., T.S., F.Z. and M.-A.W. All authors have read and agreed to the published version of the manuscript.

Funding: For the publication fee we acknowledge financial support by Deutsche Forschungsgemeinschaft within the funding programme "Open Access Publikationskosten "as well as by Heidelberg University.

Institutional Review Board Statement: The study was approved by the Institutional Review Board of Heidelberg University (S-081/2010) and was conducted in accordance with the Declaration of Helsinki.

Informed Consent Statement: Written informed consent was obtained from all patients after they were informed of the nature of the examination.

Data Availability Statement: The datasets generated and analyzed in the present study are available from the corresponding author on reasonable request.

Conflicts of Interest: The authors declare no conflict of interest.

References

1. Luime, J.; Koes, B.; Hendriksen, I.; Burdorf, A.; Verhagen, A.; Miedema, H.; Verhaar, J. Prevalence and Incidence of Shoulder Pain in the General Population; a Systematic Review. *Scand. J. Rheumatol.* **2004**, *33*, 73–81. [CrossRef]
2. Rodosky, M.W.; Harner, C.D.; Fu, F.H. The Role of the Long Head of the Biceps Muscle and Superior Glenoid Labrum in Anterior Stability of the Shoulder. *Am. J. Sport. Med.* **1994**, *22*, 121–130. [CrossRef]
3. Pagnani, M.J.; Deng, X.H.; Warren, R.F.; Torzilli, P.A.; Altchek, D.W. Effect of Lesions of the Superior Portion of the Glenoid Labrum on Glenohumeral Translation. *J. Bone Jt. Surg.* **1995**, *77*, 1003–1010. [CrossRef] [PubMed]
4. Kessler, M.A.; Burkart, A.; Weiss, M.; Imhoff, A.B. SLAP-Läsionen Als Ursache Einer Posterioren Instabilität. *Orthopade* **2003**, *32*, 642–646. [CrossRef]
5. Patzer, T.; Lichtenberg, S.; Kircher, J.; Magosch, P.; Habermeyer, P. Influence of SLAP Lesions on Chondral Lesions of the Glenohumeral Joint. *Knee Surg. Sport. Traumatol. Arthrosc.* **2010**, *18*, 982–987. [CrossRef]
6. Reinold, M.M.; Curtis, A.S. Microinstability of the Shoulder in the Overhead Athlete. *Int. J. Sport. Phys. Ther.* **2013**, *8*, 601–616.
7. Onyekwelu, I.; Khatib, O.; Zuckerman, J.D.; Rokito, A.S.; Kwon, Y.W. The Rising Incidence of Arthroscopic Superior Labrum Anterior and Posterior (SLAP) Repairs. *J. Shoulder Elb. Surg.* **2012**, *21*, 728–731. [CrossRef]
8. Weber, S.C.; Martin, D.F.; Seiler, J.G.; Harrast, J.J. Superior Labrum Anterior and Posterior Lesions of the Shoulder. *Am. J. Sport. Med.* **2012**, *40*, 1538–1543. [CrossRef]
9. Dougherty, M.C.; Kulenkamp, J.E.; Boyajian, H.; Koh, J.L.; Lee, M.J.; Shi, L.L. National Trends in the Diagnosis and Repair of SLAP Lesions in the United States. *J. Orthop. Surg.* **2020**, *28*, 230949901988855. [CrossRef] [PubMed]
10. LeVasseur, M.R.; Mancini, M.R.; Hawthorne, B.C.; Romeo, A.A.; Calvo, E.; Mazzocca, A.D. SLAP Tears and Return to Sport and Work: Current Concepts. *J. ISAKOS* **2021**, *6*, 204–211. [CrossRef]
11. Burkhart, S.; Morgan, C. SLAP Lesions in the Overhead Athlete. *Orthop. Clin. N. Am.* **2001**, *32*, 431–441. [CrossRef]
12. Schwartzberg, R.; Reuss, B.L.; Burkhart, B.G.; Butterfield, M.; Wu, J.Y.; McLean, K.W. High Prevalence of Superior Labral Tears Diagnosed by MRI in Middle-Aged Patients with Asymptomatic Shoulders. *Orthop. J. Sport. Med.* **2016**, *4*, 232596711562321. [CrossRef]
13. Chandnani, V.; Ho, C.; Gerharter, J.; Neumann, C.; Kursunoglu-Brahme, S.; Sartoris, D.J.; Resnick, D. MR Findings in Asymptomatic Shoulders: A Blind Analysis Using Symptomatic Shoulders as Controls. *Clin. Imaging* **1992**, *16*, 25–30. [CrossRef] [PubMed]
14. Pfahler, M.; Haraida, S.; Schulz, C.; Anetzberger, H.; Refior, H.J.; Bauer, G.S.; Bigliani, L.U. Age-Related Changes of the Glenoid Labrum in Normal Shoulders. *J. Shoulder Elb. Surg.* **2003**, *12*, 40–52. [CrossRef]
15. Prodromos, C.C.; Ferry, J.A.; Schiller, A.L.; Zarins, B. Histological Studies of the Glenoid Labrum from Fetal Life to Old Age. *J. Bone Jt. Surg. Am.* **1990**, *72*, 1344–1348. [CrossRef]

16. Vogel, L.A.; Moen, T.C.; Macaulay, A.A.; Arons, R.R.; Cadet, E.R.; Ahmad, C.S.; Levine, W.N. Superior Labrum Anterior-to-Posterior Repair Incidence: A Longitudinal Investigation of Community and Academic Databases. *J. Shoulder Elb. Surg.* **2014**, *23*, e119–e126. [CrossRef] [PubMed]
17. Enad, J.G.; Gaines, R.J.; White, S.M.; Kurtz, C.A. Arthroscopic Superior Labrum Anterior-Posterior Repair in Military Patients. *J. Shoulder Elb. Surg.* **2007**, *16*, 300–305. [CrossRef] [PubMed]
18. Friel, N.A.; Karas, V.; Slabaugh, M.A.; Cole, B.J. Outcomes of Type II Superior Labrum, Anterior to Posterior (SLAP) Repair: Prospective Evaluation at a Minimum Two-Year Follow-Up. *J. Shoulder Elb. Surg.* **2010**, *19*, 859–867. [CrossRef] [PubMed]
19. Stetson, W.B.; Snyder, S.J. Clinical Presentation and Follow-up of Isolated SLAP Lesions of the Shoulder (SS-04). *Arthrosc. J. Arthrosc. Relat. Surg.* **2011**, *27*, e30–e31. [CrossRef]
20. Neri, B.R.; ElAttrache, N.S.; Owsley, K.C.; Mohr, K.; Yocum, L.A. Outcome of Type II Superior Labral Anterior Posterior Repairs in Elite Overhead Athletes. *Am. J. Sport. Med.* **2011**, *39*, 114–120. [CrossRef]
21. DeFazio, M.W.; Özkan, S.; Wagner, E.R.; Warner, J.J.P.; Chen, N.C. Isolated Type II SLAP Tears Undergo Reoperation More Frequently. *Knee Surg. Sport. Traumatol. Arthrosc.* **2021**, *29*, 2570–2578. [CrossRef]
22. Chloros, G.D.; Haar, P.J.; Loughran, T.P.; Hayes, C.W. Imaging of Glenoid Labrum Lesions. *Clin. Sport. Med.* **2013**, *32*, 361–390. [CrossRef] [PubMed]
23. de Coninck, T.; Ngai, S.S.; Tafur, M.; Chung, C.B. Imaging the Glenoid Labrum and Labral Tears. *RadioGraphics* **2016**, *36*, 1628–1647. [CrossRef] [PubMed]
24. Connolly, K.P.; Schwartzberg, R.S.; Reuss, B.; Crumbie, D.; Homan, B.M. Sensitivity and Specificity of Noncontrast Magnetic Resonance Imaging Reports in the Diagnosis of Type-II Superior Labral Anterior-Posterior Lesions in the Community Setting. *J. Bone Jt. Surg.-Am. Vol.* **2013**, *95*, 308–313. [CrossRef] [PubMed]
25. Connell, D.A.; Potter, H.G.; Wickiewicz, T.L.; Altchek, D.W.; Warren, R.F. Noncontrast Magnetic Resonance Imaging of Superior Labral Lesions. *Am. J. Sport. Med.* **1999**, *27*, 208–213. [CrossRef] [PubMed]
26. Amin, M.F.; Youssef, A.O. The Diagnostic Value of Magnetic Resonance Arthrography of the Shoulder in Detection and Grading of SLAP Lesions: Comparison with Arthroscopic Findings. *Eur. J. Radiol.* **2012**, *81*, 2343–2347. [CrossRef] [PubMed]
27. Arnold, H. Non-Contrast Magnetic Resonance Imaging for Diagnosing Shoulder Injuries. *J. Orthop. Surg.* **2012**, *20*, 361–364. [CrossRef]
28. Houtz, C.G.; Schwartzberg, R.S.; Barry, J.A.; Reuss, B.L.; Papa, L. Shoulder MRI Accuracy in the Community Setting. *J. Shoulder Elb. Surg.* **2011**, *20*, 537–542. [CrossRef] [PubMed]
29. Rehnitz, C.; Klaan, B.; Burkholder, I.; von Stillfried, F.; Kauczor, H.-U.; Weber, M.-A. Delayed Gadolinium-Enhanced MRI of Cartilage (DGEMRIC) and T_2 Mapping at 3T MRI of the Wrist: Feasibility and Clinical Application. *J. Magn. Reson. Imaging* **2017**, *45*, 381–389. [CrossRef]
30. Hesper, T.; Neugroda, C.; Schleich, C.; Antoch, G.; Hosalkar, H.; Krauspe, R.; Zilkens, C.; Bittersohl, B. T2*-Mapping of Acetabular Cartilage in Patients with Femoroacetabular Impingement at 3 Tesla: Comparative Analysis with Arthroscopic Findings. *Cartilage* **2018**, *9*, 118–126. [CrossRef] [PubMed]
31. Bittersohl, B.; Miese, F.R.; Dekkers, C.; Senyurt, H.; Kircher, J.; Wittsack, H.-J.; Antoch, G.; Krauspe, R.; Zilkens, C. T2* Mapping and Delayed Gadolinium-Enhanced Magnetic Resonance Imaging in Cartilage (DGEMRIC) of Glenohumeral Cartilage in Asymptomatic Volunteers at 3 T. *Eur. Radiol.* **2013**, *23*, 1367–1374. [CrossRef] [PubMed]
32. Lee, S.-Y.; Park, H.-J.; Kwon, H.-J.; Kim, M.S.; Choi, S.H.; Choi, Y.J.; Kim, E. T2 Relaxation Times of the Glenohumeral Joint at 3.0 T MRI in Patients with and without Primary and Secondary Osteoarthritis. *Acta Radiol.* **2015**, *56*, 1388–1395. [CrossRef] [PubMed]
33. Nguyen, J.C.; Liu, F.; Blankenbaker, D.G.; Woo, K.M.; Kijowski, R. Juvenile Osteochondritis Dissecans: Cartilage T2 Mapping of Stable Medial Femoral Condyle Lesions. *Radiology* **2018**, *288*, 536–543. [CrossRef]
34. Renner, N.; Kleyer, A.; Krönke, G.; Simon, D.; Söllner, S.; Rech, J.; Uder, M.; Janka, R.; Schett, G.; Welsch, G.H.; et al. T2 Mapping as a New Method for Quantitative Assessment of Cartilage Damage in Rheumatoid Arthritis. *J. Rheumatol.* **2020**, *47*, 820–825. [CrossRef] [PubMed]
35. Eijgenraam, S.M.; Bovendeert, F.A.T.; Verschueren, J.; van Tiel, J.; Bastiaansen-Jenniskens, Y.M.; Wesdorp, M.A.; Nasserinejad, K.; Meuffels, D.E.; Guenoun, J.; Klein, S.; et al. T2 Mapping of the Meniscus Is a Biomarker for Early Osteoarthritis. *Eur. Radiol.* **2019**, *29*, 5664–5672. [CrossRef]
36. Bossuyt, P.M.; Reitsma, J.B.; Bruns, D.E.; Gatsonis, C.A.; Glasziou, P.P.; Irwig, L.; Lijmer, J.G.; Moher, D.; Rennie, D.; de Vet, H.C.W.; et al. STARD 2015: An Updated List of Essential Items for Reporting Diagnostic Accuracy Studies. *Radiology* **2015**, *277*, 826–832. [CrossRef]
37. Snyder, S.J.; Karzel, R.P.; del Pizzo, W.; Ferkel, R.D.; Friedman, M.J. SLAP Lesions of the Shoulder. *Arthrosc. J. Arthrosc. Relat. Surg.* **1990**, *6*, 274–279. [CrossRef]
38. Shrout, P.E.; Fleiss, J.L. Intraclass Correlations: Uses in Assessing Rater Reliability. *Psychol. Bull.* **1979**, *86*, 420–428. [CrossRef]
39. Alashkham, A.; Alraddadi, A.; Felts, P.; Soames, R. Histology, Vascularity and Innervation of the Glenoid Labrum. *J. Orthop. Surg.* **2018**, *26*, 230949901877090. [CrossRef]
40. Cooper, D.E.; Arnoczky, S.P.; O'Brien, S.J.; Warren, R.F.; DiCarlo, E.; Allen, A.A. Anatomy, Histology, and Vascularity of the Glenoid Labrum. An Anatomical Study. *J. Bone Jt. Surg. Am.* **1992**, *74*, 46–52. [CrossRef]
41. Bain, G.I.; Galley, I.J.; Singh, C.; Carter, C.; Eng, K. Anatomic Study of the Superior Glenoid Labrum. *Clin. Anat.* **2013**, *26*, 367–376. [CrossRef] [PubMed]

42. Cook, J.L.; Purdam, C.R. Is Tendon Pathology a Continuum? A Pathology Model to Explain the Clinical Presentation of Load-Induced Tendinopathy. *Br. J. Sport. Med.* **2009**, *43*, 409–416. [CrossRef] [PubMed]
43. Khan, K.M.; Cook, J.L.; Bonar, F.; Harcourt, P.; Astrom, M. Histopathology of Common Tendinopathies. *Sport. Med.* **1999**, *27*, 393–408. [CrossRef] [PubMed]
44. Pollard, T.C.B.; Gwilym, S.E.; Carr, A.J. The Assessment of Early Osteoarthritis. *J. Bone Jt. Surg. Br.* **2008**, *90-B*, 411–421. [CrossRef] [PubMed]
45. Liess, C.; Lüsse, S.; Karger, N.; Heller, M.; Glüer, C.-C. Detection of Changes in Cartilage Water Content Using MRI T2-Mapping in Vivo. *Osteoarthr. Cartil.* **2002**, *10*, 907–913. [CrossRef]
46. Xie, Y.; Liu, S.; qiao, Y.; Hu, Y.; Zhang, Y.; Qu, J.; Shen, Y.; Tao, H.; Chen, S. Quantitative T2 Mapping-Based Tendon Healing Is Related to the Clinical Outcomes during the First Year after Arthroscopic Rotator Cuff Repair. *Knee Surg. Sport. Traumatol. Arthrosc.* **2021**, *29*, 127–135. [CrossRef]
47. Soellner, S.T.; Goldmann, A.; Muelheims, D.; Welsch, G.H.; Pachowsky, M.L. Intraoperative Validation of Quantitative T2 Mapping in Patients with Articular Cartilage Lesions of the Knee. *Osteoarthr. Cartil.* **2017**, *25*, 1841–1849. [CrossRef]
48. Golditz, T.; Steib, S.; Pfeifer, K.; Uder, M.; Gelse, K.; Janka, R.; Hennig, F.F.; Welsch, G.H. Functional Ankle Instability as a Risk Factor for Osteoarthritis: Using T2-Mapping to Analyze Early Cartilage Degeneration in the Ankle Joint of Young Athletes. *Osteoarthr. Cartil.* **2014**, *22*, 1377–1385. [CrossRef]
49. Monu, J.U.; Pope, T.L.; Chabon, S.J.; Vanarthos, W.J. MR Diagnosis of Superior Labral Anterior Posterior (SLAP) Injuries of the Glenoid Labrum: Value of Routine Imaging without Intraarticular Injection of Contrast Material. *Am. J. Roentgenol.* **1994**, *163*, 1425–1429. [CrossRef]
50. Major, N.M.; Browne, J.; Domzalski, T.; Cothran, R.L.; Helms, C.A. Evaluation of the Glenoid Labrum With 3-T MRI: Is Intraarticular Contrast Necessary? *Am. J. Roentgenol.* **2011**, *196*, 1139–1144. [CrossRef]
51. Wuennemann, F.; Kintzelé, L.; Braun, A.; Zeifang, F.; Maier, M.W.; Burkholder, I.; Weber, M.-A.; Kauczor, H.-U.; Rehnitz, C. 3-T T2 Mapping Magnetic Resonance Imaging for Biochemical Assessment of Normal and Damaged Glenoid Cartilage: A Prospective Arthroscopy-Controlled Study. *Sci. Rep.* **2020**, *10*, 14396. [CrossRef] [PubMed]
52. Le, J.; Peng, Q.; Sperling, K. Biochemical Magnetic Resonance Imaging of Knee Articular Cartilage: T1rho and T2 Mapping as Cartilage Degeneration Biomarkers. *Ann. N. Y. Acad. Sci.* **2016**, *1383*, 34–42. [CrossRef] [PubMed]
53. Rehnitz, C.; Kuni, B.; Wuennemann, F.; Chloridis, D.; Kirwadi, A.; Burkholder, I.; Kauczor, H.-U.; Weber, M.-A. Delayed Gadolinium-Enhanced MRI of Cartilage (DGEMRIC) and T_2 Mapping of Talar Osteochondral Lesions: Indicators of Clinical Outcomes. *J. Magn. Reson. Imaging* **2017**, *46*, 1601–1610. [CrossRef] [PubMed]
54. Rehnitz, C.; Kupfer, J.; Streich, N.A.; Burkholder, I.; Schmitt, B.; Lauer, L.; Kauczor, H.-U.; Weber, M.-A. Comparison of Biochemical Cartilage Imaging Techniques at 3 T MRI. *Osteoarthr. Cartil.* **2014**, *22*, 1732–1742. [CrossRef]
55. Mosher, T.J.; Smith, H.; Dardzinski, B.J.; Schmithorst, V.J.; Smith, M.B. MR Imaging and T2 Mapping of Femoral Cartilage. *Am. J. Roentgenol.* **2001**, *177*, 665–669. [CrossRef]
56. Kaneko, Y.; Nozaki, T.; Yu, H.; Chang, A.; Kaneshiro, K.; Schwarzkopf, R.; Hara, T.; Yoshioka, H. Normal T2 Map Profile of the Entire Femoral Cartilage Using an Angle/Layer-Dependent Approach. *J. Magn. Reson. Imaging* **2015**, *42*, 1507–1516. [CrossRef]
57. Watanabe, A.; Boesch, C.; Siebenrock, K.; Obata, T.; Anderson, S.E. T2 Mapping of Hip Articular Cartilage in Healthy Volunteers at 3T: A Study of Topographic Variation. *J. Magn. Reson. Imaging* **2007**, *26*, 165–171. [CrossRef]
58. Sasaki, T.; Yodono, H.; Prado, G.L.M.; Saito, Y.; Miura, H.; Itabashi, Y.; Ootsuka, H.; Ishibashi, Y. Increased Signal Intensity in the Normal Glenoid Labrum in MR Imaging: Diagnostic Pitfalls Caused by the Magic-Angle Effect. *Magn. Reson. Med. Sci.* **2002**, *1*, 149–156. [CrossRef]
59. Kang, Y.; Choi, J.-A. T2 Mapping of Articular Cartilage of the Glenohumeral Joint at 3.0 T in Healthy Volunteers: A Feasibility Study. *Skelet. Radiol.* **2016**, *45*, 915–920. [CrossRef]
60. Lockard, C.A.; Wilson, K.J.; Ho, C.P.; Shin, R.C.; Katthagen, J.C.; Millett, P.J. Quantitative Mapping of Glenohumeral Cartilage in Asymptomatic Subjects Using 3 T Magnetic Resonance Imaging. *Skelet. Radiol* **2018**, *47*, 671–682. [CrossRef]
61. Lansdown, D.A.; Wang, K.; Cotter, E.; Davey, A.; Cole, B.J. Relationship Between Quantitative MRI Biomarkers and Patient-Reported Outcome Measures After Cartilage Repair Surgery: A Systematic Review. *Orthop. J. Sport. Med.* **2018**, *6*, 232596711876544. [CrossRef] [PubMed]
62. Jungmann, P.M.; Baum, T.; Bauer, J.S.; Karampinos, D.C.; Erdle, B.; Link, T.M.; Li, X.; Trattnig, S.; Rummeny, E.J.; Woertler, K.; et al. Cartilage Repair Surgery: Outcome Evaluation by Using Noninvasive Cartilage Biomarkers Based on Quantitative MRI Techniques? *BioMed. Res. Int.* **2014**, *2014*, 1–17. [CrossRef]
63. Stathellis, A.; Brilakis, E.; Georgoulis, J.-D.; Antonogiannakis, E.; Georgoulis, A. Treatment of SLAP Lesions. *Open Orthop. J.* **2018**, *12*, 288–294. [CrossRef] [PubMed]
64. Brockmeyer, M.; Tompkins, M.; Kohn, D.M.; Lorbach, O. SLAP Lesions: A Treatment Algorithm. *Knee Surg. Sport. Traumatol. Arthrosc.* **2016**, *24*, 447–455. [CrossRef] [PubMed]

Disclaimer/Publisher's Note: The statements, opinions and data contained in all publications are solely those of the individual author(s) and contributor(s) and not of MDPI and/or the editor(s). MDPI and/or the editor(s) disclaim responsibility for any injury to people or property resulting from any ideas, methods, instructions or products referred to in the content.

Article

Correlation of Bone Textural Parameters with Age in the Context of Orthopedic X-ray Studies

Paweł Kamiński [1,2], Rafał Obuchowicz [3,*], Aleksandra Stępień [4], Julia Lasek [5], Elżbieta Pociask [4] and Adam Piórkowski [4]

1. Clinic of Locomotor Disorders, Andrzej Frycz Modrzewski Krakow University, 30-705 Krakow, Poland
2. Małopolska Orthopedic and Rehabilitation Hospital, Modrzewiowa 22, 30-224 Krakow, Poland
3. Department of Diagnostic Imaging, Jagiellonian University Medical College, Kopernika 19, 31-501 Krakow, Poland
4. Department of Biocybernetics and Biomedical Engineering, AGH University of Science and Technology, 30-059 Krakow, Poland
5. Faculty of Geology, Geophysics and Environmental Protection, AGH University of Science and Technology, 30-059 Krakow, Poland
* Correspondence: rafalobuchowicz@su.krakow.pl

Abstract: The aim of this study was to establish a relationship between the textural parameters observed in X-ray images of bones and the age of the individual. The study utilized a meticulous visual analysis of the images to identify significant correlations between textural features and age. Five distinct regions of interest, namely the Wing of the Ilium, Neck of the Femur, Greater Trochanter, Ischium, and Shaft of the Femur, were identified on both sides of the body. Textural parameters were then measured for each of these regions. The left femoral neck showed the most noteworthy associations, with the textures generated from the histogram of oriented gradients and gray-level co-occurrence matrix exhibiting the strongest correlations (ρ -0.52, p-value 4.95×10^{-14}). The main finding of the current study is that correlation of age-dependent bone structure differences in the femoral neck area is higher than in other structures of the femur. This proposed methodology has the potential to aid in the early detection of osteoporosis, which is crucial for devising treatment plans and identifying potential risks associated with bone fragility.

Keywords: textural analysis; X-ray; radiographs; bone age; bone aging; osteoporosis

1. Introduction

Bone is a complex composite formed from both organic and inorganic components. It serves as a supportive tissue that evolved to provide a great advantage for land animals, despite being energy-consuming. From a mechanical point of view, bone tissue must possess maximal strength and stiffness (resistant to failure and deformation) with the lowest possible mass. Therefore, it has a complex internal organization, with an outer cortical zone and an internal trabecular bone [1]. This three-dimensional architecture enables it to withstand tension and compression forces that can be effectively dissipated throughout the bone without producing mechanical damage [2]. To fulfill the mechanical needs of the skeleton as a supportive tissue, bone is organized hierarchically with compact bone (approximately 80% of the skeleton) and trabecular or spongy bone (20% of the skeleton) [3]. At the microstructure level, bone is composed of osteons, which are longitudinal canals called Haversian canals surrounded by lamellae [1]. The Haversian canals house osteoblasts and blood vessels, and they are about 20 to 100 μm in diameter [4]. Single lamellae are up to 7 μm thick and up to 25 μm long. These are the locations where the inorganic phase responsible for the mechanical properties of the bone is accumulated. The inorganic phase consists of apatite-like mineral hydroxyapatite crystals ($Ca_{10}(PO_4)_6(OH)_2$) [3], which have a hexagonal lattice structure and are formed as plates with an average size of $50 \times 25 \times 3$ nm.

These structures are adjacent to collagen I, an organic material formed from protein material oriented parallel to the long axis of the bone [5]. The presence of inorganic structures embedded in collagen fibrils is responsible for the interaction with electrons emitted from the anode of the X-ray lamp [6]. Collisions with inorganic materials absorb electron energy, which is responsible for the projection of the bone, detectable by the visual system. The spatial resolution of the X-ray picture is high. For a 35×43 cm cassette and a 20×24 cm cassette, three and five line pairs per millimeter are reported, respectively [7]. The range of dimensions of bone structure accessible by X-ray imaging is up to 5 µm, which corresponds to the bone microstructure.

Osteocytes are residual, long-lived bone cells that are interconnected with each other with processes and form an important signaling network, which serves as mechanosensory units directing the response of osteoclasts-bone-depleting cells and osteoblasts-bone-forming cells [8]. Cellular action serves in constant longitudinal and transverse remodeling of the bone, where matrix turnover makes complete matrix exchange every 10 years [9]. The process of mineral exchange serves adjustments to the specific loads of the bone excreted by physical activity, but also the metabolic needs of the organism as the skeleton is a reservoir of calcium ions and takes part in the interchange of inorganic substances with the extracellular fluid (ECF) [10]. Bone turnover is precisely regulated by hormonal action throughout life, which is one of the causative factors of the differences between the skeletal systems of women and men observed from puberty to older age [11]. Pathologic changes in the regulatory process include an increase in cortical porosity, trabecular thinning, and a decrease in trabecular interconnections [12]. This normal process of bone degeneration can be markedly increased if the control of bone metabolism is dysregulated. Moreover, of importance are physical activity and dietary habits, including alcohol and calcium product consumption, but also the presence of diseases impacting hydrogen ions and calcium/phosphorus equilibrium [13–15].

It is worth noting that vitamin D and calcium deficiency may lead to secondary hyperparathyroidism, which promotes osteoclastic activation with an increase in calcium bone to extracellular fluid conversion [16]. The most important recognized regulatory factor is linked to estrogen action, which is involved in the control of bone resorption, as it inhibits osteoclast activation [17]. The processes controlling bone are very complex, and deterioration of bone architecture weakens the bone, making it susceptible to overload and a potential cause of bone trauma. Therefore, meticulous determination of the status of the bone is important at the early stages.

In the theoretical introduction above, we wish to point out that there are biology-based reasons for investigating how bone age, and hence changes in its composition and physical properties, correlate with changes in the X-ray image detectable by textural analysis. This study investigated the relationship between the textural parameters determined on the basis of radiographs of the hip bone and the age of the patients.

2. Materials and Methods

2.1. Dataset

The initial dataset comprised 3782 radiographic images of the hip and knee regions, captured using an X-ray machine and stored in PNG8 format with 8-bit color depth. The images were acquired from a group of 241 individuals of both sexes, with ages ranging from 26 to 91 years. Following an initial screening, all radiographs that did not portray the hip joint bones were excluded from the subsequent analysis. The images depicting the hip joint were obtained prior to endoprosthesis surgery or in a condition indicating the need for reoperation. In addition, images with artifacts from elements such as the mattress or endoprosthesis were also excluded. Finally, 481 radiographs from 132 patients were used for analysis, where 93 patients had a longitudinal study (several X-rays taken at intervals), and 39 patients had a single study (having only one image at one time point).

2.2. Data Acquisition

In the study X-ray machine, Del Medical EV-650, manufactured in 2008, was used. The X-ray machine was supplied with a cassette feeder (Poersch Metal Manufacturing Co., Chicago, IL 60624, USA), a portable detector DFMTS equipped with exposure tube C52 Super with an X-ray lamp RTM 101 HS manufactured by I.A.E Spa. The system is powered by a high-voltage generator (Via Sistemi Medicali). Lamp usage is carefully monitored, and the system was equipped with a new X-ray lamp (2015). System equipped with a valid technical passport to assure patient safety.

2.3. ROI Annotation

To annotate the ROIs (Regions of Interest) on the preselected images, the qMaZda software (release version 19.02) was used [18]. In each radiograph, rectangular ROIs were selected to correspond to specific anatomical structures. Where endoprostheses were present, the ROIs were refrained from being marked, resulting in a lower number of analyzed areas. A detailed description of the ROI delineation process is provided in Figure 1 and Table 1.

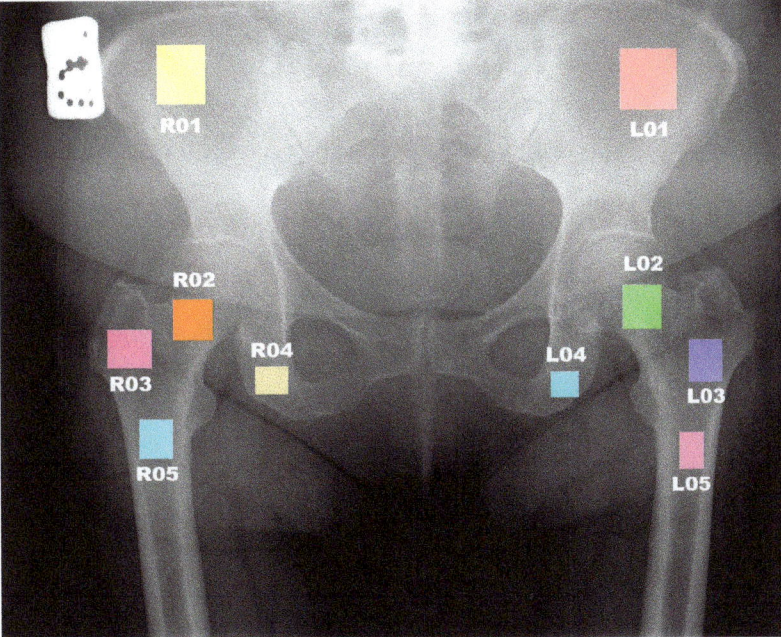

Figure 1. Regions of interest are depicted on the radiograph.

Table 1. Table of ROIs with corresponding anatomical areas.

ROI	Anatomical Structure
L 01	Wing of ilium—left side
L 02	Neck of femur—left side
L 03	Greater trochanter—left side
L 04	Ischium—left side
L 05	Shaft of femur—upper left side
R 01	Wing of ilium—right side
R 02	Neck of femur—right side
R 03	Greater trochanter—right side
R 04	Ischium—right side
R 05	Shaft of femur—upper right side

2.4. Textural Analysis

Texture analysis is a type of image processing that examines image patterns and structural features. It calculates the various statistical measurements of the grey-level intensity values of the pixels in the image and can provide information on the spatial distribution and arrangement of those pixels. Textural analysis can be used to extract contrast, entropy, and homogeneity, which express subtle changes in the X-ray image and reflects different bone tissue organization [19].

The textural analysis for each ROI was also carried out using qMaZda software, which provides a plethora of different textural parameters. The qMaZda software computes multiple textural features, including histogram-based, co-occurrence-matrix-based, run-length-matrix-based, gradient-map-based, autoregressive model-based, and Haar wavelet transform-based features. All these parameters can be calculated directly from the original image histogram or based on a normalized histogram by setting different (4 to 12) bits per pixel [18].

Initially, more than 10,000 parameters were determined for each ROI. Subsequently, the parameters that contained NaN values were eliminated. As a result, 10 datasets were generated, corresponding to each ROI, containing a total of 6836 features.

2.5. Statistical Analysis

Statistical analysis was aimed at showing which textural features correlate significantly with age (age distribution presented in Figure 2).

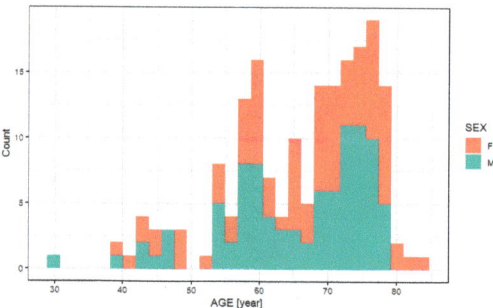

Figure 2. Age distribution, including SEX differences.

In the first step, the Shapiro–Wilk test [20] and Q-Q plot were used to evaluate the distribution of continuous variables. Continuous data were presented as mean (standard deviation, SD) or median (interquartile range, IQR) and compared using Student's t-test and Mann–Whitney–Wilcoxon U test, respectively. When one of the subgroups in the study groups had a non-normal type distribution, data were presented as median (IQR) and Mann–Whitney–Wilcoxon U test. Categorical data were presented as numbers (percentages), and Fisher's exact test was used to compare them. This determined the steps for further analysis, which was the calculation of Spearman's Rank correlation or Pearson's coefficient for each ROI. Regression models were used as quantitative methods to assess whether and how the predictor; AGE correlates with the selected textures. Further, mixed-effects regression models were used as an extension of fixed-effects regression models to account for hierarchical data structures (Tables 2 and 3 show comparison results of generated models). Such analysis takes into account intra-individual association between variables because we had a mixed data set; some data were collected for participants at several different time points. LME4 R packages were used to develop mixed-effect models.

Table 2. Summary of standard regression (fixed-effect models) for the most prominent textures.

Model	Variable	Estimate (β Coefficients)	SE	p-Value	Adjusted R2	AIC
MODEL_L02_YM6HogO8b4 fixed_regression	AGE	−0.009	0.001	2.4×10^{-14}	0.271	−161.1173
MODEL_L02_YM4GlcmH4DifEntrp Fixed_regression	AGE	−0.002	0.0003	1.55×10^{-13}	0.2565	−602.232

Table 3. Summary of mixed models for the most prominent textures.

Model	Variable	Estimate (β Coefficients)	SE	T	p-Value	Lower_2.5	Upper_97.5	AIC
MODEL_L02_YM6HogO8b4 mixed_regression	AGE	−0.008	0.001	−5.444	0	−0.011	−0.005	−159.9161
MODEL_L02_YM4GlcmH4DifEntrp mixed_regression	AGE	−0.002	0.0004	−4.998	0	−0.003	−0.001	−588.468

The idea behind regression analysis is expressed in the equation below where f(x) is the y-value we want to predict, α is the intercept (the point where the regression line crosses the y-axis at x = 0), β is the coefficient (the slope of the regression line).

$$f(x) = \alpha + \beta i x + \epsilon$$

SE is a measure that tells how much the coefficients would vary if the same regression were applied to multiple samples from the same population. Thus, a relatively small SE value indicates that the coefficients will remain very stable if the same regression model is fitted to many different samples with identical parameters. A large SE value, on the other hand, says that the model is variable and not very stable or reliable because the coefficients change substantively if the model is applied to many samples.

$$StandardError(SE) = \frac{\frac{\sum(\bar{x} - x_i)^2}{N-1}}{\sqrt{N}} = \frac{SD}{\sqrt{N}}$$

The equation below represents a formal representation of a mixed-effects regression with varying:

$$f(x) = \alpha i + \beta i x + \epsilon$$

In this model, each level of the random variable has a different intercept and a different slope. So, to predict the value of a data point, it takes the appropriate intercept (model intercept + random effect intercept) and adds the level factor of that random effect multiplied by the value of x.

The inclusion of a random effect structure with random intercepts is justified as the AIC (Akaike Information Criterion) of the model with random intercepts is substantially lower than the AIC of the model without random intercepts. The Akaike Information Criterion is a mathematical method for evaluating how well a model fits the data it was generated from. In statistics, AIC is used to compare different possible models and determine which one is the best fit for the data. The lower the AIC score, the better.

3. Results

Of the 10 anatomical areas analyzed, only ROI L 02 contained features that showed significant correlations (Table 4). The lowest correlation values were obtained when analyzing the ROI L 04 area, whose features describe the texture parameters of the ischium texture on the left side of the hip joint. The highest value for this area was characterized by the feature YM5Gab8Z4Mag, with a value of only −0.14.

Table 4. Summary of parameters with the highest Spearman's rank correlation coefficient and p-value for each ROI.

ROI	Parameter	rho Spearman	p-Value
L 01	YD4DwtHaarS4HH	0.35	1.38×10^{-9}
L 02	**YM6HogO8b4**	**−0.52**	**4.95×10^{-14}**
L 03	YS4Gab24H12Mag	−0.27	0.24×10^{-3}
L 04	YM5Gab8Z4Mag	−0.14	0.4×10^{-2}
L 05	YS5GrlmHMGLevNonUn	0.32	1.60×10^{-5}
R 01	YS6GlcmZ5SumAverg	0.26	1.60×10^{-4}
R 02	YLbpCs8n5	0.31	7.54×10^{-5}
R 03	YN8DwtHaarS1HH	0.37	4.62×10^{-6}
R 04	YD4GrlmHRLNonUni	0.17	0.53×10^{-4}
R 05	YN4Gab24Z12Mag	−0.27	0.90×10^{-3}

ROI L 02 was the most prominent, reaching as high as −0.52 in correlation with YM6HogO8b4 texture. The features determined in this area describe the textural parameters of the left femoral neck. The parameters determined in the right femoral neck area were characterized by lower values and did not coincide with the features determined on the left side (YLbpCs8n5: 0.31).

The results for the parameter YM6HogO8b4 are additionally illustrated in Figure 3 and YM4GlcmH4InvDfMom in Figure 4.

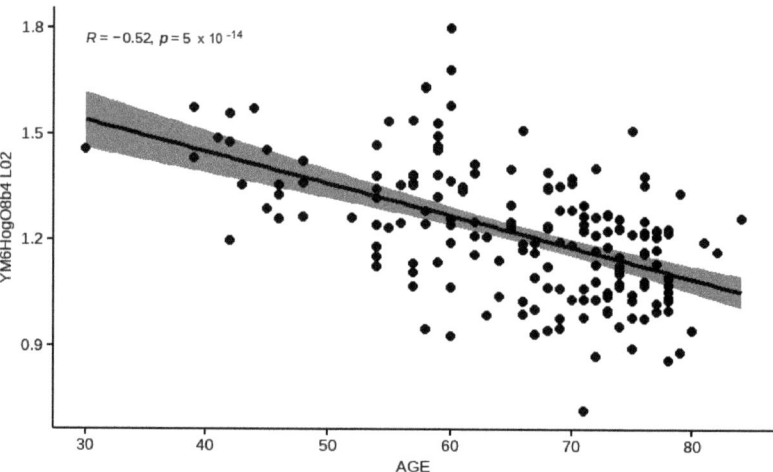

Figure 3. Correlation of YM6HogO8b4 values with age for ROI L 02. The p-value of the test is less than the significance level alpha = 0.05; it concludes that age and selected texture are significantly correlated with a correlation coefficient of −0.52 and p-value of 5×10^{-14}. This graph shows a negative correlation, which means that every time AGE increases, YM6HogO8b4 values decrease.

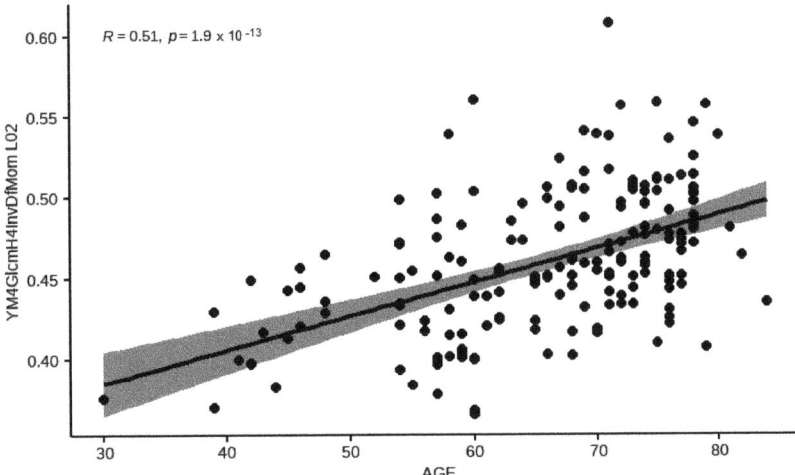

Figure 4. Correlation of YM4GlcmH4InvDfMom values with age for ROI L 02. The *p*-value of the test is less than the significance level alpha = 0.05; it concludes that age and selected texture are significantly correlated with a correlation coefficient of 0.51 and *p*-value of 1.9×10^{-13}. This graph shows a positive correlation. It means that YM4GlcmH4InvDfMom values increase with AGE.

In addition, the most relevant results for ROI L 02 are provided in Table 5.

Table 5. Texture parameters with corresponding rho Spearman correlation results and *p*-values for ROI L 02.

Parameter	rho Spearman	*p*-Value
YM6HogO8b4	−0.5194	4.95×10^{-14}
YM5HogO8b4	−0.5143	9.55×10^{-14}
YM8HogO8b4	−0.5139	1.00×10^{-13}
YM7HogO8b4	−0.5130	1.12×10^{-13}
YM4GlcmH4DifEntrp	−0.5100	1.65×10^{-13}
YM4HogO8b4	−0.5100	1.70×10^{-13}
YM4GlcmH4InvDfMom	0.5088	1.93×10^{-13}
YM4GlcmH4Contrast	−0.5085	1.99×10^{-13}
YM4HogO8b5	−0.5078	2.19×10^{-13}
YM5GlcmH4Contrast	−0.5071	2.38×10^{-13}
YM7GlcmH4Contrast	−0.5070	2.42×10^{-13}

All textural parameters of the femoral neck showing the most significant correlation with age are derived from a histogram of oriented gradients (HOG) or the gray-level co-occurrence matrix (GLCM).

HOG represents an image by calculating the distribution of gradient orientations and magnitudes in small regions of the image called cells. The "8b" in the feature name indicates the number of bins used to create the histogram. The GLCM texture feature proposed by Haralick and Shanmugam [21] is widely recognized as a useful tool for textural feature extraction [22]. It defines how often a combination of pixels occurs in an image by analyzing the spatial relationship between pixels. Another shared feature, including the other ROIs that have been analyzed, is the color component—coded as the first sign Y, which stands for the brightness component from the YUV color space. Another thing worth noting is the recurring last abbreviation defining the descriptor InvDfMom, which stands for Inverse Difference Moment. The higher levels of this parameter represent an increased pixel uniformity and homogeneity [23]. The meaning of other abbreviations can be retrieved from [18].

4. Discussion

The objective of the current investigation was to establish a relationship between alterations observed in X-ray scans of bones and the age of the individual. Such changes may not be perceptible to the imaging specialist. The utilization of mathematical algorithms to analyze the surrounding pixel environment affords an avenue for examining modifications in the bone microstructure that exceed the capabilities of human vision [24]. Our study focused on establishing correlations between bone structure in varied regions of interest within the proximal femur. X-ray appraisal is a firmly established method for assessing the skeletal system [25].

The high mineral matrix content adjacent to collagen fibrils resists X-ray propagation, which is the basis for determining the bone shape and clinical changes [26]. Bone is a dynamic organ that interacts with the endocrine system to maintain ion equilibrium and acid-base balance. This interaction relies on the action of osteoblasts and osteoclasts, which are differentiated and activated from osteogenic cells (stem cells) progenitors [12]. The lifespan of both cells is relatively short, with osteoblasts and osteoclasts surviving for three months and one month, respectively [27]. The actions of osteoblasts and osteoclasts are necessary for normal bone metabolism, including bone formation and depletion, and for remodeling bone to provide skeletal support, which varies in different locations depending on the load [28].

Although bone remodeling is a continuous process that involves the complete exchange of bone matrix every ten years, the overall bone mass is not significantly decreased [29]. However, advancing age and menopause are significant factors in reducing bone mass [30]. The gradual decrease in osteons and lamellae, as well as the organic and inorganic matrix associated with functional imbalances between osteoclast and osteoblasts, functions that favor osteoclast function, results in a gradual decline in the volume of osteons and overall bone [31]. The decrease in interconnections between bone trabeculae that form lamellae weakens the bone and makes it fragile and susceptible to pathological fractures [32]. This process of bone deterioration is ongoing in both cancellous and compact bone, which is crucial for load transmission [33]. In this study, two regions of interest (ROIs) were analyzed based on correlations of visual-based textural features. One ROI was located in the metaphysis region, where spongy osteocyte-containing bone with complex architecture is present, directed toward withstanding compression and extension forces concentrated along the main axes (lines) of support [34]. The second ROI was located in the peri-trochanteric region, where the compact bone is prevalent.

The peak of bone mass is typically reached after puberty (around 20 years) and gradually declines over one's lifetime [35]. This process, although it can be slowed by physical activity and good dietary habits, is inevitable and cannot be stopped. As trabeculae are overall of lower mass, the effect of the gradual reduction of bone mass is higher in locations with initially smaller bony mass, which is consistent with previous studies on the phenomenon of gradual depletion of bony mass [36]. Such changes are visible on traditional X-rays very late—only a loss of about 30% of the bone mass is visible on X-ray. Dual-energy X-ray absorptiometry (DEXA) is much more sensitive, but it is a less thorough examination and is performed in groups of patients at a certain risk of osteoporosis. The reduction in bone mass in the region of the trochanter is significant due to the influence of estrogen cessation [37]. Estrogens are known to be the most powerful stimuli for inhibiting the action of osteoclasts, which are known for their strong remodeling action on bone [38].

Although, for many years, the reference for diagnostic imaging of bone in humans was the interpretation of a radiologist [25], who is a specialist in diagnostic imaging, the ability of the observer to detect image details does not necessarily reflect the amount of information present in the image [24]. Therefore, many attempts have been made to evaluate bone tissue structure, which is especially susceptible to textural analysis [39]. The idea of using textural analysis for the evaluation of human tissue visualized in diagnostic imaging techniques is not new. It has been implemented for brain tissue [40–42], breast [43], and even muscle [44]. In the context of bone-based analysis, textural parameters are used, e.g., for the prediction of incident radiographic hip osteoarthritis [45], age-texture correlation analysis [46,47], and association with bone mineral density [48] and bone quality [49].

Contemporary emphasis must be placed on the role of artificial intelligence (AI), in particular deep learning (DL), in the broad field of bone analysis. It is a revolutionary tool that allows researchers to the generation of radiological reports for fractures of the proximal femur [50] and detects fractures directly on the image from different modalities [51–53]. AI-based methods have also demonstrated the potential to predict a patient's age or gender based on images of the bone [54,55]. Furthermore, neural networks can be a valuable support for bone segmentation [56,57] and the detection of a range of bone diseases [58,59].

The textural analysis presents certain benefits when compared to AI. In our theoretical overview, we elucidated the biological basis for changes in bone texture and demonstrated that there are certain specific parameters that are correlated with age. Textual analysis is more suitable for interpretation and, in this particular study, allows us to conclude that the microstructure of bone changes with age, which is accentuated in the images as an increase in the homogeneity and uniformity of pixel values. Furthermore, textural analysis can derive meaningful insights from smaller datasets compared to deep learning. Optional research may be conducted on bone corticalization [60].

This is a relatively new approach as, to the best of our knowledge, there are no similar approaches presented, excluding the work of our team [61] and the work of Dieckmayer [62], who evaluated age among different parameters with the use of deep learning methods; therefore, the approach was very different. Existing works where textures are used for bone assessment are focused on the evaluation of the presence of osteoporosis [63,64]. Textural bone assessment for osteoporosis evaluation was provided on different parts of the skeletal system, such as the jaw [65] and head [66], and with the use of different modalities as CT and MR [67]. Studies on bone mineralization were also evaluated in children [68]. However, bone mineral density was studied already with the use of textural methods, and works where age assessment was performed are lacking; therefore, we assume that our study will have an important contribution to the current literature status.

This study also has several limitations that merit discussion. First, the image acquisition was collected as digitalized images, which may have impacted the quality of the obtained images. In addition, a subset of the acquired images contained endoprostheses, resulting in a lower number of marked regions of interest (ROIs) and possibly affecting the overall distribution of the data. Another limitation of our study was the use of a broad demographic group with the inclusion of extremes of participants' age (youngest and oldest). The demographic is also limited to Caucasian origin with an extended group of participants aged 25–91; however, most of the examined group are above the sixth decade of life. Differences in bone mineral composition may influence the presented results. In future investigations, we aim to conduct more comprehensive analyses on a dataset that does not exhibit the aforementioned limitations and that includes a larger patient cohort.

5. Conclusions

In conclusion, the use of meticulous visual analysis based on textural features of X-ray images was applied, and important correlations of textural features with age were found. Implementation of textural analysis methods proved to be sensitive to changes in bone architecture. The correlation with age found in the bone shaft can be explained by the relatively lower mass of trabecular bone, even in areas of formation of compression supporting lines. The proposed method might be useful in the early diagnosis of osteoporosis. Early diagnosis of changes in bone mechanical strength might be essential in treatment planning and the diagnosis of potential threats associated with bone fragility. The most important statistical correlations were found in the femur neck. This is also the area of the highest clinical importance where most orthopedic urgencies are found. Therefore obtained results are important from a clinical point of view as they enable us to evaluate accurately areas where a potential bone loss might be a source of serious morbidities and further disabilities for the patient if not properly diagnosed.

Author Contributions: Conceptualization, P.K., R.O., A.S., J.L., E.P. and A.P.; methodology, P.K., R.O., A.S. and E.P.; software, A.S., J.L. and E.P.; validation, P.K., R.O., A.S., J.L., E.P. and A.P.; formal analysis, P.K., R.O. and A.P.; investigation, P.K., R.O., A.S., E.P. and A.P.; resources, P.K., R.O. and A.P.; data curation, A.P.; writing—original draft preparation, P.K., R.O., A.S., J.L., E.P. and A.P.; writing—review and editing, P.K., R.O., A.S., J.L., E.P. and A.P.; visualization, A.S., J.L. and E.P.; supervision, R.O., E.P. and A.P.; project administration, P.K. and A.P. All authors have read and agreed to the published version of the manuscript.

Funding: This research received no external funding.

Institutional Review Board Statement: Not applicable.

Informed Consent Statement: Not applicable.

Data Availability Statement: Data can be made available upon request by contacting the corresponding author.

Conflicts of Interest: The authors declare no conflict of interest.

Abbreviations

The meaning of texture feature abbreviations used in the article:
e.g., YM4GlcmH4Contrast
#1 {Y}: Y channel of YCbCr—luminance (also for grayscale images)
#2 {D, M, S}: method of normalization—D (no normalization), M—(min-max normalization), S—normalization to <$\mu - 3\sigma, \mu + 3\sigma$>
#3 {8, 7, 6, 5, 4}—number of depth bits (after quantization)
#4 {DwtHaar, Gab, Glcm, Grlm, Hog, Lbp}—texture name
#5 parameters of textures (direction, length}
#6 statistical function—described in detail in [61].

References

1. Downey, P.A.; Siegel, M.I. Bone Biology and the Clinical Implications for Osteoporosis. *Phys. Ther.* **2006**, *86*, 77–91. [CrossRef] [PubMed]
2. Holguin, N.; Brodt, M.D.; Sanchez, M.E.; Silva, M.J. Aging Diminishes Lamellar and Woven Bone Formation Induced by Tibial Compression in Adult C57BL/6. *Bone* **2014**, *65*, 83–91. [CrossRef]
3. Hadjidakis, D.J.; Androulakis, I.I. Bone Remodeling. *Ann. N. Y. Acad. Sci.* **2006**, *1092*, 385–396. [CrossRef] [PubMed]
4. Gartner, L.P.; Hiatt, J.L. Cartilage and Bone. In *Concise Histology*; Elsevier: Amsterdam, The Netherlands, 2011; pp. 74–93. ISBN 978-0-7020-3114-4.
5. Rho, J.-Y.; Kuhn-Spearing, L.; Zioupos, P. Mechanical Properties and the Hierarchical Structure of Bone. *Med. Eng. Phys.* **1998**, *20*, 92–102. [CrossRef]
6. McNally, E.A.; Schwarcz, H.P.; Botton, G.A.; Arsenault, A.L. A Model for the Ultrastructure of Bone Based on Electron Microscopy of Ion-Milled Sections. *PLoS ONE* **2012**, *7*, e29258. [CrossRef]
7. Huda, W.; Abrahams, R.B. X-ray-Based Medical Imaging and Resolution. *Am. J. Roentgenol.* **2015**, *204*, W393–W397. [CrossRef]
8. Bonewald, L.F. The Amazing Osteocyte. *J. Bone Miner. Res.* **2011**, *26*, 229–238. [CrossRef]
9. Parfitt, A.M. Osteonal and Hemi-Osteonal Remodeling: The Spatial and Temporal Framework for Signal Traffic in Adult Human Bone. *J. Cell. Biochem.* **1994**, *55*, 273–286. [CrossRef]
10. Di Girolamo, D.J.; Clemens, T.L.; Kousteni, S. The Skeleton as an Endocrine Organ. *Nat. Rev. Rheumatol.* **2012**, *8*, 674–683. [CrossRef]
11. Noirrit-Esclassan, E.; Valera, M.-C.; Tremollieres, F.; Arnal, J.-F.; Lenfant, F.; Fontaine, C.; Vinel, A. Critical Role of Estrogens on Bone Homeostasis in Both Male and Female: From Physiology to Medical Implications. *Int. J. Mol. Sci.* **2021**, *22*, 1568. [CrossRef]
12. Boskey, A.L.; Coleman, R. Aging and Bone. *J. Dent. Res.* **2010**, *89*, 1333–1348. [CrossRef]
13. Florencio-Silva, R.; da Silva Sasso, G.R.; Sasso-Cerri, E.; Simões, M.J.; Cerri, P.S. Biology of Bone Tissue: Structure, Function, and Factors That Influence Bone Cells. *BioMed Res. Int.* **2015**, *2015*, 421746. [CrossRef] [PubMed]
14. Kerr, D.; Morton, A.; Dick, I.; Prince, R. Exercise Effects on Bone Mass in Postmenopausal Women Are Site-Specific and Load-Dependent. *J. Bone Miner. Res.* **2009**, *11*, 218–225. [CrossRef]
15. Bonjour, J.-P.; Theintz, G.; Law, F.; Slosman, D.; Rizzoli, R. Peak Bone Mass. *Osteoporos. Int.* **1994**, *4*, S7–S13. [CrossRef]

16. Lips, P. Vitamin D Deficiency and Secondary Hyperparathyroidism in the Elderly: Consequences for Bone Loss and Fractures and Therapeutic Implications. *Endocr. Rev.* **2001**, *22*, 477–501. [CrossRef] [PubMed]
17. Khosla, S.; Oursler, M.J.; Monroe, D.G. Estrogen and the Skeleton. *Trends Endocrinol. Metab.* **2012**, *23*, 576–581. [CrossRef]
18. Szczypiński, P.M.; Strzelecki, M.; Materka, A.; Klepaczko, A. MaZda—The software package for textural analysis of biomedical images. In *Computers in Medical Activity*; Advances in Intelligent and Soft Computing; Springer: Berlin/Heidelberg, Germany, 2009; Volume 65, pp. 73–84.
19. Pociask, E.; Nurzynska, K.; Obuchowicz, R.; Bałon, P.; Uryga, D.; Strzelecki, M.; Izworski, A.; Piórkowski, A. Differential Diagnosis of Cysts and Granulomas Supported by Texture Analysis of Intraoral Radiographs. *Sensors* **2021**, *21*, 7481. [CrossRef]
20. Shapiro, S.S.; Wilk, M.B. An Analysis of Variance Test for Normality (Complete Samples). *Biometrika* **1965**, *52*, 591–611. [CrossRef]
21. Haralick, R.M.; Shanmugam, K.; Dinstein, I. Textural Features for Image Classification. *IEEE Trans. Syst. Man Cybern.* **1973**, *SMC-3*, 610–621. [CrossRef]
22. Zhang, H.; Li, Q.; Liu, J.; Shang, J.; Du, X.; McNairn, H.; Champagne, C.; Dong, T.; Liu, M. Image Classification Using RapidEye Data: Integration of Spectral and Textual Features in a Random Forest Classifier. *IEEE J. Sel. Top. Appl. Earth Obs. Remote Sens.* **2017**, *10*, 5334–5349. [CrossRef]
23. Yang, X.; Tridandapani, S.; Beitler, J.J.; Yu, D.S.; Yoshida, E.J.; Curran, W.J.; Liu, T. Ultrasound GLCM Texture Analysis of Radiation-Induced Parotid-Gland Injury in Head-and-Neck Cancer Radiotherapy: An in Vivo Study of Late Toxicity: Ultrasound Assessment of Post-RT Parotid Gland. *Med. Phys.* **2012**, *39*, 5732–5739. [CrossRef] [PubMed]
24. Julesz, B. Experiments in the Visual Perception of Texture. *Sci. Am.* **1975**, *232*, 34–43. [CrossRef]
25. Priolo, F.; Cerase, A. The Current Role of Radiography in the Assessment of Skeletal Tumors and Tumor-like Lesions. *Eur. J. Radiol.* **1998**, *27*, S77–S85. [CrossRef]
26. Fritscher, K.; Grunerbl, A.; Hanni, M.; Suhm, N.; Hengg, C.; Schubert, R. Trabecular Bone Analysis in CT and X-ray Images of the Proximal Femur for the Assessment of Local Bone Quality. *IEEE Trans. Med. Imaging* **2009**, *28*, 1560–1575. [CrossRef] [PubMed]
27. Akkus, O.; Polyakova-Akkus, A.; Adar, F.; Schaffler, M.B. Aging of Microstructural Compartments in Human Compact Bone. *J. Bone Miner. Res.* **2003**, *18*, 1012–1019. [CrossRef]
28. Ammann, P.; Rizzoli, R. Bone Strength and Its Determinants. *Osteoporos. Int.* **2003**, *14*, 13–18. [CrossRef] [PubMed]
29. Bailey, A.J.; Sims, T.J.; Ebbesen, E.N.; Mansell, J.P.; Thomsen, J.S.; Mosekilde, L. Age-Related Changes in the Biochemical Properties of Human Cancellous Bone Collagen: Relationship to Bone Strength. *Calcif. Tissue Int.* **1999**, *65*, 203–210. [CrossRef] [PubMed]
30. Karlamangla, A.S.; Burnett-Bowie, S.-A.M.; Crandall, C.J. Bone Health During the Menopause Transition and Beyond. *Obstet. Gynecol. Clin. N. Am.* **2018**, *45*, 695–708. [CrossRef] [PubMed]
31. Cao, J.J.; Wronski, T.J.; Iwaniec, U.; Phleger, L.; Kurimoto, P.; Boudignon, B.; Halloran, B.P. Aging Increases Stromal/Osteoblastic Cell-Induced Osteoclastogenesis and Alters the Osteoclast Precursor Pool in the Mouse. *J. Bone Miner. Res.* **2005**, *20*, 1659–1668. [CrossRef]
32. Chan, G.K.; Duque, G. Age-Related Bone Loss: Old Bone, New Facts. *Gerontology* **2002**, *48*, 62–71. [CrossRef]
33. Hart, N.H.; Nimphius, S.; Rantalainen, T.; Ireland, A.; Siafarikas, A.; Newton, R.U. Mechanical Basis of Bone Strength: Influence of Bone Material, Bone Structure and Muscle Action. *J. Musculoskelet. Neuronal Interact.* **2017**, *17*, 114–139. [PubMed]
34. Kersh, M.E.; Pandy, M.G.; Bui, Q.M.; Jones, A.C.; Arns, C.H.; Knackstedt, M.A.; Seeman, E.; Zebaze, R.M. The Heterogeneity in Femoral Neck Structure and Strength. *J. Bone Miner. Res. Off. J. Am. Soc. Bone Miner. Res.* **2013**, *28*, 1022–1028. [CrossRef] [PubMed]
35. Riis, B.J.; Hansen, M.A.; Jensen, A.M.; Overgaard, K.; Christiansen, C. Low Bone Mass and Fast Rate of Bone Loss at Menopause: Equal Risk Factors for Future Fracture: A 15-Year Follow-up Study. *Bone* **1996**, *19*, 9–12. [CrossRef] [PubMed]
36. Soldati, E.; Roseren, F.; Guenoun, D.; Mancini, L.; Catelli, E.; Prati, S.; Sciutto, G.; Vicente, J.; Iotti, S.; Bendahan, D.; et al. Multiscale Femoral Neck Imaging and Multimodal Trabeculae Quality Characterization in an Osteoporotic Bone Sample. *Materials* **2022**, *15*, 8048. [CrossRef] [PubMed]
37. Carpenter, R.D.; Sigurdsson, S.; Zhao, S.; Lu, Y.; Eiriksdottir, G.; Sigurdsson, G.; Jonsson, B.Y.; Prevrhal, S.; Harris, T.B.; Siggeirsdottir, K.; et al. Effects of Age and Sex on the Strength and Cortical Thickness of the Femoral Neck. *Bone* **2011**, *48*, 741–747. [CrossRef]
38. Pajamäki, I.; Sievänen, H.; Kannus, P.; Jokihaara, J.; Vuohelainen, T.; Järvinen, T.L.N. Skeletal Effects of Estrogen and Mechanical Loading Are Structurally Distinct. *Bone* **2008**, *43*, 748–757. [CrossRef]
39. Jeong, H.; Kim, J.; Ishida, T.; Akiyama, M.; Kim, Y. Computerised Analysis of Osteoporotic Bone Patterns Using Texture Parameters Characterising Bone Architecture. *Br. J. Radiol.* **2013**, *86*, 20101115. [CrossRef]
40. Kjaer, L.; Ring, P.; Thomsen, C.; Henriksen, O. Texture Analysis in Quantitative MR Imaging. Tissue Characterisation of Normal Brain and Intracranial Tumours at 1.5 T. *Acta Radiol.* **1995**, *36*, 127–135. [CrossRef]
41. Kovalev, V.; Kruggel, F. Texture Anisotropy of the Brain's White Matter as Revealed by Anatomical MRI. *IEEE Trans. Med. Imaging* **2007**, *26*, 678–685. [CrossRef]
42. Mahmoud-Ghoneim, D.; Alkaabi, M.K.; de Certaines, J.D.; Goettsche, F.-M. The Impact of Image Dynamic Range on Texture Classification of Brain White Matter. *BMC Med. Imaging* **2008**, *8*, 18. [CrossRef]

43. Holli, K.; Lääperi, A.-L.; Harrison, L.; Luukkaala, T.; Toivonen, T.; Ryymin, P.; Dastidar, P.; Soimakallio, S.; Eskola, H. Characterization of Breast Cancer Types by Texture Analysis of Magnetic Resonance Images. *Acad. Radiol.* **2010**, *17*, 135–141. [CrossRef] [PubMed]
44. Herlidou, S.; Rolland, Y.; Bansard, J.Y.; Le Rumeur, E.; de Certaines, J.D. Comparison of Automated and Visual Texture Analysis in MRI: Characterization of Normal and Diseased Skeletal Muscle. *Magn. Reson. Imaging* **1999**, *17*, 1393–1397. [CrossRef] [PubMed]
45. Hirvasniemi, J.; Gielis, W.P.; Arbabi, S.; Agricola, R.; van Spil, W.E.; Arbabi, V.; Weinans, H. Bone Texture Analysis for Prediction of Incident Radiographic Hip Osteoarthritis Using Machine Learning: Data from the Cohort Hip and Cohort Knee (CHECK) Study. *Osteoarthr. Cartil.* **2019**, *27*, 906–914. [CrossRef] [PubMed]
46. Mazur, P. The Influence of Bit-Depth Reduction on Correlation of Texture Features with a Patient's Age. In *Progress in Image Processing, Pattern Recognition and Communication Systems*; Choraś, M., Choraś, R.S., Kurzyński, M., Trajdos, P., Pejaś, J., Hyla, T., Eds.; Lecture Notes in Networks and Systems; Springer International Publishing: Cham, Switzerland, 2022; Volume 255, pp. 191–198. ISBN 978-3-030-81522-6.
47. Mazur, P.; Obuchowicz, R.; Piórkowski, A. The Influence of Age on Morphometric and Textural Vertebrae Features in Lateral Cervical Spine Radiographs. In *Information Technology in Biomedicine*; Pietka, E., Badura, P., Kawa, J., Wieclawek, W., Eds.; Advances in Intelligent Systems and Computing; Springer International Publishing: Cham, Switzerland, 2021; Volume 1186, pp. 71–80. ISBN 978-3-030-49665-4.
48. Maciel, J.G.; de Araújo, I.M.; Trazzi, L.C.; de Azevedo-Marques, P.M.; Salmon, C.E.G.; Paula, F.J.A.d.; Nogueira-Barbosa, M.H. Association of Bone Mineral Density with Bone Texture Attributes Extracted Using Routine Magnetic Resonance Imaging. *Clinics* **2020**, *75*, e1766. [CrossRef]
49. Shirvaikar, M.; Huang, N.; Dong, X.N. The Measurement of Bone Quality Using Gray Level Co-Occurrence Matrix Textural Features. *J. Med. Imaging Health Inform.* **2016**, *6*, 1357–1362. [CrossRef] [PubMed]
50. Paalvast, O.; Nauta, M.; Koelle, M.; Geerdink, J.; Vijlbrief, O.; Hegeman, J.H.; Seifert, C. Radiology Report Generation for Proximal Femur Fractures Using Deep Classification and Language Generation Models. *Artif. Intell. Med.* **2022**, *128*, 102281. [CrossRef]
51. Meena, T.; Roy, S. Bone Fracture Detection Using Deep Supervised Learning from Radiological Images: A Paradigm Shift. *Diagnostics* **2022**, *12*, 2420. [CrossRef]
52. Urakawa, T.; Tanaka, Y.; Goto, S.; Matsuzawa, H.; Watanabe, K.; Endo, N. Detecting Intertrochanteric Hip Fractures with Orthopedist-Level Accuracy Using a Deep Convolutional Neural Network. *Skelet. Radiol.* **2019**, *48*, 239–244. [CrossRef] [PubMed]
53. Wang, X.; Xu, Z.; Tong, Y.; Xia, L.; Jie, B.; Ding, P.; Bai, H.; Zhang, Y.; He, Y. Detection and Classification of Mandibular Fracture on CT Scan Using Deep Convolutional Neural Network. *Clin. Oral Investig.* **2022**, *26*, 4593–4601. [CrossRef] [PubMed]
54. Secgin, Y.; Oner, Z.; Turan, M.; Oner, S. Gender Prediction with the Parameters Obtained from Pelvis Computed Tomography Images and Machine Learning Algorithms. *J. Anat. Soc. India* **2022**, *71*, 204. [CrossRef]
55. Zhou, J.; Li, Z.; Zhi, W.; Liang, B.; Moses, D.; Dawes, L. Using Convolutional Neural Networks and Transfer Learning for Bone Age Classification. In Proceedings of the 2017 International Conference on Digital Image Computing: Techniques and Applications (DICTA), Sydney, Australia, 29 November–1 December 2017; pp. 1–6.
56. Cernazanu-Glavan, C.; Holban, S. Segmentation of Bone Structure in X-ray Images Using Convolutional Neural Network. *Adv. Electr. Comput. Eng.* **2013**, *13*, 87–94. [CrossRef]
57. Liu, X.; Han, C.; Wang, H.; Wu, J.; Cui, Y.; Zhang, X.; Wang, X. Fully Automated Pelvic Bone Segmentation in Multiparametric MRI Using a 3D Convolutional Neural Network. *Insights Imaging* **2021**, *12*, 93. [CrossRef]
58. Eweje, F.R.; Bao, B.; Wu, J.; Dalal, D.; Liao, W.; He, Y.; Luo, Y.; Lu, S.; Zhang, P.; Peng, X.; et al. Deep Learning for Classification of Bone Lesions on Routine MRI. *eBioMedicine* **2021**, *68*, 103402. [CrossRef] [PubMed]
59. He, Y.; Pan, I.; Bao, B.; Halsey, K.; Chang, M.; Liu, H.; Peng, S.; Sebro, R.A.; Guan, J.; Yi, T.; et al. Deep Learning-Based Classification of Primary Bone Tumors on Radiographs: A Preliminary Study. *eBioMedicine* **2020**, *62*, 103121. [CrossRef]
60. Kozakiewicz, M. Measures of Corticalization. *J. Clin. Med.* **2022**, *11*, 5463. [CrossRef]
61. Obuchowicz, R.; Nurzynska, K.; Pierzchala, M.; Piorkowski, A.; Strzelecki, M. Texture Analysis for the Bone Age Assessment from MRI Images of Adolescent Wrists in Boys. *J. Clin. Med.* **2023**, *12*, 2762. [CrossRef]
62. Dieckmeyer, M.; Sollmann, N.; El Husseini, M.; Sekuboyina, A.; Löffler, M.T.; Zimmer, C.; Kirschke, J.S.; Subburaj, K.; Baum, T. Gender-, Age- and Region-Specific Characterization of Vertebral Bone Microstructure Through Automated Segmenta-tion and 3D Texture Analysis of Routine Abdominal CT. *Front. Endocrinol.* **2022**, *12*, 792760. [CrossRef]
63. Lespessailles, E.; Gadois, C.; Kousignian, I.; Neveu, J.P.; Fardellone, P.; Kolta, S.; Roux, C.; Do-Huu, J.P.; Benhamou, C.L. Clinical interest of bone texture analysis in osteoporosis: A case control multicenter study. *Osteoporos. Int.* **2008**, *19*, 1019–1028. [CrossRef]
64. Zheng, K.; Makrogiannis, S. Bone texture characterization for osteoporosis diagnosis using digital radiography. In Proceedings of the 38th Annual International Conference of the IEEE Engineering in Medicine and Biology Society (EMBC), Orlando, FL, USA, 16–20 August 2016; pp. 1034–1037. [CrossRef]
65. Khojastepour, L.; Hasani, M.; Ghasemi, M.; Mehdizadeh, A.R.; Tajeripour, F. Mandibular Trabecular Bone Analysis Using Local Binary Pattern for Osteoporosis Diagnosis. *J. Biomed. Phys. Eng.* **2019**, *9*, 81–88. [CrossRef] [PubMed]
66. Kawashima, Y.; Fujita, A.; Buch, K.; Li, B.; Qureshi, M.M.; Chapman, M.N.; Sakai, O. Using texture analysis of head CT images to differentiate osteoporosis from normal bone density. *Eur. J. Radiol.* **2019**, *116*, 212–218. [CrossRef]

67. Khider, M.; Taleb-Ahmed, A.; Dubois, P.; Haddad, B. Classification of trabecular bone texture from MRI and CT scan images by multi resolution analysis. In Proceedings of the 29th Annual International Conference of the IEEE Engineering in Medicine and Biology Society, Lyon, France, 22–26 August 2007; pp. 5589–5592. [CrossRef]
68. Castellanos, N.P.; Martínez, E.; Gutierrez, J. Improving osteoporosis diagnosis in children using image texture analysis. In Proceedings of the 2011 Annual International Conference of the IEEE Engineering in Medicine and Biology Society, Boston, MA, USA, 30 August–3 September 2011. [CrossRef]

Disclaimer/Publisher's Note: The statements, opinions and data contained in all publications are solely those of the individual author(s) and contributor(s) and not of MDPI and/or the editor(s). MDPI and/or the editor(s) disclaim responsibility for any injury to people or property resulting from any ideas, methods, instructions or products referred to in the content.

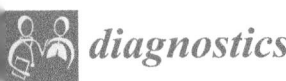

Article

Ultra-High-Resolution Photon-Counting Detector CT Arthrography of the Ankle: A Feasibility Study

Karsten Sebastian Luetkens [1,*], Jan-Peter Grunz [1], Andreas Steven Kunz [1], Henner Huflage [1], Manuel Weißenberger [2], Viktor Hartung [1], Theresa Sophie Patzer [1], Philipp Gruschwitz [1], Süleyman Ergün [3], Thorsten Alexander Bley [1] and Philipp Feldle [1]

1 Department of Diagnostic and Interventional Radiology, University Hospital Würzburg, Oberdürrbacher Straße 6, 97080 Würzburg, Germany
2 Department of Orthopaedic Surgery, University of Würzburg, König-Ludwig-Haus, Brettreichstr. 11, 97074 Würzburg, Germany
3 Institute of Anatomy and Cell Biology, University of Würzburg, Koellikerstraße 6, 97070 Würzburg, Germany
* Correspondence: luetkens_k@ukw.de

Abstract: This study was designed to investigate the image quality of ultra-high-resolution ankle arthrography employing a photon-counting detector CT. Bilateral arthrograms were acquired in four cadaveric specimens with full-dose (10 mGy) and low-dose (3 mGy) scan protocols. Three convolution kernels with different spatial frequencies were utilized for image reconstruction (ρ_{50}; Br98: 39.0, Br84: 22.6, Br76: 16.5 lp/cm). Seven radiologists subjectively assessed the image quality regarding the depiction of bone, hyaline cartilage, and ligaments. An additional quantitative assessment comprised the measurement of noise and the computation of contrast-to-noise ratios (CNR). While an optimal depiction of bone tissue was achieved with the ultra-sharp Br98 kernel ($S \leq 0.043$), the visualization of cartilage improved with lower modulation transfer functions at each dose level ($p \leq 0.014$). The interrater reliability ranged from good to excellent for all assessed tissues (intraclass correlation coefficient ≥ 0.805). The noise levels in subcutaneous fat decreased with reduced spatial frequency ($p < 0.001$). Notably, the low-dose Br76 matched the CNR of the full-dose Br84 ($p > 0.999$) and superseded Br98 ($p < 0.001$) in all tissues. Based on the reported results, a photon-counting detector CT arthrography of the ankle with an ultra-high-resolution collimation offers stellar image quality and tissue assessability, improving the evaluation of miniscule anatomical structures. While bone depiction was superior in combination with an ultra-sharp convolution kernel, soft tissue evaluation benefited from employing a lower spatial frequency.

Keywords: photon-counting CT; arthrography; ankle; cartilage; radiation dosage

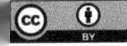

1. Introduction

The tibiotalar cartilage bears up to five times the body's weight [1], posing a risk factor for osteoarthritis, especially if these forces increase [2]. At the same time, traumatic osteochondral lesions and ligament injuries of the ankle, as well as resulting unphysiological load distributions, are frequent [3–5]; thus, assessing the stability of chondral lesions represents a crucial diagnostic imaging task, as chondral delamination and subchondral pathologies may not be visible in direct arthroscopy but can impact therapeutic concepts [6,7].

Magnetic resonance imaging (MRI) is widely recognized as the reference standard for cross-sectional imaging of soft tissue pathologies [8,9]; however, as the ankle's cartilage consists of only a thin hyaline chondral layer, averaging 1.1 mm (range 0.4–2.1 mm) [10–13], the depiction of discreet injuries continues to pose a challenge in MRI with reported sensitivities as low as 50% at 1.5 T and 75% at 3.0 T for osteochondral ankle injuries [12,14]. On the other hand, computed tomography (CT) arthrography represents a powerful, well-established, and preferable alternative for discerning osteochondral lesions, e.g., for the elbow [15]. Comparing CT to MR arthrography of the ankle joint at 1.0 and 1.5 T with regards to cartilage lesions,

Schmid et al. reported a superior level of observer agreement and reliability favoring the former [10]. Similarly, Pöhler et al. demonstrated an advantage for CT arthrography versus 3.0 T MR arthrography regarding the assessment of lesion depth in artificially induced osteochondral lesions of the talar dome while maintaining a comparable accuracy [16].

Recently, the emergence of photon-counting detector CT (PCD-CT) catalyzed further advances in depicting minute structures with unsurpassed radiation dose efficiency for CT thus far [17,18]. PCD architecture eliminates the need for a two-step conversion process of incoming X-ray photons as opposed to the current energy-integrating detector systems [19,20]. As the generated electric impulses are proportional to every photon's particular energy above a certain threshold, low-energy photons are no longer down-weighted, and contrast-to-noise ratios are significantly improved [21,22]. The current and first PCD-CT generation allows for an in-plane resolution of as little as 0.11 mm in ultra-high-resolution (UHR) mode without dose penalty, facilitating the visualization of microstructures in particular [23].

While numerous studies have analyzed the impact of PCD technology on bone imaging [24,25], to the authors' best knowledge, no thorough investigation was conducted regarding PCD-CT arthrography thus far. Aiming to address the current research gap, this study evaluates the feasibility of ankle arthrograms with the novel detector technology, establishing a clinically reproducible scan protocol in the process. We hypothesized that the PCD-CT arthrography with UHR collimation would aid the assessment of minuscule anatomical structures, such as thin cartilage layers and ligamentous stabilizers.

2. Materials and Methods

2.1. Cadaveric Specimens

The anatomical institute of the local university allocated four fresh-frozen, non-formalin-fixated cadaveric specimens to the radiology department for this investigation. During their respective lifetimes, the body donors had consented to posthumous use of their remains for study and research purposes. No additional selection criteria were imposed. The institutional review board of our university waived the need for further written informed consent and granted permission for this study.

2.2. Arthrography Procedure

A board-certified radiologist with nine years of experience in musculoskeletal imaging performed bilateral ankle arthrographies in all four cadaveric specimens. Using an ultrasound for guidance (Acuson Sequoia, Siemens Healthineers, Erlangen, Germany), each tibiotalar joint was infiltrated with a 20-gauge needle (Sterican®, Braun SE, Melsungen, Germany) on the medial side of the anterior tibial tendon in analogy to a clinical procedure. A combination of 50% iodinated contrast agent (Imeron 300®, Bracco S.p.A., Milan, Italy) and 10 mg per ml of a local anesthetic (Mecain®, Puren Pharma GmbH & Co. KG, Munich, Germany) was injected via the articular access. The injection volume was selected as high as feasible, ranging between 7 and 9 mL. Using fresh-frozen specimens instead of formalin-fixated cadavers allowed for realistic tissue properties and, subsequently, an overall procedure representative of ankle arthrograms in vivo. No particular challenges or limitations were encountered during the arthrography procedures.

2.3. Image Acquisition and Reconstruction Parameters

Directly following injection, the ankle joints were scanned using a first-generation cadmium-telluride-based PCD-CT system (Naeotom Alpha, Siemens Healthineers). All examinations were performed in UHR scan mode using a collimation of 120 × 0.2 mm. With tube potential set to 120 kVp, a full-dose and low-dose scan were acquired in each specimen with effective tube currents of 125 and 38 mAs. Resulting volume CT dose indices ($CTDI_{vol}$) amounted to 10.0 and 3.0 mGy. Detailed scan parameters are provided in Table 1. Ankles were individually scanned and reconstructed in three standardized orientations (axial, coronal, and sagittal) with an increment of 0.6 mm and a field of view of 100 mm. Matrix parameters were selected automatically to obtain optimal settings; thereby, the sharpest available non-UHR kernel (Br76), a medium-sharp UHR kernel (Br84), as well as the sharpest UHR kernel (Br98) were employed (Table 2). Preset window settings were 1400 and 300 HU (window width and center); however, observers were permitted to modify these according to personal preferences.

Table 1. Acquisition protocols. Scan parameters and resulting radiation dose of photon-counting CT arthrograms.

Scan Protocol	Full-Dose Protocol	Low-Dose Protocol
Tube voltage [kVp]	120	120
Tube current-time product [eff. mAs]	125	38
Detector collimation [mm]	120 × 0.2	120 × 0.2
Pitch factor	0.5	0.5
Rotation time [sec]	1.0	1.0
$CTDI_{vol}$ [mGy]	10	3

$CTDI_{vol}$: volume computed tomography dose index; eff. mAs: effective milliampere-seconds; kVp: kilovoltage peak; mGy: milligray; mm: millimeter; sec: second.

Table 2. Reconstruction parameters. Spatial frequencies of the employed convolution kernels at different values of the modulation transfer function. Reported data according to vendor information.

Spatial Frequency	At the 50% Value of the MTF (ρ_{50}) [Line Pairs/cm]	At the 10% Value of the MTF (ρ_{10}) [Line Pairs/cm]	At the Maximum of the MTF (ρ_{max}) [Line Pairs/cm]
Br98	39.0	42.9	20.4
Br84	22.6	27.9	10.5
Br76	16.5	21.0	7.8

Br98/84/76: vendor-specific kernel names; cm: centimeter; MTF: modulation transfer function; ρ: indicator of spatial frequency.

2.4. Subjective Image Evaluation

Seven radiologists with four to nine years of experience in musculoskeletal imaging evaluated all datasets independently using certified diagnostic monitors (RadiForce RX660, EIZO, Hakusan, Japan) in combination with standard clinical PACS software (Merlin 7.0.226222, Phönix-PACS, Freiburg, Germany). Readers were blinded to all protocol-related information. After determining whether images were suitable for diagnostic use in dichotomous fashion, observers were separately tasked with grading the image quality for bone, cartilage, and ligaments, employing a seven-point rating scale (1 = very poor; 2 = poor; 3 = fair; 4 = satisfactory; 5 = good; 6 = very good; 7 = excellent).

2.5. Objective Image Evaluation

Normed regions of interest were placed in the talus, talar cartilage, posterior tibiotalar ligament, and subcutaneous fat, noting mean density and standard deviation thereof. Due to its homogeneous texture, the standard deviation within subcutaneous fat was defined as image noise. Individual contrast-to-noise ratios were calculated for osseous tissue (CNR_{Bone}), cartilage ($CNR_{Cartilage}$), and ligaments ($CNR_{Ligament}$) with the following formula:

$$CNR = \frac{mean\ attenuation\ (bone/cartilage/ligament) - mean\ attenuation\ (fat)}{standard\ deviation\ (fat)}$$

2.6. Statistical Analysis

All statistical analyses were performed with dedicated software (SPSS Statistics Version 28, IBM, Armonk, NY, USA). For evaluating normal distribution in continuous variables, Kolmogorov–Smirnov tests were conducted. Categorical variables were reported as absolute and relative frequencies, with median values and 10–90 percentile ranges, while normally distributed metric data were presented as means ± standard deviations. Mean rank distribution in paired non-parametric variables was assessed comparatively using

Friedman tests and Bonferroni-corrected pairwise post-hoc analyses. Null hypotheses were rejected, and statistical significance was assumed if computed p-values were not greater than 0.05. Interrater agreement was tested using the intraclass correlation coefficient (ICC) for absolute agreement in a two-way random effects model. Following Koo and Li [26], ICC scores were interpreted as being associated with poor (<0.50), moderate (0.50–0.75), good (0.75–0.90), or excellent (>0.90) reliability.

3. Results

3.1. Subjective Image Quality Assessment

All datasets were deemed suitable for diagnostic assessment in a clinical routine by each of the observers. Table 3 summarizes the pooled image quality scores assigned for bone, cartilage, and ligaments. The optimal depiction of bone tissue was achieved in full-dose scans with the ultra-sharp Br98 reconstruction kernel (median value 7, range 6–7). All full-dose datasets were rated superior to the respective low-dose scans ($p < 0.001$). Figure 1 includes a side-by-side comparison of the six employed acquisition–reconstruction combinations, while highlighting hyaline cartilage lesions of various degrees. In contrast to osseous tissue, the assessment of cartilage benefited from applying reconstruction kernels with a lower spatial frequency within each dose level ($p \leq 0.014$). No significant difference was ascertained between full-dose Br98 versus low-dose Br84 and Br76 reconstructions for hyaline cartilage ($p \geq 0.186$) and ligaments ($p \geq 0.283$). Figure 2 illustrates the depiction of an intact posterior tibiofibular ligament. A pairwise comparison matrix comprising all assessed combinations of scan protocol and reconstruction settings is displayed in Table 4. Interrater reliability for bone microarchitecture visualization was excellent, indicated with an ICC of 0.938 (95% confidence interval 0.902–0.962; $p < 0.001$), while observer agreement was good for judging cartilage (0.887; 0.779–0.940; $p < 0.001$) and ligaments (0.805; 0.661–0.889; $p < 0.001$). Figure 3 exemplifies a full thickness defect located at the medial talar shoulder and a partial thickness lesion on the lateral side.

Table 3. Subjective image quality assessment. Pooled diagnostic assessability scores drawn from the subjective ratings of seven independent radiologists. Results are given as median values with 10–90 percentile ranges in parentheses.

| Scan Protocol | Full-Dose Protocol | | | Low-Dose Protocol | | | ICC |
Convolution Kernel	Br98	Br84	Br76	Br98	Br84	Br76	
Bone	7 (6–7)	6 (5–7)	5 (5–6)	4 (3–5)	5 (4–6)	5 (4–6)	0.938
Cartilage	6 (4–6.5)	6 (5–7)	7 (6–7)	4 (3–5)	5 (4–6)	5 (5–6)	0.887
Ligaments	6 (4.5–7)	6 (5–7)	6 (5–7)	4 (3–5)	5 (4–6)	5 (4–7)	0.805
Percentage of diagnostic examinations	100%	100%	100%	100%	100%	100%	

Br98/84/76: vendor-specific kernel names; ICC: intraclass correlation coefficient.

Table 4. Comparison matrix for subjective image analysis. Mean image quality ranks of protocol–kernel combinations were compared individually for bone/cartilage/ligaments in pairwise analyses.

| Bone/Cartilage/Ligaments | | Full-Dose | | | Low-Dose | | |
		Br98	Br84	Br76	Br98	Br84	Br76
Full-dose	Br98		+/−/=	+/−/=	+/+/+	+/=/=	+/=/=
	Br84	−/+/=		+/=/=	+/+/+	+/+/+	+/+/+
	Br76	−/+/=	−/=/=		+/+/+	+/+/+	+/+/+
Low-dose	Br98	−/−/−	−/−/−	−/−/−		−/−/−	−/−/−
	Br84	−/=/=	−/−/−	−/−/−	+/+/+		=/=/=
	Br76	−/=/=	−/−/−	−/−/−	+/+/+	=/=/=	

The Bonferroni procedure was performed to correct p values for multiple comparisons. "+": superior assessability; "−": inferior assessability; "=": no statistically significant difference; Br98/84/76: vendor-specific kernel names.

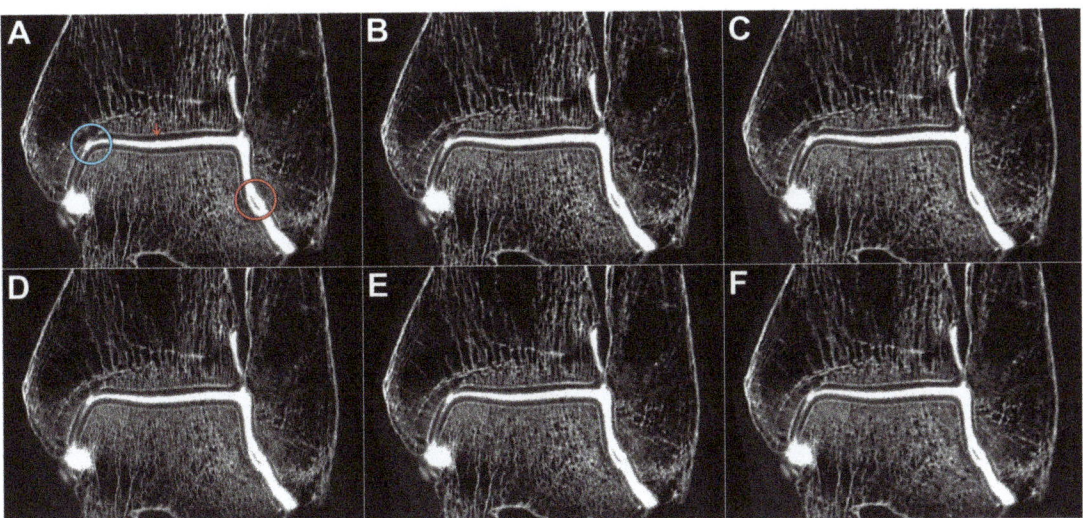

Figure 1. Photon-counting arthrographies in a cadaveric specimen performed with the full-dose (10 mGy; **A–C**) and low-dose scan protocol (3 mGy; **D–F**). Reconstructions were performed with the ultra-sharp kernel Br98 (**A/D**), medium UHR kernel Br84 (**B/E**), and non-UHR kernel Br76 (**C/F**). Please note the full thickness cartilage defect at the lateral aspect of the talus (**red circle**) versus the pseudodefect of the tibial plafond known as the "Notch of Harty" (**blue circle**). A superficial cartilage lesion of the central tibia is better visualized using means of full-dose arthrography (**red arrow**).

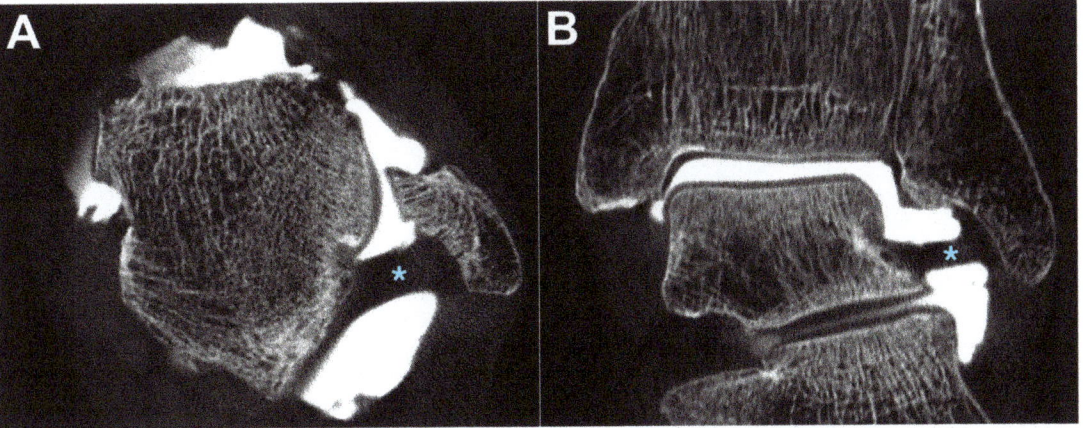

Figure 2. Depiction of an intact posterior tibiofibular ligament (**blue asterisk**) in axial (**A**) and coronal orientation (**B**). Photon-counting CT arthrography was performed with a $CTDI_{vol}$ of 10 mGy. The acquired dataset was reconstructed with the ultra-sharp Br98 kernel, which possesses the highest spatial frequency of all convolution kernels available for ultra-high-resolution imaging on a photon-counting detector.

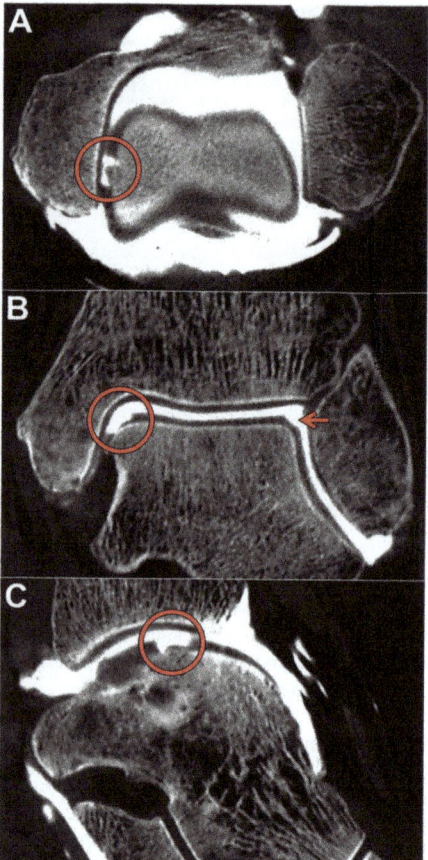

Figure 3. Tri-planar reformatting of a full-dose photon-counting CT arthrogram in axial (**A**), coronal (**B**), and sagittal orientation (**C**) using the medium BR84 kernel displays an osteochondral lesion of the medial talus shoulder (**red circle**). Additionally, a partial thickness cartilage injury of the lateral talus shoulder can be diagnosed (**red arrow**).

3.2. Objective Image Quality Assessment

Noise levels in subcutaneous fat decreased with reduced modulation transfer function ($p < 0.001$). With regards to CNR, the non-UHR Br76 kernel superseded both assessed UHR kernels based on measurements in bone, cartilage, and ligaments ($p < 0.007$). No dose-dependent difference was ascertained for any of the tissues with Br98 ($p > 0.999$); moreover, low-dose Br76 matched the quantitative metrics of full-dose Br84 ($p > 0.999$) and even superseded Br98 ($p < 0.001$) in all cases. Detailed signal and noise characteristics are provided in Table 5, while a pairwise comparison matrix thereof is exhibited in Table 6.

Table 5. Quantitative image quality assessment. Signal and noise characteristics are reported as mean ± standard deviations.

Scan Protocol	Full-Dose Protocol			Low-Dose Protocol		
Convolution Kernel	Br98	Br84	Br76	Br98	Br84	Br76
Noise$_{Fat}$ [HU]	149.5 ± 23.4	54.6 ± 10.6	38.9 ± 9.3	240.6 ± 56.2	78.4 ± 10.3	52.2 ± 7.5
CNR$_{Bone}$	3.8 ± 0.9	9.8 ± 3.0	13.5 ± 4.3	3.0 ± 3.8	6.8 ± 1.6	10.2 ± 2.6
CNR$_{Cartilage}$	3.0 ± 0.9	7.4 ± 3.5	10.2 ± 4.5	2.9 ± 4.7	5.5 ± 2.2	7.8 ± 2.3
CNR$_{Ligaments}$	1.4 ± 3.3	3.2 ± 2.4	4.3 ± 3.4	1.2 ± 1.0	2.2 ± 1.6	2.9 ± 2.2

Br98/84/76: vendor-specific kernel names; CNR: contrast-to-noise ratio; HU: Hounsfield units.

Table 6. Comparison matrix for quantitative image analysis. Contrast-to-noise ratios (CNR) were calculated based on attenuation and noise measurements in the talus, talar cartilage, posterior tibiotalar ligament, and adjacent subcutaneous fat. Mean CNR ranks of protocol–kernel combinations were compared individually for bone/cartilage/ligaments in pairwise analyses.

CNR$_{Bone}$/CNR$_{Cartilage}$/CNR$_{Ligaments}$		Full-Dose			Low-Dose		
		Br98	Br84	Br76	Br98	Br84	Br76
Full-dose	Br98		−/−/−	−/−/−	=/=/=	−/−/−	−/−/−
	Br84	+/+/+		−/−/−	+/+/=	+/+/+	=/=/=
	Br76	+/+/+	+/+/+		+/+/+	+/+/+	+/+/+
Low-dose	Br98	=/=/=	−/−/=	−/−/−		−/=/=	−/−/=
	Br84	+/+/+	−/−/−	−/−/−	+/=/=		−/−/=
	Br76	+/+/+	=/=/=	−/−/−	+/+/=	+/+/=	

The Bonferroni procedure was performed to correct p values for multiple comparisons. "+": higher contrast-to-noise ratio; "−": lower contrast-to-noise ratio; "=": no statistically significant difference; Br98/84/76: vendor-specific kernel names; CNR: contrast-to-noise ratio.

4. Discussion

This experimental multi-observer study investigated the feasibility and image quality of a photon-counting detector CT arthrography of the ankle joint with an ultra-high-resolution detector collimation. Employing two different dose levels and three convolution kernels with varying modulation transfer functions, the depictions of bone, cartilage, and ligaments were separately assessed. Our results indicate that bone depiction is superior in combination with an ultra-sharp reconstruction technique, whereas soft tissue evaluation benefits from employing lower spatial frequencies. As to be expected, higher noise levels and lower CNR were determined in dedicated low-dose studies; however, all assessed datasets were found to be of diagnostic quality.

The presented findings are in line with recent publications regarding the depiction of osseous tissue with photon-counting technology in clinical applications [17,27]. As reported previously, the incorporated low-energy threshold reduces electronic background noise, which would otherwise increase significantly in low-dose applications [28]; thereby, one of the major disadvantages of a CT arthrography compared to an MRI, i.e., radiation dose, can be minimized. As the diagnostic value of CT arthrography is generally considered to be at least equivalent to an MRI after articular contrast injection [29,30], small joint imaging focused on thin layers of hyaline cartilage in particular continues to pose a major challenge to MRI arthrograms [31]. While MRI remains the modality of choice in bone marrow imaging [32,33], CT does provide advantages in assessing the subchondral bone, which facilitates diagnostic evaluation in patients suffering from osteoarthritis. Accordingly, the only previous study investigating PCD-CT arthrography reported reliable morphological assessability of cartilage loss in a porcine knee model [34].

With regards to acquisition time, an MRI also cannot compete with CT-based approaches, plausibly posing an obstacle in pain-ridden patients. As opposed to MR arthrography, the option to perform an ultrasound-guided injection of the contrast media directly within the CT suite further minimizes the overall examination time. Although a significant amount of contrast agent in the articular cavity can still be detected for up to 120 min, following the administration thereof, an acceleration of the overall procedure optimizes contrast conditions [35].

Representing a noteworthy alternative to PCD-CT arthrography of peripheral joints, with regards to achievable spatial resolution, cone-beam CT arthrography gained increasing recognition in recent years. An experimental study evaluating arthrograms of the wrist suggested superiority of a cone-beam CT approach over a conventional energy-integrating detector CT arthrography [36]. While the present investigation does not contain a direct comparison of PCD-CT and cone-beam CT arthrography, the reported dose levels for maintaining diagnostic image quality in both studies were somewhat equivalent. These findings suggest similar dose efficiencies among both techniques, mandating further investigations in patients.

The following limitations of this study ought to be considered. First, the study cohort comprised only four cadaveric specimens; however, subjective ratings were performed by seven radiologists, aiming to alleviate this restriction to some extent. Second, to offset typical drawbacks of formalin-fixated body donor studies, e.g., the deterioration of bone quality and altered soft tissue conditions, solely fresh-frozen cadavers were included. Third, due to the experimental study design, PCD-CT arthrography findings did not incur therapeutic consequences; consequently, no comparison of diagnostic performance with other imaging modalities could be drawn. Fourth, the influence of possible motion artifacts and off-center positioning on the image quality were not assessed, warranting further evaluation in a clinical patient population. Lastly, since CNR differs with radiation exposure level, the optimal kernel choice may differ for other clinical applications.

5. Conclusions

Photon-counting detector CT arthrography of the ankle with ultra-high-resolution collimation offers stellar image quality and tissue assessability. While bone depiction was found to be superior in combination with an ultra-sharp convolution kernel, the soft tissue evaluation benefited from employing reconstructions with a lower spatial frequency.

Author Contributions: Conceptualization, K.S.L. and J.-P.G.; data curation, K.S.L., V.H., T.S.P., T.A.B. and P.F.; formal analysis, K.S.L., J.-P.G., A.S.K., P.G. and P.F.; funding acquisition, J.-P.G.; investigation, K.S.L., A.S.K., H.H., M.W., V.H. and T.S.P.; methodology, K.S.L., J.-P.G., H.H., P.G., T.A.B. and P.F.; project administration, J.-P.G. and S.E.; resources, P.G., S.E. and T.A.B.; supervision, J.-P.G., A.S.K., T.A.B. and P.F.; validation, M.W., S.E. and P.F.; visualization, K.S.L. and H.H.; writing—original draft, K.S.L.; writing—review and editing, J.-P.G., A.S.K., H.H., M.W., V.H., T.S.P., P.G., S.E., T.A.B. and P.F. All authors have read and agreed to the published version of the manuscript.

Funding: The Department of Diagnostic and Interventional Radiology receives funding from the German Research Foundation (DFG) for photon-counting CT studies. JPG [Z-3BC/02] and PG [Z-02CSP/18] were individually funded by the Interdisciplinary Center of Clinical Research Würzburg, Germany. Furthermore, this publication was supported by the Open Access Publication Fund of the University of Würzburg.

Institutional Review Board Statement: For this retrospective study, permission was obtained from the Institutional Review Board of the University of Würzburg, Germany (IRB number 20201117 04). All procedures were in accordance with the ethical standards of the institutional and national research committee and with the 1975 Declaration of Helsinki.

Informed Consent Statement: For this retrospective study, permission was obtained from the Institutional Review Board of the University of Würzburg, Germany.

Data Availability Statement: The datasets generated and/or analyzed during this study are not publicly available as CT data and DICOM headers contain patient information. Data can be obtained upon reasonable request from the corresponding author.

Conflicts of Interest: JPG, ASK, and TAB serve as research consultants for Siemens Healthineers, receiving speaker honoraria in the process. The authors of this manuscript declare no further conflicts or relationships with any companies, whose products or services may be related to the subject matter of the article.

Abbreviations

CNR	contrast-to-noise ratio
$CTDI_{vol}$	volume computed tomography dose index
PCD	photon-counting detector
UHR	ultra-high-resolution

References

1. Rodgers, M.M. Dynamic foot biomechanics. *J. Orthop. Sports Phys. Ther.* **1995**, *21*, 306–316. [CrossRef]
2. Egloff, C.; Hügle, T.; Valderrabano, V. Biomechanics and pathomechanisms of osteoarthritis. *Swiss. Med. Wkly.* **2012**, *142*, w13583. [CrossRef]
3. Huch, K.; Kuettner, K.E.; Dieppe, P. Osteoarthritis in ankle and knee joints. *Semin. Arthritis Rheum.* **1997**, *26*, 667–674. [CrossRef] [PubMed]
4. Johnson, V.L.; Giuffre, B.M.; Hunter, D.J. Osteoarthritis: What Does Imaging Tell Us about Its Etiology? *Semin. Musculoskelet Radiol.* **2012**, *16*, 410–418. [CrossRef]
5. Van Buecken, K.; Barrack, R.L.; Alexander, A.H.; Ertl, J.P. Arthroscopic treatment of transchondral talar dome frac-tures. *Am. J. Sports Med.* **1989**, *17*, 350–355, discussion 355–356. [CrossRef]
6. Grambart, S.T. Arthroscopic Management of Osteochondral Lesions of the Talus. *Clin. Podiatr. Med. Surg.* **2016**, *33*, 521–530. [CrossRef]
7. O'Loughlin, P.F.; Heyworth, B.E.; Kennedy, J.G. Current concepts in the diagnosis and treatment of osteochondral lesions of the ankle. *Am. J. Sports Med.* **2010**, *38*, 392–404. [CrossRef] [PubMed]
8. Verhagen, R.A.W.; Maas, M.; Dijkgraaf, M.G.W.; Tol, J.L.; Krips, R.; van Dijk, C.N. Prospective study on diagnostic strat-egies in osteochondral lesions of the talus. Is MRI superior to helical CT? *J. Bone Jt. Surg. Br.* **2005**, *87*, 41–46. [CrossRef]
9. Naran, K.N.; Zoga, A.C. Osteochondral lesions about the ankle. *Radiol. Clin. N. Am.* **2008**, *46*, 995–1002. [CrossRef] [PubMed]
10. Schmid, M.R.; Pfirrmann, C.; Hodler, J.; Vienne, P.; Zanetti, M. Cartilage lesions in the ankle joint: Comparison of MR arthrography and CT arthrography. *Skelet. Radiol.* **2003**, *32*, 259–265. [CrossRef]
11. Ba-Ssalamah, A.; Schibany, N.; Puig, S.; Herneth, A.M.; Noebauer-Huhmann, I.M.; Trattnig, S. Imaging articular carti-lage defects in the ankle joint with 3D fat-suppressed echo planar imaging: Comparison with conventional 3D fat-suppressed gradient echo imaging. *J. Magn. Reson. Imaging* **2002**, *16*, 209–216. [CrossRef] [PubMed]
12. Barr, C.; Bauer, J.S.; Malfair, D.; Ma, B.; Henning, T.D.; Steinbach, L.; Link, T.M. MR imaging of the ankle at 3 Tesla and 1.5 Tesla: Protocol optimization and application to cartilage, ligament and tendon pathology in cadaver specimens. *Eur. Radiol.* **2006**, *17*, 1518–1528. [CrossRef] [PubMed]
13. Shepherd, D.E.T.; Seedhom, B.B. Thickness of human articular cartilage in joints of the lower limb. *Ann. Rheum. Dis.* **1999**, *58*, 27–34. [CrossRef]
14. Do Cha, S.; Kim, H.S.; Chung, S.T.; Yoo, J.H.; Park, J.H.; Kim, J.H.; Hyung, J.W. Intra-articular lesions in chronic lateral ankle instability: Comparison of ar-throscopy with magnetic resonance imaging findings. *Clin. Orthop. Surg.* **2012**, *4*, 293–299. [CrossRef] [PubMed]
15. Waldt, S.; Bruegel, M.; Ganter, K.; Kuhn, V.; Link, T.M.; Rummeny, E.J.; Woertler, K. Comparison of multislice CT arthrography and MR arthrography for the detection of articular cartilage lesions of the elbow. *Eur. Radiol.* **2005**, *15*, 784–791. [CrossRef]
16. Pöhler, G.H.; Sonnow, L.; Ettinger, S.; Rahn, A.; Klimes, F.; Becher, C.; von Falck, C.; Wacker, F.K.; Plaass, C. High resolution flat-panel CT arthrography vs. MR arthrography of artificially created osteochondral defects in ex vivo upper ankle joints. *PLoS ONE* **2021**, *16*, e0255616. [CrossRef]
17. Bette, S.J.; Braun, F.M.; Haerting, M.; Decker, J.A.; Luitjens, J.H.; Scheurig-Muenkler, C.; Kroencke, T.J.; Schwarz, F. Visualization of bone details in a novel photon-counting dual-source CT scanner—Comparison with energy-integrating CT. *Eur. Radiol.* **2021**, *32*, 2930–2936. [CrossRef]
18. Pourmorteza, A.; Symons, R.; Henning, A.; Ulzheimer, S.; Bluemke, D.A. Dose Efficiency of Quarter-Millimeter Pho-ton-Counting Computed Tomography: First-in-Human Results. *Investig. Radiol.* **2018**, *53*, 365–372. [CrossRef]
19. Tortora, M.; Gemini, L.; D'Iglio, I.; Ugga, L.; Spadarella, G.; Cuocolo, R. Spectral Photon-Counting Computed Tomog-raphy: A Review on Technical Principles and Clinical Applications. *J. Imaging Sci. Technol.* **2022**, *8*, 4.
20. McCollough, C.H.; Boedeker, K.; Cody, D.; Duan, X.; Flohr, T.; Halliburton, S.S.; Hsieh, J.; Layman, R.R.; Pelc, N.J. Principles and applications of multienergy CT: Report of AAPM Task Group 291. *Med. Phys.* **2020**, *47*, 14157. [CrossRef]
21. Leng, S.; Bruesewitz, M.; Tao, S.; Rajendran, K.; Halaweish, A.F.; Campeau, N.G.; Fletcher, J.G.; McCollough, C.H. Photon-counting Detector CT: System Design and Clinical Applications of an Emerging Technology. *RadioGraphics* **2019**, *39*, 729–743. [CrossRef] [PubMed]

22. Flohr, T.; Petersilka, M.; Henning, A.; Ulzheimer, S.; Ferda, J.; Schmidt, B. Photon-counting CT review. *Phys. Med.* **2020**, *79*, 126–136. [CrossRef]
23. Klein, L.; Dorn, S.; Amato, C.; Heinze, S.; Uhrig, M.; Schlemmer, H.-P.; Kachelrieß, M.; Sawall, S. Effects of Detector Sampling on Noise Reduction in Clinical Photon-Counting Whole-Body Computed Tomography. *Investig. Radiol.* **2020**, *55*, 111–119. [CrossRef] [PubMed]
24. Baffour, F.I.; Rajendran, K.; Glazebrook, K.N.; Thorne, J.E.; Larson, N.B.; Leng, S.; McCollough, C.H.; Fletcher, J.G. Ultra-high-resolution imaging of the shoulder and pelvis using photon-counting-detector CT: A feasibility study in patients. *Eur. Radiol.* **2022**, *32*, 7079–7086. [CrossRef] [PubMed]
25. Grunz, J.-P.; Huflage, H.; Heidenreich, J.F.; Ergün, S.; Petersilka, M.; Allmendinger, T.; Bley, T.A.; Petritsch, B. Image Quality Assessment for Clinical Cadmium Telluride-Based Photon-Counting Computed Tomography Detector in Cadaveric Wrist Imaging. *Investig. Radiol.* **2021**, *56*, 785–790. [CrossRef]
26. Koo, T.K.; Li, M.Y. A Guideline of Selecting and Reporting Intraclass Correlation Coefficients for Reliability Re-search. *J. Chiropr. Med.* **2016**, *15*, 155–163. [CrossRef]
27. Benson, J.; Rajendran, K.; Lane, J.; Diehn, F.; Weber, N.; Thorne, J.; Larson, N.; Fletcher, J.; McCollough, C.; Leng, S. A New Frontier in Temporal Bone Imaging: Photon-Counting Detector CT Demonstrates Superior Visualization of Critical Anatomic Structures at Reduced Radiation Dose. *Am. J. Neuroradiol.* **2022**, *43*, 579–584. [CrossRef] [PubMed]
28. Baffour, F.I.; Glazebrook, K.N.; Ferrero, A.; Leng, S.; McCollough, C.H.; Fletcher, J.G.; Rajendran, K. Photon-Counting Detector CT for Musculoskeletal Imaging: A Clinical Perspective. *Am. J. Roentgenol.* **2023**, *220*, 551–560. [CrossRef]
29. Theumann, N.; Favarger, N.; Schnyder, P.; Meuli, R. Wrist ligament injuries: Value of post-arthrography computed tomography. *Skelet. Radiol.* **2001**, *30*, 88–93. [CrossRef]
30. Schmid, M.R.; Schertler, T.; Pfirrmann, C.; Saupe, N.; Manestar, M.; Wildermuth, S.; Weishaupt, D. Interosseous ligament tears of the wrist: Comparison of multi–detector row CT arthrography and MR imaging. *Radiology* **2005**, *237*, 1008–1013. [CrossRef]
31. Moser, T.; Dosch, J.-C.; Moussaoui, A.; Dietemann, J.-L. Wrist ligament tears: Evaluation of MRI and combined MDCT and MR arthrography. *Am. J. Roentgenol.* **2007**, *188*, 1278–1286. [CrossRef] [PubMed]
32. Alam, F.; Schweitzer, M.E.; Li, X.X.; Malat, J.; Hussain, S.M. Frequency and spectrum of abnormalities in the bone marrow of the wrist: MR imaging findings. *Skeletal. Radiol.* **1999**, *28*, 312–317. [CrossRef] [PubMed]
33. Saupe, N.; Pfirrmann, C.W.A.; Schmid, M.R.; Schertler, T.; Manestar, M.; Weishaupt, D. MR imaging of cartilage in cadaveric wrists: Comparison between imaging at 1.5 and 3.0 T and gross pathologic inspection. *Radiology* **2007**, *243*, 180–187. [CrossRef] [PubMed]
34. Rajendran, K.; Murthy, N.S.; Frick, M.A.; Tao, S.; Unger, M.D.; LaVallee, K.T.; Larson, N.B.; Leng, S.; Maus, T.P.; McCollough, C.H. Quantitative Knee Arthrography in a Large Animal Model of Osteo-arthritis Using Photon-Counting Detector CT. *Investig. Radiol.* **2020**, *55*, 349–356. [CrossRef]
35. Kokkonen, H.T.; Aula, A.S.; Kröger, H.; Suomalainen, J.S.; Lammentausta, E.; Mervaala, E.; Jurvelin, J.S.; Töyräs, J. Delayed Computed Tomography Arthrography of Human Knee Carti-lage In Vivo. *Cartilage* **2012**, *3*, 334–341. [CrossRef] [PubMed]
36. Luetkens, K.S.; Grunz, J.P.; Paul, M.M.; Huflage, H.; Conrads, N.; Patzer, T.S.; Gruschwitz, P.; Ergün, S.; Bley, T.A.; Kunz, A.S. One-stop-shop CT arthrography of the wrist without subject reposi-tioning by means of gantry-free cone-beam CT. *Sci. Rep.* **2022**, *12*, 14422. [CrossRef]

Disclaimer/Publisher's Note: The statements, opinions and data contained in all publications are solely those of the individual author(s) and contributor(s) and not of MDPI and/or the editor(s). MDPI and/or the editor(s) disclaim responsibility for any injury to people or property resulting from any ideas, methods, instructions or products referred to in the content.

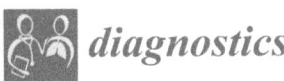

Review

Hydroxyapatite Deposition Disease: A Comprehensive Review of Pathogenesis, Radiological Findings, and Treatment Strategies

Tarek Hegazi

Department of Radiology, College of Medicine, Imam Abdulrahman Bin Faisal University, Dammam 34212, Saudi Arabia; tmhejazi@iau.edu.sa

Abstract: Hydroxyapatite deposition disease (HADD) represents a multifaceted condition characterized by the accumulation of hydroxyapatite crystals in soft tissues, leading to subsequent inflammation and discomfort. The intricate etiology of HADD is the subject of this comprehensive review, which encompasses an in-depth analysis of the four proposed pathogenic mechanisms and a deliberation on the predisposing factors that instigate the development of this disease. In order to provide a thorough understanding of the disease's progression, this manuscript delineates the stages of HADD—those preceding calcification, occurring during calcification, and following calcification—in meticulous detail. This chronology forms the basis of a complete portrayal of the evolution of HADD. Moreover, this review encompasses an examination of the radiological findings associated with HADD, furnishing an extensive discourse on imaging characteristics. The potential of HADD to mimic other diseases, thereby posing diagnostic challenges, is also articulated. The discourse continues with an investigation of HADD's differential diagnosis. This section furnishes a robust framework for distinguishing HADD from other conditions based on imaging results. To enrich the understanding of this diagnostic process, case studies illustrating real-world applications are provided. An overview of treatment modalities for HADD, including both conservative and interventional approaches, forms the concluding discussion. The pivotal role of imaging specialists in the diagnosis and management of HADD is emphasized, highlighting their vital contribution to image-guided procedures and disease monitoring.

Keywords: hydroxyapatite deposition disease; HADD; etiology; radiological findings; differential diagnosis; radiologist role

1. Introduction

Hydroxyapatite deposition disease (HADD), alternatively known as calcific tendinosis, calcific periarthritis, peritendinitis calcarea, calcific peritendinitis, calcific bursitis, and hydroxyapatite rheumatism, is a condition characterized by calcium hydroxyapatite crystal deposits in tendons, joints, and other soft tissues [1]. The disease is often asymptomatic and self-limiting, but when it is associated with an inflammatory process or when it occurs in unusual locations, it can imitate trauma, infection, or neoplasm [2], leading to misdiagnosis and unnecessary interventions [3]. It has a higher prevalence in females compared to males (2:1) [4].

Our understanding of HADD has significantly evolved over the years, with advancements in both diagnostic techniques and therapeutic approaches. Radiological imaging plays an instrumental role in the diagnosis and management of HADD. Despite the glenohumeral joint being the most common location for HADD [5], the diverse clinical presentations and locations of HADD present a considerable diagnostic and management challenge, underscoring the need for continuous research and review of the disease.

HADD's etiology is not entirely understood, but it is theorized to involve a series of stages, encompassing a precalcific stage, a calcific stage, and a postcalcific stage [6]. The

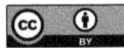

precalcific stage involves changes in the tendon cells that predispose them to calcification. The calcific stage is marked by the actual deposition of calcium hydroxyapatite crystals in the tendon [7]. The postcalcific stage involves the resolution of the calcific deposit and the healing of the tendon [8].

Comprehensive literature reviews bear vital importance in the realm of medical research. They synthesize a vast amount of research, facilitating a better understanding of the current state of knowledge, identifying research gaps, and setting directions for future studies. This comprehensive review of hydroxyapatite deposition disease aims to delve into the etiology, underscore the pivotal role of radiological findings in diagnosis, and explore the current and emerging treatment strategies for this condition.

2. Pathogenesis of HADD
2.1. Explanation of the Four Proposed Pathogenic Pathways

The precise etiology of hydroxyapatite deposition disease (HADD), a multifaceted condition, remains elusive and is an ongoing subject of investigation. The development of HADD, despite the current gap in definitive understanding, is potentially elucidated through four proposed primary pathogenic mechanisms [9] (Table 1).

Table 1. Pathogenic pathways of HADD.

Pathogenic Pathway	Key Players	Outcome
Degenerative calcification	Tendon, vascular ischemia, trauma	Deposition of calcified material
Reactive or cell-mediated calcification	Chondrocytes, phagocytosing cells	Calcium deposition and resorption of calcified material
Process similar to endochondral ossification	Cartilage, bone	Abnormal calcification within soft tissues
Erroneous differentiation of tendon-derived stem cells	Tendon-derived stem cells, chondrocytes, osteoblasts	Development of HADD due to calcium deposition

2.1.1. Degenerative Calcification

Degenerative calcification represents the first hypothesis in the potential development of HADD. According to this theory, the deposition of calcified material may be incited by localized damage to the tendon, attributable to either vascular ischemia or repetitive trauma [10].

Vascular ischemia describes a deficit in the blood supply, leading to insufficient oxygen and glucose required for cellular metabolism. For tendons, vascular ischemia could be a consequence of multiple factors such as physical injury, repetitive strain, or medical conditions that obstruct blood circulation [11]. The aftermath of vascular ischemia on a tendon potentially leads to tissue necrosis, initiating a series of biological responses including inflammation and chemical release, promoting calcification [11].

Similarly, repetitive trauma, or damage from recurring physical stress on the tendon, could stem from activities with repetitive motions like certain sports or jobs. The consequence of such trauma is often microtears in the tendon, leading to inflammation and subsequent tissue degeneration. This degenerated environment potentially facilitates calcium deposition, resulting in calcification [10].

This path of degenerative calcification indicates that HADD is a response to physical stress or injury involving tissue degeneration followed by calcification or the accumulation of calcium salts. While typically a part of the body's healing process, in HADD, this results in hydroxyapatite crystal formation, which induces pain and inflammation [11].

2.1.2. Reactive or Cell-Mediated Calcification

Reactive or cell-mediated calcification is the second theory, suggesting that chondrocytes, or the cells maintaining the cartilaginous matrix, mediate calcium deposition [12]. Chondrocytes, residing in cartilage, synthesize and maintain the cartilaginous matrix, a network of proteins and molecules that provide structure and support to the tissue. In the context of HADD, chondrocytes may contribute to calcium deposition, potentially in response to injury or inflammation [12]. In addition, this pathway involves phagocytosing cells, which absorb harmful foreign particles, bacteria, and dead or dying cells. These cells aid in the resorption of calcified material, implying that the body's cells play a part in both HADD development and resolution [13].

2.1.3. Process Similar to Endochondral Ossification

Endochondral ossification, a fundamental bodily process responsible for long bone formation and natural growth, is hypothesized to be similar to the third mechanism of HADD pathogenesis. In HADD, this process deviates pathologically, resulting in abnormal calcium deposition within the soft tissues rather than the standard transformation of cartilage into bone. This deviant calcification can occur in tendons, ligaments, and other periarticular soft tissues, leading to HADD's clinical manifestations. The specific trigger for this abnormal ossification remains elusive, but it is conjectured to be a response to tissue damage or stress, similar to the physiological injury response where bone forms to repair and strengthen the damaged area [14].

2.1.4. Erroneous Differentiation of Tendon-Derived Stem Cells

The last hypothesized mechanism involves the faulty differentiation of tendon-derived stem cells into calcium-depositing chondrocytes or osteoblasts. Stem cells, particularly tendon-derived ones, hold the capacity for self-renewal and differentiation into various cell types, including tenocytes, chondrocytes, and osteoblasts [15].

In the context of HADD, these tendon-derived stem cells are hypothesized to mis-differentiate into calcium-depositing chondrocytes or osteoblasts, contributing to disease development. This implies a dysregulation in the stem cell differentiation process, possibly due to genetic or environmental factors. The mis-differentiated cells then contribute to the formation of hydroxyapatite crystals within soft tissues, leading to HADD's clinical manifestations [15].

This pathogenic mechanism suggests that stem cells may play a part in HADD's pathogenesis, pointing to a potential novel treatment approach. However, further investigation is required to fully comprehend this mechanism and to develop effective stem cell-based treatments for HADD [15].

In conclusion, the complexity of HADD's pathogenesis likely involves multiple pathways, including processes similar to endochondral ossification and erroneous differentiation of tendon-derived stem cells. Comprehending these mechanisms is crucial for devising effective HADD treatments. Yet, further exploration is necessary to fully unravel these mechanisms and their treatment implications for HADD [15].

3. Predisposing Risk Factors for HADD

There are a number of predisposing factors that augment the likelihood of the onset of hydroxyapatite deposition disease (HADD) (Table 2). Metabolic and genetic influencers hint at a multifaceted etiology underpinning this disease [3]. Diabetes is a substantial risk factor associated with HADD. The exact contribution of diabetes to HADD is yet to be fully delineated. Nevertheless, diabetes-induced metabolic alterations, such as chronic low-grade inflammation and heightened oxidative stress, are speculated to foster the deposition of hydroxyapatite crystals within the soft tissues [16].

Another aspect to consider in the metabolic sphere are disorders pertaining to thyroid and estrogen metabolism, both of which have been associated with HADD. The thyroid gland's pivotal role in regulating metabolism and the widespread physiological consequences of its dysfunction are of interest here [17]. Similarly, estrogen, largely implicated in female reproductive health and bone metabolism, can induce abnormal calcium metabolism if imbalanced, potentially resulting in hydroxyapatite crystal deposition in soft tissues [18].

Table 2. Predisposing risk factors for HADD.

Risk Factor	Type	Possible Mechanism
Diabetes	Metabolic	Increased oxidative stress and chronic low-grade inflammation
Thyroid disorders	Metabolic	Disruptions in metabolic regulation
Estrogen metabolism disorders	Metabolic	Imbalances in hormones affecting bone health
HLA-A1 genotype	Genetic	Potential immunological component

Beyond these metabolic elements, certain genetic factors are also found to be linked with an increased HADD risk. The HLA-A1 genotype, part of the human leukocyte antigen (HLA) system that is critical to immune recognition of self and non-self cells, is one such genetic factor. The HLA-A1-HADD association hints at a potential immunological dimension to the disease, though the precise mechanism remains to be elucidated [19].

Considering these factors, the etiology of HADD is likely influenced by a complex interplay between metabolic and genetic components. These may interact with the proposed pathogenic pathways, potentially instigating the disease in susceptible individuals. Metabolic disorders like diabetes, and disorders of thyroid and estrogen metabolism, might induce cellular stress or damage, triggering the degenerative calcification pathway (16,17,18). Similarly, the HLA-A1 genotype might influence the reactive or cell-mediated calcification pathway, thus promoting hydroxyapatite crystal deposition [19].

To conclude, the emergence of HADD is thought to be influenced by the complex interplay between metabolic and genetic components. Unraveling these risk factors and their interaction with the proposed pathogenic pathways is imperative for devising efficacious preventive and therapeutic strategies for HADD. However, a comprehensive understanding of these interactions and their role in the pathogenesis of HADD demands further research [3].

4. Stages of HADD

4.1. Description of the Precalcific, Calcific, and Postcalcific Stages

The progression of hydroxyapatite deposition disease (HADD) is a temporal phenomenon that can be categorized into three primary stages: precalcific, calcific, and postcalcific [20] (Table 3).

Table 3. Stages of HADD.

Stage	Description	Symptoms	Radiographic Findings
Precalcific	Initial phase characterized by impaired perfusion and resultant focal hypoxia, triggering fibrocartilaginous transformation	Often asymptomatic	Not typically visible on radiographs
Calcific	Marked by the deposition of calcium crystals; further subdivided into formative, resting, and resorptive phases	Acute pain during resorptive phase	Visible calcifications, especially during the resorptive phase
Postcalcific	Occurs when the void from the resorptive phase of the calcific stage is replaced by granulation and scar tissue	Resolution of disease	Healing process visible, calcifications typically absent

The precalcific stage serves as the inception of HADD and is characterized by reduced perfusion and resultant localized hypoxia, triggering fibrocartilaginous transformation at the prospective calcification site. Often asymptomatic, this stage can be overlooked until the progression to the subsequent stage [12,21,22].

The calcific stage signifies the calcium crystal deposition phase and is divided into formative, resting, and resorptive phases. The formative phase sees fibrocartilage being replaced by a calcific deposit, which during the resting phase, resides without associated vascularity or inflammation for a variable duration. Eventually, the resorptive phase sees the calcium deposit being invaded by macrophages, polymorphonuclear cells, and fibroblasts that phagocytose and remove the calcium, giving the calcification an ill-defined, irregular appearance. The acute pain associated with HADD typically coincides with the resorptive phase, wherein the calcific deposit may rupture into nearby tissues, inciting an acute inflammatory response. Corresponding MRI observations report edema or a fluid signal surrounding the calcific focus [12,21,22].

The postcalcific stage is a critical juncture in HADD progression. At this stage, the body initiates the repair of calcification-induced damage. Granulation tissue, comprising new connective tissue and microscopic blood vessels, replaces the void left by the resorptive phase. This tissue matures into scar tissue over time, indicating the termination of the active disease phase. However, this does not always indicate a cessation of symptoms or treatment requirement, as the scar tissue can induce discomfort and restrict function depending on its location [12,21,22].

4.2. Explanation of the Changes in HADD over Time

The progression of HADD is a dynamic, individualized process, varying in duration and severity among individuals. Certain individuals may rapidly progress from the precalcific to the postcalcific stage, while others may stay in a single stage for an extended period with minimal disease alteration [4]. Notably, symptom severity does not necessarily align with the disease stage. The resorptive phase, despite being part of the calcific stage, is often the most acutely painful. This phase, involving the body's attempt to breakdown and remove calcium deposits, can cause significant inflammation and pain. However, the initiation of the postcalcific stage typically coincides with pain resolution and the commencement of the healing process [8].

Understanding HADD's progression, including the postcalcific stage, is critical for disease management. This knowledge can inform treatment decisions and provide patients with a better grasp of their condition. Despite the potential for significant pain and discomfort, it is crucial to remember that HADD is a self-limiting disease that typically resolves over time, particularly as the body enters and progresses through the postcalcific stage [8].

5. Radiological and Imaging Findings of HADD

Hydroxyapatite deposition disease (HADD), a condition characterized by the deposition of hydroxyapatite crystals, showcases a broad spectrum of radiological findings discernible in multiple imaging modalities. A comprehensive understanding of these findings aids in the accurate diagnosis of HADD, setting it apart from other conditions with analogous symptoms [23].

Hydroxyapatite crystals, the focal point of HADD, are predominantly radiopaque, translating to augmented density zones on radiographs. During the initial stages of HADD, these deposits appear scattered and minuscule, posing a challenge for detection. As the disease advances, these deposits merge into larger clusters, making them more visible [10].

5.1. Detailed Discussion on the Imaging Features of HADD

5.1.1. Plain Radiographs

Regarded as the first line of imaging modality for HADD diagnosis, plain radiographs capture the hallmark feature of HADD: amorphous, nebulous densities in soft tissues. These hydroxyapatite densities mainly encircle joints, particularly the shoulder (Figure 1), but can also inhabit unconventional regions like the hip, wrist, and spine.

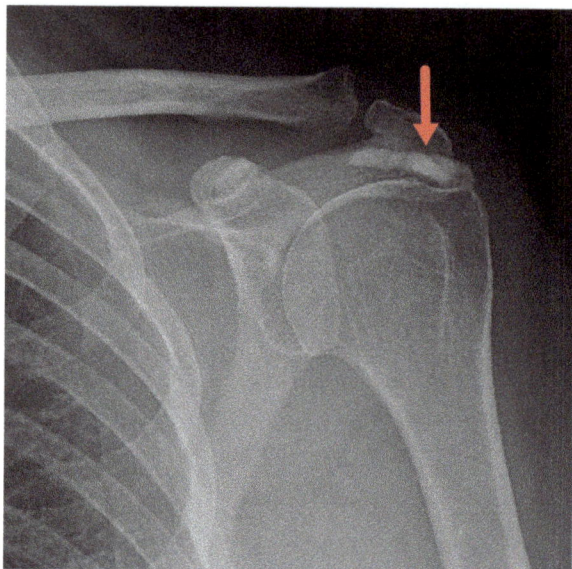

Figure 1. Frontal radiograph of the left shoulder demonstrating a well-defined calcification in the supraspinatus tendon (red arrow).

Advanced cases of HADD might exhibit these deposits in conjunction with bone erosion or cortical irregularities [3,8]. The scattered distribution of the calcified material accounts for the nebulous appearance of these deposits on radiographs, setting HADD apart from other conditions with similar radiographic findings [3,8,21]. The location of these deposits could provide valuable insights for diagnosing HADD. Instances of deposits in areas like the hip or wrist might point towards HADD in patients with discomfort in these areas.

Although rare, deposits in the spine could be indicative of HADD [24]. Progressed HADD stages might show hydroxyapatite deposits accompanied by bone erosion or cortical irregularities. Bone erosion, the dissolution of bone tissue, might occur due to the pressure exerted by the hydroxyapatite deposits on the neighboring bone tissue. Cortical irregularities, anomalies in the bone's outer layer, could be due to various factors, including HADD [24].

5.1.2. Computed Tomography

Computed tomography (CT) offers an in-depth visualization of hydroxyapatite deposits, elucidating their size, shape, and location. CT scans reveal these deposits as high-density zones within soft tissues, often associated with the inflammation around them, apparent as increased attenuation in adjacent soft tissues [23] (Figure 2). The high-density portrayal of hydroxyapatite deposits on CT scans stems from hydroxyapatite's high calcium content, which absorbs more X-rays than the surrounding soft tissues [23]. The detailed information offered by CT scans can shape treatment strategies for HADD patients, such as by guiding surgical interventions [25]. The hydroxyapatite deposits' association with surrounding inflammation can be gauged on a CT as decreased attenuation in adjacent soft tissues from the soft tissue edema. This observation can confirm the diagnosis of HADD and evaluate the disease's extent [25].

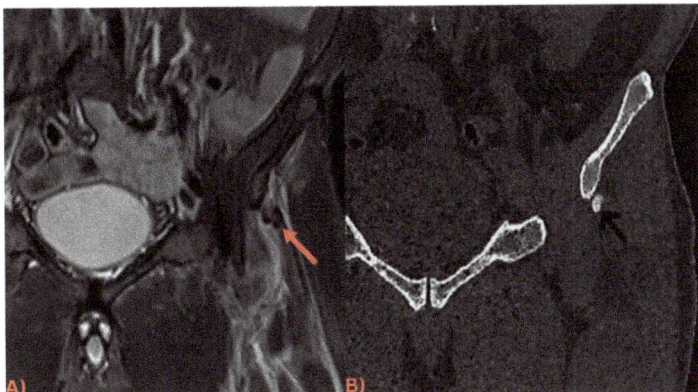

Figure 2. (**A**) Coronal short tau inversion recovery (STIR) MRI of the pelvis demonstrating an ill-defined low signal intensity focus at the origin of the left rectus femoris tendon (red arrow) with surrounding soft tissue edema. (**B**) Coronal CT image of the pelvis. Note how the calcification is more easily discernable on the CT image (black arrow).

5.1.3. Magnetic Resonance Imaging

Magnetic resonance imaging (MRI) constitutes an essential imaging modality for diagnosing soft tissue modifications linked to hydroxyapatite deposition disease (HADD) [26]. Non-invasive in nature, MRI utilizes a robust magnetic field and radio waves to generate comprehensive images of the body's internal structures, providing key insights into the hydroxyapatite deposits affiliated with HADD.

Specifically, MRI images display hydroxyapatite deposits as regions with low signal intensity across both T1- and T2-weighted images, attributable to the high mineral content of hydroxyapatite, a form of calcium phosphate crystals [27]. Consequently, this results in its manifestation in MRI images (Figure 3). Concurrently, MRI also reveals inflammation signs within surrounding soft tissues, such as edema and increased signal intensity on T2-weighted images [28] (Figure 4). Edema, a common response to inflammation or injury, indicates the body's reparative efforts, while a heightened signal intensity on T2-weighted images typifies inflammation and is present in several conditions, including HADD (Figure 5).

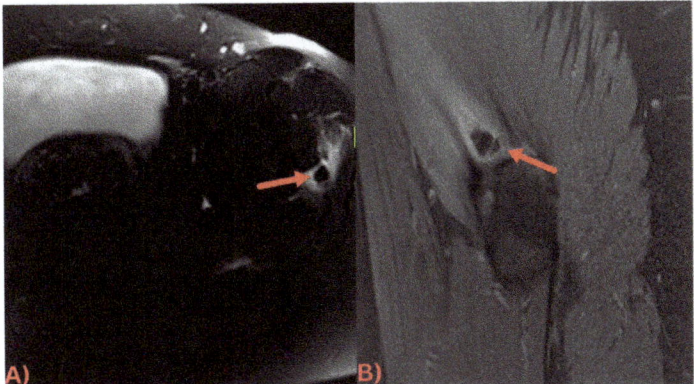

Figure 3. (**A**) Axial T2 fat-saturated MRI image and (**B**) sagittal PD fat-saturated MRI image of the left hip demonstrating a well-defined low signal intensity calcification at the insertion of the left gluteus medius tendon (red arrows) with surrounding soft tissue edema.

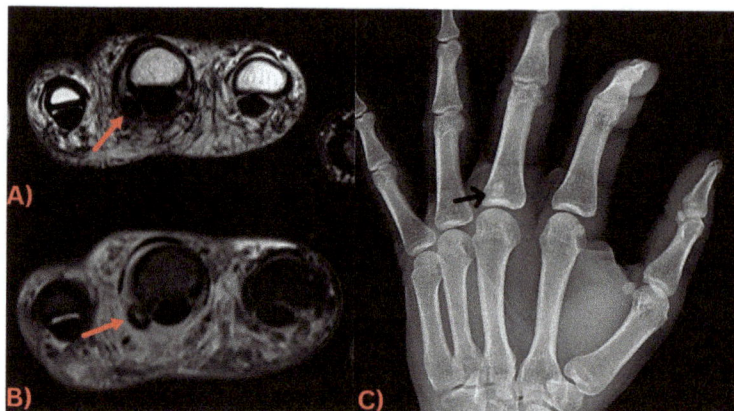

Figure 4. (**A**) Axial PD and (**B**) axial T2 fat-saturated MRI images of the hand demonstrating a well-defined globular low signal intensity focus at the volar capsule of the metacarpophalangeal joint of the middle finger (red arrows) with significant surrounding soft tissue edema. Note how this focus is more easily discernable on the (**C**) X-ray image of the hand, which clearly demonstrates that it is a focus of calcification (black arrow).

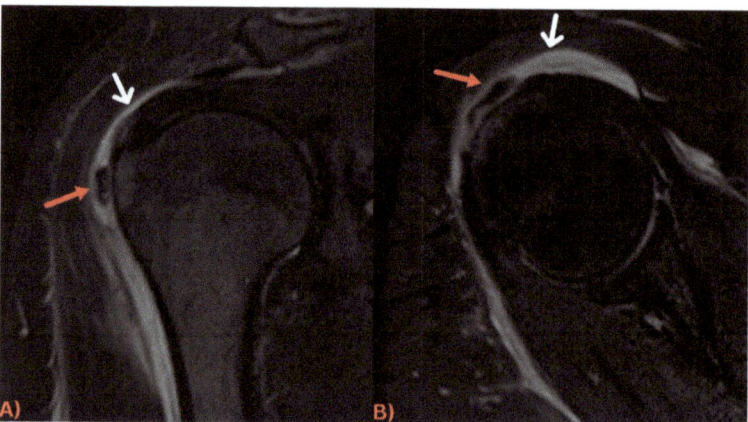

Figure 5. (**A**) Coronal PD fat-saturated MRI and (**B**) axial PD fat-saturated MRI images of the right shoulder demonstrating a few ill-defined low signal intensity calcifications (red arrows) in the subacromial/subdeltoid bursa, with fluid signal intensity within the bursa (white arrows) most suggestive of calcific bursitis.

Moreover, MRI occasionally displays the characteristic "arc and ring" pattern of the deposits, indicating a low signal intensity core of hydroxyapatite crystals encircled by a high signal intensity rim of inflammatory tissue [3]. This pattern serves as a valuable diagnostic marker in MRI readings of potential HADD patients.

Gradient recalled echo (GRE) sequences can reveal hydroxyapatite deposits as areas of signal voids or hypointensity due to the magnetic susceptibility effects of the calcified material. This is particularly useful in early-stage HADD, where the amount of hydroxyapatite deposition may be minimal and harder to detect with other imaging techniques (Figure 6).

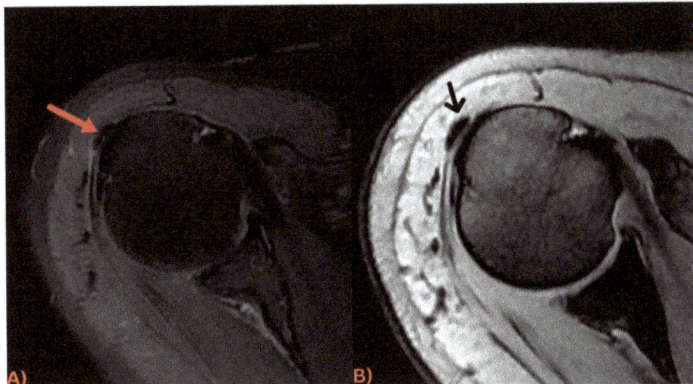

Figure 6. (**A**) Axial PD fat-saturated MRI image and (**B**) axial GRE sequence MRI of the right shoulder demonstrating a small well-defined low signal intensity calcification at the insertion of the supraspinatus tendon (red arrow). Note how the calcification is more visible and conspicuous on the GRE sequence (black arrow) due to a blooming artifact from the calcification.

5.1.4. Ultrasound

Ultrasound utilizes high-frequency sound waves to generate images of the body's internal structures. For HADD diagnosis, ultrasound is critical in identifying the size, shape, and location of hydroxyapatite deposits, which manifest as hyperechoic foci within soft tissues due to their high reflectivity [29].

These deposits may correspond to acoustic shadowing, a phenomenon where ultrasound waves are obstructed by the deposits, leading to an image shadow (Figure 7). This feature is of diagnostic value, as it differentiates hydroxyapatite deposits from other soft tissue abnormalities [30]. Furthermore, ultrasound can detect inflammation and tendon damage through increased echogenicity of the surrounding tissues and alterations in tendon size, shape, and echotexture [31].

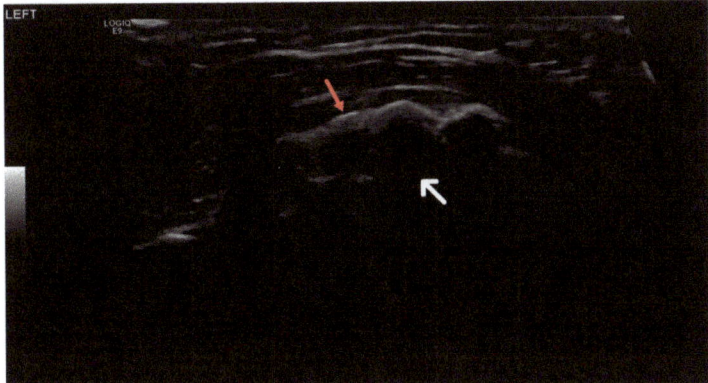

Figure 7. Ultrasound image showing calcific focus at the supraspinatus tendon insertion (red arrow) with posterior acoustic shadowing (white arrow).

Radiological findings of HADD are extensive and observable using various imaging modalities (Table 4). Combined with the patient's clinical presentation and history, these findings aid in the accurate diagnosis of HADD and differentiation from other conditions [32].

Table 4. Radiological findings in HADD.

Imaging Modality	Appearance of Hydroxyapatite Deposits	Associated Findings
Plain radiographs	Amorphous, cloud-like densities	Bone erosion or cortical irregularities
Computed tomography (CT)	High-density areas	Surrounding inflammation
Magnetic resonance imaging (MRI)	Low signal intensity areas	Surrounding inflammation, "arc and ring" pattern
Ultrasound	Hyperechoic foci	Acoustic shadowing, inflammation, tendon damage

6. HADD Can Mimic Other Diseases

HADD can mimic other diseases, such as tumoral calcinosis and aggressive neoplastic processes, presenting a diagnostic challenge.

Tumoral calcinosis, a rare condition, features large, calcified, periarticular soft tissue masses made of calcium phosphate crystals, often associated with hyperphosphatemia. Radiographs of tumoral calcinosis exhibit large, lobulated masses with a dense, amorphous calcification pattern. These can resemble the appearance of hydroxyapatite deposits in HADD, which similarly appear as amorphous, cloud-like densities in soft tissues [33].

Similarly, HADD's bone erosion can mimic bone destruction in aggressive tumors. Particularly, malignant neoplastic processes can cause substantial bone destruction and cortical irregularities, mirroring those observed in advanced HADD cases. This resemblance complicates the differentiation of HADD from malignant tumors based solely on radiological findings [25,34].

However, several elements aid in distinguishing HADD from these conditions. Characteristic calcifications, usually located around joints and associated with bone erosion or cortical irregularities, are a unique feature of HADD [24]. In comparison, calcifications in tumoral calcinosis are typically larger and more lobulated, and bone destruction in aggressive neoplastic processes is more extensive and accompanies a soft tissue mass [33].

Additionally, the localization of calcification in HADD provides diagnostic clues. They are typically located in the tendons around joints, especially the shoulder, but can also be found in unusual locations like the hip, wrist, and spine. In contrast, calcifications in tumoral calcinosis are usually found in the periarticular soft tissues, and bone destruction in aggressive neoplastic processes can occur in any bone affected by the tumor [2].

Despite the challenge posed by radiological mimicry of other diseases, a comprehensive understanding of HADD's imaging features aids in accurate diagnosis and suitable management. It is essential to consider the patient's clinical history, physical examination findings, and laboratory results along with imaging findings for the correct diagnosis. As always, correlation with clinical findings is crucial in radiology, with HADD being no exception [8].

6.1. Differentiating HADD from Other Diseases Based on Imaging Findings

Differential diagnosis is a vital component of medical practices, providing doctors the tools to distinguish diseases with comparable symptomatology or manifestation. HADD introduces unique challenges to the differential diagnosis process, as it has a propensity to mimic other conditions. This mimicry is particularly apparent in radiological findings where HADD's calcified deposits may appear to mirror diseases such as tumoral calcinosis or aggressive neoplastic processes. Thus, a comprehensive understanding of HADD's imaging traits is imperative for an accurate diagnosis and suitable treatment management [3,25,33,34].

6.1.1. The Acute Phase

Acute symptomatic HADD is often misdiagnosed as a traumatic or infectious process, especially when it affects the longus colli muscle at the cervical spine. In these scenarios, characteristic calcifications are key to differentiate HADD from infection. When individuals present with acute symptomatic HADD following minor trauma, there is a possibility that HADD's calcifications may be misinterpreted as avulsion fragments. Nevertheless, avulsion fractures typically display a linear or incompletely corticated appearance, contrasting with HADD calcification's more ambiguous or homogeneous display [35].

During HADD's acute phase, patients might exhibit symptoms similar to those of traumatic injury or infection, including pain, swelling, and a reduced motion range in the affected area. In situations where HADD affects the longus colli muscle at the cervical spine, patients might also experience neck stiffness, odynophagia (painful swallowing), and dysphagia (difficulty swallowing). In rare instances, the swelling accompanying HADD in this region can lead to airway compromise [35].

The distinguishing factor between acute symptomatic HADD and a traumatic or infectious process is the characteristic calcifications seen in imaging studies. These calcifications are calcium apatite crystal deposits within and around connective tissues, a defining feature of HADD. In radiographic images, these calcifications often exhibit an amorphous, nebulous appearance, differing considerably from the linear or incompletely corticated appearance of avulsion fragments typically seen in traumatic injuries [35].

When minor trauma occurs, the misinterpretation of HADD's calcifications as avulsion fragments might occur. Avulsion fractures result from a muscle's forceful contraction or stretch, tearing away a bone fragment. These fractures are commonly associated with sports injuries and frequently observed in younger individuals engaged in activities involving sudden accelerations or decelerations. In imaging studies, avulsion fractures usually appear as linear or incompletely corticated bone fragments, contrasting sharply with the ambiguous or homogeneous display of HADD calcification [35].

Therefore, when symptoms suggestive of a traumatic or infectious process arise, especially in minor trauma scenarios, it is crucial to consider HADD as a potential differential diagnosis. A meticulous examination of imaging studies, focusing particularly on the presence and appearance of calcifications, can assist in distinguishing HADD from other conditions, guiding appropriate management [36].

6.1.2. The Chronic Phase

Chronic symptomatic HADD frequently poses diagnostic challenges due to its similarity to other conditions like trauma's late sequela, specifically heterotopic ossification or malignancy. Heterotopic ossification denotes the aberrant formation of true bone within extraskeletal soft tissues, which typically occurs post-trauma or surgery. Its imaging characteristics can mimic HADD, but the key differentiating factor is a corticated margin's presence surrounding the heterotopic ossification, which is absent in HADD [35].

One of the challenges encountered during the process of distinguishing HADD from other diseases is the presence of bony erosion and periosteal reaction that could be mistaken for signs of a soft tissue malignancy or sarcoma [35]. These types of cancers originate in soft tissues such as fat, muscle, nerves, fibrous tissues, blood vessels, or deep-skin tissues, making the differentiation complex due to similar calcification and bone erosion patterns on imaging studies. Nevertheless, an absence of a discrete soft tissue mass, alongside calcification located at a typical HADD site, can support the differentiation between HADD and a neoplastic process.

Concluding the diagnostic perspective, the differential diagnosis of HADD relies heavily on the recognition of characteristic imaging features and an understanding of how these differ from those of other diseases [3]. This ability to distinguish HADD from other conditions based on imaging findings underpins the precision of diagnosis and tailoring of the most suitable management approach.

6.1.3. Other Conditions Acting as Differentials in HADD

Trauma

Trauma, either acute or chronic, is a significant factor that may lead to calcification within the affected soft tissues. This calcification can be easily confused with HADD. In cases of trauma, be it a singular traumatic event or an ongoing history of injury, radiological findings often reveal distinctive signs such as fracture lines, bone contusions, or other evidence that is entirely distinct from the amorphous calcifications observed in HADD. The differentiation process is vital, as it relies on a combination of the patient's history, clinical examinations, and diverse imaging modalities like X-rays, CT scans, or MRI [35]. It is worth emphasizing the significance of recognizing the exact location and pattern of calcification and the absence of systemic symptoms typically linked to HADD, as this understanding can be instrumental in determining the correct treatment approach, which significantly differs from HADD management.

Infection

Chronic infections, particularly those that infiltrate the joints or surrounding tissues, often present a clinical picture that might lead to calcifications resembling HADD. The nature of these calcifications could be bacterial, fungal, or viral, usually localized or generalized within the affected region. The importance of distinguishing infection from HADD cannot be overstated, as it is a matter of employing entirely different therapeutic strategies. This approach to diagnosis involves a detailed clinical history, laboratory markers for infection (such as elevated white blood cell counts, C-reactive protein, or culture results), and relevant imaging techniques [35]. Contrary to HADD, infections often necessitate specific treatments like antimicrobial therapy or surgical interventions, thus underlining the vital importance of accurate differentiation.

Pseudohypoparathyroidism

Pseudohypoparathyroidism (PHP) is characterized by features like short stature, obesity, round face, and intellectual disability. It may also cause calcifications within soft tissues that resemble HADD [14]. However, the diagnosis process involves the observation of unique laboratory findings, such as low calcium and high phosphate levels and specific skeletal abnormalities on radiological examinations such as shortening of the fourth metacarpal. Further assessment may include a detailed family history and identifying additional features related to Albright's hereditary osteodystrophy, making the management of PHP remarkably different from HADD.

Hyperparathyroidism

Hyperparathyroidism can also induce generalized calcifications within soft tissues, creating confusion with HADD. The hallmarks of this disorder include increased levels of PTH, leading to disturbances in calcium and phosphate metabolism. Differentiating this condition from HADD relies on laboratory findings, such as elevated serum calcium and PTH levels, and radiological imaging that might reveal calcification in various parts of the body [15]. Proper differentiation from HADD is crucial, as its management might necessitate measures, like medication, dietary modification, or even surgical intervention, that are tailored to the underlying cause.

CPPD (Chondrocalcinosis)

Calcium pyrophosphate deposition disease (CPPD) sets itself apart from HADD due to its more defined calcification patterns. Unlike HADD's typical amorphous calcifications, CPPD manifests in acute or chronic joint pain and is often linked with underlying metabolic disorders. Specific radiographic findings and the involvement of certain joints, predominantly affecting areas like the knees or wrists, further support its differentiation from HADD. The treatment approach for CPPD, encompassing NSAIDs, corticosteroids, or colchicine, varies markedly from that for HADD.

In summary, the complexity of conditions like trauma, infections, PHP, hyperparathyroidism, and CPPD necessitates a nuanced understanding to differentiate them from HADD. Through careful examination, clinical expertise, and the use of appropriate diagnostic tools, the proper treatment and management approach for each condition can be effectively implemented.

7. Treatment of HADD

In the treatment of HADD, a myriad of strategies have been utilized, combining conservative and interventional approaches [37]. These methods are employed considering the disease's severity, the deposit location, and the patient's overall health status.

The first line of defense in managing HADD often consists of conservative treatment approaches. These include rest, physical therapy, and administration of non-steroidal anti-inflammatory drugs (NSAIDs) [38]. The importance of rest as a fundamental component of this approach cannot be overstated, providing the body an opportunity to heal and recover naturally, thus reducing HADD-induced inflammation and pain [37].

Physical therapy, a significant element in HADD management, works towards improving joint function, increasing range of motion, and strengthening muscles surrounding the affected joint [39]. NSAIDs, often employed to reduce inflammation and alleviate pain, function by inhibiting the production of certain inflammation-causing chemicals in the body [40].

In instances where conservative treatment strategies fail to offer sufficient relief, interventional treatments are considered. These include extracorporeal shock wave therapy (ESWT) and surgical intervention [41]. ESWT, a non-invasive procedure, uses sound waves to break up hydroxyapatite deposits, facilitating their resorption. Particularly effective in cases where deposits are near the skin surface, this therapy represents an innovative approach to treatment [42,43].

Surgical intervention, reserved typically for severe cases, involves arthroscopic or open surgery to remove deposits [44,45]. The decision to proceed with surgery requires careful evaluation of the patient's overall health status, the severity of their symptoms, and their response to conservative treatment. It is of paramount importance that patients work closely with their healthcare provider in developing a treatment plan tailored to their specific needs and circumstances [46].

Role of the Imaging Specialist in the Treatment of HADD

The role of the imaging specialist in the treatment of HADD is indeed crucial. Imaging specialists play a key role in the diagnosis of HADD, as the disease is primarily identified through imaging studies. They are responsible for identifying the hydroxyapatite deposits and differentiating HADD from other conditions that may present with similar imaging findings [1,47].

The imaging specialist's role begins with the initial diagnosis. Using imaging modalities such as X-ray, CT, MRI, and ultrasound, imaging specialists can identify the characteristic calcifications associated with HADD. These deposits typically appear as areas of increased density or signal in these imaging studies, allowing the imaging specialist to differentiate HADD from other conditions that may present with similar symptoms but different imaging findings [47].

In addition to identifying the hydroxyapatite deposits, imaging specialists also play a crucial role in assessing the extent of the disease. They can determine the size and location of the deposits as well as any associated soft tissue changes or bone erosion. This information is vital for planning the appropriate treatment strategy [47].

Imaging specialists also play a significant role in the treatment of HADD through image-guided procedures. For instance, they may perform image-guided needle aspiration or lavage to remove the deposits. This procedure involves using imaging guidance to insert a needle into the affected area and aspirate the calcific deposits (Figure 8). This can help to alleviate symptoms and promote healing [48].

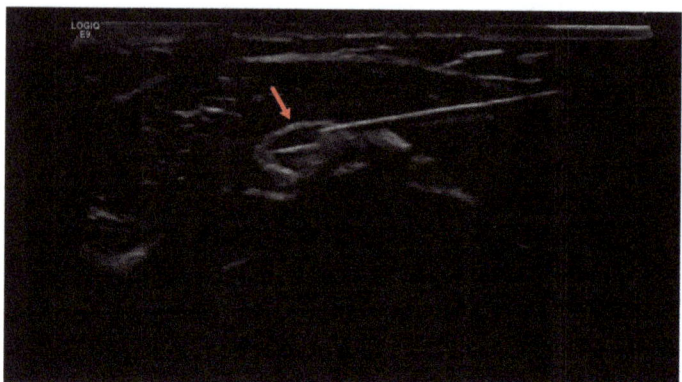

Figure 8. Ultrasound image showing a percutaneous calcific lavage procedure with a needle within the calcific focus during the irrigation (red arrow).

In addition, imaging specialists may guide the placement of corticosteroid injections to reduce inflammation. These injections can be administered directly into the bursae or soft tissues surrounding the affected joint, providing immediate relief from pain and inflammation. The precise placement of these injections is crucial to ensure their effectiveness and minimize potential side effects, and the expertise of the imaging specialist is invaluable [41].

Furthermore, imaging specialists play a key role in monitoring the progress of the disease and the effectiveness of treatment. Through follow-up imaging studies, they can assess whether the hydroxyapatite deposits are decreasing in size or disappearing altogether, indicating a positive response to treatment. They can also identify any potential complications or new areas of calcification [47].

Therefore, the role of the imaging specialist in the treatment of HADD extends beyond the initial diagnosis. They are integral to the treatment and management of the disease, providing valuable insights through their expertise in imaging studies and image-guided procedures. Their contributions are essential to ensuring the most effective treatment strategy for each individual patient, ultimately leading to better patient outcomes [1,47].

Imaging specialists are integral to multidisciplinary approaches to managing HADD. Collaborating with healthcare professionals like rheumatologists, orthopedic surgeons, and physical therapists, they provide key imaging findings that guide treatment strategies. For example, the extent of hydroxyapatite deposition can inform decisions about surgical intervention, while signs of inflammation can help tailor therapeutic interventions. Additionally, imaging specialists aid in patient education, explaining imaging results to help patients better understand their condition and fostering improved treatment adherence and outcomes.

8. Future Recommendations

Hydroxyapatite deposition disease (HADD) is a convoluted medical condition, with significant advances in its comprehension and administration observed over the years. Yet, several areas remain unexplored and necessitate further scientific scrutiny and inquiry.

A prime area that calls for an intensified probe lies in the pathogenesis of HADD. The deposition of hydroxyapatite crystals in soft tissues, a pivotal phenomenon in HADD, still leaves researchers speculating about its precise mechanisms. Although four potential pathways have been proposed, their exact implications remain elusive. Therefore, it is crucial to shed light on these mechanisms. Doing so could pave the way for innovative therapeutic strategies that prevent or reverse these processes. Expounding the interactions between genetic, environmental, and cellular factors in HADD pathogenesis could further elucidate this intricate disease process.

Simultaneously, the role of imaging specialists in the diagnostic and management process of HADD is another area that requires further exploration. Recent advancements in artificial intelligence (AI) can be a potential game-changer in this respect. AI promises transformative tools capable of enhancing image analysis, boosting diagnostic precision, and even offering prognostic capabilities for disease progression [49]. Consequently, future studies exploring AI applications in HADD diagnosis and treatment could be pivotal. For instance, machine learning algorithms can be designed to recognize HADD's imaging features, distinguish it from other conditions, and even predict the outcomes of treatment approaches [50].

Furthermore, the scope of imaging specialists' roles could transcend diagnosis and treatment. As subject matter experts in HADD imaging findings, imaging specialists are strategically positioned to educate patients about their condition, demystify imaging results, and promote apt treatment strategies, thus evolving into patient advocates.

9. Conclusions

In conclusion, HADD's complexity is manifested in its diagnostic and treatment challenges. It can present itself in various bodily locations and imitate other conditions, necessitating a profound understanding of its radiological findings for precise diagnosis. A blend of conservative and interventionist approaches formulates the treatment plan, which is tailored to the disease severity and the overall health status of the patient. The pivotal role of radiologists in diagnosing and treating HADD underscores the importance of a multidisciplinary approach to managing this disease. Notwithstanding the substantial strides made in HADD comprehension and management, several areas still demand intensified research. Pioneering research in these areas, especially in demystifying HADD pathogenesis and AI's role in radiology, could potentially usher in an era of enhanced diagnostic tools and treatment strategies. This would significantly boost outcomes for patients grappling with HADD.

Funding: This research received no external funding.

Institutional Review Board Statement: Not applicable.

Informed Consent Statement: Not applicable.

Data Availability Statement: Not applicable.

Conflicts of Interest: The author declares no conflict of interest.

References

1. Bonavita, J.A.; Dalinka, M.K.; Schumacher, H.R., Jr. Hydroxyapatite deposition disease. *Radiology* **1980**, *134*, 621–625. [CrossRef] [PubMed]
2. Flemming, D.J.; Murphey, M.D.; Shekitka, K.M.; Temple, H.T.; Jelinek, J.J.; Kransdorf, M.J. Osseous involvement in calcific tendinitis: A retrospective review of 50 cases. *Am. J. Roentgenol.* **2003**, *181*, 965–972. [CrossRef] [PubMed]
3. Hongsmatip, P.; Cheng, K.Y.; Kim, C.; Lawrence, D.A.; Rivera, R.; Smitaman, E. Calcium hydroxyapatite deposition disease: Imaging features and presentations mimicking other pathologies. *Eur. J. Radiol.* **2019**, *120*, 108653. [CrossRef] [PubMed]
4. Benvenuto, P.; Locas, S. Hydroxyapatite deposition disease: A common disease in an uncommon location. *Intern. Emerg. Med.* **2020**, *15*, 333–334. [CrossRef] [PubMed]
5. Louwerens, J.K.; Sierevelt, I.N.; van Hove, R.P.; van den Bekerom, M.P.; van Noort, A. Prevalence of calcific deposits within the rotator cuff tendons in adults with and without subacromial pain syndrome: Clinical and radiologic analysis of 1219 patients. *J. Shoulder Elb. Surg.* **2015**, *24*, 1588–1593. [CrossRef] [PubMed]
6. Hayes, C.W.; Conway, W.F. Calcium hydroxyapatite deposition disease. *RadioGraphics* **1990**, *10*, 1031–1048. [CrossRef]
7. Haake, M.; Deike, B.; Thon, A.; Schmitt, J. Bedeutung der exakten Fokussierung extrakorporaler Stoßwellen (ESWT) bei der Therapie der Tendinitis calcarea. Eine prospektive randomisierte Studie—Importance of Accurately Focussing Extracorporeal Shock Waves in the Treatment of Calcifying Tendinitis. A Prospective Randomized Study. *Biomed. Eng. Biomed. Tech.* **2001**, *46*, 69–74. [CrossRef]
8. Siegal, D.S.; Wu, J.S.; Newman, J.S.; Del Cura, J.L.; Hochman, M.G. Calcific tendinitis: A pictorial review. *Can. Assoc. Radiol. J.* **2009**, *60*, 263–272. [CrossRef]
9. Oliva, F.; Via, A.G.; Maffulli, N. Physiopathology of intratendinous calcific deposition. *BMC Med.* **2012**, *10*, 95. [CrossRef]

10. Bosworth, B.M. Calcium deposits in the shoulder and subacromial bursitis: A survey of 12,122 shoulders. *J. Am. Med. Assoc.* **1941**, *116*, 2477–2482. [CrossRef]
11. Bishop, W.A. Calcification of the supraspinatus tendon: Cause, pathologic picture and relation to the scalenus anticus syndrome. *Arch. Surg.* **1939**, *39*, 231–246. [CrossRef]
12. Uhthoff, H.K.; Loehr, J.W. Calcific tendinopathy of the rotator cuff: Pathogenesis, diagnosis, and management. *J. Am. Acad. Orthop. Surg.* **1997**, *5*, 183–191. [CrossRef] [PubMed]
13. Uhthoff, H.K.; Sarkar, K.; A Maynard, J. Calcifying tendinitis: A new concept of its pathogenesis. *Clin. Orthop. Relat. Res.* **1976**, *118*, 164–168. [CrossRef]
14. Benjamin, M.; Rufai, A.; Ralphs, J.R. The mechanism of formation of bony spurs (enthesophytes) in the Achilles tendon. *Arthritis Rheum.* **2000**, *43*, 576–583. [CrossRef]
15. Rui, Y.-F.; Lui, P.P.-Y.; Chan, L.-S.; Chan, K.-M.; Fu, S.-C.; Li, G. Does erroneous differentiation of tendon-derived stem cells contribute to the pathogenesis of calcifying tendinopathy? *Chin. Med J.* **2011**, *124*, 606–610.
16. E Mavrikakis, M.; Drimis, S.; A Kontoyannis, D.; Rasidakis, A.; Moulopoulou, E.S.; Kontoyannis, S. Calcific shoulder periarthritis (tendinitis) in adult onset diabetes mellitus: A controlled study. *Ann. Rheum. Dis.* **1989**, *48*, 211–214. [CrossRef]
17. Harvie, P.; Pollard, T.C.; Carr, A.J. Calcific tendinitis: Natural history and association with endocrine disorders. *J. Shoulder Elb. Surg.* **2007**, *16*, 169–173. [CrossRef]
18. Wright, V.; Haq, A.M. Periarthritis of the shoulder. I. Aetiological considerations with particular reference to personality factors. *Ann. Rheum. Dis.* **1976**, *35*, 213–219. [CrossRef]
19. Sengar, D.P.S.; McKendry, R.J.; Uhthoff, H.K. Increased frequency of HLA-A1 in calcifying tendinitis. *Tissue Antigens* **1987**, *29*, 173–174. [CrossRef]
20. Uhthoff, H.K.; Sarkar, K. Calcifying tendinitis. *Bailliere's Clin. Rheumatol.* **1989**, *3*, 567–581. [CrossRef]
21. Reddy, G.; Hodgson, N.; Peach, C.; Phillips, N.J. Plain radiographic evidence of stages of calcifying tendinitis of supraspinatus tendon of shoulder. *Emerg. Med. J.* **2015**, *32*, 582–583. [CrossRef] [PubMed]
22. Doumas, C.; Vazirani, R.M.; Clifford, P.D.; Owens, P. Acute calcific periarthritis of the hand and wrist: A series and review of the literature. *Emerg. Radiol.* **2007**, *14*, 199–203. [CrossRef] [PubMed]
23. Freire, V.; Moser, T.P.; Lepage-Saucier, M. Radiological identification and analysis of soft tissue musculoskeletal calcifications. *Insights Imaging* **2018**, *9*, 477–492. [CrossRef] [PubMed]
24. Kraemer, E.J.; El-Khoury, G.Y. Atypical calcific tendinitis with cortical erosions. *Skelet. Radiol.* **2000**, *29*, 690–696. [CrossRef]
25. Hayes, C.; Rosenthal, D.; Plata, M.; Hudson, T.; Hayes, D.R.C.; Flemming, D.J.; Murphey, M.D.; Shekitka, K.M.; Temple, H.T.; Jelinek, J.J.; et al. Calcific tendinitis in unusual sites associated with cortical bone erosion. *Am. J. Roentgenol.* **1987**, *149*, 967–970. [CrossRef]
26. Zubler, C.; Mengiardi, B.; Schmid, M.R.; Hodler, J.; Jost, B.; Pfirrmann, C.W.A. MR arthrography in calcific tendinitis of the shoulder: Diagnostic performance and pitfalls. *Eur. Radiol.* **2007**, *17*, 1603–1610. [CrossRef]
27. Merolla, G.; Singh, S.; Paladini, P.; Porcellini, G. Calcific tendinitis of the rotator cuff: State of the art in diagnosis and treatment. *J. Orthop. Traumatol.* **2016**, *17*, 7–14. [CrossRef]
28. Abreu, M.R.; Recht, M. MR imaging of the rotator cuff and rotator interval. In *Musculoskeletal Diseases 2017–2020: Diagnostic Imaging*; Springer: Cham, Switzerland, 2017; pp. 203–214. [CrossRef]
29. Farin, P.U.; Jaroma, H. Sonographic findings of rotator cuff calcifications. *J. Ultrasound Med.* **1995**, *14*, 7–14. [CrossRef]
30. Chiou, H.J.; Chou, Y.H.; Wu, J.J.; Hsu, C.C.; Huang, D.Y.; Chang, C.Y. Evaluation of calcific tendonitis of the rotator cuff: Role of color Doppler ultrasonography. *J. Ultrasound Med.* **2002**, *21*, 289–295. [CrossRef]
31. Le Goff, B.; Berthelot, J.-M.; Guillot, P.; Glémarec, J.; Maugars, Y. Assessment of calcific tendonitis of rotator cuff by ultrasonography: Comparison between symptomatic and asymptomatic shoulders. *Jt. Bone Spine* **2010**, *77*, 258–263. [CrossRef]
32. Chianca, V.; Albano, D.; Messina, C.; Midiri, F.; Mauri, G.; Aliprandi, A.; Catapano, M.; Pescatori, L.C.; Monaco, C.G.; Gitto, S.; et al. Rotator cuff calcific tendinopathy: From diagnosis to treatment. *Acta Biomed.* **2018**, *89* (Suppl. 1), 186.
33. Del Bravo, V.; Liuzza, F.; Perisano, C.; Chalidis, B.; Marzetti, E.; Colelli, P.; Maccauro, G. Gluteal Tumoral Calcinosis. *HIP Int.* **2012**, *22*, 585–591. [CrossRef]
34. Malghem, J.; Omoumi, P.; Lecouvet, F.; Berg, B.V. Intraosseous migration of tendinous calcifications: Cortical erosions, subcortical migration and extensive intramedullary diffusion, a SIMS series. *Skelet. Radiol.* **2015**, *44*, 1403–1412. [CrossRef] [PubMed]
35. Beckmann, N.M. Calcium Apatite Deposition Disease: Diagnosis and Treatment. *Radiol. Res. Pract.* **2016**, *2016*, 4801474. [CrossRef] [PubMed]
36. Carroll, R.E.; Sinton, W.; Garcia, A. Acute calcium deposits in the hand. *J. Am. Med. Assoc.* **1955**, *157*, 422–426. [CrossRef]
37. Cho, N.S.; Lee, B.G.; Rhee, Y.G. Radiologic course of the calcific deposits in calcific tendinitis of the shoulder: Does the initial radiologic aspect affect the final results? *J. Shoulder Elb. Surg.* **2010**, *19*, 267–272. [CrossRef]
38. Harmon, P.H. Methods and results in the treatment of 2,580 painful shoulders: With special reference to calcific tendinitis and the frozen shoulder. *Am. J. Surg.* **1958**, *95*, 527–544. [CrossRef]
39. Singh, J.R.; Yip, K. Gluteus maximus calcific tendonosis: A rare cause of sciatic pain. *Am. J. Phys. Med. Rehabil.* **2015**, *94*, 165–167. [CrossRef]
40. Hurt, G.; Baker, C.L. Calcific tendinitis of the shoulder. *Orthop. Clin.* **2003**, *34*, 567–575. [CrossRef]

41. de Witte, P.B.; Selten, J.W.; Navas, A.; Nagels, J.; Visser, C.P.; Nelissen, R.G.; Reijnierse, M. Calcific tendinitis of the rotator cuff: A randomized controlled trial of ultrasound-guided needling and lavage versus subacromial corticosteroids. *Am. J. Sport. Med.* **2013**, *41*, 1665–1673. [CrossRef]
42. Bannuru, R.R.; Flavin, N.E.; Vaysbrot, E.; Harvey, W.; McAlindon, T. High-energy extracorporeal shock-wave therapy for treating chronic calcific tendinitis of the shoulder: A systematic review. *Ann. Intern. Med.* **2014**, *160*, 542–549. [CrossRef]
43. Kim, Y.S.; Lee, H.J.; Kim, Y.V.; Kong, C.G. Which method is more effective in treatment of calcific tendinitis in the shoulder? Prospective randomized comparison between ultrasound-guided needling and extracorporeal shock wave therapy. *J. Shoulder Elb. Surg.* **2014**, *23*, 1640–1646. [CrossRef]
44. Jerosch, J.; Strauss, J.; Schmiel, S. Arthroscopic treatment of calcific tendinitis of the shoulder. *J. Shoulder Elb. Surg.* **1998**, *7*, 30–37. [CrossRef]
45. Seil, R.; Litzenburger, H.; Kohn, D.; Rupp, S. Arthroscopic Treatment of Chronically Painful Calcifying Tendinitis of the Supraspinatus Tendon. *Arthrosc. J. Arthrosc. Relat. Surg.* **2006**, *22*, 521–527. [CrossRef]
46. Suzuki, K.; Potts, A.; Anakwenze, O.; Singh, A. Calcific tendinitis of the rotator cuff: Management options. *J. Am. Acad. Orthop. Surg.* **2014**, *22*, 707–717. [CrossRef]
47. Hussain, J.; Jawhar, O.D.; Judge, S.D.; Joshi, V.; Stavrakis, C.D.; Brooks, M. Calcific Tendinosis: What the General Radiologist Needs to Know. *Contemp. Diagn. Radiol.* **2021**, *44*, 1–7. [CrossRef]
48. Aina, R.; Cardinal, E.; Bureau, N.J.; Aubin, B.; Brassard, P. Calcific Shoulder Tendinitis: Treatment with Modified US-guided Fine-Needle Technique. *Radiology* **2001**, *221*, 455–461. [CrossRef]
49. Oren, O.; Gersh, B.J.; Bhatt, D.L. Artificial intelligence in medical imaging: Switching from radiographic pathological data to clinically meaningful endpoints. *Lancet Digit. Heal.* **2020**, *2*, e486–e488. [CrossRef]
50. Sm, C.M. Artificial intelligence in radiology—Are we treating the image or the patient? *Indian J. Radiol. Imaging* **2018**, *28*, 137–139. [CrossRef]

Disclaimer/Publisher's Note: The statements, opinions and data contained in all publications are solely those of the individual author(s) and contributor(s) and not of MDPI and/or the editor(s). MDPI and/or the editor(s) disclaim responsibility for any injury to people or property resulting from any ideas, methods, instructions or products referred to in the content.

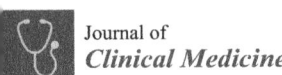

Article

Is Corticalization in Radiographs Related to a Higher Risk of Bone Loss around Dental Implants in Smoking Patients? A 5-Year Observation of Radiograph Bone-Texture Changes

Tomasz Wach [1,*], Piotr Hadrowicz [2], Grzegorz Trybek [3,4], Adam Michcik [5] and Marcin Kozakiewicz [1]

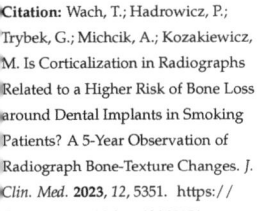

1. Department of Maxillofacial Surgery, Medical University of Lodz, 113 Żeromskiego Str., 90-549 Lodz, Poland; marcin.kozakiewicz@umed.lodz.pl
2. Department of Otolaryngology, Hospital in Sosnowiec, Zegadłowicza 3, 41-200 Sosnowiec, Poland; phadrowicz@gmail.com
3. Department of Oral Surgery, Pomeranian Medical University in Szczecin, 70-111 Szczecin, Poland; g.trybek@gmail.com
4. 4th Military Clinical Hospital in Wroclaw, ul. Rudolfa Weigla 5, 50-981 Wroclaw, Poland
5. Department of Maxillofacial Surgery, Medical University of Gdansk, 80-210 Gdańsk, Poland; adammichcik@gumed.edu.pl
* Correspondence: tomasz.wach@umed.lodz.pl; Tel.: +48-42-639-3422

Abstract: Background: Currently, the topic of dental implants is widely researched. However, still compromising are the factors that can affect implant loss as a consequence of marginal bone loss. One of the factors is smoking, which has a devastating effect on human health and bone structure. Oral health and jaw condition are also negatively affected by smoking. The aim of this study was to evaluate the peri-implant jawbone corticalization phenomenon in tobacco smokers. Methods: A total of 2196 samples from 768 patients with an implant in the neck area were checked, and texture features were analyzed. The corticalization phenomenon was investigated. All analyses were performed in MaZda Software. The influence of corticalization was investigated as a factor on bone structure near the implant neck. The statistical analysis included a feature distribution evaluation, mean (t-test) or median (W-test) comparison, analysis of regression and one-way analysis of variance or Kruskal–Wallis test as no normal distribution or between-group variance was indicated for the significant differences in the investigated groups. Detected differences or relationships were assumed to be statistically significant when $p < 0.05$. Results: The research revealed that MBL was correlated with smoking after 5 years (0.42 mm ± 1.32 mm 0 mm ± 1.25 mm), the Corticalization Index was higher in the smoker group on the day of surgery, and it became higher after 5y of observation (185.98 ± 90.8 and 243.17 ± 155.47). The implant-loss frequency was higher in the group of smokers, too, compared to non-smokers (6.74% and 2.87%). The higher the torque value during the implant placement, the higher the Corticalization Phenomenon Index. Conclusions: The research revealed a correlation between smoking and changes in bone structure in radio textures near the implants. The corticalization phenomenon is important, may be detected immediately after implant placement and may be one of the indicators of the implant success rate.

Keywords: bone remodeling; dental implant; smoking; torque; marginal bone loss; intraoral radiographs; radiomics; texture analysis

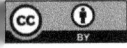

1. Introduction

Tobacco smoking has a devastating effect on human health and is one of the leading risks of early death. Smoking was the second risk factor for deaths in the world in 2019. Nearly 7.69 million people died because of this addiction [1–3]. There are many health disorders caused by smoking. For example, it increases the risk of many types of cancer and heart and lung diseases and increases the risk of pregnancy complications, oral cavity diseases, neuroticism (also in groups of e-cigarette smokers) and more [4–9]. Marginal bone loss is strongly connected with smoking and also with the degree of smoking [10–14]. On the other hand, it is not stated that tobacco smoking is an absolute contraindication for implant placement, but it is still associated with decreased dental implant surveys [14,15].

Bone metabolism is also disturbed directly and indirectly. Smoking directly decreases osteogenesis and angiogenesis and, through this, increases osteoclast cell activity and bone resorption occur. Indirectly, it causes decreased parathormone levels, estrogen production and levels of oxidants. It increases the level of cortisol, as well as free radicals. All of the above have an indirect negative effect on the balance of osteoblasts/osteoclasts activity [16–18], such as bisphosphonates' action [19–21]. Spine densitometry is one of the methods used to check and control the metabolism of human bone [22,23]. Previous studies observed a warning relation between marginal bone loss and the transformation of the bone surrounding dental implants toward corticalization [24,25]. The coexistence of these two phenomena may have an adverse effect on the long-term success of dental implant treatment.

This raised the question of whether a known negative factor (tobacco smoking) increases corticalization.

The aim of this study was to evaluate peri-implant jawbone corticalization in tobacco smokers.

2. Materials and Methods

This research is the result of analyses of prospective radiological data of oral implantological treatment of patients with dental loss.

The inclusion criteria were as follows: at least 18 years of age, bleeding upon gingival probing < 20%, probing depth ≤ 3 mm, good oral hygiene, regular follow-ups, two-dimensional radiographs taken during regular checks, laboratory tests to check vitamin levels and ions and hormones levels—parathormone (PTH, where the norm is 10 to 60 pg/mL); thyrotropin (TSH), where the norm is 0.23–4.0 µU/mL; calcium in serum (Ca^{2+}), where the norm is 9–11 mg/dL; glycated hemoglobin (HbA1c), where the norm is <5%; and vitamin 25(OH)D3 (D3), where the norm is 31–50 ng/mL. Patients smoking 1 or more cigarettes per day were qualified to be in the smoker group.

Spine densitometry, where the T-score can be examined, was also considered. The T-score shows the ratio between bone mineral density (BMD) of the examined patient and the average BMD for young patients. The normal value for normal bone is >-1.0, osteopenia is indicated by values between -1.0 and -2.5, and scores <-2.5 indicate osteoporosis (Table 1).

Table 1. Inclusion criteria for the research.

Inclusion Criteria
18 years of age
Bleeding upon gingival probing < 20%
Probing depth ≤ 3 mm
Good oral hygiene
Regular follow-ups
Two-dimensional radiographs taken during the regular check
Laboratory test: • PTH, where the norm is from 10 to 60 pg/mL; • TSH, where the norm is 0.23–4.0 µU/mL; • Calcium in serum (Ca^{2+}), where the norm is 9–11 mg/dL; • HbA1c, where the norm is <5%; • Vitamin 25(OH)D3 (D3), where the norm is 31–50 ng/mL.
Spine densitometry
Smoking 1 or more cigarettes per day

The exclusion criteria included a lack of or defective X-ray images in the visual assessment, lack of laboratory tests, uncontrolled internal co-morbidity (diabetes mellitus, thyroid dishormonoses, rheumatoid disease and other immunodeficiencies), a history of oral radiation therapy, past or current use of cytostatic drugs, soft and bone tissue augmentation, and low-quality or lack of follow-up radiographs. Finally, 2196 samples of a dental implant neck area (768 patients) were included in this study and analyzed (the average number of implants per patient was 2.86) (Table 2).

Table 2. Exclusion criteria for the research.

Exclusion Criteria
Lack of X-ray images
Defective X-ray images in the visual assessment
Lack of laboratory tests
Uncontrolled internal co-morbidity: • Diabetes mellitus; • Thyroid dishormonoses; • Rheumatoid disease; • Other immunodeficiencies.
History of oral radiation therapy
Past or current use of cytostatic drugs
Soft and bone tissue augmentation
Low-quality or lack of follow-up radiographs

Additionally, the following factors were considered: confidence level of 95%, margin error of 5%, population of 37 million and a fraction of 28.8%. In that case, the minimal sample size is 323 patients. Taking into account the amount of 768 patients, the error is on the level of 3%.

The limitation of the study is that the laboratory tests have not been carried out 3 months after the research (Table 3).

Table 3. Limitation of the research.

Limitations of the Study
Laboratory tests have not been carried out 3 months after the research.

Twenty-two types of dental implants were used in this study: AB Dental Devices I5 (www.ab-dent.com Ashdod, Israel; accessed on 21 July 2022); ADIN Dental Implants Touareg (www.adin-implants.com Afula, Israel; accessed on 21 July 2022); Alpha Bio ARRP (www.alpha-bio.net Petah-Tikva, Israel; accessed on 21 July 2022); Alpha Bio ATI (www.alpha-bio.net Petah-Tikva, Israel; accessed on 21 July 2022); Alpha Bio DFI (www.alpha-bio.net Petah-Tikva, Israel); Alpha Bio OCI (www.alpha-bio.net Petah-Tikva, Israel; accessed on 21 July 2022); Alpha Bio SFB (www.alpha-bio.net Petah-Tikva, Israel; accessed on 21 July 2022); Alpha Bio SPI (www.alpha-bio.net Petah-Tikva, Israel; accessed on 21 July 2022); Argon K3pro Rapid (www.argon-dental.de Bingen am Rhein, Germany; accessed on 21 July 2022); Bego Semados RI (www.bego-implantology.com Bremen, Germany; accessed on 21 July 2022); Dentium Super Line (www.dentium.com Gyeonggi-do, South Korea; accessed on 21 July 2022); Friadent Ankylos C/X (www.dentsplysirona.com Warszawa, Poland; accessed on 21 July 2022); Implant Direct InterActive (www.implantdirect.com Thousand Oaks, United States of America; accessed on 21 July 2022); Implant Direct Legacy 3 (www.implantdirect.com Thousand Oaks, United States of America; accessed on 21 July 2022); MIS BioCom M4 (www.mis-implants.com Bar-Lev Industrial Park, Israel; accessed on 21 July 2022); MIS C1 (www.mis-implants.com Bar-Lev Industrial Park, Israel; accessed on

21 July 2022); MIS Seven (www.mis-implants.com Bar-Lev Industrial Park, Israel; accessed on 21 July 2022); MIS UNO One Piece (www.mis-implants.com Bar-Lev Industrial Park, Israel; accessed on 21 July 2022); Osstem Implant Company GS III (www.en.osstem.com Seoul, South Korea; accessed on 21 July 2022); SGS Dental P7N (www.sgs-dental.com Schaan, Liechtenstein; accessed on 21 July 2022); TBR Implanté (www.tbr.dental Toulouse, France; accessed on 21 July 2022); and Wolf Dental Conical Screw-Type (www.wolf-dental. com Osnabrück, Germany; accessed on 21 July 2022) (Table 4).

Table 4. The implant types used and their features.

Implant Name	Titanium Alloy No.	Insertion Level	Connection Type	Connection Shape	Neck Shape	Neck Microthread	Body Shape	Body Thread	Apex Shape	Apex Hole	Apex Groove
AB Dental Devices I5	Grade 5	Bone level	Internal	Hexagon	Straight	No	Tapered	Square	Flat	No hole	Yes
ADIN Dental Implants Touareg	Grade 5	Bone level	Internal	Hexagon	Straight	Yes	Tapered	Square	Flat	No hole	Yes
Alpha Bio ATI	Grade 5	Bone level	Internal	Hexagon	Straight	Yes	Straight	Square	Flat	No hole	Yes
Alpha Bio OCI	Grade 5	Bone level	Internal	Hexagon	Straight	No	Straight	No Threads	Dome	Round	No
Alpha Bio DFI	Grade 5	Bone level	Internal	Hexagon	Straight	Yes	Tapered	Square	Flat	No hole	Yes
Alpha Bio SFB	Grade 5	Bone level	Internal	Hexagon	Straight	No	Tapered	V-shaped	Flat	No hole	Yes
Alpha Bio SPI	Grade 5	Bone level	Internal	Hexagon	Straight	Yes	Tapered	Square	Flat	No hole	Yes
Argon Medical Prod. K3pro Rapid	Grade 4	Subcrestal	Internal	Conical	Straight	Yes	Tapered	V-shaped	Dome	No hole	Yes
Bego Semados RI	Grade 4	Bone level	Internal	Hexagon	Straight	Yes	Tapered	Reverse buttress	Cone	No hole	Yes
Dentium Super Line	Grade 5	Bone level	Internal	Conical	Straight	No	Tapered	Buttress	Dome	No hole	Yes
Friadent Ankylos C/X	Grade 4	Subcrestal	Internal	Conical	Straight	No	Tapered	V-shaped	Dome	No hole	Yes
Implant Direct InterActive	Grade 5	Bone level	Internal	Conical	Straight	Yes	Tapered	Reverse buttress	Dome	No hole	Yes
Implant Direct Legacy 3	Grade 5	Bone level	Internal	Hexagon	Straight	Yes	Tapered	Reverse buttress	Dome	No hole	Yes
MIS BioCom M4	Grade 5	Bone level	Internal	Hexagon	Straight	No	Straight	V-shaped	Flat	No hole	Yes
MIS C1	Grade 5	Bone level	Internal	Conical	Straight	Yes	Tapered	Reverse buttress	Dome	No hole	Yes
MIS Seven	Grade 5	Bone level	Internal	Hexagon	Straight	Yes	Tapered	Reverse buttress	Dome	No hole	Yes
Osstem Implant Company GS III	Grade 5	Bone level	Internal	Conical	Straight	Yes	Tapered	V-shaped	Dome	No hole	Yes
SGS Dental P7N	Grade 5	Bone level	Internal	Hexagon	Straight	Yes	Tapered	V-shaped	Flat	No hole	Yes
TBR Implanté	Grade 5	Bone level	Internal	Octagon	Straight	No	Straight	No threads	Flat	Round	Yes
Wolf Dental Conical Screw-Type	Grade 4	Bone level	Internal	Hexagon	Straight	No	Tapered	V-shaped	Cone	No Hole	Yes

Surgery was performed under local anesthesia Artycaine + Adrenaline 1:100,000 by one surgeon (M.K) following the manufacturer-recommended protocols for dental implant placements. The healing process was carried out under a closed mucoperiosteal flap, unloaded in two-stage implants. Implants were loaded after 3 months of healing from the surgery.

Standardized intraoral radiographs were taken immediately after surgery (00M) every 3 months in the first year of healing, every 6 months in the second year and every year until 5 years of observation (5y). Radiographs were taken using the DIGORA OPTIME radiography system (TYPE DXR-50, SOREDEX, Helsinki, Finland). The RTG images were taken in a standardized way [26] with the following parameters: 7 mA, 70 mV, and 0.1 s (the focus apparatus was from Instrumentarium Dental, Tuusula, Finland). Positioners were used to take images repeatably with a 90° angle of X-ray beam to the surface of phosphor plate.

Radiologically recorded peri-implant bone structure was studied by digital texture analysis using the Corticalization Index previously proposed [25,27] (as version 1 (CI)). It consists of the product of a measure that evaluates the number of long series of pixels of similar optical density with the mean optical density of the studied site (in the numerator) and the magnitude of the chaotic arrangement of the texture pattern, i.e., differential entropy (in the denominator).

Marginal bone loss (MBL) was measured on radiological images [28] (Figure 1) by only one researcher. Texture of X-ray images was analyzed in MaZda 4.6 freeware invented by University of Technology in Lodz [29,30] to test measures of corticalization in peri-implant environment of trabecular bone (representing original bone before implant-dependent alterations) and soft tissue (representing product of marginal bone loss). MaZda provides both first-order (mean optical density) and second-order (Differential Entropy: DifEntr, Long-Run Emphasis Moment: LngREmph) data. Due to the fact that the second-order data are given for four directions in the image, and in the present study, the authors do not wish to search for directional features, the arithmetic mean of these four primary data was included for further analysis. The regions of interest (ROIs) were marked near the neck area (Figure 2) and normalized ($\mu \pm 3\sigma$) to share the same mean (μ) and standard deviation (σ) of optical density within the ROI. To eliminate noise, [26] further worked on data reduced to 6 bits. For analysis in a co-occurrence matrix, a spacing of 5 pixels was chosen. In the formulas that follow, p(i) is a normalized histogram vector (i.e., histogram whose entries are divided by the total number of pixels in ROI), i = 1, 2,..., Ng, and Ng denotes the number of optical density levels. Mean optical density feature (only a first-order feature) was calculated as below:

$$\text{Mean Optical Density} = \sum_{i=1}^{Ng} i p(i)$$

Second-order features:

$$\text{DifEntr} = -\sum_{i=1}^{Ng} p_{x-y}(i) \log(p_{x-y}(i))$$

where Σ is the sum; Ng is the number of levels of optical density in the radiograph; i and j are the optical density of pixels with a 5-pixel distance from one another; p is probability; and log is common logarithm [31]. The differential entropy calculated in this way is a measure of the overall scatter of bone structure elements in a radiograph. Its high values are typical for cancellous bone [32–35]. Next, the last primary texture feature was calculated:

$$\text{LngREmph} = \frac{\sum_{i=1}^{Ng} \sum_{k=1}^{Nr} k^2 p(i,k)}{\sum_{i=1}^{Ng} \sum_{k=1}^{Nr} p(i,k)}$$

where Σ is the sum; Nr is the number of series of pixels with density level i and length k; Ng is the number of levels for image optical density; Nr is the number of pixels in series; and p is probability [36,37]. This texture feature describes thick, uniformly dense, radio-opaque bone structures in intra-oral radiograph images [33,35].

$$\text{CI} = \frac{\text{LngREmph} \cdot \text{Mean Optical Density}}{\text{DifEntr}}$$

Statistical analysis includes feature distribution evaluation, mean (*t*-test) or median (W-test) comparison, analysis of regression and one-way analysis of variance or Kruskal–Wallis test as non-normal distribution or between-group variance indicated on significant differences in investigated groups. Detected differences or relationships were assumed to be statistically significant when $p < 0.05$. Statgraphics Centurion version 18.1.12 (StatPoint Technologies, Warrenton, VA, USA) was used for statistical analyses.

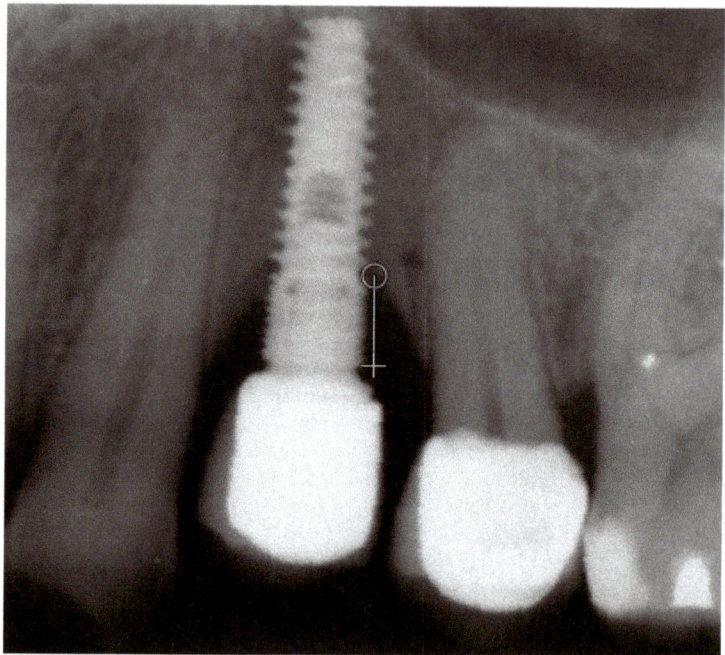

Figure 1. Measuring of marginal bone loss on the radiographic images 5 years after the functional loading. White line indicates the implant platform to the bottom of the bone loss cavity.

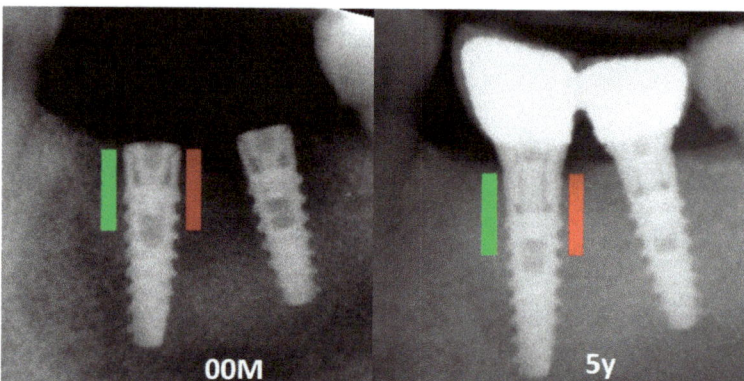

Figure 2. Marking an ROI. ROIs were marked near the implant neck area. Green area—mesial implant neck area; red area—distal implant neck area; Abbreviations: ROI—region of interest; 00M—0 months of observation; 5y—five years of observation.

3. Results

3.1. All Samples

Statistical examination revealed that the initial MBL for the mandible and maxilla in the non-smoker group of samples was lower than in the group with smokers, respectively (mean 0 mm ± 0.85 mm; 0 mm ± 1.13 mm), which was statistically significant ($p < 0.05$). MBL after 5 years of observation was also correlated with nicotinismus according to statistics where $p < 0.05$, meaning there was statistical significance: MBL for non-smokers (mean 0 mm ± 1.25 mm) and MBL for smokers (mean 0.42 mm ± 1.32 mm). Corticalization

Index for smokers and non-smokers was calculated immediately after the implant insertion and 5 years after the implantation; respectively, 185.98 ± 90.8 and 163.97 ± 151.9 for 00M; 243.17 ± 155.47 and 220.32 ± 184.97 after the 5 years. p value was lower than 0.05, which means it was statistically significant. Implant loss depending on MBL appearance after five years of observation was checked along with the value and analyzed for smokers and non-smoker group: 1.69 mm ± 1.73 mm and 0 mm ± 1.24 mm. p value was lower than 0.05. Implant loss frequency was checked. In a group of smokers, 6.74% of implants were lost; in a group of non-smoking patients, 2.87% of implants were lost, where the p value was lower than 0.05 (Table 5, Figure 3).

Table 5. Table presents values for marginal bone loss, values of Corticalization Index and implant loss frequency. Values were calculated for all the implantations for smokers and non-smokers. 00M—the observation period immediately after the implantation; 5y—the observation period 5 years after the implantation.

	Observation Period	Smoker	Non-Smoker	p Value
Smoking/Marginal Bone Loss	00M	0 mm ± 1.13 mm	0 mm ± 0.85 mm	$p < 0.05$
	5y	0.42 mm ± 1.32 mm	0 mm ± 1.25 mm	$p < 0.05$
Smoking/Corticalization Index	00M	185.98 ± 90.8	163.97 ± 151.9	$p < 0.05$
	5y	243.17 ± 155.47	220.32 ± 184.97	$p = 0.85$
Implant Loss to Marginal Bone Loss	5y	1.69 mm ± 1.73 mm	0 mm ± 1.24 mm	$p < 0.05$
Implant Loss Frequency	5y	6.74%	2.87%	$p < 0.05$

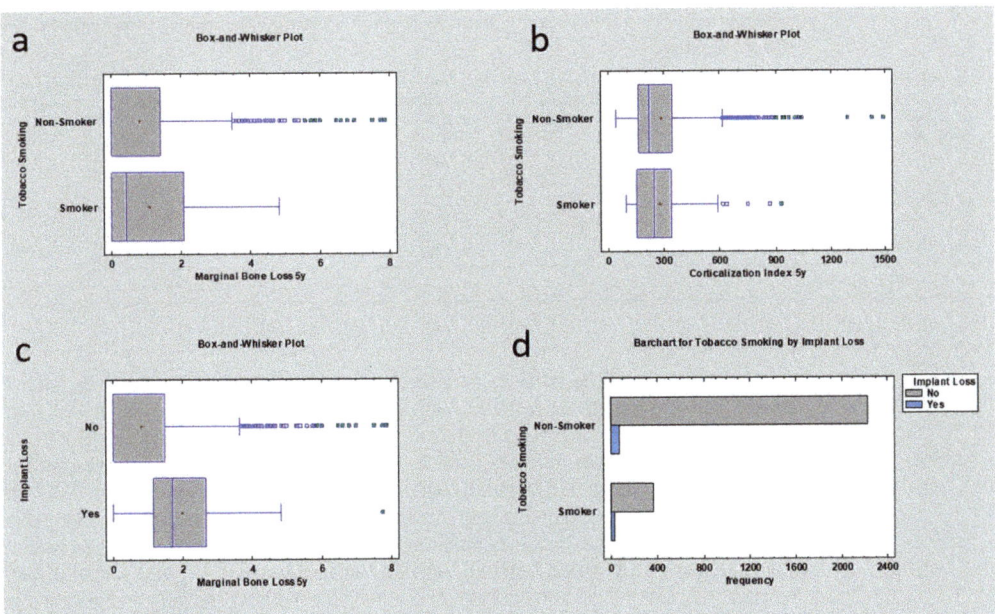

Figure 3. Dependences for all samples: (**a**) dependence of marginal bone loss from tobacco smoking after the dental implant insertion after 5 years of observation. The higher marginal bone loss was observed in the tobacco smoker group; (**b**) dependence of Corticalization Index from tobacco smoking after 5 years from implant insertion—there was no statistical difference; (**c**) dependence of implant loss from marginal bone loss after 5 years from functional loading—the higher marginal bone loss, the higher probability of implant loss; (**d**) frequency of implant loss depending on smoker or non-smoker group—the higher frequency was in the smoker group.

3.2. Mandible Group

Research revealed that the initial MBL for implants in the mandible in the non-smoker group was lower than in the group with smokers, respectively (mean 0 mm ± 0.88 mm; 0 mm ± 1.83 mm), which was statistically significant ($p < 0.05$). MBL after 5 years of observation was also correlated with nicotinismus according to statistics where $p < 0.05$, which means that there was statistical significance: MBL for non-smokers (mean 0 mm ± 1.09 mm) and MBL for smokers (mean 1.10 mm ± 1.46 mm). Corticalization Index for smokers and non-smokers in the mandible implants group was calculated after the implant insertion and 5 years after the implantation, respectively, 195.81 ± 68.8 and 193.27 ± 136.54 for 00M; 263.87 ± 130.7 and 298.02 ± 200.1 after the 5 years. p value was higher than 0.05, which means it was not statistically significant. Implant loss depended on MBL appearance after five years of observation in a group of mandible-inserted implants; the value was checked and analyzed for smokers and non-smoker group: 2.36 mm ± 0.94 mm and 0 mm ± 1.13 mm. p value was lower than 0.05. The relation between implant loss and the occurrence of corticalization was analyzed. Respectively, for smokers and non-smokers, values for initial corticalization were 183.62 ± 18 and 194.10 ± 131.65; 5 years after the implantation, values were 438.18 ± 341.70 for smokers and 292.40 ± 193.95 for non-smokers, and the p value was higher than 0.05. Implant loss frequency was also checked for mandible implants in relation to smoking. In a group of smokers, 1.66% of implants were lost; in a group of non-smoking patients, 1.25% of implants were lost; the relationship was weak, but the p value was still lower than 0.05 (Table 6, Figure 4).

Table 6. Table presents values for marginal bone loss, values of Corticalization Index and implant loss frequency. Values were calculated for implants in mandible for smokers and non-smokers. 00M—the observation period immediately after the implantation; 5y—the observation period 5 years after the implantation.

	Observation Period	Smoker	Non-Smoker	p Value
Smoking/Marginal Bone Loss	00M	0 mm ± 1.83 mm	0 mm ± 0.88 mm	$p < 0.05$
	5y	1.10 mm ± 1.46 mm	0 mm ± 1.09 mm	$p < 0.05$
Smoking/Corticalization Index	00M	195.81 ± 68.8	193.27 ± 136.54	$p = 0.85$
	5y	263.87 ± 130.7	298.02 ± 200.1	$p = 0.68$
Implant Loss to Marginal Bone Loss	5y	2.36 mm ± 0.94 mm	0 mm ± 1.13 mm	$p < 0.05$
Implant Loss Frequency	5y	1.66%	1.25%	$p < 0.05$

3.3. Maxilla Group

Implants in the maxilla were also examined separately. Statistics showed that the initial MBL for implants in the maxilla in the non-smoker group was lower than in the group with smokers, respectively (mean 0 mm ± 0.82 mm; 0 mm ± 2.38 mm), which was statistically significant ($p < 0.05$). MBL after 5 years of observation was also correlated with nicotinismus according to statistics where $p < 0.05$, meaning there was statistical significance: MBL for non-smokers (mean 0 mm ± 1.29 mm) and MBL for smokers (mean 1.42 mm ± 1.34 mm). The Corticalization Index for smokers and non-smokers in the maxilla implants group was calculated after implant insertion and 5 years after implantation; respectively, 173.50 ± 92.80 and 146.56 ± 109.65 for 00M, where the p value was lower than 0.05; 207.06 ± 153.50 and 193.68 ± 151.10 after 5 years. The p value was higher than 0.05, meaning there was no statistical significance. Implant loss, depending on MBL appearance after five years of observation in the group of maxilla inserted implants, was checked and analyzed for smokers and non-smoker groups: 1.42 mm ± 1.34 mm and 0 mm ± 1.29 mm. p value was lower than 0.05. In this group, the relation between implant loss and the occurrence of corticalization was also analyzed. Respectively, for smokers and non-smokers, values for initial corticalization were 173.56 ± 70.82 and 147.20 ± 109.40; and 5 years after implantation, 235.15 ± 268.71 for smokers and 193.67 ± 147.98 for non-smokers. The *p* value was higher than 0.05. Implant loss frequency was also checked for maxilla implants in relation to smoking. In the group of smokers, 4.34% of implants were lost; conversely, in the group of non-smoking patients, 1.49% of implants were lost. The relationship between smoking and implant loss was weak, but the *p* value was still lower than 0.05 (Table 7, Figure 5).

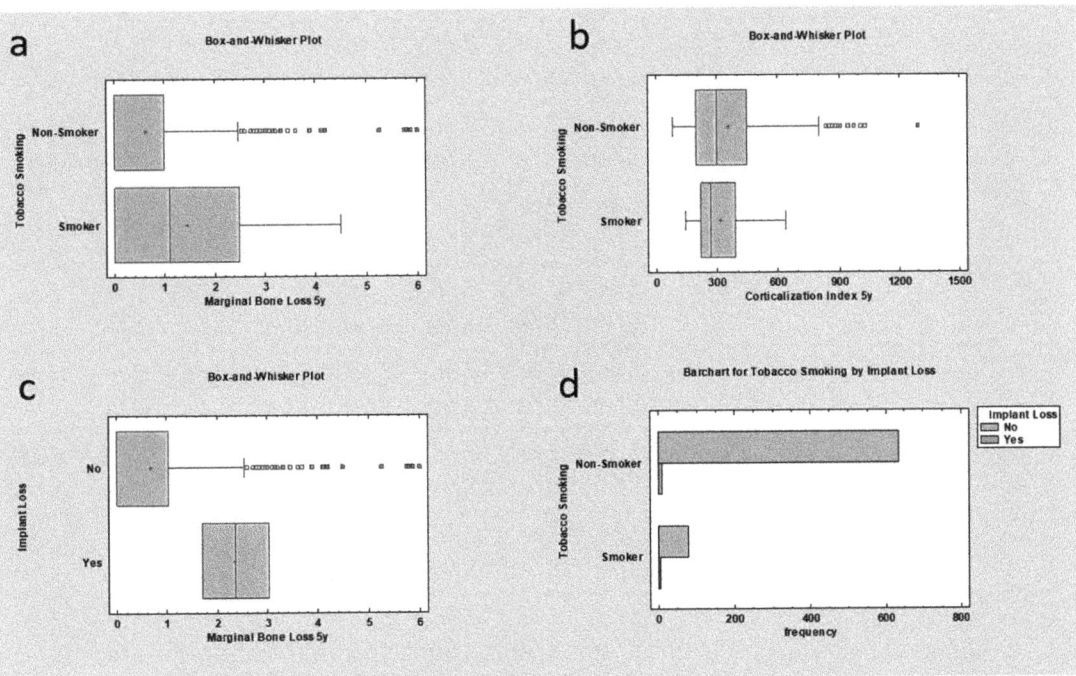

Figure 4. Dependencies for mandible samples: (**a**) dependence of marginal bone loss on tobacco smoking after the dental implant insertion after 5 years of observation. Higher marginal bone loss was observed in the tobacco smoker group; (**b**) dependence of the Corticalization Index on tobacco smoking 5 years after implant insertion—there was no statistical difference; (**c**) dependence of implant loss on marginal bone loss 5 years after functional loading—the higher the marginal bone loss, the higher probability of implant loss; (**d**) frequency of implant loss depending on the smoker or non-smoker group—the higher frequency was in the smoker group.

Table 7. This table presents values for marginal bone loss, Corticalization Index and implant loss frequency. Values were calculated for implants in maxilla for smokers and non-smokers. 00M—the observation period immediately after implantation; 5y—the observation period 5 years after implantation.

	Observation Period	Smoker	Non-Smoker	*p* Value
Smoking/Marginal Bone Loss	00M	0 mm ± 2.38 mm	0 mm ± 0.82 mm	$p < 0.05$
	5y	1.42 mm ± 1.34 mm	0 mm ± 1.29 mm	$p < 0.05$
Smoking/Corticalization Index	00M	173.50 ± 92.80	146.56 ± 109.65	$p < 0.05$
	5y	207.06 ± 153.50	193.68 ± 151.10	$p = 0.81$
Implant Loss to Marginal Bone Loss	5y	1.42 mm ± 1.34 mm	0 mm ± 1.29 mm	$p < 0.05$
Implant Loss Frequency	5y	4.34%	1.49%	$p < 0.05$

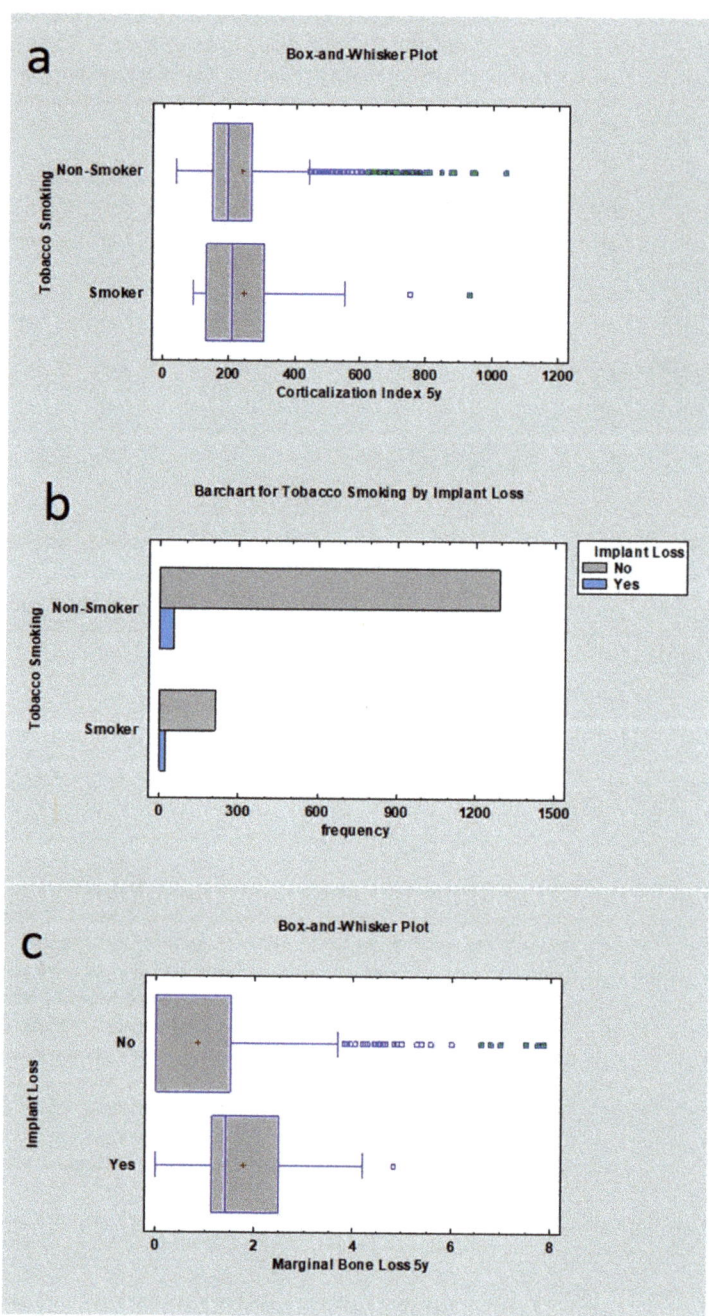

Figure 5. Dependencies for maxilla samples: (**a**) dependence of the Corticalization Index on tobacco smoking 5 years after implant insertion—there was no statistical difference; (**b**) frequency of implant loss depending on the smoker or non-smoker group—the higher frequency was in the smoker group; (**c**) dependence of implant loss on marginal bone loss a 5 years after functional loading—the higher the marginal bone loss, the higher the probability of implant loss.

3.4. Corticalization vs. Torque

The study also revealed a correlation between the Corticalization Index and the torque used during implant insertion (when the torque value was increasing), and the probability of occurrence of the corticalization phenomenon was also higher. The p value was lower than 0.05 (Figure 6).

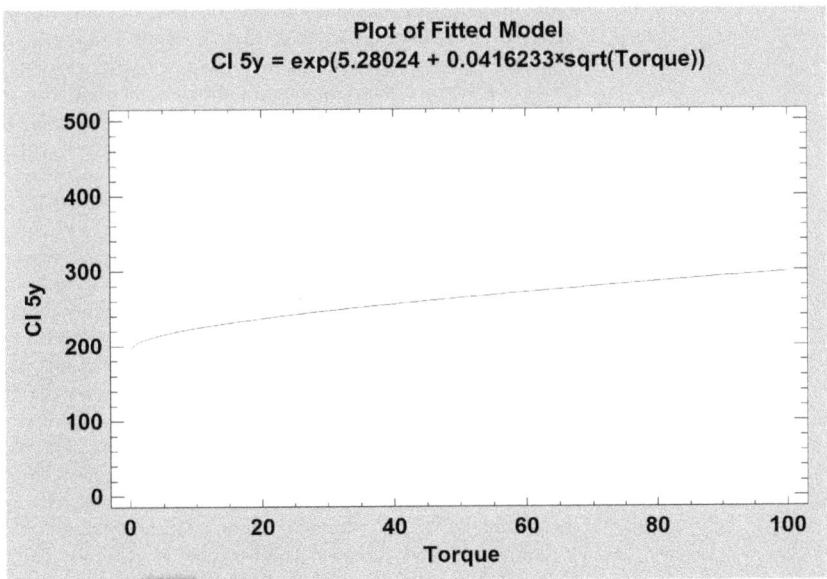

Figure 6. Dependence of the Corticalization Index on torque value after dental implant insertion, following 5 years of observation. The higher the torque during dental implantation, the higher the Corticalization Index after 5 years.

4. Discussion

The question that arises is the following: Is corticalization in radiographs associated with a higher risk of bone loss around dental implants in smoking patients? Until now, there have been no publications that can confirm or deny this. In this research, 768 patients with dental implants were studied, and 2196 samples of the neck implant area were analyzed. The study showed that the Corticalization Index is real and changes throughout the healing period, and the value of this index varies depending on the groups analyzed (smoking and non-smoking patients). The presented research shows that there is a close correlation between smoking and changes in bone structure. This correlation was calculated and discovered at the pixel level, taking into account texture features. Marginal bone loss has been analyzed many times, but no one has ever checked the bone structure and its relations to nicotinism at the pixel level [38–40].

Taking into account the corticalization phenomenon in all analyzed implants, a higher index was observed in the group of smokers already at the time of implantation (Table 5). A higher index of corticalization was observed in the group of smokers on the day of surgery, and a smaller index was observed in the group where patients did not smoke (bone changes at the pixel level were observed before implant placement, this may confirm that the tobacco smoking habit leads to undesirable changes in bone morphology). The Corticalization Index increases throughout the healing process. It was also observed in the mandible and maxilla separately, but in the case of the maxilla, the difference was greater. Corticalization is a process that changes the structure of the bone, where the trabecular bone is replaced by cortical bone. Remodeling depends on resorption and new bone formation [41–43].

Cancellous bone is composed of trabeculae with marrow between them. Corticalization is the process that changes trabecular bone into denser tissue—cortical [44].

Marginal bone loss is also correlated with nicotinismus, a fact that is commonly known and confirmed in this research. This study affirmed that marginal bone loss around dental implants is associated with tobacco smoking, as analyzed through radiographs and texture features in a large group of implants. Further research showed that MBL is higher in implants that were inserted in the maxilla in the smoker group, as opposed to implants inserted in the mandible. It can be concluded that smoking has an influence on bone structure before implantation and leads to a higher value of the Corticalization Index. The effect of this correlation may result in marginal bone loss. After five years of observation, the research showed that the higher the MBL, the greater the probability of implant loss in the smoking patients' group, which is indirectly correlated with the occurrence of the corticalization phenomenon [24,25,27].

Directly in statistics, there is no statistical significance between smoking and corticalization, but a similarity can be suspected. The Corticalization Index is consistent after 5 years. Smoking is a factor that can change the structure of bone tissue at the cellular level. Changes depend on disturbances in angiogenesis, impaired vascularization and nutrition of bone cells, with an impact on bone metabolism and osteogenesis. If the tissue is not nourished, it atrophies [45–48]. The study presented shows a close relationship between smoking and MBL and also between smoking and implant failure after 5 years of observation. The research emphasizes the impact of smoking on dental implant loss, mainly in the maxilla. Implant loss frequency was almost two times higher than in the case of mandible implants. All these correlations were detected at the pixel level using only texture features and by calculating and analyzing the Corticalization Index.

Additionally, the appearance of corticalization after 5 years of observation was also correlated with the increasing torque value during the implantation procedure. Recent studies have proved that a high value of torque during implant insertion leads to MBL [49–51]. There is a probability that condensed bone around the dental implant, caused by a high torque value, is not a desirable effect. Currently, the popular preparation method and implantation technique is osseodensification [52–54]. Osseodensification around dental implants increases the primary stability of the implant, but if corticalization may lead to peri-implantitis, marginal bone loss, and consequently dental implant loss, what will be the long-term consequences of densifying bone tissue next to the implant body? This phenomenon should be a focus of future research.

Taking into account the types of implants, it can be stated that not only the design of the dental implant affects the corticalization phenomenon. There is a relationship between bone condition, prosthetic restoration and also the surgeon's experience and preferences [24,55,56].

The corticalization phenomenon, as analyzed in this research, is closely related to smoking, marginal bone loss and implant loss. This phenomenon may be indicated before implant placement and also before marginal bone loss during the control periods when RTG images are taken. Considering the clinical relevance of this research, if there are enough studies about this phenomenon and it becomes well-known, it may become a useful tool for prognosis, contraindications and marginal bone loss prevention. Until now, there have been many tools, as mentioned above, but never at the pixel level [57–59].

Two-dimensional RTG images were taken in a defined period of observation. If the general condition of the patient changes, it may have an impact on bone structure. This can also be observed in the textures of RTG images. A limitation of this study was that laboratory tests were not checked after the implant insertion throughout the observation period. This should be taken into consideration in future research [60].

5. Conclusions

The higher Corticalization Index that occurs is related to tobacco smoking, even as early as the day of surgery. This is the latest study that confirms the close and non-beneficial impact of the corticalization phenomenon on the implant region, leading to peri-implantitis. This research demonstrated and proved that smoking tobacco has an impact on bone structure, which can be identified at the pixel level without clinical examination, using only two-dimensional radiographs.

The corticalization phenomenon may not be directly related to implant loss after 5 years of observation, but a relationship is observed between corticalization and marginal bone loss after 5 years, which may lead to peri-implantitis and implant loss.

The uniqueness of this research is that all these dependencies can be diagnosed by analyzing texture features in RTG images.

Author Contributions: Conceptualization, T.W. and G.T.; data curation, P.H. and T.W.; formal analysis, T.W.; funding acquisition, M.K.; investigation, P.H. and T.W.; methodology, T.W.; resources, T.W.; software T.W.; supervision, M.K.; validation, M.K.; visualization, A.M. and T.W.; writing—original draft, T.W.; writing—review and editing, T.W., M.K. and G.T. All authors have read and agreed to the published version of the manuscript.

Funding: This research was funded by the Medical University of Lodz (grant numbers 503/5-061-02/503-51-001-18, 503/5-061-02/503-51-001-17, and 503/5-061-02/503-51-002-18).

Institutional Review Board Statement: This study was conducted according to the guidelines of the Declaration of Helsinki and approved by the Institutional Ethics Committee of the Medical University of Lodz, PL (protocol no. RNN 485/11/KB and date of approval: 14 June 2011).

Informed Consent Statement: Informed consent was obtained from all subjects involved in the study.

Data Availability Statement: The data on which this study is based will be made available upon request at https://www.researchgate.net/profile/Tomasz-Wach.

Conflicts of Interest: The authors declare no conflict of interest.

References

1. Reitsma, M.B.; Kendrick, P.J.; Ababneh, E.; Abbafati, C.; Abbasi-Kangevari, M.; Abdoli, A.; Abedi, A.; Abhilash, E.S.; Abila, D.B.; Aboyans, V.; et al. Spatial, temporal, and demographic patterns in prevalence of smoking tobacco use and attributable disease burden in 204 countries and territories, 1990–2019: A systematic analysis from the Global Burden of Disease Study 2019. *Lancet* **2021**, *397*, 2337–2360. [CrossRef] [PubMed]
2. Yanbaeva, D.G.; Dentener, M.A.; Creutzberg, E.C.; Wesseling, G.; Wouters, E.F.M. Systemic Effects of Smoking. *Chest* **2007**, *131*, 1557–1566. [CrossRef] [PubMed]
3. Onor, I.O.; Stirling, D.L.; Williams, S.R.; Bediako, D.; Borghol, A.; Harris, M.B.; Darensburg, T.B.; Clay, S.D.; Okpechi, S.C.; Sarpong, D.F. Clinical effects of cigarette smoking: Epidemiologic impact and review of pharmacotherapy options. *Int. J. Environ. Res. Public Health* **2017**, *14*, 1147. [CrossRef] [PubMed]
4. Afolalu, E.F.; Spies, E.; Bacso, A.; Clerc, E.; Abetz-Webb, L.; Gallot, S.; Chrea, C. Impact of tobacco and/or nicotine products on health and functioning: A scoping review and findings from the preparatory phase of the development of a new self-report measure. *Harm Reduct. J.* **2021**, *18*, 79. [CrossRef] [PubMed]
5. Wyszyńska-Pawelec, G.; Gontarz, M.; Zapała, J.; Szuta, M. Minor Salivary Gland Tumours of Upper Aerodigestive Tract: A Clinicopathological Study. *Gastroenterol. Res. Pract.* **2012**, *2012*, 780453. [CrossRef] [PubMed]
6. Trybek, G.; Preuss, O.; Aniko-Wlodarczyk, M.; Kuligowski, P.; Gabrysz-Trybek, E.; Suchanecka, A. The effect of nicotine on oral health. *Balt. J. Health Phys. Act.* **2018**, *10*, 7–13. [CrossRef]
7. Suchanecka, A.; Chmielowiec, K.; Chmielowiec, J.; Trybek, G.; Masiak, J.; Michałowska-Sawczyn, M.; Nowicka, R.; Grocholewicz, K.; Grzywacz, A. Vitamin D Receptor Gene Polymorphisms and Cigarette Smoking Impact on Oral Health: A Case-Control Study. *Int. J. Environ. Res. Public Health* **2020**, *17*, 3192. [CrossRef]
8. Grzywacz, A.; Suchanecka, A.; Chmielowiec, J.; Chmielowiec, K.; Szumilas, K.; Masiak, J.; Balwicki, Ł.; Michałowska-Sawczyn, M.; Trybek, G. Personality Traits or Genetic Determinants—Which Strongly Influences E-Cigarette Users? *Int. J. Environ. Res. Public Health* **2020**, *17*, 365. [CrossRef]
9. Aredo, J.V.; Luo, S.J.; Gardner, R.M.; Sanyal, N.; Choi, E.; Hickey, T.P.; Riley, T.L.; Huang, W.-Y.; Kurian, A.W.; Leung, A.N.; et al. Tobacco Smoking and Risk of Second Primary Lung Cancer. *J. Thorac. Oncol.* **2021**, *16*, 968–979. [CrossRef]
10. Ali, A.; Al Attar, A.; Chrcanovic, B.R. Frequency of Smoking and Marginal Bone Loss around Dental Implants: A Retrospective Matched-Control Study. *J. Clin. Med.* **2023**, *12*, 1386. [CrossRef]
11. Lindquist, L.; Carlsson, G.; Jemt, T. Association between Marginal Bone Loss around Osseointegrated Mandibular Implants and Smoking Habits: A 10-year Follow-up Study. *J. Dent. Res.* **1997**, *76*, 1667–1674. [CrossRef] [PubMed]

12. Chrcanovic, B.R.; Albrektsson, T.; Wennerberg, A. Smoking and dental implants: A systematic review and meta-analysis. *J. Dent.* **2015**, *43*, 487–498. [CrossRef] [PubMed]
13. Radi, I.A.E.; Elsayyad, A.A. Smoking Might Increase the Failure Rate and Marginal Bone Loss around Dental Implants. *J. Evid.-Based Dent. Pract.* **2022**, *22*, 101804. [CrossRef]
14. Dinesh; Nazeer, J.; Singh, R.; Suri, P.; Mouneshkumar, C.; Bhardwaj, S.; Iqubal, M. Evaluation of marginal bone loss around dental implants in cigarette smokers and nonsmokers. A comparative study. *J. Fam. Med. Prim. Care* **2020**, *9*, 729–734. [CrossRef]
15. Mumcu, E.; Beklen, A. The effect of smoking on the marginal bone loss around implant-supported prostheses. *Tob. Induc. Dis.* **2019**, *17*, 43. [CrossRef] [PubMed]
16. Al-Bashaireh, A.M.; Haddad, L.G.; Weaver, M.; Chengguo, X.; Kelly, D.L.; Yoon, S. The Effect of Tobacco Smoking on Bone Mass: An Overview of Pathophysiologic Mechanisms. *J. Osteoporos.* **2018**, *2018*, 1206235. [CrossRef]
17. Yoon, V.; Maalouf, N.M.; Sakhaee, K. The effects of smoking on bone metabolism. *Osteoporos. Int.* **2012**, *23*, 2081–2092. [CrossRef]
18. Bonfiglio, R.; Tarantino, U.; Weng, W.; Li, H.; Zhu, S. An Overlooked Bone Metabolic Disorder: Cigarette Smoking-Induced Osteoporosis. *Genes* **2022**, *13*, 806. [CrossRef]
19. Wiesner, A.; Szuta, M.; Galanty, A.; Paśko, P. Optimal Dosing Regimen of Osteoporosis Drugs in Relation to Food Intake as the Key for the Enhancement of the Treatment Effectiveness—A Concise Literature Review. *Foods* **2021**, *10*, 720. [CrossRef]
20. Drake, M.T.; Clarke, B.L.; Khosla, S. Bisphosphonates: Mechanism of Action and Role in Clinical Practice. *Mayo Clin. Proc.* **2008**, *83*, 1032–1045. [CrossRef]
21. Lomashvili, K.A.; Monier-Faugere, M.-C.; Wang, X.; Malluche, H.H.; O'Neill, W.C. Effect of bisphosphonates on vascular calcification and bone metabolism in experimental renal failure. *Kidney Int.* **2009**, *75*, 617–625. [CrossRef] [PubMed]
22. Miller, P.D.; Zapalowski, C.; Kulak, C.A.M.; Bilezikian, J.P. Bone Densitometry: The Best Way to Detect Osteoporosis and to Monitor Therapy. *J. Clin. Endocrinol. Metab.* **1999**, *84*, 1867–1871. [CrossRef]
23. Chun, K.J. Bone densitometry. *Semin. Nucl. Med.* **2011**, *41*, 220–228. [CrossRef] [PubMed]
24. Kozakiewicz, M.; Wach, T. Exploring the Importance of Corticalization Occurring in Alveolar Bone Surrounding a Dental Implant. *J. Clin. Med.* **2022**, *11*, 7189. [CrossRef]
25. Kozakiewicz, M.; Skorupska, M.; Wach, T. What Does Bone Corticalization around Dental Implants Mean in Light of Ten Years of Follow-Up? *J. Clin. Med.* **2022**, *11*, 3545. [CrossRef] [PubMed]
26. Kozakiewicz, M.; Bogusiak, K.; Hanclik, M.; Denkowski, M.; Arkuszewski, P. Noise in subtraction images made from pairs of intraoral radiographs: A comparison between four methods of geometric alignment. *Dentomaxillofacial Radiol.* **2008**, *37*, 40–46. [CrossRef]
27. Kozakiewicz, M. Measures of Corticalization. *J. Clin. Med.* **2022**, *11*, 5463. [CrossRef]
28. Kwiatek, J.; Jaroń, A.; Trybek, G. Impact of the 25-Hydroxycholecalciferol Concentration and Vitamin D Deficiency Treatment on Changes in the Bone Level at the Implant Site during the Process of Osseointegration: A Prospective, Randomized, Controlled Clinical Trial. *J. Clin. Med.* **2021**, *10*, 526. [CrossRef]
29. Szczypiński, P.M.; Strzelecki, M.; Materka, A.; Klepaczko, A. MaZda-A software package for image texture analysis. *Comput. Methods Programs Biomed.* **2009**, *94*, 66–76. [CrossRef]
30. Szczypiński, P.M.; Strzelecki, M.; Materka, A.; Klepaczko, A. MaZda—The Software Package for Textural Analysis of Biomedical Images. In *Computers in Medical Activity*; Springer: Berlin/Heidelberg, Germany, 2009; pp. 73–84. [CrossRef]
31. Linkevicius, T.; Puisys, A.; Linkevicius, R.; Alkimavicius, J.; Gineviciute, E.; Linkeviciene, L. The influence of submerged healing abutment or subcrestal implant placement on soft tissue thickness and crestal bone stability. A 2-year randomized clinical trial. *Clin. Implant. Dent. Relat. Res.* **2020**, *22*, 497–506. [CrossRef]
32. Wach, T.; Kozakiewicz, M. Are recent available blended collagen-calcium phosphate better than collagen alone or crystalline calcium phosphate? Radiotextural analysis of a 1-year clinical trial. *Clin. Oral Investig.* **2021**, *25*, 3711–3718. [CrossRef] [PubMed]
33. Kozakiewicz, M.; Szymor, P.; Wach, T. Influence of General Mineral Condition on Collagen-Guided Alveolar Crest Augmentation. *Materials* **2020**, *13*, 3649. [CrossRef] [PubMed]
34. Kozakiewicz, M.; Wach, T. New Oral Surgery Materials for Bone Reconstruction—A Comparison of Five Bone Substitute Materials for Dentoalveolar Augmentation. *Materials* **2020**, *13*, 2935. [CrossRef] [PubMed]
35. Wach, T.; Kozakiewicz, M. Fast-Versus Slow-Resorbable Calcium Phosphate Bone Substitute Materials—Texture Analysis after 12 Months of Observation. *Materials* **2020**, *13*, 3854. [CrossRef] [PubMed]
36. Haralick, R.M. Statistical and structural approaches to texture. *Proc. IEEE* **1979**, *67*, 786–804. [CrossRef]
37. Materka, A.S.M. Texture analysis methods—A review, COST B11 report. In *MC Meeting and Workshop*; Technical University of Lodz, Institute of Electronics: Belgium, Brussels, 1998.
38. Bahrami, G.; Væth, M.; Kirkevang, L.; Wenzel, A.; Isidor, F. The impact of smoking on marginal bone loss in a 10-year prospective longitudinal study. *Community Dent. Oral Epidemiol.* **2016**, *45*, 59–65. [CrossRef]
39. Jansson, L.; Lavstedt, S. Influence of smoking on marginal bone loss and tooth loss—A prospective study over 20 years. *J. Clin. Periodontol.* **2002**, *29*, 750–756. [CrossRef]
40. Afshari, Z.; Yaghini, J.; Naseri, R. Levels of Smoking and Peri-Implant Marginal Bone Loss: A Systematic Review and Meta-Analysis. *J. Évid. Based Dent. Pr.* **2022**, *22*, 101721. [CrossRef]
41. Filipowska, J.; Tomaszewski, K.A.; Niedźwiedzki, Ł.; Walocha, J.A.; Niedźwiedzki, T. The role of vasculature in bone development, regeneration and proper systemic functioning. *Angiogenesis* **2017**, *20*, 291–302. [CrossRef]

42. Siddiqui, J.A.; Partridge, N.C. Physiological Bone Remodeling: Systemic Regulation and Growth Factor Involvement. *Physiology* **2016**, *31*, 233–245. [CrossRef]
43. Lin, D.; Li, Q.; Li, W.; Swain, M. Dental implant induced bone remodeling and associated algorithms. *J. Mech. Behav. Biomed. Mater.* **2009**, *2*, 410–432. [CrossRef] [PubMed]
44. Mustapha, A.D.; Salame, Z.; Chrcanovic, B.R. Smoking and Dental Implants: A Systematic Review and Meta-Analysis. *Medicina* **2021**, *58*, 39. [CrossRef] [PubMed]
45. Monier-Faugere, M.C.; Chris Langub, M.; Malluche, H.H. Chapter 8—Bone Biopsies: A Modern Approach. In *Metabolic Bone Disease and Clinically Related Disorders*, 3rd ed.; Avioli, L.V., Krane, S.M., Eds.; Academic Press: San Diego, CA, USA, 1998; pp. 237–280. Available online: https://www.sciencedirect.com/science/article/pii/B9780120687008500098 (accessed on 2 September 2007).
46. Tarantino, U.; Cariati, I.; Greggi, C.; Gasbarra, E.; Belluati, A.; Ciolli, L.; Maccauro, G.; Momoli, A.; Ripanti, S.; Falez, F.; et al. Skeletal System Biology and Smoke Damage: From Basic Science to Medical Clinic. *Int. J. Mol. Sci.* **2021**, *22*, 6629. [CrossRef] [PubMed]
47. Robling, A.; Duijvelaar, K.; Geevers, J.; Ohashi, N.; Turner, C. Modulation of appositional and longitudinal bone growth in the rat ulna by applied static and dynamic force. *Bone* **2001**, *29*, 105–113. [CrossRef] [PubMed]
48. Chang, C.-J.; Jou, I.-M.; Wu, T.-T.; Su, F.-C.; Tai, T.-W. Cigarette smoke inhalation impairs angiogenesis in early bone healing processes and delays fracture union. *Bone Jt. Res.* **2020**, *9*, 99–107. [CrossRef]
49. Wach, T.; Skorupska, M.; Trybek, G. Are Torque-Induced Bone Texture Alterations Related to Early Marginal Jawbone Loss? *J. Clin. Med.* **2022**, *11*, 6158. [CrossRef]
50. Aldahlawi, S.; Demeter, A.; Irinakis, T. The effect of implant placement torque on crestal bone remodeling after 1 year of loading. *Clin. Cosmet. Investig. Dent.* **2018**, *10*, 203–209. [CrossRef]
51. Barone, A.; Alfonsi, F.; Derchi, G.; Tonelli, P.; Toti, P.; Marchionni, S.; Covani, U. The Effect of Insertion Torque on the Clinical Outcome of Single Implants: A Randomized Clinical Trial. *Clin. Implant. Dent. Relat. Res.* **2015**, *18*, 588–600. [CrossRef]
52. Mahesh, L.; Poonia, N. *Osseodensification with Densah Burs*; Jaypee Digital: London, UK, 2018; p. 287. [CrossRef]
53. El-Hawary, H. A Novel Osseodensification Technique for Dental Implant Placement in Osteoporotic Patients (A Clinical Prospective Study). *Egypt. J. Oral Maxillofac. Surg.* **2020**, *11*, 118–123. [CrossRef]
54. Lahens, B.; Lopez, C.D.; Neiva, R.F.; Bowers, M.M.; Jimbo, R.; Bonfante, E.A.; Morcos, J.; Witek, L.; Tovar, N.; Coelho, P.G. The effect of osseodensification drilling for endosteal implants with different surface treatments: A study in sheep. *J. Biomed. Mater. Res. Part B Appl. Biomater.* **2018**, *107*, 615–623. [CrossRef]
55. Van de Velde, T.; Collaert, B.; Sennerby, L.; De Bruyn, H. Effect of Implant Design on Preservation of Marginal Bone in the Mandible. *Clin. Implant. Dent. Relat. Res.* **2009**, *12*, 134–141. [CrossRef] [PubMed]
56. Ormianer, Z.; Matalon, S.; Block, J.; Kohen, J. Dental Implant Thread Design and the Consequences on Long-Term Marginal Bone Loss. *Implant. Dent.* **2016**, *25*, 471–477. [CrossRef] [PubMed]
57. Raikar, S.; Talukdar, P.; Kumari, S.; Panda, S.K.; Oommen, V.M.; Prasad, A. Factors affecting the survival rate of dental implants: A retrospective study. *J. Int. Soc. Prev. Community Dent.* **2017**, *7*, 351–355. [CrossRef] [PubMed]
58. Yang, Y.; Hu, H.; Zeng, M.; Chu, H.; Gan, Z.; Duan, J.; Rong, M. The survival rates and risk factors of implants in the early stage: A retrospective study. *BMC Oral Health* **2021**, *21*, 293. [CrossRef]
59. Tolstunov, L. Implant Zones of the Jaws: Implant Location and Related Success Rate. *J. Oral Implant.* **2007**, *33*, 211–220. [CrossRef]
60. Health, B.A. Report of the Surgeon General. Available online: http://www.surgeongeneral.gov/library (accessed on 31 December 2004).

Disclaimer/Publisher's Note: The statements, opinions and data contained in all publications are solely those of the individual author(s) and contributor(s) and not of MDPI and/or the editor(s). MDPI and/or the editor(s) disclaim responsibility for any injury to people or property resulting from any ideas, methods, instructions or products referred to in the content.

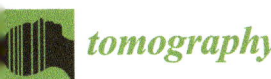

Article

Detection and Quantitative Assessment of Arthroscopically Proven Long Biceps Tendon Pathologies Using T2 Mapping

Patrick Stein [1,*], Felix Wuennemann [1,2], Thomas Schneider [1], Felix Zeifang [3,4], Iris Burkholder [5], Marc-André Weber [6], Hans-Ulrich Kauczor [1] and Christoph Rehnitz [1]

1. Diagnostic and Interventional Radiology, University Hospital Heidelberg, Im Neuenheimer Feld 420, 69120 Heidelberg, Germany
2. Institute of Diagnostic and Interventional Radiology & Neuroradiology, Helios Dr. Horst Schmidt Clinics Wiesbaden, Ludwig-Erhard-Straße 100, 65199 Wiesbaden, Germany
3. Center for Orthopedics, Trauma Surgery and Spinal Cord Injury, University Hospital Heidelberg, Schlierbacher Landstraße 200A, 69118 Heidelberg, Germany
4. Ethianum Clinic Heidelberg, Voßstraße 6, 69115 Heidelberg, Germany
5. Department of Nursing and Health, University of Applied Sciences of the Saarland, 66117 Saarbruecken, Germany
6. Institute of Diagnostic and Interventional Radiology, Pediatric Radiology and Neuroradiology, University Medical Center Rostock, Ernst-Heydemann-Straße 6, 18057 Rostock, Germany
* Correspondence: patrick.stein@med.uni-heidelberg.de

Abstract: This study evaluates how far T2 mapping can identify arthroscopically confirmed pathologies in the long biceps tendon (LBT) and quantify the T2 values in healthy and pathological tendon substance. This study comprised eighteen patients experiencing serious shoulder discomfort, all of whom underwent magnetic resonance imaging, including T2 mapping sequences, followed by shoulder joint arthroscopy. Regions of interest were meticulously positioned on their respective T2 maps, capturing the sulcal portion of the LBT and allowing for the quantification of the average T2 values. Subsequent analyses included the calculation of diagnostic cut-off values, sensitivities, and specificities for the detection of tendon pathologies, and the calculation of inter-reader correlation coefficients (ICCs) involving two independent radiologists. The average T2 value for healthy subjects was measured at 23.3 ± 4.6 ms, while patients with tendinopathy displayed a markedly higher value, at 47.9 ± 7.8 ms. Of note, the maximum T2 value identified in healthy tendons (29.6 ms) proved to be lower than the minimal value measured in pathological tendons (33.8 ms), resulting in a sensitivity and specificity of 100% (95% confidence interval 63.1–100) across all cut-off values ranging from 29.6 to 33.8 ms. The ICCs were found to range from 0.93 to 0.99. In conclusion, T2 mapping is able to assess and quantify healthy LBTs and can distinguish them from tendon pathology. T2 mapping may provide information on the (ultra-)structural integrity of tendinous tissue, facilitating early diagnosis, prompt therapeutic intervention, and quantitative monitoring after conservative or surgical treatments of LBT.

Keywords: T2 mapping; long biceps tendon; tendinopathy; arthroscopy

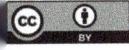

1. Introduction

Shoulder pain is a common clinical issue and a known cause of disability, which can lead to significant functional impairment and thereby compromise the overall quality of patients' lives [1,2]. Pathologies of the long biceps head tendon (LBT) are a significant source of shoulder pain, not only because of their association with other shoulder injuries, but also because of their tendency to become chronic [3,4]. In addition to middle-aged or older adults, overhead athletes are also known to be at risk for developing LBT tendinopathy, making them particularly susceptible to chronic shoulder pain given their usually young age [5,6].

In addition to clinical examination, imaging techniques, especially non-contrast magnetic resonance imaging (MRI), are central to the evaluation of the shoulder joint. While a variety of common shoulder pathologies can be detected via MRI with relatively high diagnostic accuracy, several studies have reported suboptimal diagnostic performance regarding pathologies of the LBT, which are usually visualized in more advanced stages of tendinopathy or rupture [7–10]. In an arthroscopy-controlled study, Dubrow et al. reported a sensitivity of only 56.3% for non-contrast MRI in detecting complete LBT tears [11]. The diagnostic performance in detecting partial tears was even lower, with a sensitivity of 27.7%. As reported by Tadros et al. and De Maeseneer et al., even the additional performance of MR arthrography did not show improvement in the detection of LBT pathologies, with sensitivities ranging from 15 to 38% [12,13]. In addition, the visualization of LBT may be difficult in conventional 2D MRI sequences due to the arcuate course of the tendon through the glenoid joint in conjunction with its typically small size when using slice thicknesses of 3 mm, making it susceptible to imaging artifacts such as the partial volume effect. Early LBT pathologies can only be detected to a very limited extent by means of common morphological MRI sequences, and a diagnostic tool for early diagnosis is lacking, which appear to be even more problematic, as tendon degeneration seems to be a chronically progressive process [14,15].

Functional MRI sequences, such as T2 or T2* mapping, have mainly been used for the evaluation of ultrastructural changes affecting the collagen network of articular cartilage and have been shown to detect and quantify early degenerative changes in various joints [16–18]. Because changes in proteoglycans, and thus, water content are known histologic signs of early osteoarthritis (OA), quantitative MRI sequences with measurements of the T2 relaxation time have been investigated in previous studies of OA and its progression [19,20]. In view of the promising results, these sequences were also included in a multicenter longitudinal study called the Osteoarthritis Initiative, which found an association between elevated T2 values and knee pain along with early signs of OA [21]. In addition to joint degeneration, Kasar et al. reported increased T2 values in the sacroiliac joints of patients with active and even inactive axial spondyloarthropathies, making T2 mapping sequences potentially useful for detecting inflammation-related tissue changes [22]. Since microscopic mucoid degeneration and disruption of the 3D collagen network in tendinopathic LBT specimens have been reported as histopathological correlates of hyperintense signal changes in T2-weighted sequences, T2 mapping might also be a viable tool for assessing and especially quantifying damages to tendinous structures [23]. To our knowledge, T2 mapping has rarely been systematically studied for the assessment of LBTs or tendons in general, and the few existing studies have not yet validated this technique using arthroscopy [24,25].

Thus, the purpose of this study was to investigate the ability of T2 mapping to detect arthroscopically proven pathologies of the long biceps tendon and to quantify the correlating T2 values for damaged and healthy tendons.

2. Materials and Methods

2.1. Participants and Inclusion

Over a period of three months, this study enrolled 19 consecutive patients with shoulder pain who were referred to our radiology department for preoperative MRI assessments between September and November 2017. MRI and shoulder arthroscopy were indicated when the patient complained of significant shoulder pain, severe enough to interfere with activities of daily living, and for which conservative therapy, including physical therapy and analgesic medications, did not improve the overall pain level. In patients with negative MRI examination, the indication for exploratory shoulder arthroscopy was based on the combination of symptom severity, clinical examination, and ineffective conservative therapy. Patients with endoprosthetic joint replacement or osteosynthetic material at the proximal humerus, advanced osteoarthritis (OA; Kellgren–Lawrence score >1), a previous shoulder joint surgery, or an age of less than 18 years were excluded from the study. In addition, one patient was excluded who mistakenly underwent a routine MRI protocol without T2 mapping sequences, leaving 18 patients for inclusion in the study. The study was approved by the Institutional Review Board of Heidelberg University (S-081/2010) and was conducted in accordance with the Declaration of Helsinki. Written informed consent was obtained from all patients after they were informed of the nature of the examination.

2.2. Study Design

After enrollment, each participant underwent the index test, which included a T2 mapping MRI sequence at 3 Tesla. Subsequently, the reference examination, a shoulder arthroscopy, was performed within a maximum period of 6 days (mean: 4 days). Based on the arthroscopy findings, the study population was divided into two subgroups: "healthy subjects" and "patients with confirmed LBT pathology". With respect to item 5 from the latest version of the STARD guidelines published by the EQUATOR network (Centre for Statistics in Medicine (CSM), NDORMS, University of Oxford, Oxford, UK) in 2015, this study can, therefore, be defined as a prospective observational study [26].

2.3. MRI Protocol and T2 Mapping

Each participant underwent imaging with a 3-Tesla MRI system with a 70 cm wide gantry and an 18-channel imaging matrix (Magnetom Verio, Siemens Healthineers, Erlangen, Germany). The examination was conducted in the supine position with the shoulder joints kept stabilized in external rotation to ensure that the joint was positioned as isocentrically as possible. A standard house-internal MRI protocol was used to morphologically assess the joint structures, including the proton density-weighted fat-saturated sequences as well as the T1- and T2-weighted sequences without fat saturation. For the acquisition of the oblique coronal views, the sequences were acquired perpendicular to the glenoid fossa, whereas the oblique sagittal sequences were aligned parallel to the glenoid articular surface. A manufacturer-supplied oblique coronal multiecho spin-echo T2 mapping sequence (syngo MapIT, Siemens Healthineers, Erlangen, Germany) was used as the primary sequence of interest. In this sequence, a pixel-by-pixel, monoexponential, non-negative least squares analysis was conducted to determine the T2 relaxation times from the T2 parameters. This analysis resulted in a color-coded T2 map, which could then be used for subsequent analysis.

The MRI protocol used in this study represents our in-house standard protocol augmented by the T2 mapping study sequence, and is based on a previous study by our research group investigating the diagnostic performance of T2 mapping with respect to the detection of superior labral anterior to posterior (SLAP) lesions [27]. For more details on the MRI study protocol and the T2 mapping sequence, see Table 1.

2.4. Image Analysis and Definition of LBT Pathologies

A picture archiving and communication system (Centricity PACS, v. 4.0; GE Healthcare IT Solutions, Barrington, IL, USA) was used to evaluate the morphologic sequences by two independent radiologists with 19 (CR) and 6 (FW) years of experience in musculoskeletal MRI. Both gained experience in the MRI evaluation of the shoulder joint through several training courses as well as by participation in previous studies with functional and quantitative MRI imaging techniques for (fibro)cartilaginous structures. The parameters for slice selection, magnification, and windowing were set by both radiologists, and the ambient light was minimized during the reading sessions. To ensure objectivity, the patients' names, clinical data, arthroscopy results, and ratings from the other reader were blinded for both radiologists. As all study participants were informed about the additional study sequence and their upcoming shoulder arthroscopy, they were not blinded.

Table 1. In-house shoulder MRI protocol and T2 mapping study sequence.

No.	Sequence	Orientation	Repetition Time (TR; ms)	EchoTime (TE; ms)	Acquisition Matrix	Flip Angle	Echo Train Length	No. of Slices	TA (min)	Slices (mm)
1	PD FS TSE	axial	3660	24	384 × 346	176	7	27	04:32	3
2	PD FS TSE	oblique coronal	2490	24	384 × 307	160	7	19	03:37	3
3	PD FS TSE	oblique sagittal	3950	23	320 × 256	140	7	29	04:49	3
4	PD TSE	oblique coronal	1670	23	384 × 307	160	5	19	03:24	3
5	T1 SE	oblique coronal	787	10	384 × 346	90	1	19	04:51	3
6	T2 TSE	oblique sagittal	5640	88	384 × 307	150	15	29	02:33	3
7	T2 MapIt	oblique coronal	2140	13.8, 27.6, 41.4, 55.2, 69	320 × 320	180	1	16	06:50	3

TA = time of acquisition, PD = proton-density, FS = fat-saturated, TSE = turbo spin-echo. Note: Differences in the values of the acquisition matrix and flip angle were caused by differences in the imaged volume among the respective slice orientations.

Proton density-weighted, fat-saturated sequences were utilized to classify the LBT as either normal or damaged. Focal or longitudinal changes in signal intensity, a significantly increased tendon diameter, marked fraying or contour irregularities, and partial or complete tears of tendon substance were defined as LBT tendinopathy. If none of these diagnostic features were present, the LBT was considered normal.

2.5. Placement of Regions of Interest

First, an oblique coronally orientated proton-density-weighted fat-saturated sequence dissecting the bicipital groove was used to identify the LBT and decide upon the optimal position for the placement of the region of interest (ROI). The ROI was placed in the section in which the largest longitudinal diameter of the sulcal part of the LBT was depicted and no partial volume effect was present (Figure 1). To further reduce the possible effects of artifacts or imperfect ROI placement, each measurement was performed three times, and the average T2 relaxation times were used for analysis. In order to obtain precise measurements, the regions of interest (ROIs) were carefully placed on the first echo images acquired using a multi-echo-spin-echo T2-weighted sequence. Subsequently, the ROI was duplicated onto a color-coded parametric T2 map after visual comparison with the proton-density-weighted fat-saturated sequences and further adjusted, if necessary, to exclude artifacts or non-tendinous structures, such as the humeral cortex or deltoid muscle.

2.6. Arthroscopy

Two experienced orthopedic surgeons performed shoulder arthroscopy on all patients. The operations were performed under general anesthesia with the patients seated at an angle of 30–90° above the horizontal plane and the head fixed in a headrest. During the arthroscopy, both the labroligamentous and cartilaginous joint structures were assessed. A standardized questionnaire was used to evaluate the intra-articular portion of the LBT, including its extension into the sulcal portion. If medically indicated, a ventral approach was made for surgical intervention. The diagnosis of LBT tendinopathy was defined by a marked fraying of the tendon substance or significant changes in the tendon diameter. Partial tears were defined as a disruption of a single or multiple tendon fibers, whereas complete tears were defined as a disruption of the entire thickness of the LBT. In terms of the statistical calculations, partial and complete tears were also considered tendinopathic changes.

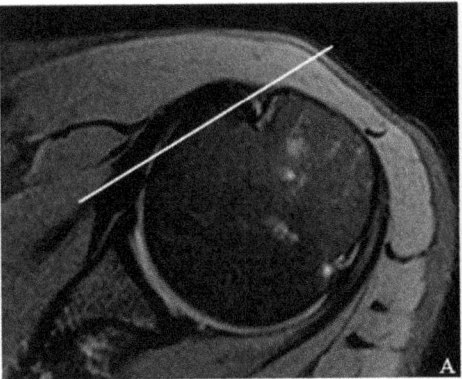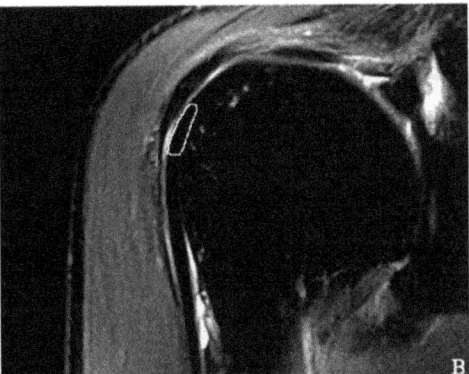

Figure 1. Axial (**A**) and oblique coronal (**B**) proton-density-weighted sequences showing the slice positioning (white line in (**A**)) used to place the region of interest (ROI). As outlined by the white circle in (**B**), the sulcal portion of the long biceps tendon was chosen as the primary region of interest and subsequently transferred onto a color-coded T2 map.

2.7. Statistical Analysis

The analysis of the patient's demographic data was carried out in a descriptive manner, while the analysis of the continuous variables was summarized as the mean values, median, and associated extrema. The frequency and percentage were calculated for the qualitative variables. For comparison of the patients' ages between the groups with and without LBT tendinopathy, the Wilcoxon two-sample test was used.

For analysis of the T2 mapping values of the sulcal part of the LBT, three measurements were performed by the two readers and repeated within a time interval of 7 days for calculation of the intra-rater agreement. Statistical analysis of the T2 imaging was carried out descriptively using summary statistics and interpreted exploratively. A comparison of the groups with and without lesions was performed using a two-sample t-test. The p-values were presented as two-sided p-values, and the level of significance was set to 5%. To assess whether the T2 mapping values were normally distributed, the Shapiro–Wilk test was used.

We performed an analysis of the diagnostic performance of T2 mapping for tendinopathic changes in the LBT or LBT lesions and reported the estimates and exact 95% confidence intervals for the sensitivity, specificity, positive predictive values, and negative predictive values. As complete separation of the data occurred, no ROC curves were plotted for the accuracy assessment.

As the raters were viewed as a random selection of observers drawn from a larger pool of possible observers, the intraclass correlation coefficient (ICC) was utilized to assess both the inter- and intra-reader agreement. In order to gauge interrater reliability, we employed a two-way random-effect model considering the subject and rater as random effects to estimate the ICC and 95% confidence intervals, following the methodology outlined by Shrout and Fleiss [28]. Data analysis was carried out using SAS for Windows (version 9.4; SAS Institute Inc., Cary, NC, USA) and R version 3.5.1 (www.cran.r-project.org, accessed on 10 May 2022) by a qualified statistician who was independent of the study.

3. Results

3.1. Demographics and Arthroscopic Evaluation of the Long Biceps Tendon

A total of 12 (66.7%) out of the 18 patients included were male, and 6 (33.3%) were female. The mean patient age was 52.4 ± 14.72 (range, 22.0–67.0) years. On average, patients with LBT tendinopathy were slightly younger than the healthy subjects (46.3 ± 17.2 (range: 22–64) years vs 60.0 ± 5.0 (range: 52–67) years). Out of the eight patients with arthroscopically proven LBT tendinopathy, seven (87.5%) were male and only one (12.5%)

was female. In Table 2, an overview of the patients' demographic characteristics is presented, categorized by whether LBT tendinopathy was present or not.

Table 2. Demographic characteristics for patients with and without LBT lesion.

		LBS Tendinopathy		p-Value
		No (N = 10)	Yes (N = 8)	
Sex	Male	5 (50.0%)	7 (87.5%)	
	Female	5 (50.0%)	1 (12.5%)	
Age (years)	n	10	8	0.1274
	Mean	46.3	60.0	
	SD	17.24	5.01	
	Median	54.0	59.5	
	Min	22.0	52.0	
	Max	64.0	67.0	

SD = standard deviation, Min = minimum, Max = maximum.

A total of 10 persons (55.6%) had healthy long biceps tendons, whereas 8 patients (44.4%) showed tendinopathic changes. Out of the eight patients with pathologic long biceps tendons, the majority showed minor lesions or partial tears (n = 7; 87.5%), whereas one patient (12.5%) was diagnosed with a complete tear. Using the conventional morphological MRI sequence, all eight patients with arthroscopically proven tendinopathy were detected by both readers.

3.2. T2 Mapping of the Long Biceps Tendon

In matching the arthroscopy results, eight LBT lesions were detected in the MRI, and no additional lesions were found intraoperatively. The mean T2 values show a significant difference between the patients with LBT tendinopathy, with 47.9 ± 7.8 ms, and the healthy subjects, with 23.3 ± 4.6 ms ($p < 0.001$). In the subgroup of healthy individuals, the maximum T2 value measured was 29.6 ms, which was found to be lower than the minimum T2 value recorded in patients with confirmed LBT tendinopathy (33.8 ms). This difference led to a complete separation of the T2 mapping values between the normal and pathological tendon substance, as depicted in Figure 2. As a result, all cut-off values between 29.6 ms and 33.8 ms showed sensitivities and positive predictive values of 100%, with 95% confidence intervals (CIs) (63.1–100.0%), along with specificities and negative predictive values of 100%, with 95% CIs (69.2–100.0%). For a more comprehensive view, Table 3 illustrates the mean T2 mapping parameters for patients with LBT tendinopathy and for healthy individuals.

Table 3. T2 mapping values (ms) for normal and damaged LBT.

		Overall	Population without Lesion	Population with Lesion	p-Value (t Value)
	n	18	10	8	
T2 values (ms)	Mean	34.2	23.3	47.9	<0.001 (−8.33)
	SD	13.97	4.61	7.84	
	Median	29.0	24.2	48.2	
	Min	15.8	15.8	33.8	
	Max	61.4	29.6	61.4	

SD = standard deviation, Min = minimum, Max = maximum.

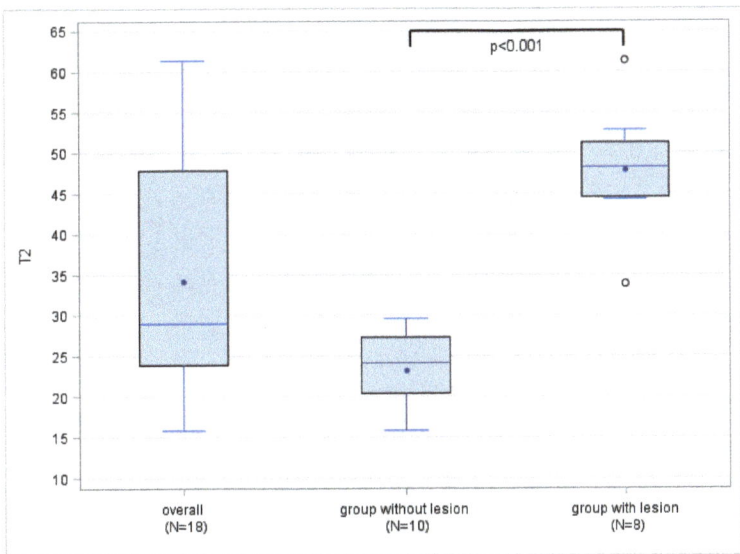

Figure 2. Boxplots of overall T2 mapping values (ms) in healthy labrum and patients with LBT lesion. Note the complete separation of T2 values between patients with LBT lesions and healthy subjects.

In correlation with the statistical results, there was also a visual difference between the healthy subjects and the individuals with proven LBT pathologies in the color-coded T2 maps (Figures 3–5).

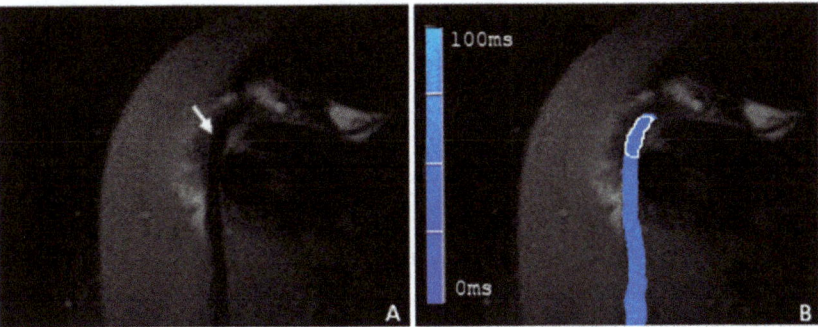

Figure 3. (**A**) A coronal proton-density-weighted fat-saturated magnetic resonance image of a 59-year-old man with morphologically normal-appearing and arthroscopically proven healthy tendon of the long biceps head (arrow). (**B**) A merged image of the proton-density-weighted images and the corresponding color-coded T2 maps with the placed ROI in the sulcal portion of the LBT (white frame). The average T2 mapping value was 21.3 ms.

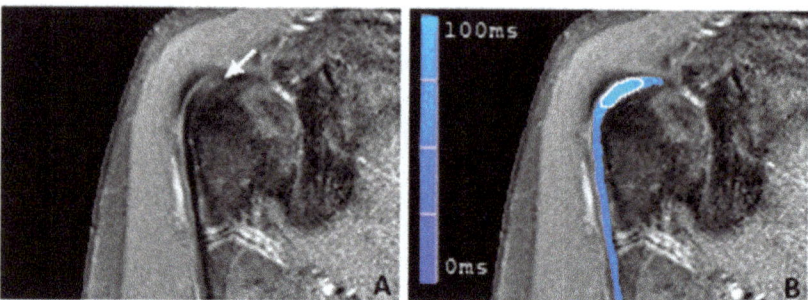

Figure 4. (**A**) A coronal proton-density-weighted fat-saturated magnetic resonance image of a 58-year-old man with focal hyperintensity of the sulcal portion of the LBT (arrow). (**B**) A merged image of the proton-density-weighted images and the corresponding color-coded T2 maps with the placed ROI in the sulcal portion of the LBT (white frame). Note the elevated average T2 mapping value of 44.7 ms. During the arthroscopy, a partial tear of the LBT was found.

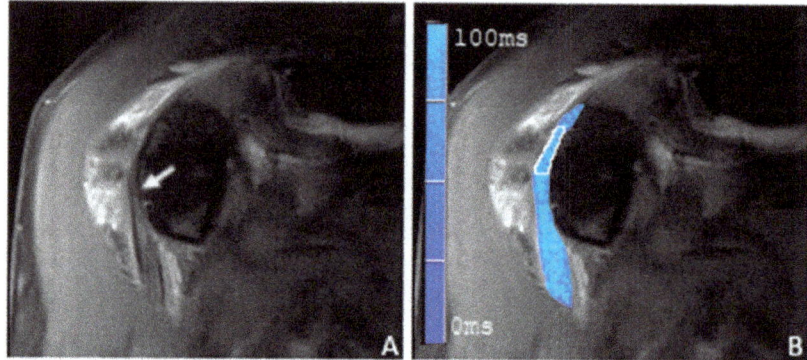

Figure 5. (**A**) A coronal proton-density-weighted fat-saturated magnetic resonance image of a 57-year-old man with longitudinal hyperintensity of the sulcal and the partially depicted extraarticular portion of the LBT with a markedly increased tendon diameter (arrow). (**B**) A merged image of the proton-density-weighted images and the corresponding color-coded T2 maps with the placed ROI in the sulcal portion of the LBT (white frame). Note the elevated average T2 mapping value of 52.8 ms. During the arthroscopy, a longitudinal partial tear was found.

3.3. Inter- and Intra-Reader Agreement

The calculation of the intra-class correlation coefficient (ICC) showed a near-perfect inter-reader agreement of 0.99 (95% confidence interval (CI): 0.98–1.00). The intra-reader agreement for the two respective readers was also almost perfect, with 0.93 (95% CI: 0.86–0.97) for reader 1 and 0.96 (95% CI: 0.97–0.99) for reader 2.

4. Discussion

Although pathologies of the long biceps tendon (LBT) are a well-known cause of shoulder pain, limited mobility, and associated impairments in daily living, common diagnostic tools have proven to be low in accuracy, particularly regarding the evaluation of early tendon damage. When detected by conventional MRI or MR arthrography, most LBT pathologies are visualized at more advanced stages of rupture or tendinopathy [7–9]. Despite the fact that tendon degeneration appears to have a chronically progressive course, diagnostic tools for early detection, although desirable, are not yet present [14]. T2 mapping as a functional and quantitative MRI sequence has been successfully used to evaluate the ultrastructural integrity of the 3D collagen network and water content of articular cartilage in several joints [16,17,29]. However, to our knowledge, its applicability to tendinous structures has not yet systematically evaluated nor validated using arthroscopy as the gold standard.

Therefore, the aim of this study was to evaluate the ability of T2 mapping to identify and quantify pathologies of the LBT and to distinguish them from healthy tendons using arthroscopy as the gold standard. As one major finding, the mean T2 values showed a significant difference between the healthy subjects (23.3 ± 4.6 ms) and patients with LBT tendinopathy (47.9 ± 7.8 ms; $p < 0.001$). Additionally, the maximum T2 value in healthy subjects (29.6 ms) was lower than the minimum T2 value in damaged tendons (33.8 ms; $p < 0.001$). Therefore, these two findings, resulting in sensitivities, specificities, and positive and negative predictive values of 100% for all cut-off values between 29.6 and 33.8 ms (95% CI: 63.1–100.0%), demonstrate the ability of T2 mapping to evaluate tendinous tissues and to distinguish between healthy and damaged tendons. A previous study by our working group focused on the T2 mapping of SLAP lesions in the glenoid labrum [27]. The mean T2 values found in the pathological specimens differed to some extent from those reported in this study (37.7 ± 10.6 ms for SLAP lesions vs. 47.9 ± 7.8 ms for LBT pathologies), which could be explained by the different histological composition, being fibrocartilaginous for the glenoid labrum and mainly collagenous for the LBT. Nevertheless, as in this study, complete statistical separation of the T2 values was found between the healthy subjects and the patients with SLAP lesions. These significant differences in T2 relaxation time may reflect damages to the ultrastructural integrity of the collagen network and the associated biochemical repair mechanisms. In a histopathological correlation study, Buck et al. analyzed cadaveric tendon specimens from the LBT and compared the histological findings to the associated signal changes in MRI [23]. In addition to significant changes in the tendon diameter, the study group found mucoid degeneration with subsequent alterations in the water content as the main histopathological correlate for T2-signal hyperintensities in MRI. Another study showed that collagen network disorganization and myxoid/mucoid degeneration were the major histological correlates of tendon degeneration in 45 LBT specimens obtained from tenodesis [30]. These biochemical and histological processes are in line not only with the increased T2 relaxation times of the LBT shown in our study but also with several other studies describing an increase in the T2 values in damaged tendons other than the LBT or in the focal lesions of articular cartilage [31,32]. In a systematic review, Baum et al. described T2 mapping as a promising, non-invasive method for the biochemical evaluation of articular cartilage and fibrocartilaginous structures, like the menisci underlining the broad spectrum of potential clinical utility [33].

While T2 hyperintensities are well-known radiological correlates of tendon or cartilage damage using morphological MRI sequences, the novel aspect of T2 mapping lies in its ability to quantify the actual T2 relaxation times and thereby provide objectifiable measures. Thus, several areas of potential clinical use can be inferred. First, by providing cut-off values, quantification of the T2 relaxation times may help to increase diagnostic accuracy in the detection of tendon lesions. While the complete statistical separation between healthy and pathological tendon substance described in this study may be partially due to the small study population, future studies with larger sample sizes might show a gradual increase in T2 values with progressing degrees of degeneration and ascribe certain stages of degeneration to the associated levels of increased T2 relaxation times. In an analogy using area-under-the-curve calculations, Li et al. reported a diagnostic cut-off value of 49.5 ms for discriminating between healthy subjects and early stages of osteoarthritis in the articular cartilage of the knee ($n = 79$), with a resulting sensitivity of 91.2% and specificity of 92.3% [34]. However, larger sample sizes and additional studies of T2 mapping in tendinous tissue are needed to define reasonable cut-off values and thereby improve the diagnostic performance of MRI for detecting damage to the LBT.

Since there are currently no valid tools for the early detection of degenerative changes in collagen networks, T2 mapping, with its ability to detect and quantify ultrastructural damages and biochemical remodeling processes, holds promise for clinical use in the early detection of tendon pathologies. While explicit studies on early degenerative changes in the LBT are missing, several studies describe the general process of tendon degeneration as chronically progressive [15,35]. Analyzing the histopathological changes of 891 tendon specimens obtained from repair surgeries at various anatomic sites, Kannus et al. found that almost all (97%) tendons showed evidence of previous degeneration before tendon rupture occurred [36]. The study group also found similar degenerative changes in 34% of cadaveric tendon specimens from a young control group, indicating that tendon degeneration is a common finding in people older than 35 years. Although explicit studies on tendinous collagen networks are lacking, several studies have reported the ability of T2 mapping to sensitively detect early matrix degeneration in articular cartilage and predict its progression into manifest osteoarthritis (OA) [37,38]. Comparing normal controls and subjects with various risk factors for the development of OA but no radiographic signs of OA, Joseph et al. found higher and more heterogeneously distributed T2 values in subjects with OA risk factors than in the normal control group [39]. A similar but longitudinal study over a 24-month period reported higher T2 values in patients with risk factors for but without radiographic signs of OA compared to a normal control group [40]. As our study demonstrated the ability of T2 mapping to detect structural damage to the LBT, the aforementioned results may also be applicable to the T2 mapping of tendinous tissues. However, none of these studies used MRI for morphological correlation, and future studies need to further investigate the extent to which T2 mapping can detect early tendon degeneration, and thus, could serve as a valid tool for early detection in patients at risk for developing chronic tendinopathy. In particular, histological correlation studies using ex vivo human or animal models could be considered to further investigate the relationship between elevated T2 mapping values and histological changes. Additionally, diffusion-weighted sequences have also been described as a valid tool for the assessment of microstructural changes in musculoskeletal radiology. The combination of these sequences with quantitative T2 sequences might improve the detection of beginning histopathological changes even further than each of these techniques alone. The recently reported reduction in acquisition time using deep-learning-based reconstruction techniques in T2-weighted MR imaging may further enhance this advantage by allowing for the acquisition of additional information without negatively impacting the clinical workflow [41].

Another novel aspect yielded by the quantification of T2 relaxation times lies in its potential use for monitoring degenerative changes under conservative therapy or postoperative healing processes after tendon repair. Histological studies describe tendon healing as three overlapping phases consisting of an acute inflammatory phase with increased cellularity and vascularity and consequently increased water content, which, after a few days, transitions into the remodeling phase, in which the synthesis of glycosaminoglycans begins and the water content remains high. The last phase is described as the maturation/consolidation phase, during which the repair tissue changes from cellular to fibrous, and later, to scar-like tissue with a gradually decreasing water content [42]. Since T2 mapping evaluates the ultrastructural composition of collagen networks and changes in water content, it might provide objectifiable measures as correlates for these histological mechanisms. By evaluating the rotator cuff tendons after surgical repair over a 12-month period using T2 mapping, Xie et al. found gradually decreasing T2 values reaching the level of the healthy controls as a possible indicator of complete tendon healing [25]. The study group also described a correlation between lower T2 values and satisfactory clinical outcome after one-year follow-up. Another study focusing on the T2 values of knee cartilage after meniscal allograft transplantation reported similar results, with significantly increased T2 values in the early postoperative period that returned to baseline levels after one year [43]. Further studies correlating the longitudinal progression of T2 values with the clinical outcome after tendon, ligament, or cartilage repair could confirm these findings, thus qualifying T2 mapping as a method to further improve the clinical evaluation of postoperative healing processes by relating objectifiable measures to the common clinical examination.

In addition to the biochemical and histological factors discussed above, it is important to recognize that T2 mapping values may be influenced by several other variables that should be recognized as potential confounders. In addition to age-related changes in the composition of the tendon matrix and differences in mechanical loading, and consequently, water content along the entire tendon length, artificial signal changes, such as partial volume effects and the "magic angle" artifact, are known causes of variations in the T2 signal in various collagenous tissues [44,45]. The "magic angle" artifact is known to lead to a prolongation of T2 relaxation times in collagen fibers oriented at an angle of 55° to the magnetic field [46,47]. Because of its curved course through the glenohumeral joint, such imaging artifacts are particularly pronounced in the LBT. Buck et al. found signal changes caused by the "magic angle" artifact to be most eminent before the entrance of the LBT into the intertubercular groove [23]. They described the artificial signal intensity to be lower than T2 hyperintensities caused by histologically correlated mucoid degeneration. For this reason, and considering that the artifact of the "magic angle" can also lead to signal changes in healthy tendons, the significant differentiation in T2 values between the healthy subjects and the patients with confirmed tendinopathy observed in our study cannot be attributed to artificial factors only. The observed differentiation could possibly be due to the precise positioning of the region of interest (ROI) and the limited size of our study population. It is likely that future studies with larger cohorts will demonstrate overlap and a more gradual increase in T2 values, reflecting the progressive nature of LBT tendinopathy.

As evidenced by the almost perfect intra- and inter-reader agreement observed in the T2 values between the healthy and damaged long biceps tendons, T2 mapping demonstrates potential for reliable clinical utilization. The intraclass correlation coefficients (ICCs) for intra-reader agreement ranged from 0.93 to 0.96 (95% CI 0.86–0.99), while inter-reader agreement reached ICCs of up to 0.99 (95% CI 0.98–1.00). In concordance with this, previous studies on T2 mapping of the glenohumeral joint in healthy subjects have shown comparable intraclass correlation coefficients (ICCs), with good to excellent agreement among investigators [48,49]. Nevertheless, it is important to acknowledge that the small sample size and the limited number of confirmed LBT lesions ($n = 8$) in our study could potentially contribute to statistical artifacts, which may have influenced these findings to some extent.

Our study has some limitations. As a major limitation, the small sample size has to be mentioned, as it has important statistical implications. In studies investigating a small number of participants, extreme values can have a disproportionate impact on confidence interval (CI) calculations, resulting in wider ranges. For this study, the 95% CI for sensitivity and specificity ranged from 63.1% to 100%, indicating the potential effect of the small sample size on the precision of these measures. Furthermore, this study recruited patients from a specialized referral center, which makes it highly selective and prone to sampling errors. The higher prevalence of LBT lesions in this specific population may have led to improved test performance. Given these statistical limitations, the results may apply only to our specific study cohort, giving this study the characteristics of a pilot or preliminary study. To address this concern, further studies with larger sample sizes are necessary. These larger studies would also provide the opportunity to more accurately differentiate lesion severity and potentially identify different T2 values for the respective lesion grades.

Another limitation to consider is the possibility of human error in the manual placement of regions of interest (ROIs), which can lead to variability and subjective judgments. Although all patients were positioned for MRI examination in the same way and a standardized slice orientation was used for ROI placement (Figure 1), the exact position of ROI placement differed slightly among the subjects because of small interindividual variations in anatomy. Despite our efforts to mitigate potential errors arising from the imprecise placement of the region of interest (ROI) by averaging T2 values obtained from three different measurements, there is still room for improvement. Additionally, it has to be mentioned that the long acquisition time of the T2 mapping sequences (Table 1) is susceptible to motion artifacts, which in turn, could influence T2 mapping values. In future studies, the utilization of 3D T2 mapping sequences with voxel-wise analysis of T2 relaxation times would be highly advantageous. This advanced approach would enable the most precise acquisition of T2 values, enhancing the accuracy and reliability of the results. In addition, 3D sequences could also reduce the potential impact of the partial volume effect in the imaging of the LBT, which could be better visualized than with conventional 2D sequences due to its arcuate course combined with its usually small size. Examination of the LBT using dynamic modalities, such as ultrasound, could also contribute to a better assessment of tendon substance and reveal correlations between sonographic findings and elevated T2 values. Furthermore, because the intertubercular portion of the LBT may be partially invisible to arthroscopy, it is possible that small tendon portions captured within the ROI may have missed arthroscopic correlation. However, in correspondence with orthopedic surgeons and careful review of the surgical protocols, all lesions found during the arthroscopy were longitudinally distributed along the course of the tendon, and thus, were reliably detectable.

Additionally, it is important to note that, to the best of our knowledge, this study represents the first systematic evaluation of T2 mapping specifically for the LBT. As a result, there are no suitable studies available for direct comparison of the quantified T2 relaxation times in this context. The few existing studies on the T2 mapping of tendinous structures have reported similar results, with T2 relaxation times around 30 ms for healthy supraspinatus tendons, for instance [24,25]. However, further research is required to validate the T2 mapping values specifically for the long biceps tendon, as observed in our study.

Finally, it should be mentioned that the T2 values analyzed in this study and the resulting diagnostic parameters are representative only of a field strength of 3.0 Tesla. Some studies comparing cardiac and uterine T2 mapping sequences at 1.5 and 3.0 Tesla found significant field strength-dependent differences in the mean T2 values [50,51]. While explicit studies on the cartilaginous tissue of tendinous structures are lacking, this effect might also be applicable to musculoskeletal imaging.

5. Conclusions

T2 mapping effectively detects and quantifies long biceps tendon (LBT) pathologies, as evidenced by the significantly higher T2 values observed in arthroscopically confirmed tendinopathy compared to provenly healthy tendons. Additionally, the high diagnostic performance values and strong inter-rater reliability (ICC) among radiologists further support this finding. Thus, T2 mapping has the potential to provide valuable insights into the (ultra-)structural integrity of the tendinous collagen network and may, therefore, serve as a valuable tool for early diagnosis, facilitating the prompt initiation of therapy. Additionally, by providing objectifiable measures, it may enable longitudinal quantitative monitoring during conservative therapy or after surgical treatment.

Author Contributions: Conceptualization, C.R., P.S. and F.W.; methodology, P.S., F.W., C.R., I.B. and T.S.; validation, C.R. and M.-A.W.; formal analysis, I.B., P.S., F.W. and C.R.; data interpretation, P.S., C.R., I.B., H.-U.K., T.S., F.Z. and M.-A.W.; writing—original draft preparation, P.S. and C.R.; writing—review and editing, P.S., C.R., F.W., I.B., H.-U.K., T.S., F.Z. and M.-A.W. All authors have read and agreed to the published version of the manuscript.

Funding: For the publication fee, we acknowledge the financial support from Deutsche Forschungsgemeinschaft (DFG) within the funding program "Open Access Publikationskosten", and from Heidelberg University.

Institutional Review Board Statement: This study was approved by the Institutional Review Board of Heidelberg University (S-081/2010) and conducted in accordance with the Declaration of Helsinki.

Informed Consent Statement: Written informed consent was obtained from all patients after they were informed of the nature of the examination.

Data Availability Statement: The datasets generated and analyzed in the present study are available from the corresponding author upon reasonable request.

Conflicts of Interest: The authors declare no conflict of interest.

References

1. Gartsman, G.M.; Brinker, M.R.; Khan, M. Early Effectiveness of Arthroscopic Repair for Full-Thickness Tears of the Rotator Cuff: An Outcome Analysis. *J. Bone Jt. Surg. Am.* **1998**, *80*, 33–40. [CrossRef]
2. Beaton, D.E.; Richards, R.R. Measuring Function of the Shoulder. A Cross-Sectional Comparison of Five Questionnaires. *J. Bone Jt. Surg. Am.* **1996**, *78*, 882–890. [CrossRef] [PubMed]
3. Raney, E.B.; Thankam, F.G.; Dilisio, M.F.; Agrawal, D.K. Pain and the Pathogenesis of Biceps Tendinopathy. *Am. J. Transl. Res.* **2017**, *9*, 2668–2683. [PubMed]
4. Szabó, I.; Boileau, P.; Walch, G. The Proximal Biceps as a Pain Generator and Results of Tenotomy. *Sport. Med. Arthrosc. Rev.* **2008**, *16*, 180–186. [CrossRef] [PubMed]
5. Kelly, M.P.; Perkinson, S.G.; Ablove, R.H.; Tueting, J.L. Distal Biceps Tendon Ruptures. *Am. J. Sport. Med.* **2015**, *43*, 2012–2017. [CrossRef]
6. Eakin, C.L.; Faber, K.J.; Hawkins, R.J.; Hovis, D.W. Biceps Tendon Disorders in Athletes. *J. Am. Acad. Orthop. Surg.* **1999**, *7*, 300–310. [CrossRef]
7. Lee, R.W.; Choi, S.-J.; Lee, M.H.; Ahn, J.H.; Shin, D.R.; Kang, C.H.; Lee, K.W. Diagnostic Accuracy of 3T Conventional Shoulder MRI in the Detection of the Long Head of the Biceps Tendon Tears Associated with Rotator Cuff Tendon Tears. *Skelet. Radiol.* **2016**, *45*, 1705–1715. [CrossRef]
8. Malavolta, E.A.; Assunção, J.H.; Guglielmetti, C.L.B.; de Souza, F.F.; Gracitelli, M.E.C.; Ferreira Neto, A.A. Accuracy of Preoperative MRI in the Diagnosis of Disorders of the Long Head of the Biceps Tendon. *Eur. J. Radiol.* **2015**, *84*, 2250–2254. [CrossRef]
9. Baptista, E.; Malavolta, E.A.; Gracitelli, M.E.C.; Alvarenga, D.; Bordalo-Rodrigues, M.; Ferreira Neto, A.A.; de Barros, N. Diagnostic Accuracy of MRI for Detection of Tears and Instability of Proximal Long Head of Biceps Tendon: An Evaluation of 100 Shoulders Compared with Arthroscopy. *Skelet. Radiol.* **2019**, *48*, 1723–1733. [CrossRef]
10. Rol, M.; Favard, L.; Berhouet, J. Diagnosis of Long Head of Biceps Tendinopathy in Rotator Cuff Tear Patients: Correlation of Imaging and Arthroscopy Data. *Int. Orthop.* **2018**, *42*, 1347–1355. [CrossRef]
11. Dubrow, S.A.; Streit, J.J.; Shishani, Y.; Robbin, M.R.; Gobezie, R. Diagnostic Accuracy in Detecting Tears in the Proximal Biceps Tendon Using Standard Nonenhancing Shoulder MRI. *Open Access J. Sport. Med.* **2014**, *5*, 81–87. [CrossRef] [PubMed]
12. De Maeseneer, M.; Boulet, C.; Pouliart, N.; Kichouh, M.; Buls, N.; Verhelle, F.; De Mey, J.; Shahabpour, M. Assessment of the Long Head of the Biceps Tendon of the Shoulder with 3T Magnetic Resonance Arthrography and CT Arthrography. *Eur. J. Radiol.* **2012**, *81*, 934–939. [CrossRef] [PubMed]
13. Tadros, A.S.; Huang, B.K.; Wymore, L.; Hoenecke, H.; Fronek, J.; Chang, E.Y. Long Head of the Biceps Brachii Tendon: Unenhanced MRI versus Direct MR Arthrography. *Skelet. Radiol.* **2015**, *44*, 1263–1272. [CrossRef]
14. Cook, J.L.; Purdam, C.R. Is Tendon Pathology a Continuum? A Pathology Model to Explain the Clinical Presentation of Load-Induced Tendinopathy. *Br. J. Sport. Med.* **2009**, *43*, 409–416. [CrossRef] [PubMed]
15. Riley, G. Chronic Tendon Pathology: Molecular Basis and Therapeutic Implications. *Expert. Rev. Mol. Med.* **2005**, *7*, 1–25. [CrossRef] [PubMed]
16. Rehnitz, C.; Klaan, B.; Burkholder, I.; von Stillfried, F.; Kauczor, H.-U.; Weber, M.-A. Delayed Gadolinium-Enhanced MRI of Cartilage (DGEMRIC) and T_2 Mapping at 3T MRI of the Wrist: Feasibility and Clinical Application. *J. Magn. Reson. Imaging* **2017**, *45*, 381–389. [CrossRef] [PubMed]
17. Lee, S.-Y.; Park, H.-J.; Kwon, H.-J.; Kim, M.S.; Choi, S.H.; Choi, Y.J.; Kim, E. T2 Relaxation Times of the Glenohumeral Joint at 3.0 T MRI in Patients with and without Primary and Secondary Osteoarthritis. *Acta Radiol.* **2015**, *56*, 1388–1395. [CrossRef]
18. Nguyen, J.C.; Liu, F.; Blankenbaker, D.G.; Woo, K.M.; Kijowski, R. Juvenile Osteochondritis Dissecans: Cartilage T2 Mapping of Stable Medial Femoral Condyle Lesions. *Radiology* **2018**, *288*, 536–543. [CrossRef]
19. Quatman, C.E.; Hettrich, C.M.; Schmitt, L.C.; Spindler, K.P. The Clinical Utility and Diagnostic Performance of Magnetic Resonance Imaging for Identification of Early and Advanced Knee Osteoarthritis. *Am. J. Sport. Med.* **2011**, *39*, 1557–1568. [CrossRef]
20. Crema, M.D.; Roemer, F.W.; Marra, M.D.; Burstein, D.; Gold, G.E.; Eckstein, F.; Baum, T.; Mosher, T.J.; Carrino, J.A.; Guermazi, A. Articular Cartilage in the Knee: Current MR Imaging Techniques and Applications in Clinical Practice and Research. *RadioGraphics* **2011**, *31*, 37–61. [CrossRef]
21. Eckstein, F.; Wirth, W.; Nevitt, M.C. Recent Advances in Osteoarthritis Imaging—The Osteoarthritis Initiative. *Nat. Rev. Rheumatol.* **2012**, *8*, 622–630. [CrossRef] [PubMed]
22. Kasar, S.; Ozturk, M.; Polat, A.V. Quantitative T2 Mapping of the Sacroiliac Joint Cartilage at 3T in Patients with Axial Spondyloarthropathies. *Eur. Radiol.* **2022**, *32*, 1395–1403. [CrossRef] [PubMed]
23. Buck, F.M.; Grehn, H.; Hilbe, M.; Pfirrmann, C.W.A.; Manzanell, S.; Hodler, J. Degeneration of the Long Biceps Tendon: Comparison of MRI with Gross Anatomy and Histology. *AJR Am. J. Roentgenol.* **2009**, *193*, 1367–1375. [CrossRef] [PubMed]

24. Anz, A.W.; Lucas, E.P.; Fitzcharles, E.K.; Surowiec, R.K.; Millett, P.J.; Ho, C.P. MRI T2 Mapping of the Asymptomatic Supraspinatus Tendon by Age and Imaging Plane Using Clinically Relevant Subregions. *Eur. J. Radiol.* **2014**, *83*, 801–805. [CrossRef]
25. Xie, Y.; Liu, S.; Qiao, Y.; Hu, Y.; Zhang, Y.; Qu, J.; Shen, Y.; Tao, H.; Chen, S. Quantitative T2 Mapping-Based Tendon Healing Is Related to the Clinical Outcomes during the First Year after Arthroscopic Rotator Cuff Repair. *Knee Surg. Sport. Traumatol. Arthrosc.* **2021**, *29*, 127–135. [CrossRef]
26. Bossuyt, P.M.; Reitsma, J.B.; Bruns, D.E.; Gatsonis, C.A.; Glasziou, P.P.; Irwig, L.; Lijmer, J.G.; Moher, D.; Rennie, D.; de Vet, H.C.W.; et al. STARD 2015: An Updated List of Essential Items for Reporting Diagnostic Accuracy Studies. *Radiology* **2015**, *277*, 826–832. [CrossRef]
27. Stein, P.; Wuennemann, F.; Schneider, T.; Zeifang, F.; Burkholder, I.; Weber, M.-A.; Kauczor, H.-U.; Rehnitz, C. 3-Tesla T2 Mapping Magnetic Resonance Imaging for Evaluation of SLAP Lesions in Patients with Shoulder Pain: An Arthroscopy-Controlled Study. *J. Clin. Med.* **2023**, *12*, 3109. [CrossRef]
28. Shrout, P.E.; Fleiss, J.L. Intraclass Correlations: Uses in Assessing Rater Reliability. *Psychol. Bull.* **1979**, *86*, 420–428. [CrossRef]
29. Renner, N.; Kleyer, A.; Krönke, G.; Simon, D.; Söllner, S.; Rech, J.; Uder, M.; Janka, R.; Schett, G.; Welsch, G.H.; et al. T2 Mapping as a New Method for Quantitative Assessment of Cartilage Damage in Rheumatoid Arthritis. *J. Rheumatol.* **2020**, *47*, 820–825. [CrossRef]
30. Simon, M.J.K.; Yeoh, J.; Nevin, J.; Nimmo, M.; Regan, W.D. Histopathology of Long Head of Biceps Tendon Removed during Tenodesis Demonstrates Degenerative Histopathology and Not Inflammatory Changes. *BMC Musculoskelet. Disord.* **2022**, *23*, 185. [CrossRef]
31. Golditz, T.; Steib, S.; Pfeifer, K.; Uder, M.; Gelse, K.; Janka, R.; Hennig, F.F.; Welsch, G.H. Functional Ankle Instability as a Risk Factor for Osteoarthritis: Using T2-Mapping to Analyze Early Cartilage Degeneration in the Ankle Joint of Young Athletes. *Osteoarthr. Cartil.* **2014**, *22*, 1377–1385. [CrossRef] [PubMed]
32. Zarins, Z.A.; Bolbos, R.I.; Pialat, J.B.; Link, T.M.; Li, X.; Souza, R.B.; Majumdar, S. Cartilage and Meniscus Assessment Using T1rho and T2 Measurements in Healthy Subjects and Patients with Osteoarthritis. *Osteoarthr. Cartil.* **2010**, *18*, 1408–1416. [CrossRef] [PubMed]
33. Baum, T.; Joseph, G.B.; Karampinos, D.C.; Jungmann, P.M.; Link, T.M.; Bauer, J.S. Cartilage and Meniscal T2 Relaxation Time as Non-Invasive Biomarker for Knee Osteoarthritis and Cartilage Repair Procedures. *Osteoarthr. Cartil.* **2013**, *21*, 1474–1484. [CrossRef] [PubMed]
34. Li, Z.; Wang, H.; Lu, Y.; Jiang, M.; Chen, Z.; Xi, X.; Ding, X.; Yan, F. Diagnostic Value of T1ρ and T2 Mapping Sequences of 3D Fat-Suppressed Spoiled Gradient (FS SPGR-3D) 3.0-T Magnetic Resonance Imaging for Osteoarthritis. *Medicine* **2019**, *98*, e13834. [CrossRef] [PubMed]
35. Kannus, P.; Paavola, M.; Paakkala, T.; Parkkari, J.; Järvinen, T.; Järvinen, M. Pathophysiologie Des Sehnenüberlastungsschadens. *Radiologe* **2002**, *42*, 766–770. [CrossRef]
36. Kannus, P.; Józsa, L. Histopathological Changes Preceding Spontaneous Rupture of a Tendon. A Controlled Study of 891 Patients. *J. Bone Jt. Surg.* **1991**, *73*, 1507–1525. [CrossRef]
37. Joseph, G.B.; Baum, T.; Alizai, H.; Carballido-Gamio, J.; Nardo, L.; Virayavanich, W.; Lynch, J.A.; Nevitt, M.C.; McCulloch, C.E.; Majumdar, S.; et al. Baseline Mean and Heterogeneity of MR Cartilage T2 Are Associated with Morphologic Degeneration of Cartilage, Meniscus, and Bone Marrow over 3years—Data from the Osteoarthritis Initiative. *Osteoarthr. Cartil.* **2012**, *20*, 727–735. [CrossRef]
38. Prasad, A.P.; Nardo, L.; Schooler, J.; Joseph, G.B.; Link, T.M. T1ρ and T2 Relaxation Times Predict Progression of Knee Osteoarthritis. *Osteoarthr. Cartil.* **2013**, *21*, 69–76. [CrossRef]
39. Joseph, G.B.; Baum, T.; Carballido-Gamio, J.; Nardo, L.; Virayavanich, W.; Alizai, H.; Lynch, J.A.; McCulloch, C.E.; Majumdar, S.; Link, T.M. Texture Analysis of Cartilage T2 Maps: Individuals with Risk Factors for OA Have Higher and More Heterogeneous Knee Cartilage MR T2 Compared to Normal Controls—Data from the Osteoarthritis Initiative. *Arthritis Res. Ther.* **2011**, *13*, R153. [CrossRef]
40. Baum, T.; Stehling, C.; Joseph, G.B.; Carballido-Gamio, J.; Schwaiger, B.J.; Müller-Höcker, C.; Nevitt, M.C.; Lynch, J.; McCulloch, C.E.; Link, T.M. Changes in Knee Cartilage T2 Values over 24 Months in Subjects with and without Risk Factors for Knee Osteoarthritis and Their Association with Focal Knee Lesions at Baseline: Data from the Osteoarthritis Initiative. *J. Magn. Reson. Imaging* **2012**, *35*, 370–378. [CrossRef]
41. Wessling, D.; Herrmann, J.; Afat, S.; Nickel, D.; Othman, A.E.; Almansour, H.; Gassenmaier, S. Reduction in Acquisition Time and Improvement in Image Quality in T2-Weighted MR Imaging of Musculoskeletal Tumors of the Extremities Using a Novel Deep Learning-Based Reconstruction Technique in a Turbo Spin Echo (TSE) Sequence. *Tomography* **2022**, *8*, 1759–1769. [CrossRef] [PubMed]
42. Sharma, P.; Maffulli, N. Biology of Tendon Injury: Healing, Modeling and Remodeling. *J. Musculoskelet. Neuronal Interact.* **2006**, *6*, 181–190. [PubMed]
43. Park, S.-Y.; Lee, S.H.; Lee, M.H.; Chung, H.W.; Shin, M.J. Changes in the T2 Value of Cartilage after Meniscus Transplantation over 1 Year. *Eur. Radiol.* **2017**, *27*, 1496–1504. [CrossRef] [PubMed]
44. Liess, C.; Lüsse, S.; Karger, N.; Heller, M.; Glüer, C.-C. Detection of Changes in Cartilage Water Content Using MRI T2-Mapping in Vivo. *Osteoarthr. Cartil.* **2002**, *10*, 907–913. [CrossRef] [PubMed]

45. Rehnitz, C.; Kupfer, J.; Streich, N.A.; Burkholder, I.; Schmitt, B.; Lauer, L.; Kauczor, H.-U.; Weber, M.-A. Comparison of Biochemical Cartilage Imaging Techniques at 3 T MRI. *Osteoarthr. Cartil.* **2014**, *22*, 1732–1742. [CrossRef]
46. Mosher, T.J.; Smith, H.; Dardzinski, B.J.; Schmithorst, V.J.; Smith, M.B. MR Imaging and T2 Mapping of Femoral Cartilage. *Am. J. Roentgenol.* **2001**, *177*, 665–669. [CrossRef]
47. Kaneko, Y.; Nozaki, T.; Yu, H.; Chang, A.; Kaneshiro, K.; Schwarzkopf, R.; Hara, T.; Yoshioka, H. Normal T2 Map Profile of the Entire Femoral Cartilage Using an Angle/Layer-Dependent Approach. *J. Magn. Reson. Imaging* **2015**, *42*, 1507–1516. [CrossRef]
48. Lockard, C.A.; Wilson, K.J.; Ho, C.P.; Shin, R.C.; Katthagen, J.C.; Millett, P.J. Quantitative Mapping of Glenohumeral Cartilage in Asymptomatic Subjects Using 3 T Magnetic Resonance Imaging. *Skelet. Radiol.* **2018**, *47*, 671–682. [CrossRef]
49. Kang, Y.; Choi, J.-A. T2 Mapping of Articular Cartilage of the Glenohumeral Joint at 3.0 T in Healthy Volunteers: A Feasibility Study. *Skelet. Radiol.* **2016**, *45*, 915–920. [CrossRef]
50. Baeßler, B.; Schaarschmidt, F.; Stehning, C.; Schnackenburg, B.; Maintz, D.; Bunck, A.C. A Systematic Evaluation of Three Different Cardiac T2-Mapping Sequences at 1.5 and 3T in Healthy Volunteers. *Eur. J. Radiol.* **2015**, *84*, 2161–2170. [CrossRef]
51. Zhu, L.; Lu, W.; Wang, F.; Wang, Y.; Wu, P.-Y.; Zhou, J.; Liu, H. Study of T2 Mapping in Quantifying and Discriminating Uterine Lesions under Different Magnetic Field Strengths: 1.5 T vs. 3.0 T. *BMC Med. Imaging* **2023**, *23*, 1. [CrossRef]

Disclaimer/Publisher's Note: The statements, opinions and data contained in all publications are solely those of the individual author(s) and contributor(s) and not of MDPI and/or the editor(s). MDPI and/or the editor(s) disclaim responsibility for any injury to people or property resulting from any ideas, methods, instructions or products referred to in the content.

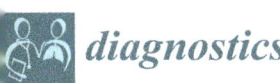

Article

Detecting Bone Marrow Edema of the Extremities on Spectral Computed Tomography Using a Three-Material Decomposition

Marie Schierenbeck [1], Martin Grözinger [2], Benjamin Reichardt [3], Olav Jansen [1], Hans-Ulrich Kauczor [4], Graeme M. Campbell [5] and Sam Sedaghat [4,*]

1. Department for Radiology and Neuroradiology, University Hospital Schleswig-Holstein Campus Kiel, 24105 Kiel, Germany
2. German Cancer Research Center, University Hospital Heidelberg, 69120 Heidelberg, Germany
3. Department of Interventional Radiology and Neuroradiology, Klinikum Hochsauerland, 59821 Arnsberg, Germany
4. Department of Diagnostic and Interventional Radiology, University Hospital Heidelberg, 69120 Heidelberg, Germany
5. Clinical Science, Philips GmbH Market DACH, 22335 Hamburg, Germany
* Correspondence: samsedaghat1@gmail.com

Abstract: Background: Detecting bone marrow edema (BME) as a sign of acute fractures is challenging on conventional computed tomography (CT). This study evaluated the diagnostic performance of a three-material decomposition (TMD) approach for detecting traumatic BME of the extremities on spectral computed tomography (SCT). Methods: This retrospective diagnostic study included 81 bone compartments with and 80 without BME. A TMD application to visualize BME was developed in collaboration with Philips Healthcare. The following bone compartments were included: distal radius, proximal femur, proximal tibia, distal tibia and fibula, and long bone diaphysis. Two blinded radiologists reviewed each case independently in random order for the presence or absence of BME. Results: The interrater reliability was 0.84 ($p < 0.001$). The different bone compartments showed sensitivities of 86.7% to 93.8%, specificities of 84.2% to 94.1%, positive predictive values of 82.4% to 94.7%, negative predictive values of 87.5% to 93.3%, and area under the curve (AUC) values of 85.7% to 93.1%. The distal radius showed the highest sensitivity and the proximal femur showed the lowest sensitivity, while the proximal femur presented the highest specificity and the distal tibia presented the lowest specificity. Conclusions: Our TMD approach provides high diagnostic performance for detecting BME of the extremities. Therefore, this approach could be used routinely in the emergency setting.

Keywords: bone marrow edema; fracture; computed tomography; trauma; extremity

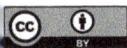

1. Introduction

Bone fractures are common conditions that present in the routine emergency setting. The accurate diagnosis of fractures after acute trauma is essential for adequate consecutive treatment. This can be challenging in the case of detecting occult fractures. Acute trauma can cause microfractures in the trabecular bone, leading to bone marrow edema (BME) and microhemorrhages, eventually causing a reduction in fat components [1]. Although BME is not specific to fractures, the presence of BME in acutely injured bone indicates the presence of a fracture [2,3]. To appreciate the importance of BME as an indirect sign of a fracture, Baumbach et al. developed a workflow for BME management and decision-making, placing the presence of BME at the beginning of their decision algorithm [3]. The changes in the fluid content of the bones causing BME are best diagnosed with magnetic resonance imaging (MRI), which reveals reduced signal intensity on T1-weighted (w) images and increased signal intensity on fat-suppressed T2w or proton density-weighted

(PDw) images [4,5]. MRI is often performed to identify BME, which many authors consider highly specific for acute trauma [6,7]. Therefore, it is not surprising that MRI has become a standard imaging modality for assessing bone marrow edema in the emergency setting [5]. However, contraindications, such as implemented medical devices, ferromagnetic materials, claustrophobia, or severe back pain, often restrict the use of MRI [8,9]. Additionally, MRI examinations are time-consuming and usually not immediately available in an emergency setting [10]. Patients with acute trauma of the extremities often require immediate operative treatment. Therefore, computed tomography (CT) is often the imaging modality of choice in emergency situations, as the examination times are faster, hence the susceptibility to patients' motion is reduced [8,11]. With traditional CT scanners, which are based on a single-energy X-ray tube and detector, the diagnosis of BME is often very challenging, as for low-contrast tissues like bone marrow, the discrimination from normal bone is aggravated by a superposition of the X-rays and the overlying trabecular bone [12–15]. An advanced technique using dual-energy computed tomography (DECT) has been employed for many years to provide additional information on different tissue characteristics. Different approaches for DECT, such as rapid kilovoltage (kV) switching or two X-ray sources, have already been described in the literature [7]. The kV-switching method uses a single X-ray tube with the ability to rapidly change the energy levels [10]. A major disadvantage of using a DECT system was previously seen in higher radiation doses [16]. However, further developments have led to significantly reduced radiation doses [17]. Apart from these source-based systems, there is also a detector-based approach for material separation by their energy-dependent X-ray absorption characteristics. A novel technique called dual-layer spectral CT (SCT), using one X-ray tube and two different detector layers, was introduced recently, which registers different energy spectra of the polychromatic X-ray spectrum [7,18,19]. The top layer absorbs low-energy spectra and the bottom layer absorbs high-energy spectra [12]. This allows for the simultaneous absorption of the polychromatic X-ray beam's high- and low-energy spectra. In this way, the discrimination of tissues by different atomic weights and electron densities is acquired [7,13,18,19]. Various post-processing approaches and other image reconstruction methods using SCT have already been described in the literature [7,13,18,19]. Post-processing SCT image reconstructions allow for the visualization of different tissues, leading to selective imaging of tissue changes in different clinical scenarios. BME using SCT and DECT has already been investigated in several studies [4,11,14,20,21]. Also, BME of the extremities has been described in previous studies using DECT [22,23], and one of these studies also used a three-material decomposition (TMD) approach [22]. However, no study has addressed the detection of BME of the extremities using SCT. Therefore, the applicability of TMD on SCT to detect BME in extremity bones is an interesting and relatively novel issue to investigate. In summary, this study evaluated the diagnostic performance of a TMD approach to visualize BME of the extremities using SCT.

2. Materials and Methods

Study design and IRB approval: This is a retrospective monocentric study. The study was approved by the local institutional review board (IRB) of our institution. Informed consent was waived due to the retrospective design of the study and the inclusion of patients who had undergone their examinations during routine clinical examinations. The study was conducted between 2019 and 2022.

Patients: Our institutional picture archiving and communication system (PACS) was screened for patients who underwent SCT of the extremities within the study period. First, the patients who presented with extremity fractures were identified. In the second step, control patients without any fractures of the extremities were included. All available spectral-based images (SBI) from the patients were downloaded and reconstructed for the subsequent BME analysis (as indicated under the subheading SCT and BME imaging). Before the main evaluation took place, we performed a two-step pre-evaluation. First, we screened all fracture sites for the number of occurrences. From this list, we excluded all fracture sites with a low number (n). In the second step, we reconstructed all available SBI datasets from the remaining patients and pre-evaluated the performance of our TMD approach. Our pre-evaluation of the TMD tool showed that small edemas, as well as smaller bone structures (carpal or tarsal bones), could not be reliably identified using our TMD approach. Therefore, small edemas and small bone structures were excluded. Patients who underwent CT examinations other than SCT (e.g., dual-energy CT) were excluded as well. Also, patients who presented with foreign materials causing artifacts, those aged under 18 years, those with pathological fractures, and those with infections of the extremities were excluded. We performed a pre-selection of fractures based on the most common kinds of fractures scanned with SCT. According to our pre-selection, the following body compartments remained for evaluation: distal radius, proximal femur, proximal and distal tibia, and long bone diaphysis (humerus, femur, tibia, radius). As patients' baseline data, age and sex were included. All other patient-related data were not evaluated. Figure 1 shows a flowchart of the study selection process based on the inclusion and exclusion criteria.

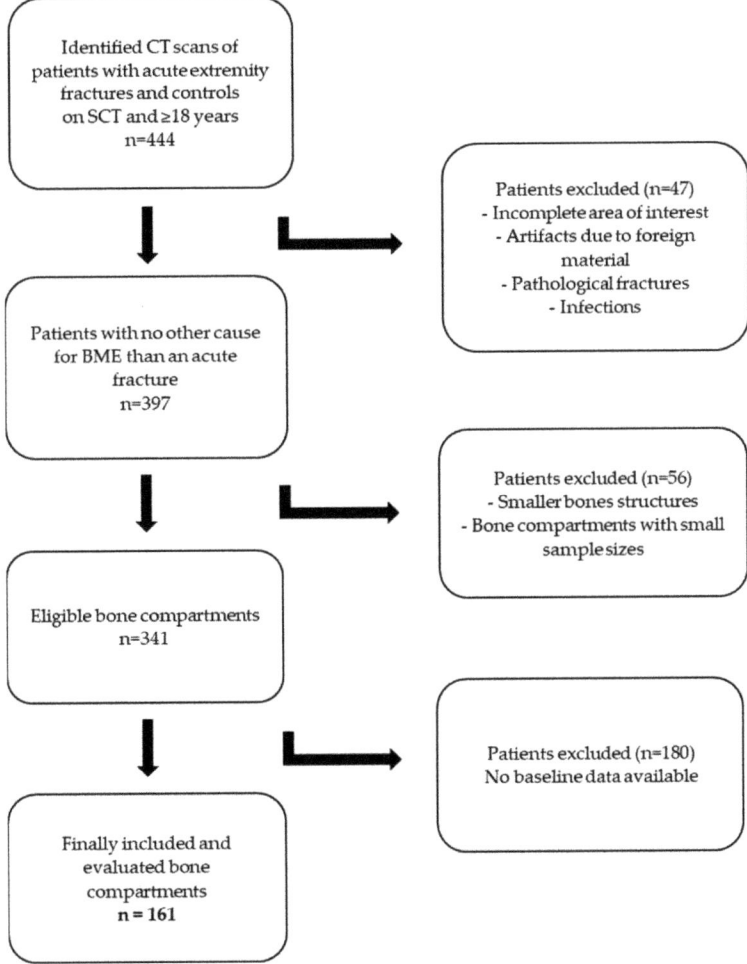

Figure 1. Flowchart of the study selection process based on the inclusion and exclusion criteria.

SCT and BME imaging: The patients were examined using dual-layer spectral computed tomography (Spectral IQON®, Philips Healthcare, Best, The Netherlands) without i.v. contrast application. CT images were acquired using a tube voltage of 120 kV, an automated attenuation-based dose modulation (DoseRight, Philips Healthcare), a rotation time of 0.27 s, a collimation of 64 × 0.625, and a slice thickness of 1 mm. Spectral-based image (SBI) data, which contain information on energy-dependent absorption, were reconstructed. For further image reconstructions, a post-processing platform (IntelliSpace, Philips Healthcare) was used. A plug-in was implemented to generate the evaluated TMD tool using the following process: The dual-layer attenuation data were decomposed into photo-electric (PE) and Compton-scatter (CS) attenuation, which provides the basis for the TMD method. PE and CS values for three materials (water, fat, and bone mineral) in pure form were set as inputs to the algorithm, after which the volume fraction of each material in each voxel was calculated, knowing the total PE and CS attenuation of that voxel. This resulted in a BME tool, where the voxel values represent the water volume fraction in each voxel. This method assumes that the sum of the volume fractions of each material is equal to one. TMD images were reconstructed using iDose level 2 (Philips Healthcare, The Netherlands) and Spectral level 2 (Philips Healthcare, The Netherlands). The density maps for the water volume fractions were generated in different orientations (according to the original CT image) and with a section thickness of 3 mm. The reconstruction resulted in grayscale images, simulating the contrast of MR images.

Image Analysis: Datasets of bones with and without BME were reconstructed and prepared by M.S. for consecutive review and analysis. The images were downloaded from our institutional PACS and saved in DICOM (digital imaging and communications in medicine) files. Two radiologists (readers) with 5 and 15 years of experience in musculoskeletal radiology evaluated the prepared datasets. The radiologists were blinded to the data and reviewed the TMD images independently in a random order. They indicated the presence of BME using a binary classification (0 no edema visible, 1 edema visible). Only clearly visible BME had to be rated as "1" according to the binary rating. The radiologists were allowed to scroll through the reformations and adjust the window for personal convenience. The cases were randomly chosen. MRI was used as a baseline to determine the presence or absence of BME.

Statistical analysis: Data were provided as mean values with standard deviation (SD). Interrater reliability was calculated with weighted Cohen's κ statistics. The diagnostic performance (sensitivity, specificity, positive predictive value, and negative predictive value) was assessed using contingency tables and then calculated. The area under the curve (AUC) was also derived from the receiver operating characteristic (ROC) curve analysis. From the BME ratings of the readers, mean values between the ratings were calculated and used for the determination of the diagnostic performance. Statistical significance for all tests was set at $p < 0.05$. Statistical analysis was performed using the IBM-SPSS version 28.0 software package (IBM, Armonk, NY, USA).

3. Results

3.1. Baseline Data

This study included 161 bone compartments—81 bone compartments with and 80 bone compartments without BME. The fracture locations are shown in Table 1. The locations presented with total numbers between $n = 29$ and $n = 35$. The mean age of the patients was 59.5 years (SD 21.9); 51% of the patients were male and 49% were female. The inter-rater reliability was 0.84 ($p < 0.001$).

Table 1. Overview of cases with and without bone marrow edema (BME) (*n* = number).

Location	BME (*n*)	No BME (*n*)	Total (*n*)
Distal radius	16	14	30
Proximal femur	15	17	32
Proximal tibia	20	15	35
Distal tibia	16	19	35
Long bone diaphysis	14	15	29
Total	81	80	161

True/false positive/negative results using the TMD approach

Altogether, 73 of the 81 BME were correctly identified. Only 16 cases were falsely classified as positive or negative (*n* = 8 each). Out of the 80 bones without BME, 72 were correctly classified. Altogether, 90% of the bone compartments were correctly classified by the two readers.

Calculated diagnostic performance using the TMD approach

Table 2 presents the diagnostic performance values of the TMD tool.

The different bone compartments showed sensitivities of 86.7% to 93.8%, specificities of 84.2% to 94.1%, positive predictive values of 82.4% to 94.7%, negative predictive values of 87.5% to 93.3%, and area under the curve (AUC) values of 85.7% to 93.1%.

The distal radius showed the highest sensitivity (93.8%) and the proximal femur showed the lowest sensitivity (86.7%), while the proximal femur presented the highest specificity (94.1%) and the distal tibia presented the lowest specificity (84.2%). The highest AUC was seen in the long bone diaphysis (93.1%), while the distal tibia showed the lowest AUC (85.7%). There was no diagnostic value lower than 80%.

3.2. Examples

Figures 2 and 3 show examples of BME on TMD images in different locations. Figure 2 presents an example of a fractured proximal tibia on conventional CT images and the TMD tool, whereas Figure 3 shows a fractured distal radius.

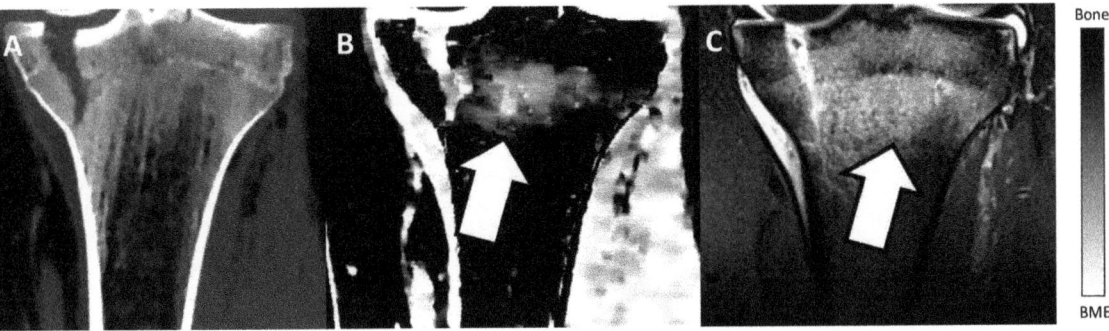

Figure 2. Fractured proximal tibia of a patient on a conventional CT image (**A**), on the TMD tool (**B**), and the corresponding MRI (**C**). The BME (white arrow) is visible on the TMD tool and the corresponding MRI, but it is not detectable on the conventional CT image. Additionally, a bar chart shows the density/intensity levels between normal bone and BME.

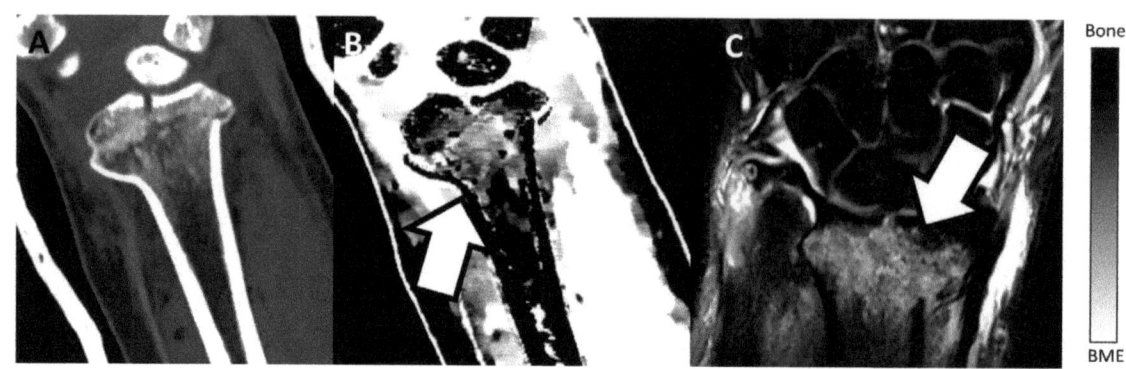

Figure 3. Fractured distal radius of a patient on a conventional CT image (**A**), on the TMD tool (**B**), and the corresponding MRI (**C**). The TMD tool and the corresponding MRI clearly show a BME (white arrow), whereas the conventional CT image does not depict the BME. Additionally, a bar chart shows the density/intensity levels between normal bone and BME.

Table 2. Diagnostic performance showing sensitivity, specificity, positive predictive value (PPV), negative predictive value (NPV), and area under the curve (AUC) (all in %) (combined for both readers).

	Sensitivity	Specificity	PPV	NPV	AUC
Distal radius	93.8%	85.7%	88.2%	92.3%	90.0%
Proximal femur	86.7%	94.1%	92.9%	88.9%	90.6%
Proximal tibia	90.0%	93.3%	94.7%	87.5%	91.4%
Distal tibia	87.5%	84.2%	82.4%	88.9%	85.7%
Long bone diaphysis	92.9%	93.3%	92.9%	93.3%	93.1%

4. Discussion

This study investigated the diagnostic performance of a TMD approach for detecting BME of the extremities on SCT. Although extremity fractures are commonly seen after trauma, there is still a lack of studies systematically addressing extremity fractures [24]. Additionally, many extremity fracture studies are outdated or include only a few patient samples [25]. Most upper extremity fractures in older patients are caused by a fall and a subsequent direct fracture impact [26]. Also, many other fracture mechanisms exist, such as stress fractures [27,28].

BME plays an essential role in diagnosing acute fractures [29,30]. Although BME is not a specific characteristic of acute fractures and it might appear in both symptomatic and asymptomatic individuals [2], BME is routinely seen in acute traumatic bone. Therefore, BME is often regarded as an indirect sign of acute fractures [3,29,30].

Radiological diagnostics is one of the major pillars for identifying traumatic fractures. Radiography is usually performed first, followed by CT. Computed tomography is nowadays established as an imaging modality that provides reliable fracture diagnostics [31,32]. However, the utilization of conventional CT is unrewarding for detecting BME, as superposition aggravates the discrimination of low-contrast tissues [12,13]. This is a well-known problem for radiologists and other clinical disciplines. However, many radiologists try to provide some vague information about fracture age, mainly based on their personal experience [33]. This could cause radiologists to be accused of misdiagnosis or failure to diagnose [34], although they only wanted to help their patients. Consequently, radiologists should try to reduce errors as much as possible. Reducing errors will improve patient care and reduce healthcare costs [34]. Therefore, in routine clinical settings, MRI is often used in undefined cases to detect BME. Nevertheless, MRI examinations are often not immediately available in the emergency setting and additionally, many patients are ineligible for MRI [7,10]. Although only a few fractures are missed in the emergency setting [35], occult fractures still cause a major problem for radiologists. Occult fractures are often difficult to detect on CT, leading to misdiagnosis or further diagnostics. Therefore, in an emergency, where time saves lives, it is preferable to detect occult fractures, indicated by BME, on-site without needing additional MRI [36,37].

Depending on the hardware setup, there are different ways to generate spectral information based on dual-energy CT [7]. Dual-energy with dual-source CT, using either different X-ray sources or rapid kV switching [7], has been available and clinically tested for many years [10,38]. The SCT consists of two detector layers, which simultaneously collect low-energy and high-energy data, consecutively allowing for the separation of these different energy spectra [1,13,18,19]. This relatively novel technique makes multiple reconstructions of various structures within the human body possible. One of the many advantages of SCT compared to DECT is that SCT allows for the analysis of spectral information without requiring specific predefined protocols [7]. The idea of a three-material decomposition for BME visualization is not new, and a similar approach has already been investigated for DECT [22]. Accordingly, Yadav et al. assessed the diagnostic accuracy of DECT in detecting bone marrow edema in patients with trauma of the lower limb. They included both virtual non-contrast (VNC) and TMD approaches, and eventually found sensitivities and specificities of 94.1% and 91.3%, respectively [22]. However, there is no previous study that evaluates a TMD approach for use in the extremity bones on SCT. Our TMD approach was developed in collaboration with the manufacturer. Also, "self-made" approaches using the same technique are possible, especially when there is no SCT available. Post-processing tools, such as our TMD approach, enhance the quality of imaging and allow for more accurate diagnostics of targeted tissues. The potential of many SCT reconstructions and applications has yet to be fully utilized. Previous studies on BME detection in SCT mainly focused on post-processing imaging using CaSupp, which relies primarily on suppressing calcium as a central component of bones and consecutively making BME visible [4,13,14,39]. In contrast to this, our approach allows for the direct visualization of BME on SCT, compared to CaSupp. Our TMD method enables BME depiction by evaluating each voxel's water volume fraction. Additionally, previous SCT studies mainly focused on vertebral fractures rather than fractures outside the vertebrae [7,11,13,21,37,39]. However, fractures of the extremities, with their various locations, are among the most common fracture sites [40,41].

In this study, we achieved high diagnostic performance of the TMD tool in identifying BME in major bone structures of the extremities, subsequently allowing for an accurate evaluation of the fracture acuity. Despite the high diagnostic performance of our TMD tool, the interrater reliability was also high, allowing for the reliable and objective detection of BME. Nevertheless, we performed a pre-selection and pre-evaluation of the included fractures. The pre-evaluation revealed that our TMD approach could only be used for major bone compartments of the extremities. Small bone structures and small edemas can be hard to identify using our approach.

Taking our results into account, our TMD approach could be used in the routine emergency setting for major bone compartments of the extremities and acute fractures in these compartments. Consequently, patients with clinically acute extremity fractures could be identified earlier and more precisely compared to conventional CT, in which BME is typically not visible. This could be very helpful, especially in occult fractures. Also, time-consuming MRI for fracture evaluation could recede into the background, eventually leading to a more time-effective treatment of trauma patients. Baumbach et al. presented an algorithm and decision tree for BME evaluation [3]. Acute fractures thereby presented a main point of their algorithm, with BME among the first appearances and features to be reviewed. The first step was described to be the pain, followed by an MRI, which shows the BME as an indirect sign of an acute fracture. Thereafter, comes CT or X-ray. By using our TMD approach, CT could rank more importantly in the algorithm as a first-line diagnostic tool. However, our TMD tool cannot fully replace MRI, and our approach is still a concept/prototype at the time of this study. Further development and exciting features, such as color-mapping or quantitative voxel-based analysis, could improve the performance of our tool. Future studies should test our approach by including many more patients. Also, automated post-processing TMD reconstruction after trauma CT, without any further manual reconstruction, could be an interesting aim for future studies.

This study has some limitations. First, we performed a retrospective study. Future studies could perform the same study in a prospective design and include many more patients. Second, we excluded other BME-causing conditions, such as metabolic diseases or malignancies. However, in the emergency setting, these types of patients could still be encountered. Therefore, future studies could focus on the evaluation of trauma-related and non-trauma-related BME. Third, many eligible patients did not undergo MRI baseline examinations, and they had to be excluded from this study. In fact, MRI examinations are often not performed in an emergency setting to avoid treatment delays, leading to a lack of baseline MRI data. Fourth, we did not include smaller bone structures, such as carpal and tarsal bones, as a pre-evaluation of our tool revealed difficulties in depicting BME in those smaller bone compartments. Future studies should use our TMD approach and optimize it for smaller bone structures. Lastly, the developed and evaluated TMD tool is still a concept or prototype. For future developments, an easy-to-handle interface [42] or an automated approach could be very helpful in making our TMD approach broadly usable in clinics.

5. Conclusions

We developed and tested a novel TMD approach for making BME of the extremities more visible on SCT. Our TMD approach revealed high diagnostic accuracy in detecting BME of the extremities, with sensitivities and specificities ranging from 86.7% to 93.8% and 84.2% to 94.1%, respectively. Our approach could facilitate diagnostics of acute extremity fractures, especially in occult fractures, consecutively leading to a faster onset of therapy. However, the presented TMD tool is not suitable for small bone structures, as BME is usually not visible in those bone compartments. Further studies could focus on testing the proposed TMD tool in larger cohorts or routine clinical settings and could include additional body compartments not evaluated in this study.

Author Contributions: Conceptualization, M.S., G.M.C. and S.S.; methodology, M.S., O.J., G.M.C. and S.S.; software, M.S., O.J., G.M.C. and S.S.; validation, all authors; formal analysis, M.S., M.G., B.R. and S.S.; investigation, M.S., M.G., B.R. and S.S.; resources, M.S., O.J., H.-U.K., G.M.C. and S.S.; data curation, M.S., G.M.C. and S.S.; writing—original draft preparation, M.S. and S.S.; writing—review and editing, all authors; visualization, M.S., G.M.C. and S.S.; supervision, O.J. and S.S.; project administration, G.M.C. and S.S.; funding acquisition, O.J., H.-U.K. and S.S. All authors have read and agreed to the published version of the manuscript.

Funding: This research received no external funding.

Institutional Review Board Statement: The study was conducted in accordance with the Declaration of Helsinki and approved by the Ethics Committee of University Hospital Schleswig-Holstein Kiel.

Informed Consent Statement: Patient consent was waived due to the retrospective design of the study.

Data Availability Statement: Data cannot be provided due to ethical reasons.

Conflicts of Interest: G.C. works for Philips Healthcare. The other authors declare no conflict of interest.

References

1. D'Angelo, T.; Albrecht, M.H.; Caudo, D.; Mazziotti, S.; Vogl, T.J.; Wichmann, J.L.; Martin, S.; Yel, I.; Ascenti, G.; Koch, V.; et al. Virtual non-calcium dual-energy CT: Clinical applications. *Eur. Radiol. Exp.* **2021**, *5*, 38. [CrossRef] [PubMed]
2. Tarantino, U.; Greggi, C.; Cariati, I.; Manenti, G.; Primavera, M.; Ferrante, P.; Iundusi, R.; Gasbarra, E.; Gatti, A. Reviewing Bone Marrow Edema in Athletes: A Difficult Diagnostic and Clinical Approach. *Medicina* **2021**, *57*, 1143. [CrossRef] [PubMed]

3. Baumbach, S.F.; Pfahler, V.; Bechtold-Dalla Pozza, S.; Feist-Pagenstert, I.; Fürmetz, J.; Baur-Melnyk, A.; Stumpf, U.C.; Saller, M.M.; Straube, A.; Schmidmaier, R.; et al. How We Manage Bone Marrow Edema-An Interdisciplinary Approach. *J. Clin. Med.* **2020**, *9*, 551. [CrossRef]
4. Kellock, T.T.; Nicolaou, S.; Kim, S.S.Y.; Al-Busaidi, S.; Louis, L.J.; O'Connell, T.W.; Ouellette, H.A.; McLaughlin, P.D. Detection of bone marrow edema in nondisplaced hip fractures: Utility of a virtual noncalcium dual-energy CT application. *Radiology* **2017**, *284*, 798–805. [CrossRef] [PubMed]
5. Reddy, T.; McLaughlin, P.D.; Mallinson, P.I.; Reagan, A.C.; Munk, P.L.; Nicolaou, S.; Ouellette, H.A. Detection of occult, undisplaced hip fractures with a dual-energy CT algorithm targeted to detection of bone marrow edema. *Emerg. Radiol.* **2015**, *22*, 25–29. [CrossRef]
6. Mandalia, V.; Henson, J.H.L. Traumatic bone bruising—A review article. *Eur. J. Radiol.* **2008**, *67*, 54–61. [CrossRef] [PubMed]
7. Schwaiger, B.J.; Gersing, A.S.; Hammel, J.; Mei, K.; Kopp, F.K.; Kirschke, J.S.; Rummeny, E.J.; Wörtler, K.; Baum, T.; Noël, P.B. Three-material decomposition with dual-layer spectral CT compared to MRI for the detection of bone marrow edema in patients with acute vertebral fractures. *Skelet. Radiol.* **2018**, *47*, 1533–1540. [CrossRef]
8. Abbassi, M.; Jain, A.; Shin, D.; Arasa, C.A.; Li, B.; Anderson, S.W.; LeBedis, C.A. Quantification of bone marrow edema using dual-energy CT at fracture sites in trauma. *Emerg. Radiol.* **2022**, *29*, 691–696. [CrossRef]
9. de Bakker, C.M.J.; Walker, R.E.A.; Besler, B.A.; Tse, J.J.; Manske, S.L.; Martin, C.R.; French, S.J.; Dodd, A.E.; Boyd, S.K. A quantitative assessment of dual energy computed tomography-based material decomposition for imaging bone marrow edema associated with acute knee injury. *Med. Phys.* **2021**, *48*, 1792–1803. [CrossRef]
10. Mallinson, P.I.; Coupal, T.M.; McLaughlin, P.D.; Nicolaou, S.; Munk, P.L.; Ouellette, H.A. Dual-energy CT for the musculoskeletal system. *Radiology* **2016**, *281*, 690–707. [CrossRef]
11. Kaup, M.; Wichmann, J.L.; Scholtz, J.-E.; Beeres, M.; Kromen, W.; Albrecht, M.H.; Lehnert, T.; Boettcher, M.; Vogl, T.J.; Bauer, R.W. Dual-energy CT–based display of bone marrow edema in osteoporotic vertebral compression fractures: Impact on diagnostic accuracy of radiologists with varying levels of experience in correlation to MR imaging. *Radiology* **2016**, *280*, 510–519. [CrossRef] [PubMed]
12. Rassouli, N.; Etesami, M.; Dhanantwari, A.; Rajiah, P. Detector-based spectral CT with a novel dual-layer technology: Principles and applications. *Insights Imaging* **2017**, *8*, 589–598. [CrossRef] [PubMed]
13. Neuhaus, V.; Lennartz, S.; Abdullayev, N.; Hokamp, N.G.; Shapira, N.; Kafri, G.; Holz, J.A.; Krug, B.; Hellmich, M.; Maintz, D.; et al. Bone marrow edema in traumatic vertebral compression fractures: Diagnostic accuracy of dual-layer detector CT using calcium suppressed images. *Eur. J. Radiol.* **2018**, *105*, 216–220. [CrossRef] [PubMed]
14. Pache, G.; Krauss, B.; Strohm, P.; Saueressig, U.; Blanke, P.; Bulla, S.; Schäfer, O.; Helwig, P.; Kotter, E.; Langer, M.; et al. Dual-energy CT virtual noncalcium technique: Detecting posttraumatic bone marrow lesions—Feasibility study. *Radiology* **2010**, *256*, 617–624. [CrossRef] [PubMed]
15. Wortman, J.R.; Uyeda, J.W.; Fulwadhva, U.P.; Sodickson, A.D. Dual-energy CT for abdominal and pelvic trauma. *Radiographics* **2018**, *38*, 586–602. [CrossRef] [PubMed]
16. McCollough, C.H.; Leng, S.; Yu, L.; Fletcher, J.G. Dual- and Multi-Energy CT: Principles, Technical Approaches, and Clinical Applications. *Radiology* **2015**, *276*, 637–653. [CrossRef]
17. Grajo, J.R.; Sahani, D.V. Dual-Energy CT of the Abdomen and Pelvis: Radiation Dose Considerations. *J. Am. Coll. Radiol.* **2018**, *15*, 1128–1132. [CrossRef]
18. Langguth, P.; Aludin, S.; Horr, A.; Campbell, G.M.; Lebenatus, A.; Ravesh, M.S.; Schunk, D.; Austein, F.; Larsen, N.; Syrek, H.; et al. Iodine uptake of adrenal glands: A novel and reliable spectral dual-layer computed tomographic-derived biomarker for acute septic shock. *Eur. J. Radiol.* **2022**, *156*, 110492. [CrossRef]
19. Sedaghat, S.; Langguth, P.; Larsen, N.; Campbell, G.; Both, M.; Jansen, O. Diagnostische Wertigkeit der Dual-Layer-Spektral-CT zur Detektion von posttraumatischen prävertebralen Hämatomen der Halswirbelsäule unter Verwendung von Elektronendichtebildern. *Rofo* **2021**, *193*, 1445–1450.
20. Wang, C.-K.; Tsai, J.-M.; Chuang, C.-M.; Wang, M.-T.; Huang, K.-Y.; Lin, R.-M. Bone marrow edema in vertebral compression fractures: Detection with dual-energy CT. *Radiology* **2013**, *269*, 525–533. [CrossRef]
21. Petritsch, B.; Kosmala, A.; Weng, A.M.; Krauss, B.; Heidemeier, A.; Wagner, R.; Heintel, T.M.; Gassenmaier, T.; Bley, T.A. Vertebral Compression Fractures: Third-Generation Dual-Energy CT for Detection of Bone Marrow Edema at Visual and Quantitative Analyses. *Radiology* **2017**, *284*, 161–168. [CrossRef]
22. Yadav, H.; Khanduri, S.; Yadav, P.; Pandey, S.; Yadav, V.K.; Khan, S. Diagnostic accuracy of dual energy CT in the assessment of traumatic bone marrow edema of lower limb and its correlation with MRI. *Indian J. Radiol. Imaging* **2020**, *30*, 59–63. [CrossRef] [PubMed]
23. Yang, S.J.; Jeon, J.Y.; Lee, S.-W.; Jeong, Y.M. Added value of color-coded virtual non-calcium dual-energy CT in the detection of acute knee fractures in non-radiology inexpert readers. *Eur. J. Radiol.* **2020**, *129*, 109102. [CrossRef] [PubMed]
24. Karl, J.W.; Olson, P.R.; Rosenwasser, M.P. The Epidemiology of Upper Extremity Fractures in the United States, 2009. *J. Orthop. Trauma* **2015**, *29*, e242–e244. [CrossRef] [PubMed]
25. Beerekamp, M.S.H.; de Muinck Keizer, R.J.O.; Schep, N.W.L.; Ubbink, D.T.; Panneman, M.J.M.; Goslings, J.C. Epidemiology of extremity fractures in the Netherlands. *Injury* **2017**, *48*, 1355–1362. [CrossRef] [PubMed]

26. Palvanen, M.; Kannus, P.; Parkkari, J.; Pitkäjärvi, T.; Pasanen, M.; Vuori, I.; Järvinen, M. The injury mechanisms of osteoporotic upper extremity fractures among older adults: A controlled study of 287 consecutive patients and their 108 controls. *Osteoporos. Int.* **2000**, *11*, 822–831. [CrossRef]
27. Milner, C.E.; Hamill, J.; Davis, I. Are knee mechanics during early stance related to tibial stress fracture in runners? *Clin. Biomech.* **2007**, *22*, 697–703. [CrossRef]
28. Jacobs, J.M.; Cameron, K.L.; Bojescul, J.A. Lower extremity stress fractures in the military. *Clin. Sports Med.* **2014**, *33*, 591–613. [CrossRef]
29. Zbijewski, W.; Sisniega, A.; Stayman, J.W.; Thawait, G.; Packard, N.; Yorkston, J.; Demehri, S.; Fritz, J.; Siewerdsen, J.H. Dual-Energy Imaging of Bone Marrow Edema on a Dedicated Multi-Source Cone-Beam CT System for the Extremities. *Proc. SPIE Int. Soc. Opt. Eng.* **2015**, *9412*, 94120V.
30. Boks, S.S.; Vroegindeweij, D.; Koes, B.W.; Hunink, M.G.M.; Bierma-Zeinstra, S.M.A. Follow-up of occult bone lesions detected at MR imaging: Systematic review. *Radiology* **2006**, *238*, 853–862. [CrossRef]
31. Dubreuil, T.; Mouly, J.; Ltaief-Boudrigua, A.; Martinon, A.; Tilhet-Coartet, S.; Tazarourte, K.; Pialat, J.B. Comparison of Cone-Beam Computed Tomography and Multislice Computed Tomography in the Assessment of Extremity Fractures. *J. Comput. Assist Tomogr.* **2019**, *43*, 372–378. [CrossRef]
32. Falkowski, A.L.; Kovacs, B.K.; Schwartz, F.R.; Benz, R.M.; Stieltjes, B.; Hirschmann, A. Comparison of 3D X-ray tomography with computed tomography in patients with distal extremity fractures. *Skelet. Radiol.* **2020**, *49*, 1965–1975. [CrossRef] [PubMed]
33. Prosser, I.; Maguire, S.; Harrison, S.K.; Mann, M.; Sibert, J.R.; Kemp, A.M. How old is this fracture? Radiologic dating of fractures in children: A systematic review. *AJR Am. J. Roentgenol.* **2005**, *184*, 1282–1286. [CrossRef]
34. Pinto, A.; Brunese, L. Spectrum of diagnostic errors in radiology. *World J. Radiol.* **2010**, *2*, 377–383. [CrossRef] [PubMed]
35. Wei, C.-J.; Tsai, W.-C.; Tiu, C.-M.; Wu, H.-T.; Chiou, H.-J.; Chang, C.-Y. Systematic analysis of missed extremity fractures in emergency radiology. *Acta Radiol.* **2006**, *47*, 710–717. [CrossRef] [PubMed]
36. Gosangi, B.; Mandell, J.C.; Weaver, M.J.; Uyeda, J.W.; Smith, S.E.; Sodickson, A.D.; Khurana, B. Bone Marrow Edema at Dual-Energy CT: A Game Changer in the Emergency Department. *Radiographics* **2020**, *40*, 859–874. [CrossRef]
37. Cavallaro, M.; D'Angelo, T.; Albrecht, M.H.; Yel, I.; Martin, S.S.; Wichmann, J.L.; Lenga, L.; Mazziotti, S.; Blandino, A.; Ascenti, G.; et al. Comprehensive comparison of dual-energy computed tomography and magnetic resonance imaging for the assessment of bone marrow edema and fracture lines in acute vertebral fractures. *Eur. Radiol.* **2022**, *32*, 561–571. [CrossRef]
38. Kalender, W.A.; Perman, W.H.; Vetter, J.R.; Klotz, E. Evaluation of a prototype dual-energy computed tomographic apparatus. I. Phantom studies. *Med. Phys.* **1986**, *13*, 334–339. [CrossRef]
39. Wang, M.-Y.; Zhang, X.-Y.; Xu, L.; Feng, Y.; Xu, Y.-C.; Qi, L.; Zou, Y.F. Detection of bone marrow oedema in knee joints using a dual-energy CT virtual non-calcium technique. *Clin. Radiol.* **2019**, *74*, 815.e1–815.e7. [CrossRef]
40. Court-Brown, C.M.; Caesar, B. Epidemiology of adult fractures: A review. *Injury* **2006**, *37*, 691–697. [CrossRef]
41. Melton, L.J. Epidemiology of Fractures. In *Osteoporosis in Men*; Elsevier: Amsterdam, The Netherlands, 1999; pp. 1–13.
42. Sedaghat, S. Success Through Simplicity: What Other Artificial Intelligence Applications in Medicine Should Learn from History and ChatGPT. *Ann. Biomed. Eng.* **2023**, *ahead of print*. [CrossRef] [PubMed]

Disclaimer/Publisher's Note: The statements, opinions and data contained in all publications are solely those of the individual author(s) and contributor(s) and not of MDPI and/or the editor(s). MDPI and/or the editor(s) disclaim responsibility for any injury to people or property resulting from any ideas, methods, instructions or products referred to in the content.

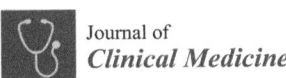

Article

Changes in Parameters after High Tibial Osteotomy: Comparison of EOS System and Computed Tomographic Analysis

Hyun-Jin Yoo [†], Jae-Kyu Choi [†], Youn-Moo Heo, Sung-Jun Moon and Byung-Hak Oh *

Department of Orthopedic Surgery, College of Medicine, Konyang University, 158 Gwanjeodong-ro, Seo-gu, Daejeon 35365, Republic of Korea; yoo15love@gmail.com (H.-J.Y.); 400852@kyuh.ac.kr (J.-K.C.); hurym1973@hanmail.net (Y.-M.H.); 400911@kyuh.ac.kr (S.-J.M.)
* Correspondence: sebslab@hanmail.net; Tel.: +82-42-600-9964; Fax: +82-42-545-2373
[†] These authors contributed equally to this work.

Abstract: Unintended rotation of the distal tibia occurs during medial open-wedge high tibial osteotomy (MOWHTO). Computed tomography (CT) is the standard method of measuring lower limb alignment; however, the new low-dose EOS system allows three-dimensional limb modeling with automated measurements of lower limb alignment. This study investigated the differences between the changes in lower limb alignment profiles obtained using the EOS system and CT in patients who underwent MOWHTO. We investigated whether any factors contributed to the degree of deformation. Thirty patients were prospectively enrolled between October 2019 and February 2023. Changes in femoral and tibial torsion, femorotibial rotation, and posterior tibial slope were measured using pre- and post-MOWHTO CT and EOS images. We found no significant difference in pre- and postoperative tibial torsion or posterior tibial slope between CT and EOS. No variables showed a significant correlation with changes in the tibial torsion or posterior tibial slope. This study confirmed the possibility that the EOS system could replace CT in measuring changes in several parameters pre- and postoperatively. Furthermore, we confirmed that the distal tibia tended to be internally rotated after MOWHTO; however, we found no significantly related parameters related to deformation caused by MOWHTO.

Keywords: EOS imaging; computed tomography; rotational alignment; osteotomy; malalignment

1. Introduction

Medial open-wedge high tibial osteotomy (MOWHTO) is a surgical technique widely performed in relatively young and active adults with medial compartment osteoarthritis, varus deformities of the knee joints, or anterior cruciate ligament deficiency [1–5]. This surgical procedure transfers mechanical loading from the damaged medial compartment to the intact lateral compartments. In addition, MOWHTO can delay or prevent deterioration of the medial compartment of the knee joint, thereby delaying the need for knee joint arthroplasty. Several studies have reported relatively satisfactory short- and mid-term results of this surgical method [6–8].

Accurate alignment correction in MOWHTO is essential for achieving satisfactory clinical outcomes. Surgeons performing MOWHTO have focused on correcting lower limb alignment in the coronal plane [9]. However, when MOWHTO is performed, three-dimensional (3D) structural deformation occurs in the coronal, axial, and sagittal planes [10]. Various studies have reported that MOWHTO causes unintended rotation of the distal tibia and alteration of the posterior tibial slope [11–14]. MOWHTO can also adversely affect the ankle and knee joints, causing patellofemoral arthritis, pes planus, and gait abnormalities [15–17].

Therefore, many studies on alignment changes after MOWHTO have been conducted and various discussions have been made on how to measure alignment of lower extremities as interest in the alignment of lower limbs before and after HTO has increased [10,14,18–23]. Various methods including clinical, sonographic, fluoroscopic, and magnetic resonance imaging have been proposed to measure the rotation of lower extremities, but none of them have been widely used routinely [24–27]. In recent years, computed tomography (CT) has become the gold-standard radiographic method for evaluating alignment [9,28].

However, a biplanar low-dose EOS system (EOS Imaging, Paris, France) has recently been developed to analyze lower limb alignment [29]. The EOS system enables significantly lower radiation exposure than conventional radiographs. Simultaneously, the EOS system captures whole-body anteroposterior (AP) and lateral two-dimensional radiographs in a scaled environment, allowing 3D reconstruction of the bone structures of the spine and lower extremities using stereoscopic radiography [30]. Thus, various clinical parameters of the lower extremities and spine, including the femoral and tibial torsions, can be measured using the 3D model [31,32].

Some studies have reported that the rotation of the lower extremities can be evaluated using the EOS system; however, few studies have investigated the use of the EOS system in assessing other factors, such as rotation after MOWHTO [33,34]. Therefore, we aimed to investigate the differences between the changes in lower limb alignment and rotation profiles obtained using the EOS system and CT in patients who underwent MOWHTO. We hypothesized that there would be no differences in the changes in lower limb alignment and rotation profiles between the EOS system and CT. Furthermore, we investigated whether other factors contributed to the amount of rotational deformation and slope changes.

2. Materials and Methods

2.1. Patients

This prospective study was approved by the Institutional Review Board (IRB no. 2023-02-012). We prospectively included all patients who underwent MOWHTO between October 2019 and February 2023. Patients with severe lower extremity deformities such as traumas, fractures, or prosthetic implants in the lower extremity were excluded. In total, 97 patients (97 knees) met the criteria; however, 60 patients (60 knees) did not undergo pre- or postoperative CT. Furthermore, seven patients (seven knees) did not undergo EOS imaging studies as part of the preoperative work-up or to evaluate changes in lower limb alignment postoperatively. A flowchart of this study is shown in Figure 1.

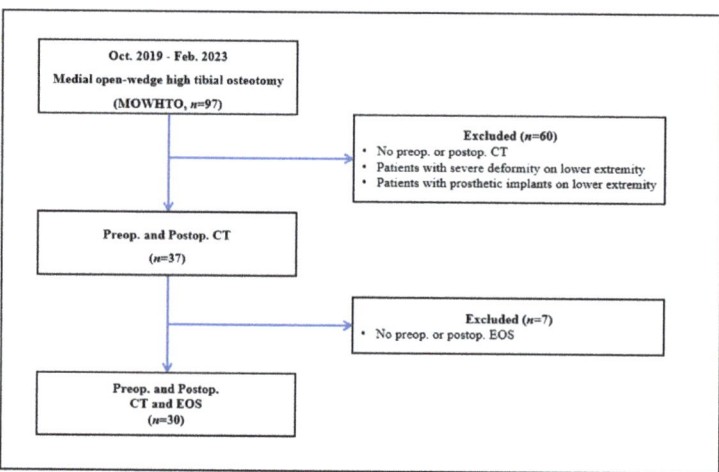

Figure 1. Flowchart of the study.

2.2. Evaluation Methods

During the scan, the patients were instructed to touch both hands to their cheeks while holding their breath. We obtained standing AP and lateral images, including the entire lower extremity, and created images using the EOS imaging system. The images were stored on an institutional picture archiving and communication system (PACS) network. Subsequently, anatomical landmark identification was performed manually on the digital AP and lateral EOS two-dimensional radiographs using PACS workstation software tools (sterEOS; Biospace Med, Paris, France) (Figure 2A,B) [35]. Three-dimensional images were reconstructed by radiology technicians with several years of experience in musculoskeletal radiology who were trained in using sterEOS software. Various parameters of the lower extremities were calculated using these images by the computer-aided program (Figure 2C,D).

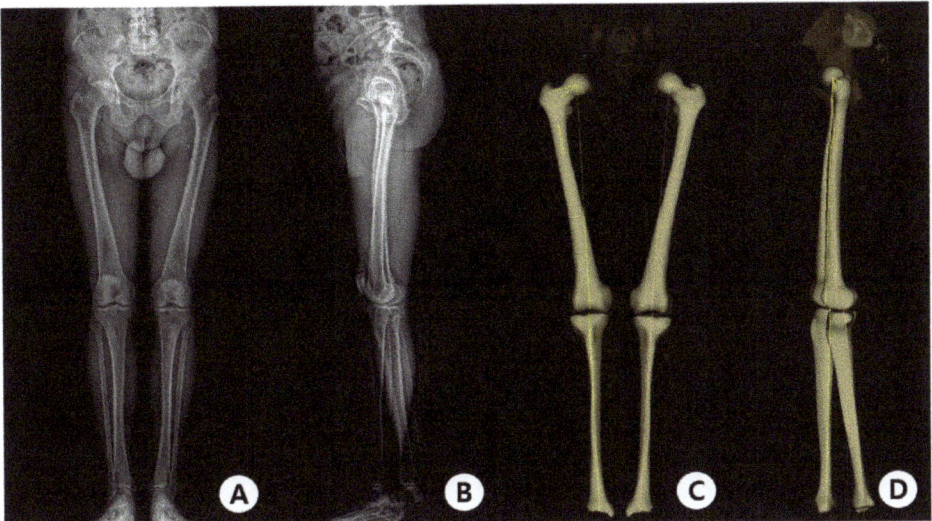

Figure 2. (**A**,**B**) Anteroposterior and lateral radiographs acquired for 3D reconstruction; (**C**,**D**) The 3D reconstruction images made by the EOS imaging system.

In addition, a helical CT machine (Aquilion Prime, Canon Medical Systems, Otawara, Japan) was used to obtain axial images of lower extremities with a voltage source of 120 kV, and slices were acquired at 3 mm intervals. The CT scan captured the whole lower extremity, and the threshold was defined from −1000 HU to 1000 HU to highlight the bone. Patients were instructed to straighten their legs while lying down, and radiologists fixed their legs with a device to prevent them from moving while undergoing CT. Furthermore, a simple radiographic evaluation was performed using weight-bearing lower extremity AP radiographs.

Measurements were performed using our institution's PACS workstation (M6, INFINITT Healthcare Co., Ltd., Seoul, Republic of Korea). These were conducted by two senior orthopedists who were mainly involved in the care of lower extremities, including the hip and knee joints.

2.3. Measurement of Parameters and Clinical Outcomes

The femoral neck anteversion was computed as the angle between the femoral neck axis and the axis tangential to the posterior condyles on the transverse femoral plane [36]. The angle was positive when the femoral neck was anteverted. Moreover, the axis adapted to the posterior tibial plateau rim and the bimalleolar axis was defined as tibial torsion [37,38]. Femorotibial rotation was the angle between the axis of the posterior condyles of the femur and the posterior tibial plateau rim. The values were positive when the distal fragment externally rotated during tibial torsion and femorotibial rotation.

Images of the EOS and CT measurements are described in Figure 3A,B and Figure 4A–D, respectively. The posterior tibial slope measurements were performed in the sagittal plane. The tibial axis was determined according to the method described by Lipps et al. (Figure 3C). The angle between the proximal posterior tibial axis and the osteotomy axis of the tibial tuberosity was defined as the angle of the tuberosity osteotomy axis (Figure 5A,B) [14,39]. Furthermore, the hip–knee–ankle angle (HKAA), the angle between the lines from the knee joint center to the femoral head center and the ankle joint center, was calculated from the weight-bearing AP long-leg view. When the knee had a varus deformity, the angle had a positive value. In addition, the medial angle between the articular line of the proximal tibia and the anatomical axis of the tibia was defined as the medial proximal tibial angle.

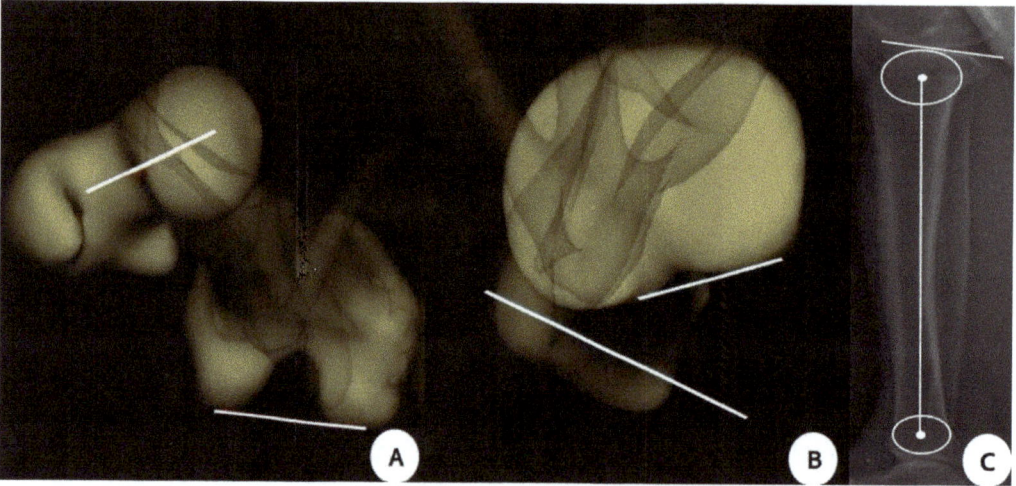

Figure 3. EOS measurements. (**A**) Femoral torsion; (**B**) Tibial torsion; (**C**) Posterior tibial slope on the sagittal plane of the EOS.

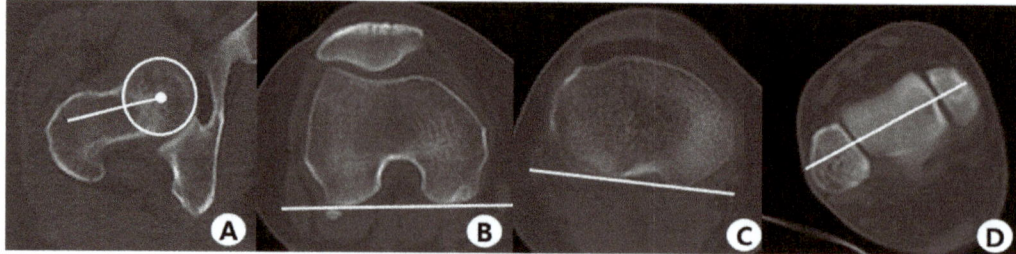

Figure 4. Axial computed tomography. (**A**) Femoral neck axis; (**B**) The line adapted to the posterior contour of the medial and lateral femoral condyles; (**C**) The line adapted to the posterior contour of the proximal tibial head; (**D**) The bimalleolar axis.

The Western Ontario and McMaster Universities Osteoarthritis Index (WOMAC), Hospital for Special Surgery (HSS) score, and range of motion of the involved knees were used to evaluate functional outcomes in this study. Additionally, patient-reported outcomes were collected twice in the clinic by a single orthopedic surgeon, once preoperatively and once 1 year postoperatively.

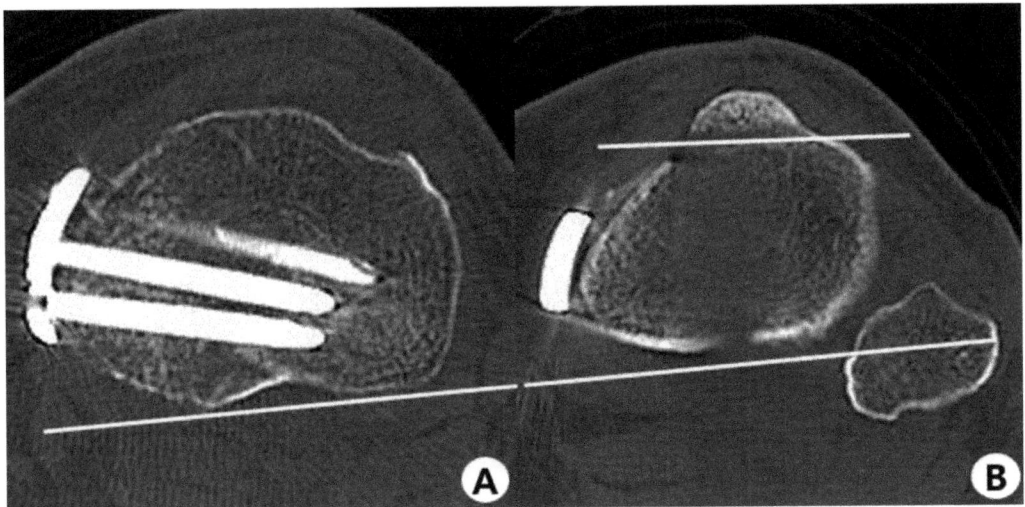

Figure 5. Measurement of the tibial osteotomy angle. (**A**) The line adapted to the posterior tibial plateau; (**B**) The line of the osteotomy at the level of the tibial tuberosity axis.

2.4. Surgical Technique

All operations were performed by a single senior surgeon. A 5 cm anteromedial skin incision was made medial to the tibial tuberosity. Subsequently, the pes anserinus tendon was released, and the superficial medial collateral ligament was exposed and detached with a Cobb elevator. To protect the neurovascular structures of the knee, the Cobb elevator was inserted, and subperiosteal dissection on the posteromedial and posterolateral aspect of the tibia was performed. Diagnostic arthroscopy was performed in all patients for meniscal procedures such as repair or meniscectomy before MOWHTO, and lateral retinacular release was performed after the arthroscopic procedure. Guidewires were inserted approximately 3.5 cm below the medial joint line and directed obliquely toward the tip of the fibula head. Biplane osteotomy was performed at the medial tibial cortex using an oscillating saw. The osteotomes were carefully advanced to approximately 1 cm into the lateral cortex without breakage. The osteotomy site was carefully widened to the planned width using a chisel. When the expected osteotomy width was reached, we checked whether the mechanical axis passed the 62.5% point of the tibial plateau using the cable method. Stabilization of the osteotomy site was achieved using a metal plate with a metal block (Ohtofix, Ohtomedical Co., Ltd., Goyang, Republic of Korea).

2.5. Statistical Analysis

The normality of the distribution was confirmed by performing the Kolmogorov–Smirnov test. The rotational alignment and slope of the lower extremity were measured by two orthopedists in CT taken before surgery. The average value of the values measured by two orthopedists was determined as the preoperative rotational alignment and slope values, and the CT images taken after the surgery were also measured in the same way. The change between the values of each variable before and after surgery was calculated. The amount of change in variables of EOS before and after surgery was also calculated. Student's *t*-tests were then performed to compare changes in femoral torsion, tibial torsion, femorotibial rotation, and posterior tibial slope between the CT and EOS groups. In addition, pre- and postoperative comparisons of functional outcomes, tibial slope, tibial rotation, femorotibial rotation, the HKAA, and the medial proximal tibial angle were performed using paired *t*-tests. Pearson's correlation coefficients were calculated to investigate the association between the variables and the changes in tibial torsion and posterior tibial slope after

MOWHTO in patients with pre- and postoperative CT, regardless of the EOS system. All statistical analyses were performed using SPSS version 20.0 (IBM Corp., Armonk, NY, USA), and statistical significance was set at $p < 0.05$.

3. Results

All patients were diagnosed with medial compartment osteoarthritis with varus malalignment. The population consisted of 22 females (73%) and 8 males (27%), with a mean age of 59.9 years at the time of surgery. There were 16 and 14 left and right knees, respectively. Furthermore, the mean preoperative flexion contracture was 4.0 degrees, while the average correction angle calculated using the Dugdale and Noyes method was 8.27 (4.0–15.0 degrees). MOWHTO was combined with medial meniscus repair in 19 knees (63%) and partial medial meniscectomy in 11 knees (37%). Additionally, 2/25 (7%) patients underwent simultaneous MOWHTO and allogeneic mesenchymal stem cell transplantation (Table 1).

Table 1. Patient demographics.

Parameters	Knees ($n = 30$)
Sex	
Male	8 (27)
Female	22 (73)
Age (years)	59.9
Height (cm)	159.8
Weight (kg)	67.7
Body mass index (kg/m^2)	26.41
Side	
Left	16 (53)
Right	14 (47)
Flexion contracture (°)	4.0
Correction angle (°)	8.25 (4–15)
Concomitant surgery	
Medial meniscus repair	19 (63)
Partial medial meniscectomy	11 (37)
Allogenic mesenchymal stem cell transplantation	2 (7)

Data are presented as n (%) or mean (range).

The mean differences in femoral torsion between pre- and post-MOWHTO when using CT and the EOS system were 0.17° ± 2.73° and −2.96° ± 9.24°, respectively; however, there were no statistically significant results between these values ($p = 0.142$). In addition, the mean differences between pre- and postoperative tibial torsion when using CT and EOS were −3.59° ± 2.64° and −3.39° ± 7.34°, respectively ($p = 0.894$). Furthermore, the mean difference of the femorotibial rotation when using CT was 2.61° ± 3.63°, while that for the EOS system was 2.46° ± 10.58° ($p = 0.947$). When the posterior tibial slope was measured before and after MOWHTO, the change observed when using the EOS system was 1.07° greater than that in CT, which was not statistically significant ($p = 0.227$) (Table 2).

The clinical and radiological outcomes after MOWHTO are described in Table 3. We observed that the posterior tibial slope increased by 0.82° ± 1.92° after MOWHTO ($p = 0.035$). Additionally, the tibial rotation showed a change of −3.59° ± 2.64° between the pre- and postoperative measurements, which was statistically significant ($p < 0.001$). Similarly, the femorotibial rotation showed a statistically significant change of 2.61° ± 3.63° between the pre- and postoperative measurements ($p < 0.001$). Furthermore, the mean HKAA changed from varus (6.29° ± 2.33°) to valgus (−1.11° ± 2.10°) after MOWTHO, which was statistically significant ($p < 0.001$). In terms of clinical outcomes, the WOMAC scores decreased in all categories after MOWHTO. The total WOMAC and WOMAC pain scores had statistically significant outcomes: p-values of 0.008 and 0.007, respectively. The HSS score also increased postoperatively by 8.75 ± 3.58 ($p < 0.001$).

Table 2. Measurement of the lower extremity rotation and posterior tibial slope using the EOS system and CT.

	CT			EOS System			p-Value
	Before MOWHTO (SD)	After MOW1HTO (SD)	Change (SD)	Before MOWHTO (SD)	After MOWHTO (SD)	Change (SD)	
Femoral torsion (°)	14.42 (5.87)	14.59 (6.47)	0.17 (2.73)	17.39 (7.28)	14.96 (9.50)	−2.96 (9.24)	0.142
Tibial torsion (°)	25.16 (6.86)	21.57 (5.21)	−3.59 (2.64)	26.29 (7.97)	22.89 (6.37)	−3.39 (7.34)	0.894
Femorotibial rotation (°)	0.87 (3.66)	3.48 (5.14)	2.61 (3.63)	−1.64 (7.50)	0.82 (9.49)	2.46 (10.58)	0.947
Posterior tibial slope (°)	12.10 (3.33)	12.92 (3.66)	0.82(1.91)	12.75 (4.26)	14.64 (4.53)	1.89 (2.10)	0.227

CT, computed tomography; SD, standard deviation; MOWHTO, medial open-wedge high tibial osteotomy.

Table 3. Clinical and radiologic outcomes after MOWHTO.

	Preop. (SD)	Postop. (SD)	Change (SD)	p-Value
Radiologic outcomes				
Tibial slope (°)	12.10 (3.33)	12.92 (3.66)	0.82 (1.92)	0.035 *
Tibial rotation (°)	25.16 (6.86)	21.57 (5.21)	−3.59 (2.64)	<0.001 *
Femorotibial rotation (°)	0.87 (3.66)	3.48 (5.14)	2.61 (3.63)	<0.001 *
HKAA (°)	6.29 (2.33)	−1.11 (2.10)	−7.39 (2.74)	<0.001 *
MPTA (°)	84.54 (2.15)	89.89 (3.29)	5.36 (3.88)	<0.001 *
Clinical outcomes (POD 1Y)				
ROM (o)	131.64 (7.68)	132.46 (7.39)	0.82 (2.73)	0.129
WOMAC score				
Total	44.50 (8.68)	41.21 (4.97)	−3.29 (5.99)	0.008 *
Pain	9.04 (3.92)	7.54 (2.44)	−1.50 (2.69)	0.007 *
Function	30.21 (6.75)	28.61 (4.32)	−1.61 (4.93)	0.102
Stiffness	5.21 (1.15)	5.07 (1.22)	−0.14 (0.91)	0.424
HSS score	71.18 (6.37)	79.93 (7.13)	8.75 (3.58)	<0.001 *

SD, standard deviation; MOWHTO, medial open-wedge high tibial osteotomy; POD, postoperative duration; HKAA, hip–knee–ankle angle; MPTA, medial proximal tibial angle; Y, year; ROM, range of motion; WOMAC, Western Ontario and McMaster Universities Osteoarthritis Index; HSS, Hospital for Special Surgery; * Statistical significance was set at $p < 0.05$.

Using Pearson's correlation analysis in 37 patients, the correlations between the change in tibial torsion and posterior tibial slope (difference between pre- and postoperative values) and each independent variable were assessed (Table 4). No variables showed a significant correlation between the changes in the tibial torsion or posterior tibial slope.

Table 4. Correlations of the changes in tibial torsion and posterior slope with other parameters.

	Change in Tibial Torsion		Change in Posterior Tibial Slope	
	Pearson's Correlation Coefficient (r)	p	Pearson's Correlation Coefficient (r)	p
Correction angle (°)	0.150	0.377	0.186	0.269
TOA (°)	−0.060	0.730	0.027	0.878
Flexion contracture (°)	−0.205	0.224	−0.125	0.462
Change of tibial torsion	1.0		0.000	0.998
Change of posterior tibial slope	0.000	0.998	1.0	
Change of clinical outcomes (POD 1Y)				
ROM (°)	0.173	0.306	−0.036	0.834
WOMAC score				

Table 4. Cont.

	Change in Tibial Torsion		p	Change in Posterior Tibial Slope	p
	Pearson's Correlation Coefficient (r)			Pearson's Correlation Coefficient (r)	
Total	0.104		0.538	−0.130	0.445
Pain	0.110		0.515	−0.156	0.358
Function	0.05		0.769	−0.056	0.742
Stiffness	0.172		0.309	−0.050	0.770
HSS score	−0.113		0.505	0.250	0.135

TOA, tuberosity osteotomy angle; POD, postoperative duration; ROM, range of motion; WOMAC, Western Ontario and McMaster Universities Osteoarthritis Index; HSS, Hospital for Special Surgery.

4. Discussion

The main finding of this study was that there was no significant difference between the CT and EOS systems when measuring the changes in femoral rotation, femorotibial rotation, tibial rotation, and posterior tibial slope. This suggests that the EOS system developed for evaluating lower extremity alignment may replace CT, the gold standard for measuring lower extremity profiles. Additionally, we confirmed that the distal tibia was internally rotated as a result of MOWHTO; however, there was no significant correlation between the degree of internal rotation and various parameters and functional results.

Since the development of the EOS system, studies comparing the EOS system with CT for evaluating lower extremity alignment have been published. Folinais et al. reported that rotation parameters measured using the EOS system strongly correlated with the values measured by CT. Buck et al. reported that measuring femoral and tibial torsion using 3D models based on the EOS system could replace standard CT measurements in patients with knee osteoarthritis [33,34]. Similarly, Hecker et al. reported that posterior tibial slope measurements using the EOS 3D imaging system were as reliable and reproducible as those obtained using CT [40]. Previous cross-sectional studies have also reported that EOS can replace CT; however, our study is novel in that we examined the differences between the EOS system and CT before and after surgery and found that the EOS system can replace CT for these measurements.

It was reported that the difference between EOS and CT was about 3 degrees on average in the femoral torsion in the study comparing EOS and CT [33,34]. In the femoral torsion values in Table 2, the CT showed the result as anteversion, and the EOS showed the opposite result (CT: 0.17°/EOS system: −2.96°). Research that MOWHTO affects femoral torsion has not been confirmed yet, and it is thought that MOWHTO does not affect the alignment of femoral torsion. Therefore, the different results were thought to be due to the differences in the diagnostic methods, i.e., the CT and EOS systems.

Some studies have reported coronal realignment, unintended rotation of the distal fragment in the axial plane, and increases in the posterior tibial slope occurring after HTO surgery [9,10,14,23]. These unintended deformities can adversely affect the knee and ankle joints and contribute to patellofemoral joint arthritis. Therefore, care should be taken by surgeons when performing HTO. Our study also showed that the distal fragment was internally rotated, and the posterior tibial slope was increased after MOWHTO, as shown in Table 3. Therefore, because realignment of the axial and sagittal planes could occur during surgery, particular care was taken during MOWHTO. However, we cannot rule out the possibility that statistically significant realignment occurred during technical aspects such as plate fixation (performed with the distal bone fragment slightly extended) or as the bone fragments were fixed with reduction forceps to improve the contact of the anterior surface in biplane osteotomy. Notably, Suh et al. reported that the increase in posterior tibial slope was lower in uniplane medial-opening HTO than in biplane HTO, suggesting that the use of biplane MOWHTO in our study may have also affected the increase in posterior tibial slope [41].

Many studies have confirmed the occurrence of realignment after MOWHTO; however, factors that cause greater deformation have not been reported [9,10,14,23,25,42]. Hinterwimme et al. reported that distal tibial rotation was not related to the correction angle; instead, they assumed that rotation of the distal tibia would occur because of the influence of the 3D anatomic complexity of the tibia and the state of peripheral soft tissue, especially the semitendinosus and gracilis tendons [10]. Moreover, Jang et al. reported that a greater opening width and tuberosity osteotomy angle during MOWHTO showed a tendency for greater internal rotation of the distal tibia [14]. Similarly, Kim et al. reported that the distal tibial fragment was externally rotated after MOWHTO, and this degree was related to the opening gap width [42]. In line with these previous studies, we confirmed the relationship between the correction angle, tibial osteotomy angle, and preoperative flexion contracture with the degree of realignment; however, these results were not statistically significant. In addition, we confirmed that the degree of deformation did not affect functional outcomes in the first year after surgery; this result was also not statistically significant (Table 4).

As tibial rotation changes after high tibial osteotomy, several studies have reported that the posterior tibial slope also changes after high tibial surgery. The axis of the osteotomy hinge has been studied as a significant determinant in determining the change in the posterior tibial slope during MOWHTO [13,19,20,22,23,43]. Theoretically, the internally rotated osteotomy hinge axis may decrease the posterior tibial slope, and the externally rotated hinge axis may increase the posterior tibial slope. Wang et al. reported that the posterolateral osteotomy axis increased the posterior tibial slope after MOWHTO more than the lateral osteotomy axis [23]. Claire et al. reported that the distalization–flexion position of the hinge axis also increased the posterior tibial slope in addition to the external rotation of the osteotomy axis [20]. Therefore, MOWHTO should be performed in a way that the axis of osteotomy rotates internally and angulates proximalization–extension simultaneously to prevent changes in the posterior tibial slope, but this is challenging. The surgeon also paid much attention to not changing the posterior tibial slope in this study, but the result showed that the angle increased by an average of about 0.8 degrees after MOWHTO, which was a statistically significant change before and after surgery. Therefore, it is necessary to pay more attention to the determination of the hinge axis of osteotomy, keeping in mind that the posterior tibial slope may change after MOWHTO.

Research using computer simulation is a research method that is more convenient and can obtain faster results than research conducted in a laboratory or on patients. Various in silico studies have also been reported by realizing bones or surgical instruments as images using 3D CT reconstruction in orthopedics [44–48]. Recently, a finite element analysis on the pressure applied to the knee cartilage according to the correction angle after HTO surgery has been published. The study reported that the desired alignment was achieved under a valgus hypercorrection of 4.5° that significantly unloads the medial compartment, loads the lateral compartment, and arrests the progression of osteoarthritis [49]. In addition to this, it is possible to conduct research (using computer stimulation) on how much rotation of the distal tibia occurs and how the slope changes due to the influence of the correction angle, osteotomy axis, opening gap width, and soft tissue. It is also necessary to study the change in pressure applied to the knee joint and ankle joint by considering the change in the mechanical axis due to high tibial osteotomy and the rotation and slope change of the tibia by various factors simultaneously. It will be helpful to find the optimal correction angle and osteotomy axis when performing HTO surgery by considering both the slope and rotation as well as the change in mechanical axis.

An advantage of the EOS system is the reconstruction of 3D data based on biplanar radiographs (Figure 2); therefore, it is regarded as a new diagnostic method for femoral and tibial torsion measurements that can replace preoperative radiographs and CT. Visualization of the spinal geometry is enabled by the 3D reconstruction by the EOS system in the horizontal plane view from above, which provides the surgeon with more information in orthopedic surgery, especially in scoliosis surgery. The EOS system can help patients with multiple abnormalities, especially when they are present simultaneously [50]. In addition, because the radiation exposure of the EOS system is significantly lower than that of X-ray or CT, alignment measurement using EOS imaging is advantageous for children and adolescents, especially patients who need various orthopedic imaging studies [51]. Dietrich et al. reported that the radiation dose is 50% lower in the EOS system than in X-ray imaging for the entire lower limb [52]. CT involves a fairly high radiation dose because of the broad scanning area. In addition, EOS imaging and various parameters can be acquired simultaneously [53].

The EOS system can be used in various ways, including preoperative planning and postoperative alignment evaluation in spine and lower extremity surgery. Orfeuvre et al. published a study using the EOS system to evaluate postoperative nonunion in patients with femur shaft fractures who underwent intramedullary nailing [54]. Peeters et al. evaluated pedicle size using the EOS system in scoliosis patients [55]. Evaluating pelvic tilt and the position of the acetabulum using the EOS system after total hip arthroplasty was studied by Loppini et al. [56].

The EOS system's 3D model reconstruction requires accurate landmarks of the bone and is influenced by the standing position before taking an image [57]. In this study, the correct standing position was achieved by standing with one foot slightly anterior to the other. If this is not performed, superimposed knees can negatively affect the identification of the anatomical landmarks of the femur and tibia on the lateral image [35]. However, Cho et al. evaluated the reliability of lower extremity alignment measurements using the EOS imaging system as the patient stood with feet placed parallel in an even weight-bearing posture. They confirmed a significant difference in the tibial and femorotibial rotation [58]. Therefore, we used the adjusted standing position in our implementation of the EOS system.

Our study has a few limitations. First, the number of enrolled patients was relatively low and the patient population lacked diversity; however, the study was conducted only with pure data, and it was statistically reasonable. Second, only two orthopedists interpreted the CT results, which can introduce bias. Third, the follow-up period of 1 year was short. However, this study had the advantage of being a prospective study, unlike other previous studies that compared the EOS system and CT, which were retrospective. We also simultaneously compared the EOS system and CT and investigated the postoperative outcomes of MOWHTO.

In conclusion, this study confirmed the possibility that the EOS system could replace CT in measuring changes in several parameters pre- and postoperatively. Furthermore, we confirmed that the distal tibia tended to be internally rotated after MOWHTO; however, we found no significantly related parameters related to deformation caused by MOWHTO.

Author Contributions: Conceptualization, B.-H.O.; Methodology, H.-J.Y., Y.-M.H. and B.-H.O.; Formal analysis, H.-J.Y.; Investigation, J.-K.C. and S.-J.M.; Data curation, J.-K.C. and S.-J.M.; Writing—original draft, H.-J.Y. and J.-K.C.; Writing—review & editing, H.-J.Y., J.-K.C. and B.-H.O.; Visualization, B.-H.O.; Supervision, H.-J.Y. and Y.-M.H.; Project administration, Y.-M.H. and B.-H.O. All authors have read and agreed to the published version of the manuscript.

Funding: This research received no external funding.

Institutional Review Board Statement: This prospective study was conducted in accordance with the Declaration of Helsinki and approved by the Institutional Review Board of (Konyang University Hospital) (IRB no. 2023-02-011).

Informed Consent Statement: Informed consent was obtained from all subjects involved in the study.

Data Availability Statement: Deidentified data are available on reasonable request from the corresponding author.

Conflicts of Interest: The authors declare no conflict of interest.

References

1. Lee, D.C.; Byun, S.J. High tibial osteotomy. *Knee Surg. Rel. Res.* **2012**, *24*, 61–69. [CrossRef] [PubMed]
2. Amendola, A.; Fowler, P.J.; Litchfield, R.; Kirkley, S.; Clatworthy, M. Opening wedge high tibial osteotomy using a novel technique–early results and complications. *J. Knee Surg.* **2004**, *17*, 164–169. [CrossRef] [PubMed]

3. Jakob, R.; Murphy, S. Tibial osteotomy for varus gonarthrosis: Indication, planning, and operative technique. *Instr. Course Lect.* **1992**, *41*, 87–93. [PubMed]
4. Koshino, T.; Murase, T.; Saito, T. Medial opening-wedge high tibial osteotomy with use of porous hydroxyapatite to treat medial compartment osteoarthritis of the knee. *J. Bone Joint Surg. Am.* **2003**, *85*, 78–85. [CrossRef]
5. Gomoll, A.H. High tibial osteotomy for the treatment of unicompartmental knee osteoarthritis: A review of the literature, indications, and technique. *Phys. Sportsmed.* **2011**, *39*, 45–54. [CrossRef]
6. Bauer, G.C.; Insall, J.; Koshino, T. Tibial osteotomy in gonarthrosis (osteo-arthritis of the knee). *J. Bone Joint Surg. Am.* **1969**, *51*, 1545–1563. [CrossRef]
7. Insall, J.N.; Joseph, D.M.; Msika, C. High tibial osteotomy for varus gonarthrosis. A long-term follow-up study. *J. Bone Joint Surg. Am.* **1984**, *66*, 1040–1048. [CrossRef]
8. Yasuda, K.; Majima, T.; Tsuchida, T.; Kaneda, K. A ten- to 15-year follow-up observation of high tibial osteotomy in medial compartment osteoarthrosis. *Clin. Orthop. Relat. Res.* **1992**, *282*, 186–195. [CrossRef]
9. Kendoff, D.; Lo, D.; Goleski, P.; Warkentine, B.; O'Loughlin, P.F.; Pearle, A.D. Open wedge tibial osteotomies influence on axial rotation and tibial slope. *Knee Surg. Sports Traumatol. Arthrosc.* **2008**, *16*, 904–910. [CrossRef]
10. Hinterwimmer, S.; Feucht, M.J.; Paul, J.; Kirchhoff, C.; Sauerschnig, M.; Imhoff, A.B.; Beitzel, K. Analysis of the effects of high tibial osteotomy on tibial rotation. *Int. Orthop.* **2016**, *40*, 1849–1854. [CrossRef]
11. Kawai, R.; Tsukahara, T.; Kawashima, I.; Yamada, H. Tibial rotational alignment after opening-wedge and closing-wedge high tibial osteotomy. *Nagoya J. Med. Sci.* **2019**, *81*, 621–628. [PubMed]
12. Kuwashima, U.; Takeuchi, R.; Ishikawa, H.; Shioda, M.; Nakashima, Y.; Schroter, S. Comparison of torsional changes in the tibia following a lateral closed or medial open wedge high tibial osteotomy. *Knee* **2019**, *26*, 374–381. [CrossRef] [PubMed]
13. Nha, K.W.; Kim, H.J.; Ahn, H.S.; Lee, D.H. Change in posterior tibial slope after open-wedge and closed-wedge high tibial osteotomy: A meta-analysis. *Am. J. Sports Med.* **2016**, *44*, 3006–3013. [CrossRef] [PubMed]
14. Jang, K.M.; Lee, J.H.; Park, H.J.; Kim, J.L.; Han, S.B. Unintended rotational changes of the distal tibia after biplane medial open-wedge high tibial osteotomy. *J. Arthroplast.* **2016**, *31*, 59–63. [CrossRef] [PubMed]
15. McLaren, C.; Wootton, J.R.; Heath, P.D.; Jones, C.H. Pes planus after tibial osteotomy. *Foot Ankle* **1989**, *9*, 300–303. [CrossRef]
16. Lee, S.H.; Lee, O.S.; Teo, S.H.; Lee, Y.S. Change in gait after high tibial osteotomy: A systematic review and meta-analysis. *Gait Posture* **2017**, *57*, 57–68. [CrossRef]
17. Gaasbeek, R.; Welsing, R.; Barink, M.; Verdonschot, N.; van Kampen, A. The influence of open and closed high tibial osteotomy on dynamic patellar tracking: A biomechanical study. *Knee Surg. Sports Traumatol. Arthrosc.* **2007**, *15*, 978–984. [CrossRef]
18. Baumgarten, K.M.; Meyers, K.N.; Fealy, S.; Wright, T.M.; Wickiewicz, T.L. The coronal plane high tibial osteotomy. Part II: A comparison of axial rotation with the opening wedge high tibial osteotomy. *HSS J.* **2007**, *3*, 155–158. [CrossRef]
19. Ducat, A.; Sariali, E.; Lebel, B.; Mertl, P.; Hernigou, P.; Flecher, X.; Zayni, R.; Bonnin, M.; Jalil, R.; Amzallag, J.; et al. Posterior tibial slope changes after opening- and closing-wedge high tibial osteotomy: A comparative prospective multicenter study. *Orthop. Traumatol. Surg. Res.* **2012**, *98*, 68–74. [CrossRef]
20. Eliasberg, C.D.; Hancock, K.J.; Swartwout, E.; Robichaud, H.; Ranawat, A.S. The Ideal Hinge Axis Position to Reduce Tibial Slope in Opening-Wedge High Tibial Osteotomy Includes Proximalization-Extension and Internal Rotation. *Arthroscopy* **2021**, *37*, 1577–1584. [CrossRef]
21. Jacobi, M.; Villa, V.; Reischl, N.; Demey, G.; Goy, D.; Neyret, P.; Gautier, E.; Magnussen, R.A. Factors influencing posterior tibial slope and tibial rotation in opening wedge high tibial osteotomy. *Knee Surg. Sports Traumatol. Arthrosc.* **2015**, *23*, 2762–2768. [CrossRef] [PubMed]
22. Moon, S.W.; Park, S.H.; Lee, B.H.; Oh, M.; Chang, M.; Ahn, J.H.; Wang, J.H. The Effect of Hinge Position on Posterior Tibial Slope in Medial Open-Wedge High Tibial Osteotomy. *Arthroscopy* **2015**, *31*, 1128–1133. [CrossRef] [PubMed]
23. Wang, J.H.; Bae, J.H.; Lim, H.C.; Shon, W.Y.; Kim, C.W.; Cho, J.W. Medial open wedge high tibial osteotomy: The effect of the cortical hinge on posterior tibial slope. *Am. J. Sports Med.* **2009**, *37*, 2411–2418. [CrossRef] [PubMed]
24. Clementz, B.G.; Magnusson, A. Fluoroscopic measurement of tibial torsion in adults. A comparison of three methods. *Arch. Orthop. Trauma Surg.* **1989**, *108*, 150–153. [CrossRef]
25. Schneider, B.; Laubenberger, J.; Jemlich, S.; Groene, K.; Weber, H.M.; Langer, M. Measurement of femoral antetorsion and tibial torsion by magnetic resonance imaging. *Br. J. Radiol.* **1997**, *70*, 575–579. [CrossRef]
26. Hudson, D.; Royer, T.; Richards, J. Ultrasound measurements of torsions in the tibia and femur. *J. Bone Joint Surg. Am.* **2006**, *88*, 138–143.
27. Tamari, K.; Tinley, P.; Briffa, K.; Breidahl, W. Validity and reliability of existing and modified clinical methods of measuring femoral and tibiofibular torsion in healthy subjects: Use of different reference axes may improve reliability. *Clin. Anat.* **2005**, *18*, 46–55. [CrossRef]
28. Amanatullah, D.F.; Ollivier, M.P.; Pallante, G.D.; Abdel, M.P.; Clarke, H.D.; Mabry, T.M.; Taunton, M.J. Reproducibility and precision of CT scans to evaluate tibial component rotation. *J. Arthroplast.* **2017**, *32*, 2552–2555. [CrossRef]
29. Dubousset, J.; Charpak, G.; Skalli, W.; Kalifa, G.; Lazennec, J.Y. EOS stereo-radiography system: Whole-body simultaneous anteroposterior and lateral radiographs with very low radiation dose. *Rev. Chir. Orthop. Reparatrice Appar. Mot.* **2007**, *93* (Suppl. S6), 141–143. (In French) [CrossRef]

30. Kalifa, G.; Charpak, Y.; Maccia, C.; Fery-Lemonnier, E.; Bloch, J.; Boussard, J.M.; Attal, M.; Dubousset, J.; Adamsbaum, C. Evaluation of a new low-dose digital x-ray device: First dosimetric and clinical results in children. *Pediatr. Radiol.* **1998**, *28*, 557–561. [CrossRef]
31. Li, Q.; Weng, W.J.; Wang, W.J.; Sun, M.H. Introduction of EOS imaging system and its current research status in evaluating clinical value of lower limb force line. *China J. Orthop. Traumatol.* **2019**, *32*, 875–878.
32. Peeters, C.M.M.; Bos, G.; Kempen, D.H.R.; Jutte, P.C.; Faber, C.; Wapstra, F.H. Assessment of spine length in scoliosis patients using EOS imaging: A validity and reliability study. *Eur. Spine J.* **2022**, *31*, 3527–3535. [CrossRef] [PubMed]
33. Folinais, D.; Thelen, P.; Delin, C.; Radier, C.; Catonne, Y.; Lazennec, J.Y. Measuring femoral and rotational alignment: EOS system versus computed tomography. *Orthop. Traumatol. Surg. Res.* **2013**, *99*, 509–516. [CrossRef] [PubMed]
34. Yan, W.; Xu, X.; Xu, Q.; Yan, W.; Sun, Z.; Jiang, Q.; Shi, D. Femoral and tibial torsion measurements based on EOS imaging compared to 3D CT reconstruction measurements. *Ann. Transl. Med.* **2019**, *7*, 460. [CrossRef] [PubMed]
35. Chaibi, Y.; Cresson, T.; Aubert, B.; Hausselle, J.; Neyret, P.; Hauger, O.; de Guise, J.A.; Skalli, W. Fast 3D reconstruction of the lower limb using a parametric model and statistical inferences and clinical measurements calculation from biplanar X-rays. *Comput. Methods Biomech. Biomed. Eng.* **2012**, *15*, 457–466. [CrossRef]
36. Reikeras, O.; Bjerkreim, I.; Kolbenstvedt, A. Anteversion of the acetabulum and femoral neck in normals and in patients with osteoarthritis of the hip. *Acta Orthop. Scand.* **1983**, *54*, 18–23. [CrossRef]
37. Liodakis, E.; Doxastaki, I.; Chu, K.; Krettek, C.; Gaulke, R.; Citak, M.; Kenawey, M. Reliability of the assessment of lower limb torsion using computed tomography: Analysis of five different techniques. *Skelet. Radiol.* **2012**, *41*, 305–311. [CrossRef]
38. Reikeras, O.; Hoiseth, A. Torsion of the leg determined by computed tomography. *Acta Orthop. Scand.* **1989**, *60*, 330–333. [CrossRef]
39. Lipps, D.B.; Wilson, A.M.; Ashton-Miller, J.A.; Wojtys, E.M. Evaluation of different methods for measuring lateral tibial slope using magnetic resonance imaging. *Am. J. Sports Med.* **2012**, *40*, 2731–2736. [CrossRef]
40. Hecker, A.; Lerch, T.D.; Egli, R.J.; Liechti, E.F.; Klenke, F.M. The EOS 3D imaging system reliably measures posterior tibial slope. *J. Orthop. Surg. Res.* **2021**, *16*, 388. [CrossRef]
41. Suh, D.W.; Nha, K.W.; Han, S.B.; Cheong, K.; Kyung, B.S. Biplane medial opening-wedge high tibial osteotomy increases posterior tibial slope more than uniplane osteotomy. *J. Knee Surg.* **2022**, *35*, 1229–1235. [CrossRef] [PubMed]
42. Kim, J.H.; Kim, H.Y.; Lee, D.H. Opening gap width influences distal tibial rotation below the osteotomy site following open wedge high tibial osteotomy. *PLoS ONE* **2020**, *15*, e0227969. [CrossRef] [PubMed]
43. Jo, H.S.; Park, J.S.; Byun, J.H.; Lee, Y.B.; Choi, Y.L.; Cho, S.H.; Moon, D.K.; Lee, S.H.; Hwang, S.C. The effects of different hinge positions on posterior tibial slope in medial open-wedge high tibial osteotomy. *Knee Surg. Sports Traumatol. Arthrosc.* **2018**, *26*, 1851–1858. [CrossRef] [PubMed]
44. Salaha, Z.F.M.; Ammarullah, M.I.; Abdullah, N.; Aziz, A.U.A.; Gan, H.S.; Abdullah, A.H.; Abdul Kadir, M.R.; Ramlee, M.H. Biomechanical Effects of the Porous Structure of Gyroid and Voronoi Hip Implants: A Finite Element Analysis Using an Experimentally Validated Model. *Materials* **2023**, *16*, 3298. [CrossRef]
45. Hayatbakhsh, Z.; Farahmand, F. Effects of plate contouring quality on the biomechanical performance of high tibial osteotomy fixation: A parametric finite element study. *Proc. Inst. Mech. Eng. H* **2022**, *236*, 356–366. [CrossRef] [PubMed]
46. Pan, C.S.; Wang, X.; Ding, L.Z.; Zhu, X.P.; Xu, W.F.; Huang, L.X. The best position of bone grafts in the medial open-wedge high tibial osteotomy: A finite element analysis. *Comput. Methods Programs Biomed.* **2023**, *228*, 107253. [CrossRef]
47. Ammarullah, M.I.; Hartono, R.; Supriyono, T.; Santoso, G.; Sugiharto, S.; Permana, M.S. Polycrystalline Diamond as a Potential Material for the Hard-on-Hard Bearing of Total Hip Prosthesis: Von Mises Stress Analysis. *Biomedicines* **2023**, *11*, 951. [CrossRef] [PubMed]
48. Prakoso, A.T.; Basri, H.; Adanta, D.; Yani, I.; Ammarullah, M.I.; Akbar, I.; Ghazali, F.A.; Syahrom, A.; Kamarul, T. The Effect of Tortuosity on Permeability of Porous Scaffold. *Biomedicines* **2023**, *11*, 427. [CrossRef]
49. Trad, Z.; Barkaoui, A.; Chafra, M.; Tavares, J.M.R. Finite element analysis of the effect of high tibial osteotomy correction angle on articular cartilage loading. *Proc. Inst. Mech. Eng. H* **2018**, *232*, 553–564. [CrossRef]
50. Thelen, P.; Delin, C.; Folinais, D.; Radier, C. Evaluation of a new low-dose biplanar system to assess lower-limb alignment in 3D: A phantom study. *Skelet. Radiol.* **2012**, *41*, 1287–1293. [CrossRef]
51. Dubousset, J.; Charpak, G.; Dorion, I.; Skalli, W.; Lavaste, F.; Deguise, J.; Kalifa, G.; Ferey, S. A new 2D and 3D imaging approach to musculoskeletal physiology and pathology with low-dose radiation and the standing position: The EOS system. *Bull. Acad. Natl. Med.* **2005**, *189*, 287–297; discussion 297–300. (In French)
52. Dietrich, T.J.; Pfirrmann, C.W.; Schwab, A.; Pankalla, K.; Buck, F.M. Comparison of radiation dose, workflow, patient comfort and financial break-even of standard digital radiography and a novel biplanar low-dose X-ray system for upright full-length lower limb and whole spine radiography. *Skelet. Radiol.* **2013**, *42*, 959–967. [CrossRef]
53. Flecher, X.; Ollivier, M.; Argenson, J.N. Lower limb length and offset in total hip arthroplasty. *Orthop. Traumatol. Surg. Res.* **2016**, *102* (Suppl. S1), S9–S20. [CrossRef] [PubMed]
54. Orfeuvre, B.; Tonetti, J.; Kerschbaumer, G.; Barthelemy, R.; Moreau-Gaudry, A.; Boudissa, M. EOS stereographic assessment of femoral shaft malunion after intramedullary nailing. A prospective series of 48 patients at 9 months' follow-up. *Orthop. Traumatol. Surg. Res.* **2021**, *107*, 102805. [CrossRef] [PubMed]

55. Peeters, C.M.M.; Van Houten, L.; Kempen, D.H.R.; Wapstra, F.H.; Jutte, P.C.; van den Akker-Scheek, I.; Faber, C. Assessment of pedicle size in patients with scoliosis using EOS 2D imaging: A validity and reliability study. *Eur. Spine J.* **2021**, *30*, 3473–3481. [CrossRef]
56. Loppini, M.; Pisano, A.; Ruggeri, R.; Della Rocca, A.; Grappiolo, G. Pelvic tilt and functional acetabular position after total hip arthroplasty: An EOS 2D/3D radiographic study. *Hip Int.* **2023**, *33*, 365–370. [CrossRef]
57. Moon, H.S.; Choi, C.H.; Jung, M.; Lee, D.Y.; Kim, J.H.; Kim, S.H. The effect of knee joint rotation in the sagittal and axial plane on the measurement accuracy of coronal alignment of the lower limb. *BMC Musculoskelet. Disord.* **2020**, *21*, 470. [CrossRef]
58. Cho, B.W.; Lee, T.H.; Kim, S.; Choi, C.H.; Jung, M.; Lee, K.Y.; Kim, S.H. Evaluation of the reliability of lower extremity alignment measurements using EOS imaging system while standing in an even weight-bearing posture. *Sci. Rep.* **2021**, *11*, 22039. [CrossRef] [PubMed]

Disclaimer/Publisher's Note: The statements, opinions and data contained in all publications are solely those of the individual author(s) and contributor(s) and not of MDPI and/or the editor(s). MDPI and/or the editor(s) disclaim responsibility for any injury to people or property resulting from any ideas, methods, instructions or products referred to in the content.

MDPI
St. Alban-Anlage 66
4052 Basel
Switzerland
www.mdpi.com

MDPI Books Editorial Office
E-mail: books@mdpi.com
www.mdpi.com/books

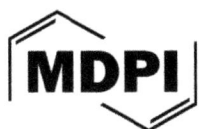

Disclaimer/Publisher's Note: The statements, opinions and data contained in all publications are solely those of the individual author(s) and contributor(s) and not of MDPI and/or the editor(s). MDPI and/or the editor(s) disclaim responsibility for any injury to people or property resulting from any ideas, methods, instructions or products referred to in the content.

www.ingramcontent.com/pod-product-compliance
Lightning Source LLC
LaVergne TN
LVHW070232100526
838202LV00015B/2119